**Greek and Latin Roots of Medical
and Scientific Terminologies**

T0393745

Greek and Latin Roots of Medical and Scientific Terminologies

Todd A. Curtis
Department of Classics
The University of Texas at Austin
TX, USA

WILEY Blackwell

Copyright © 2025 by John Wiley & Sons, Inc. All rights reserved, including rights for text and data mining and training of artificial technologies or similar technologies.

Published by John Wiley & Sons, Inc., Hoboken, New Jersey.
Published simultaneously in Canada.

No part of this publication may be reproduced, stored in a retrieval system, or transmitted in any form or by any means, electronic, mechanical, photocopying, recording, scanning, or otherwise, except as permitted under Section 107 or 108 of the 1976 United States Copyright Act, without either the prior written permission of the Publisher, or authorization through payment of the appropriate per-copy fee to the Copyright Clearance Center, Inc., 222 Rosewood Drive, Danvers, MA 01923, (978) 750-8400, fax (978) 750-4470, or on the web at www.copyright.com. Requests to the Publisher for permission should be addressed to the Permissions Department, John Wiley & Sons, Inc., 111 River Street, Hoboken, NJ 07030, (201) 748-6011, fax (201) 748-6008, or online at http://www.wiley.com/go/permission.

Trademarks: Wiley and the Wiley logo are trademarks or registered trademarks of John Wiley & Sons, Inc. and/or its affiliates in the United States and other countries and may not be used without written permission. All other trademarks are the property of their respective owners. John Wiley & Sons, Inc. is not associated with any product or vendor mentioned in this book.

Limit of Liability/Disclaimer of Warranty: While the publisher and author have used their best efforts in preparing this book, they make no representations or warranties with respect to the accuracy or completeness of the contents of this book and specifically disclaim any implied warranties of merchantability or fitness for a particular purpose. No warranty may be created or extended by sales representatives or written sales materials. The advice and strategies contained herein may not be suitable for your situation. You should consult with a professional where appropriate. Further, readers should be aware that websites listed in this work may have changed or disappeared between when this work was written and when it is read. Neither the publisher nor authors shall be liable for any loss of profit or any other commercial damages, including but not limited to special, incidental, consequential, or other damages.

For general information on our other products and services or for technical support, please contact our Customer Care Department within the United States at (800) 762-2974, outside the United States at (317) 572-3993 or fax (317) 572-4002.

Wiley also publishes its books in a variety of electronic formats. Some content that appears in print may not be available in electronic formats. For more information about Wiley products, visit our web site at www.wiley.com.

Library of Congress Cataloging-in-Publication Data
Names: Curtis, Todd (Todd Anthony), author.
Title: Greek and Latin roots of medical and scientific terminologies / Todd
    A. Curtis.
Description: Hoboken, New Jersey : Wiley-Blackwell, 2025. | Includes index.
Identifiers: LCCN 2024020696 (print) | LCCN 2024020697 (ebook) | ISBN
    9781118358634 (paperback) | ISBN 9781118358498 (adobe pdf) | ISBN
    9781118358559 (epub)
Subjects: LCSH: Greek language–Terms and phrases. | Greek
    language–Medical Greek. | Latin language–Terms and phrases. | Latin
    language–Medical Latin. | Medicine–Terminology. | English
    language–Foreign elements–Greek. | English language–Foreign
    elements–Latin.
Classification: LCC PA455.M4 C87 2024 (print) | LCC PA455.M4 (ebook) |
    DDC 610.1/4–dc23/eng/20240524
LC record available at https://lccn.loc.gov/2024020696
LC ebook record available at https://lccn.loc.gov/2024020697

Cover image: © Wellcome Collection. Attribution 4.0 International (CC BY 4.0)
Cover design: Wiley

Set in 9.5/12.5pt STIXTwoText by Straive, Pondicherry, India
SKY10093881_121624

Contents

To the Student

Who Is This Textbook Written For?

This textbook is primarily for college students interested in learning the language of medicine. Its approach to medico-scientific terminology is linguistic rather than scientific, making it useful also to students with nonprofessional interests in the language of medicine and science. Although this textbook concerns Greek and Latin words, no background knowledge of these languages is required.

What Will You Learn?

This textbook takes an etymological approach to teaching the language of medicine. Thus, instead of focusing on learning the current definitions of medical and scientific terms found in dictionaries, you will be learning the literal meanings of the Greek and Latin words and word elements that form medical terms. These word elements are the building blocks for over 90% of the terms you will encounter in medicine and science. Learning the original meanings of these word elements will help you memorize the words. More importantly, you will be able to decipher the meanings of medical terms that are unfamiliar to you. By the end of this course, you will have learned most of the words and word elements used in medicine and science, and therefore, you will be able to easily recognize the literal meanings of compound terms, such as **poikiloderma**, by breaking these terms down into their Greek and Latin word elements (e.g. Gr. *poikilo*, irregular + Gr. *derma*, skin).

You will also gain a basic understanding of the Latin grammar that is used in anatomical and biological Latin. Thus, you will be able to recognize how the inflectional endings of Latin words reveal their grammatical usage in biological taxonomies (e.g. *nervi digiti* = nerves **of the finger**; *nervi digitorum* = nerves **of the fingers**).

Lastly, you will learn the history of the ancient Greek and Roman worlds, with particular attention to ancient Greek medicine. This kind of information is not only interesting in respect to the origins of western medicine, but it is also quite useful in recognizing why the literal meanings of certain loan words in modern medicine are somewhat misleading because they are ensconced in the ancient Greek medical concepts of disease (e.g. **cholera**, **gonorrhea**, and **melancholia**). It also will help you to make sense of the eponyms commonly used in medicine and science, such as **Hippocratic facies**, **Galenicals**, and **Promethium**.

What Information Is in the Vocabulary Tables?

The following is the tabular format for the majority of the vocabulary in this textbook:

Greek or Latin word element	Current usage	Etymology	Examples
DERM/O (dĕr-mō)	Skin	L. *dermis, -is*, f. dermis fr. Gr. *derma, dermatos*, skin	Ecto**derm, derma**tocele
DERMAT/O (dĕr-mă-tō)			Loan word: **Dermis** (dĕr′mĭs) pl. **Dermes** (dĕr′mēz″)
-DERM (dĕrm)			

Greek or Latin word element	Current usage	Etymology	Examples
CUT/O **(kū-tō)** **CUTANE/O** **(kū-tā-nē-ō)**	Skin	L. *cutis*, -*is*, f. skin, hide	**Cut**icle, trans**cutane**ous Loan word: **Cutis** (kūt′ĭs) pl. **Cutes** (kūt′ēz″)

The first column (**Greek or Latin Word Element**) provides you with the combining form, prefix, or suffix that are commonly used in medical terminology. The phonetic spelling of each word element is provided to help with the pronunciation of medical terms.

The second column (**Current Usage**) provides you with the current medical and scientific usages of the word elements in the first column. Learning the information in these first two columns is fundamental to your success.

The third column (**Etymology**) reveals the original form of the Greek or Latin words used to form the corresponding word elements. The abbreviation **Gr.** stands for 'Greek'. The **L.** stands for Latin. The first word represents the nominative singular form (e.g. Gr. *derma*; L. *cutis*) of the Greek or Latin word, and the second word is the genitive singular form (e.g. Gr. *dermatos*; L. -*is*). Most of the roots are derived from the genitive form of the word so that is why it is included. This information is followed by the original meaning of the word. The anatomical Latin term is often derived from a Greek word. In these cases, the anatomical Latin term is presented first, followed by the Greek word that it is derived from (e.g. L. *dermis*, -*is*, f. dermis fr. Gr. *derma*, *dermatos*, skin, hide). The **fr.** stands for "from." In general, it is not necessary to memorize whether the term is Greek or Latin, and the original meaning of the term may differ from its current usage. This column, therefore, is included primarily for your information.

The fourth column (**Examples**) reveals how the word element appears in compound terms (e.g. ectoderm, dermatocele). The word element will appear in bold font in the term. The loan words (i.e. words that are spelled, more or less, the same as in the parent language) are in bold at the bottom of the column. The plural form of the loan word is revealed in the parenthesis (e.g. pl. *dermes*; pl. *cutes*). The plural form of the loan word is not included if medical English does not use this form.

What Is the Best Way to Learn the Word Elements in This Textbook?

It is important to bear in mind that this is a language course. Primary focus should be placed on learning the meanings of word elements to help one recognize the literal meanings of compound medico-scientific terminology. Like other language courses, memorization is key to this process. Here are some recommendations to help you study effectively:

1) It is best to consider this a language course. As with learning modern languages, your goal is to create a working vocabulary. Like modern languages, learning medical and scientific terminology requires continued and frequent practice. Learning a language is also a cumulative process. Therefore, the combining forms, roots, prefixes, and suffixes that you have already learned from previous chapters will show up again in subsequent chapters.

2) It is advisable to create your own flashcards. Write the Latin or Greek word on one side and the literal meaning of this word on the other side. Unlike scientific facts, learning a language requires repetition and time for it to properly percolate in your mind. It is better to see a word multiple times each day for multiple days rather than to look at it just once the night before the test. When learning lists of vocabulary, always focus on what you do not know. There are numerous websites and apps that will help you create electronic notecards and memorize these terms.

3) You should begin the study of your notecards by trying to give the meaning of the Greek or Latin word element/loan word on the card (e.g. DERM/O = ?). Once you have a good understanding of the vocabulary using this method, the best way to know if you have a word element memorized is if you can give the Greek and/or Latin word element in response to the English definition/meaning (e.g. Skin = ?). This also will allow you to recognize that multiple word elements can mean the same thing (e.g. Skin = DERM/O, DERMAT/O, CUTANE/O, CORI/O). As stated earlier, while of interest to classicists, it is not necessary to distinguish whether a word element comes from Greek or Latin because it is of little use to developing a working vocabulary, which is the primary goal of this textbook.

4) Repeatedly saying the Greek and Latin word elements aloud to yourself will help you to memorize and confidently pronounce medical terms, which is why this textbook includes the phonetic spelling of each word element: DERM/O (dĕr-mō).

5) Lastly, repeated practical application of the vocabulary will help you memorize the terms more effectively. For example, you can try to figure out the literal meanings of compound terms (word analysis) that you encounter in your medical dictionary. You can also try to create technical words (word synthesis) for things you encounter in everyday life. Your textbook and the companion website provide you with practice via the word analysis and synthesis questions. They also provide questions in which the word elements and loan words are presented in medical and scientific contexts. **It is strongly recommended that you make use of the companion website because all of the review questions that test your knowledge of word analysis and synthesis, anatomical Latin and loan words, as well as word elements in context for Chapters 2–15 are found on the website.** When you attempt to answer these questions, do not look in the textbook or online for help. If you don't know the answer, you should write down your best guess. After doing this, check your answer. This uncomfortable yet necessary process will reveal what you actually know and what you need to work on. It will also help you commit the vocabulary to long term memory.

To the Instructor

This is a college-level textbook for medical terminology courses taught by classicists. Most medical terminology textbooks on the market today are designed to be taught by healthcare professionals. Because this textbook's approach is linguistic rather than scientific, it better utilizes a classicist's knowledge of Greek and Latin. Furthermore, this textbook allows classicists to teach medical terminology as a true classical civilizations course by presenting medico-scientific terms in their historical context, namely ancient Greek medicine. Having taught this course for over a decade, it has been my experience that pre-medical and pre-allied healthcare students' retention and interest in medical terminology are greatly enhanced by this approach. Although emphasis is placed on ancient medical theories and practices, an instructor need not be a specialist in ancient medicine to use this textbook. Because ancient physicians developed much of their technical vocabulary from everyday Greek and Latin words, there are ample opportunities for the instructor to link medical terms to the history, literature, and mythology of the Greco-Roman world.

I have avoided the typical format used by medical and scientific terminology textbooks written by classicists. These textbooks tend to focus on making a distinction between Latin-based vocabulary and Greek-based vocabulary. The problem with the Latin/Greek arrangement is that it places unnecessary emphasis on whether a root is Greek or Latin, which has little practical value to non-classical students. Instead, I have chosen to use the human anatomical system arrangement because it dovetails with the orientation commonly used in medical and biological courses. This approach fosters the development of a working vocabulary through the recognition and implementation of these word elements in the students' studies. Unlike most medical terminology books, this textbook also provides a basic understanding of Latin grammar to help students make sense of the Latin phrases used in scientific nomenclatures. For the most part, I have kept this to binomial Latin phrases and loan words because the grammar for these types of terms are easier to master.

This textbook is designed so that it can be used as a short course or long course. Unit I contains five chapters, which can be taught in a self-standing short course format (e.g. a five-week summer school format), or it can be combined with Unit II, which allows the textbook to be used in the typical 15-week semester long course format. Unit I provides the basics of Latin and Greek word elements and grammar in respect to diagnostic, therapeutic, chemical, pharmaceutical, and biological terms. Unit II covers the terminology associated with the systems of the body. Each chapter is broken up into manageable sections with accompanying exercises, which provide students with immediate feedback. The explanations of ancient medico-scientific theories/practices, etymological notes, images, tables of vocabulary, and review exercises place emphasis on students recognizing the multivalent nature of Greek and Latin word elements. The historical readings allow students to recognize how the history of Greek medicine is relevant both to the practice and language of modern medicine. **It is strongly recommended that you make use of the companion website because all of the review questions that test the student's knowledge of word analysis and synthesis, anatomical Latin and loan words, as well as word elements in context for Chapters 2–15 are found on the website.**

The pedagogical approach that I have used to teach medical terminology is derived from Lesley Dean-Jones' "Teaching Medical Terminology as a Classics Course." *The Classical Journal* 93, no. 3 (February-March 1998): 290–296. I also have deeply benefited from Oscar Nybakken's *Greek and Latin in Scientific Terminology*. Ames: Iowa State University Press, 1962. Although written in 1960, Nybakkens' text continues to be an indispensable tool for any instructor intending to teach a classical approach to medical and scientific terminology. John Scarborough's *Medical and Biological Terminologies Classical Origins*. Norman: University of Oklahoma Press has provided me with a wealth of historical and etymological information that I have used in teaching medical terminology and in writing this textbook. Similar to Barbara A. Gylys' *Medical Terminology Simplified: A Programmed Learning Approach to Body Systems*

(1993) and Marjorie Canfield Willis' *Medical Terminology: A Programmed Learning Approach to the Language of Health Care* (2008), I have used programmed approach to make the etymological and medical information in each chapter more engaging and memorable. In respect to medical dictionaries, I have found *Taber's Cyclopedic Medical Dictionary* to be one of the best medical sources for reliable etymologies, pronunciations, and clear-cut medical definitions. The phonetic spellings in this book are derived from Donald Venes, ed., *Taber's Medical Dictionary, 24th edition*. Philadelphia: F.A. Davis Company, 2021. Lastly, the cursory treatment of the grammar of anatomical and scientific Latin taught in this textbook can be supplemented by an introductory Latin course or the textbook that I have written specifically for this subject, *Anatomical Latin: A Programmed Approach to Learning the Grammar and Vocabulary of Anatomical Latin.*

Acknowledgments

The inspiration for this textbook came from Lesley Dean-Jones, who has been my mentor and colleague at the University of Texas at Austin for the past decade. Thanks to the medical terminology students whom I have taught at UT, particularly Bridget Coonrod, Sarah Doski, and Austin Ivery, whose feedback was instrumental to the creation of this textbook. Special thanks to Ellyn Hillberry and Joonmo Chun for their help formatting and proofreading earlier versions of the chapters and appendix. With deep gratitude, I would like to thank my mother, Dixie Curtis, and my wonderful wife, Emerald Curtis, for their patience, encouragement, help, and feedback on this textbook. I love you. Lastly, I would be remiss not to thank my Lord and Savior, Jesus Christ, for making all of this possible.

About the Companion Website

This book is accompanied by a companion website.

www.wiley.com/go/Curtis

The website includes:

Student website: Final Review for chapters 2–15
Instructor website: Answers for chapters 2–15

Unit I

Basics of Medical and Scientific Terminology

1

The Historical Origins of Greek and Latin in Medical Terminology

CHAPTER LEARNING OBJECTIVES
1) Why are most medical and scientific terms derived from Greek? When did Greek begin to be used in medicine? How is it related to modern medical terminology?
2) What are the historical origins of the use of Latin in medical terminology? What is Medieval Latin? What is New Latin? How is Latin used in modern medical and scientific terminology?
3) Who is Asclepius? What is Asclepius' relationship to ancient Greek medicine? What is the Rod of Asclepius? What is the Caduceus of Hermes?
4) Why were ancient Greek physicians important to European medical schools of the medieval and Renaissance periods? Who is Hippocrates? What is the Hippocratic Corpus? Who is Galen? How are Hippocrates and Galen relevant to modern medicine and medical terminology?

The vast majority of technical and scientific terms used in medical terminology are derived from ancient Greek and Latin. It has been estimated that over 90% of our medical terms come from these two classical languages. Far from becoming obsolete due to the advances in modern medicine, these two so-called dead languages continue to function as the primary word-stock for creating new terms for the ever-changing vocabulary of medicine. This raises the question as to how Greek and Latin became the dominant languages of medicine.

Historical Origins of Greek in Medical Terminology

Unlike everyday English, which draws more heavily upon Latin, over two-thirds of our modern medical and scientific terms are derived from ancient Greek words, making Greek the language of medicine. The predominance of Greek in medical terminology is a result of ancient Greek medicine's longstanding influence on Western medicine and civilization. The origins of this influence can be traced back to the 5th and 4th century BC, a period of time in which the Greek-speaking world saw radical developments in government, architecture, theater, art, philosophy, and science. During this time, a large number of medical texts were written by various Greek authors. These ancient medical texts addressed a wide array of subjects, ranging from broad theories on the nature of the human body and disease to technical works dedicated to explaining the treatment of specific kinds of maladies, such as hemorrhoids and bone fractures. Over time, a collection of these texts came to be known as the Hippocratic Corpus because many of them, at one time or another, were perceived as representing the teachings of Hippocrates (c. 460–c. 375 BC), the famous physician from the Greek island of Cos. That said, of the 60 or so texts making up the Hippocratic Corpus, it is unclear which, if any, of these texts were written by Hippocrates. Nevertheless, the belief that these works were "Hippocratic" led to them being studied, expounded upon, and spread throughout the ancient world, and thereby, becoming a fundamental source of terminologies for the practice and study of medicine.

Greek and Latin Roots of Medical and Scientific Terminologies, First Edition. Todd A. Curtis.
© 2025 John Wiley & Sons, Inc. Published 2025 by John Wiley & Sons, Inc.
Companion website: www.wiley.com/go/Curtis

Greek continued to be the language of medicine even after the Latin-speaking Romans conquered Greece. This is because most of the doctors practicing in the Roman Empire were Greek, and therefore, they wrote in Greek. Some of these physicians' writings, particularly the works of Galen of Pergamum (129–c. 216 AD), became an integral part of medical education in medieval and Renaissance universities. The study of such ancient Greek medical texts via Latin translations in early European medical schools ultimately led to our continued usage of ancient Greek terms for disease in modern medicine. While we continue to use Greek disease terms, such as "cholera," "eczema," and "gonorrhea," it is important to bear in mind that their original meanings do not correspond to their current clinical usage because the origins of such terms are ensconced within ancient medical concepts of disease.

Because ancient physicians developed much of their technical vocabulary from everyday Greek words, most Greek speakers had a basic understanding of what these medical terms meant. For example, when the Alexandrian anatomist Herophilus (335–280 BC) chose the Greek word ἀμνειός (*amneios,* which appears as "amnion" in modern anatomical terminology) for the membrane surrounding the fetus in the womb, his audience would have recognized it as a word for "lambskin," thus giving them a basic understanding of the appearance and protective function of the membrane. Or when Galen used the anatomical term σταφυλή (*staphyle*) for what we call the uvula, his audience would have understood the word picture of a "cluster of grapes," which is what the Greek word originally meant. Today, medical terms such as amnion and staphylectomy appear completely foreign and technical to most English speakers; their potential meanings have been obscured by the boundaries of language and culture. However, when you learn the original meanings of these Greek words, the multivalent nature of word elements in medical terminology becomes far less baffling and technical. For example, if one recognized that the word element STAPHYL- is derived from the Greek word for "a cluster of grapes," *staphyle*, it becomes apparent why STAPHYL- is used today for both the "uvula" and a "type of bacteria" (the uvula looks like a hanging cluster of grapes, and staphylococci bacteria form grapelike clusters, see Figs. 1.1 and 1.2).

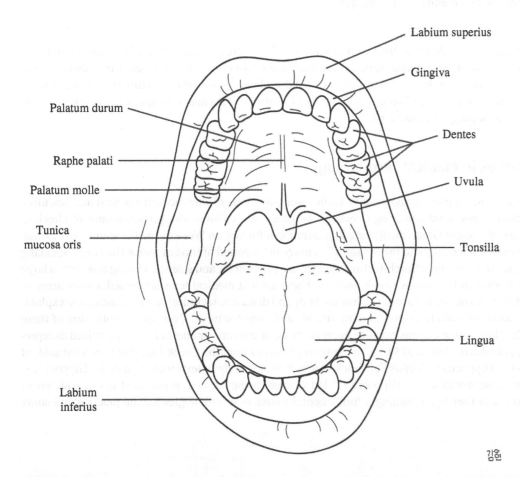

Fig. 1.1 The uvula hanging like a cluster of grapes in the oral cavity. *Source:* Line drawing by Chloe Kim.

Fig. 1.2 Clustering of *Staphylococcus aureus* under a scanning electron microscope (SEM). *Source:* Janice Haney Carr/U.S. Department of Health & Human Services/Wikimedia Commons/Public domain.

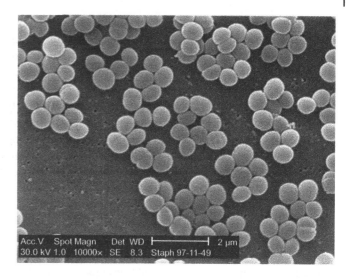

Historical Origins of Latin in Medical Terminology

Rome's conquest of Greek lands in the 2nd century BC and the subsequent opportunity for employment led to a large influx of Greek physicians into the Roman world. Over time, the traditional medicine of the Romans was supplanted by Greek medical theories and practices. Greek medical terms began to be translated into Latin, the language of ancient Rome. The translation of Greek medical thought into Latin was pivotal to ancient Greek medicine's longstanding influence because Latin would later become the universal language of scholarly exchange in government, religion, science, literature, law, and medicine for much of Europe well into the 17th century.

One of the ways Latin-speaking medical authors conveyed Greek medical terms into Latin was by transliterating them. Transliteration is the movement of a word from one language into another. For example, when faced with the Greek term for "arm," βραχίων, they first changed the Greek letters into their Latin equivalents, *brachion*, and then they removed the Greek ending "*on*" replacing it with the Latin ending "*um*," *brachium*, in order to fit Latin grammar. Many of the Greek terms found in modern medical terminology have been Latinized in this way, and therefore, they adhere to the laws of Latin grammar.

Another way in which Latin medical authors dealt with Greek medical terms was to replace the Greek medical term with a Latin word having an equivalent meaning. For example, the Latin word for "brain," *cerebrum*, was often used instead of the transliterated Greek term for the "brain" *enkephalos* (ἐγκέφαλος). Because many of these Latin terms did not supplant their Greek equivalents, there are a large number of Greek and Latin synonyms used in modern medical terminology. For instance, a reconstructive surgery of the lip can be termed either a labioplasty or a cheiloplasty because the word elements from the Latin *labium* and the Greek word *cheilos* are both used in medicine for the English equivalent of "lip."

Much like their Greek counterparts, Latin medical terms are quite descriptive, having a tendency to be derived from words for everyday objects such as musical instruments (*tibia* = flute), sounds (*murmur* = humming), tools (*fibula* = brooch), plants (*glans* = acorn), and animals (*cancer* = crab). Consequently, the Latin equivalents also often retain the ancient medical concepts of disease associated with the Greek term. Aulus Cornelius Celsus (1st century AD), the author of a Latin encyclopedia of Greek medicine, used the Latin term for a "crab," *cancer*, in place of the Greek term for "crab," *karkinos*, to maintain the metaphor of a burrowing, gnawing, and grasping crab, which was used in antiquity to describe a variety of diseases causing pernicious ulcers. Today, both of these Latin and Greek words are associated with very specific cellular pathologies that metastasize (e.g. cancer and carcinogen). In medical dictionaries, words that are derived from **classical Greek** have the abbreviation **Gr.** before the word, and words that have a **classical Latin** origin have **L.** before the word.

The Middle Ages or the medieval period (c. 5th–14th century AD) saw a sharp decline in the knowledge of the Greek language in the West, and therefore, ancient Greek medical texts were far less accessible to Europeans. Although ancient Greek medical theories continued to be used in Christian monasteries and among learned physicians, their knowledge of Greek medical texts was limited to a small number of Greek texts and parts of more complete works that had been translated into Latin. Conversely, in the Greek-speaking East, also known as the Byzantine Empire, access to ancient Greek medical texts continued, and these texts were later translated into Syriac and Arabic, forming the foundation for the learned approach to medicine found in the medieval Islamic period (900–1300 AD). European understanding of ancient Greek medicine was transformed by gaining access to these Arabic sources. This started around the 11th century, when learned figures such as Constantinus Africanus began to translate scripts of Greco-Arabic medicine into Latin. By the 12th century, much of the writings of Aristotle, Hippocrates, Galen, and the Arabic medical authors known in Europe as Avicenna (Ibn Sina, 980–1037 AD), Rhazes (Al-Razi 865–925 AD), Isaac Judaeus (Israeli ben Solomon, c. 832–932 AD), and Algizar (Al Jazzar, 895–979 AD) were available in Latin. These Greco-Arabic texts, particularly the writings of Galen, became the curricula for the 13th century medical schools in Italy, and these Italian medical schools served as the blueprint for later medical schools throughout Europe. The new Latin that was formed to translate these Arabic sources is referred to as "**Medieval Latin**," and it is abbreviated **ML.** in the etymologies of medical dictionaries.

With the Renaissance (c. 15th–17th century AD) came a renewed interest in recovering classical Latin and Greek culture. Renaissance Humanists' desire to rediscover and assimilate the language and ideas found in ancient Greek and Roman texts bolstered Latin as the universal language of scholarly exchange and opened the door for knowledge of ancient Greek to be valued as a sign of a strong education. Thus, medico-scientific authors continued to write in Latin up to the 19th century, many revealing at least a rudimentary knowledge of Greek words. The Latin and Latinized Greek terms that medico-scientific authors such as Andreas Vesalius, William Harvey, Giovanni Morgagni, and Aloysius Galvani used for the purpose of expressing their discoveries are the source of much of our modern anatomical terminology. Terms that were coined during this period are termed "**New Latin**" and abbreviated **NL.** in most dictionaries. The Latin used for the familiar binomial of "genus" and "species" devised by Carolus Linnaeus (1707–1778 AD) used today in the classification of living organisms also falls under the category of New Latin.

Renaissance Humanist reforms in education of the 16th century resulted in a preference for Latin and Greek words when forming new English words. The effect of this movement is evident in early English medical books, such as Andrew Boorde's *The Breviarie of Health* (1547 AD), which contains anglicized forms of Latin and Latinized Greek terms (e.g. "vein" from the Latin *vena*, "artery" from the Latinized Greek word *arteria*). Despite the radical changes in our understanding of disease and the body, scientists and physicians continue to pull from the same word-stock that ancient physicians used in the Greco-Roman world. For this reason, modern medical English contains numerous Greek and Latin words whose modern usages have no classical equivalents, such as the Latin word for "poison," *virus*, being used today for "a small infectious agent that replicates inside living cells." The preference for using Greek and Latin words also has led to medical terminology making extensive use of Greek and Latin word elements to form compound terms such as periodontosis (Greek *peri-*, around; Greek *odous*, tooth; *-osis*, condition) and microdentism (Greek *micros*, small; Latin *dens*, tooth; *-ism*, condition).

By the 18th century, the growing movement for the use of national languages in science greatly reduced the amount of medical material written in Latin. As medico-scientific authors increasingly turned to their respective vernacular to express their ideas, Latin began to function less as language and more as a code for technical phrases in medicine, such as *nihil per os* (NPO = nothing by mouth) and *bis in die* (BID = twice a day). The rise of the vernacular and the demise of classical language as a subject in academia ultimately led to a gulf between the technical language of medicine and everyday English.

That said, the rise of the vernacular did not lead to the complete death of Latin. International codes of scientific nomenclatures prescribe that all anatomical and biological terms must be written in grammatically correct Latin (e.g. *flexor pollicis longus* [the long flexor muscle of the thumb], *Toxicodendron radicans* [poison ivy], and *Rana macrocnemis* [a long-legged wood frog]). Up until very recently, the International Botanical Congress demanded that not only the names but even the descriptions of newly discovered plants had to be written in Latin. For this reason, Latin continues to function as *lingua franca* (universal language) of biological and anatomical classification systems. Thus, every newly discovered organism and anatomical structure is given a Latin name. This includes organisms and structures whose vernacular names are derived from an individual or place not found in Latin. In these cases, the vernacular name is Latinized. For instance, the Latin used for the genus and species of a type of cockroach in the United States, *periplaneta americana*, is derived from terms not found in the Latin of the ancient Romans. The term *periplaneta* is a Latinization of two Greek words (*peri*, around + *planan*, to wander) and the modern Latin adjective *americana*, which is derived from the Latin name of the famous explorer of the New World, Amerigo Vespucci (1454–1512 AD). Because Latin is the language of anatomical and biological classification systems, a basic understanding of Latin grammar is still quite useful when one is faced with such terms.

Asclepius and the Symbols of Medicine

In addition to medical terms, the influence of ancient Greek culture is also evident in our medical symbols. The image of a single snake entwined around a knotty staff has been used as a symbol of medicine for well over 2000 years. Owing to its association with the Greek god of medicine, it is called the **Rod of Asclepius**. According to Greek mythology,

Asclepius (also spelled Aesculapius) was the child of the god Apollo and a human princess named Coronis (or in some myths Arsinoë). Having become enraged over Coronis' love for a mortal named Ischys, Apollo killed Coronis before she could give birth to Asclepius. After her body was laid on a funeral pyre to be burned, Apollo came to his senses and rescued his son from the flames by cutting Asclepius out of Coronis' womb. Apollo then gave Asclepius to the centaur Chiron, the friend and patron of heroes. Chiron educated Asclepius in the art of medicine teaching him the uses of herbs and how to perform surgery. In some myths, Asclepius became so skilled in medicine that he was not only able to prevent death, but he could also bring the dead back to life. Because of the audacity of Asclepius allowing mortals to cheat death, or in some accounts, because he was stirred by Hades' fear that Asclepius' healing powers would lead to a lack of souls in the underworld, Zeus killed Asclepius with a thunderbolt. At the request of Apollo and in reward for Asclepius' benefactions to mankind, Asclepius was later elevated to the pantheon of gods through apotheosis (deification).

To ancient Greek doctors, Asclepius was more than merely the patron deity of medicine; he was also the progenitor of a line of physicians. According to legend, Asclepius fathered two sons, Machaon and Podalirius, whom he taught his art of medicine. Their descendants were considered to be the ancestors of a family of Greek physicians called the Asclepiades, from whom Hippocrates was reputed to have descended. In the *Iliad*, Machaon and Podalirius served in Agamemnon's army during the Trojan War. Machaon is said to have healed Menelaus with remedies his father received from Chiron. Later commentators on Homer suggested that each brother had his own expertise, Machaon specializing in surgery on wounds and Podalirius in diet and healing herbs. This distinction can be seen on the arms of the Royal College of Surgeons of England, where Machaon is observed holding a broken arrow assumedly removed from his patient's body and Podalirius appears with the healing staff of Asclepius (Fig. 1.3).

Fig. 1.3 Machaon (left) and Podalirius (right) on the title page for the *Annals of the Royale College of Surgeons of England*, Volume 1, July to December 1947. According to the Royale College of Surgeon's website (https://www.rcseng.ac.uk/about-the-rcs/history-of-the-rcs/coat-of-arms/accessed6/17/19): "The original coat of arms featured the sons of Aesculapius (Greek god of healing); two brothers who were surgeons at the siege of Troy. On the left side is Machaon who is depicted holding the broken dart reportedly extracted from the side of King Menelaus and which symbolises the healing of wounds. On the right side is Podalirus, a physician, who was originally featured holding a surgeon's knife.... The motto – QUAE PROSUNT OMNIBUS ARTES – means: "the arts which are of service to all." *Source:* Wellcome Collection/CC BY 4.0.

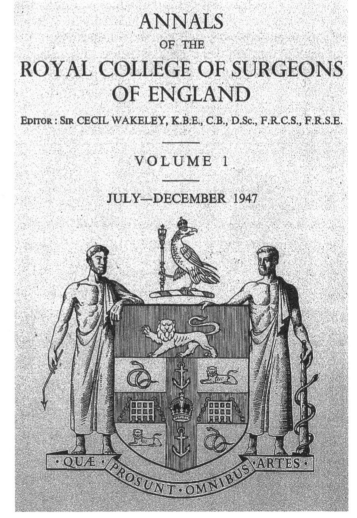

ANNALS
OF THE
ROYAL COLLEGE OF SURGEONS
OF ENGLAND

EDITOR : SIR CECIL WAKELEY, K.B.E., C.B., D.Sc., F.R.C.S., F.R.S.E.

VOLUME 1

JULY—DECEMBER 1947

The healing cult of Asclepius was a common feature in the Greco-Roman world. Sanctuaries to Asclepius, known as **Asclepeia** (singular **Asclepeion**), appeared throughout the Mediterranean world, flourishing well into the Christian era. Those suffering with illnesses would either simply pray to Asclepius, or if able, go to Asclepius' sanctuary to be healed. In order to receive healing dreams, the suppliants would go through a process of purifications culminating in the act of "incubation," which involved lying down in a sacred building in the sanctuary known as the *abaton* ("the untrodden place"). According to the ancient testimonies, Asclepius would appear in their dreams, healing them, or he would advise them what to do if they wanted to be cured. These ancient testimonies reveal that Asclepius' cures were, albeit miraculous in nature, often through medical means. For instance, in one account, a man lacking one of his eyes had a dream in which Asclepius poured a salve in his eye socket and when day came, he departed with sight in both his eyes. Some of the ancient accounts of healing attributed to Asclepius describe how a snake cured the suppliant by licking the injured part, which partially explains why the snake is associated with Asclepius' staff and medicine.

The **Caduceus of Hermes** is often confused with the Rod of Asclepius (Fig. 1.4). The caduceus is a herald's wand used by messenger gods such as Hermes, who in the Roman world was known as Mercury. When used as a symbol of medicine, the Caduceus of Hermes is depicted as a winged staff with two snakes entwined around it. Its use as a medical emblem came much later. One of the first instances of the Caduceus of Hermes' association with medicine came in the 16th century AD. Johann Froben (1460–1527 AD), whose printed editions included medical texts, used a caduceus with entwined snakes surmounted by a dove as a printer's device (Fig. 1.5). William Butts (1506–1583 AD), the physician to Henry VIII, and John Caius (1510–1573 AD), the physician to Edward I, were the first doctors to use this symbol. That said, it was rarely used as a symbol of medicine until the 19th century, when the publisher of medical texts, John Churchill (1810–1875 AD), made use of this image. Thanks in part to its adoption in 1902 as a symbol of the U.S. Army Corps, the Caduceus of Hermes is widely used in the United States, albeit less frequently than the Rod of Asclepius. Some have objected to the Caduceus of Hermes being used as a symbol of medicine. They maintain that the Rod of Asclepius is the appropriate symbol because of its longstanding association with medicine. Their criticisms are also based on an awareness of Hermes' role in Greek mythology as the god of merchants, as well as the conductor of the souls of the dead to the realm of Hades. Thus, using the Caduceus of Hermes could be seen as an advertisement that one's approach to medicine is mercantile in nature, or even worse, that it will lead to a patients' soul being conducted to the underworld.

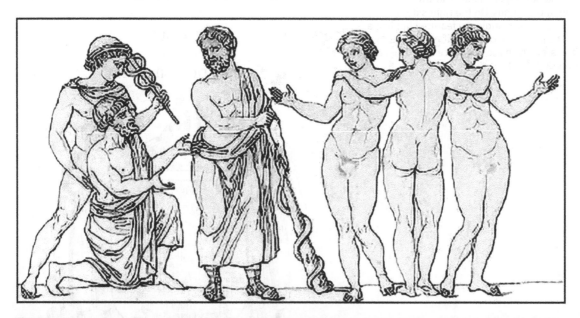

Fig. 1.4 Hermes (Mercury) and a merchant approach a disapproving Asclepius. Hermes (left) is holding his caduceus and Asclepius (right) is holding his iconic snake-entwined staff. The naked Graces to the right of Asclepius are sometimes interpreted as representing Asclepius' retinue of healing goddesses, Hygeia (Health), Panacea (Cure-all), and Iaso (Curing). *Source:* Millin, 1811/Soyer/ Public domain.

Fig. 1.5 The printer's symbol for Johann Froben's 1538 edition of the Hippocratic Corpus. *Source:* Hieronymus Froben and Nicolaus Episcopius/Wikimedia Commons/Public domain.

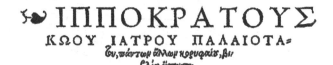

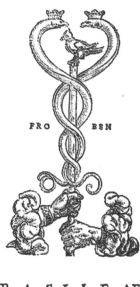

Famous Ancient Greek Physicians

A large collection of physicians gained prominence in the Greek and Roman world. Although there was a general lack of consensus among these ancient Greek physicians with respect to their pathophysiological theories and corresponding treatments, their writings were considered to be essential to the practice of medicine for centuries. And despite many of these physicians being pagan with respect to their religious beliefs, medieval Islamic medicine and physicians in the Christian world embraced Greek medicine because they considered ancient Greek medicine's teleological understanding of nature as being consistent with the religious teachings of these monotheistic faiths.

The above frontispiece (Fig. 1.6) is from Thomas Linacre's Latin translation (Paris, S. de Colines, 1530 AD) of Galen's medical treatise *De methodo medendi*. This frontispiece reveals a Renaissance perception of ancient Greek medicine representing the pillars of medicine. Dressed somewhat as contemporaries and standing among the pillars of medicine are some of the great medical authorities from Greek and Roman antiquity: Hippocrates of Cos (c. 460–c. 375 BC), Galen of Pergamum (129-c. 216 AD), Paul of Aegina (death c. 642 AD), Oribasius of Pergamum (c. 320–400 AD), Asclepiades of Bithynia (c. 1st century BC), and Dioscorides of Anazarbus (c. 1st century AD). The base portrays the dissection of a human body, which reflects Galen's conception that the study of human anatomy was fundamental to medicine. At the top, there is an image of Jesus Christ healing a leper, which is described in the Bible, Matthew 8 : 1–3. The collective symbolism is that Jesus is the great physician and Greek medicine should be considered consistent with Christian conceptions of *servus dei* (servant of god) and the *sacra congregatio* (sacred congregation). As to the Galenic text to which this frontispiece is attached, *De method medendi* (*Therapeutic Method*) was one of the most highly read medical texts in the Middle Ages and Renaissance, and it was an integral part of the medical curriculum up to the 17th century.

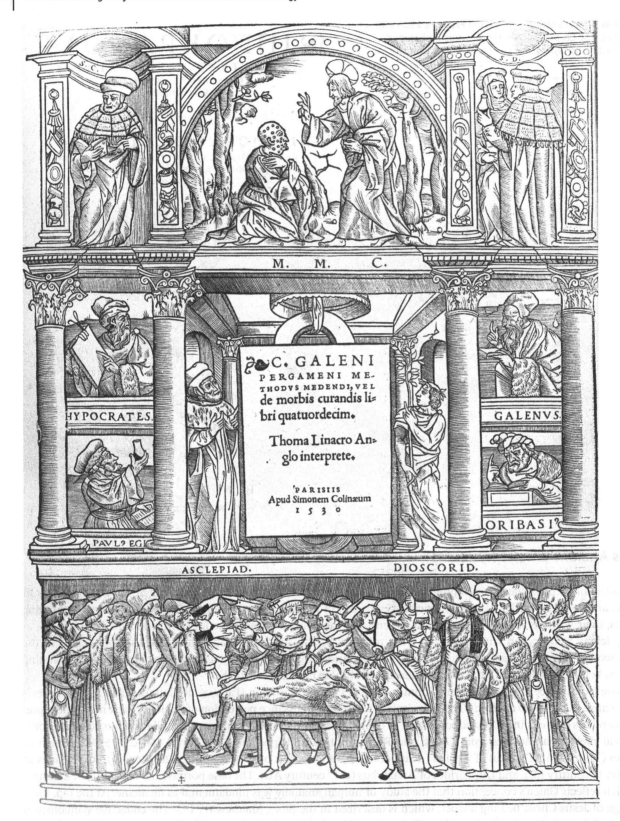

Fig. 1.6 Frontispiece is from Thomas Linacre's Latin translation (Paris, S. de Colines, 1530) of Galen's medical treatise *De methodo medendi. Source:* Wellcome Collection/CC BY 4.0.

Hippocrates

Of all the noteworthy physicians from the Greco-Roman world, **Hippocrates** is undoubtedly the most famous. However, very little is known about his life and actual teachings. He was often referred to as "Hippocrates of Cos." The title was used to distinguish him from other Greek men with the name Hippocrates. The title "of Cos" indicated that he was born on the Greek island of Cos, which is located along the coast of present-day Turkey. It is on this island that he is said to have taught his influential approach to medicine. By the 4th century BC, Hippocrates was well known for his teachings and was held up as a paragon of the art of medicine by his contemporaries Plato and Aristotle. Over time, fanciful accounts of Hippocrates' life and teachings reinforced the notion that he was an impeccable physician deserving of the title "Father of Medicine." Like other physicians, he was called an "Asclepiad" after the Greek hero and god of medicine, Asclepius. In later legends about Hippocrates' life, this epithet was taken to mean that he was actually a direct descendent of Asclepius. Because there has been disagreement among physicians over what were Hippocrates' actual doctrines, what is truly Hippocratic medicine continues to be reinvented by physicians throughout the centuries in support of their own approaches to medicine.

The belief in "Hippocratic medicine" led to the study of the writings of Hippocrates in medicine that continued even up to the 19th century, when the medically trained author, Emile Littré, produced a French translation of the Hippocratic Corpus to serve as a textbook for French doctors. However, radical changes in disease theory, particularly the notion of cellular pathologies, made Littré's work obsolete before it was published. Hippocrates is still considered the founder of scientific medicine and a paragon of medical ethics. Even to this day, the various oaths that numerous medical students vow upon graduation are often called the "Hippocratic Oath" based on the belief that Hippocrates himself had penned the ethical principles found in a 5th century BC medical oath.

Galen

Of equal importance, although less well known outside of medical historians, is the ancient Greek physician known as **Galen**. Galen was born around 129 AD in Pergamum, an influential Greek city on the coast of what is now called Turkey. After the death of his father, Galen traveled to Smyrna, Corinth, and Alexandria to study medicine under the best physicians. Upon his return to Pergamum, he took up the commission of physician to a troupe of gladiators. Galen eventually traveled to Rome in 162 AD, where he made a name for himself as a physician and philosopher. His medical skill and knowledge caught the eye of the famous emperor Marcus Aurelius, who later appointed him as his court physician. Galen used this opportunity to research and write extensively on a wide variety of subjects pertaining to medicine, anatomy, philosophy, and rhetoric. His writings were disseminated throughout the Roman world, and over time, they eclipsed the writings of other ancient physicians.

Based on the longevity of the influence of his theories, Galen is arguably the most influential physician in the history of medicine. His philosophical approach to medicine made him a figure of equal importance to Aristotle in scientific matters in medieval and Renaissance universities. His interpretations of Hippocratic treatises were largely responsible for the adoption of the theory of the four humors (i.e. blood, phlegm, and yellow and black bile) becoming the standard view of human physiology for centuries. Translations and interpretations of Galenic works made by Arab and Syrian scholars formed the basis for Medieval Islamic medicine, which continues to be practiced in India in the form of Unani medicine. Galen's writings formed the backbone of medical education in European universities up to the Renaissance (Fig. 1.7). The 16th and 17th centuries saw the decline of Galenic medicine. Galen's writings on anatomy had remained largely unchallenged until the Renaissance anatomist Andreas Vesalius printed his famous *De humani corporis fabrica* (*On the Material of the Human Body*) in 1543 AD, revealing how Galenic anatomy was at times erroneous because it was largely dependent on animal dissection rather than human dissection. William Harvey's seminal work on the circulation of blood, as well as other advancements made during the Enlightenment, began the collapse of Galenic medicine, opening the way for radically different approaches to human physiology and disease that we benefit from today. Modern medical terms such as "Galen anastomosis" (an anastomosis between the superior and inferior laryngeal nerve) and "the vein of Galen" (a short vein between the cerebral hemispheres of the brain) continue to give testimony to the far-reaching influence of Galen.

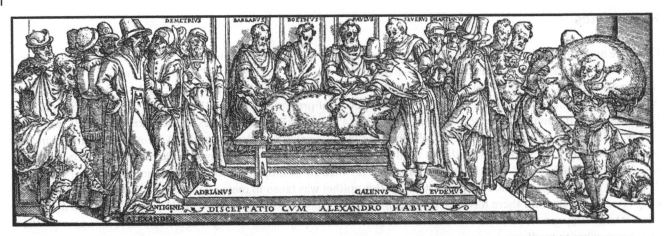

Fig. 1.7 Image is from the title page of the 1565 Junta edition of Galen's writings. The image is a Renaissance artist's depiction of one of Galen's famous anatomical demonstrations. Here Galen demonstrates the vocal function of recurrent laryngeal nerve by severing it on a squealing pig, and thus leaving the pig voiceless. The collection of figures labeled in the audience includes the names of Roman consuls, lawyers, and philosophers whom Galen claimed attended his anatomical demonstrations. *Source:* Wellcome Collection/Public domain.

Some Suggested Readings

Conrad, Lawrence I. *The Western Medical Tradition: 800 BC to AD 1800*. Cambridge: Cambridge University Press, 1995.

Craik, Elizabeth M. *The "Hippocratic" Corpus: Context and Content*. New York: Routledge, 2015.

Edelstein, Emma J. and Ludwig Edelstein. *Asclepius: A Collection and Interpretation of the Testimonies*. Baltimore: Johns Hopkins University Press, 1945.

Hankinson, Robert J., ed. *The Cambridge Companion to Galen*. Cambridge: Cambridge University Press, 2008.

Jackson, Ralph. *Doctors and Diseases in the Roman Empire*. London: British Museum, 1988.

Jouanna, Jacques. *Hippocrates*. Translated by M. B. DeBevoise. Baltimore: Johns Hopkins University Press, 2001.

Nutton, Vivian. *Ancient Medicine*. Second Edition. London: Routledge: Sciences of Antiquity, 2013.

Pormann, Peter and Emilie Savage-Smith. *Medieval Islamic Medicine*. Washington: Georgetown University Press, 2007.

Siraisi, Nancy. *Medieval and Early Renaissance Medicine: An Introduction to Knowledge and Practice*. Chicago: The University of Chicago Press, 1990.

Temkin, Owsei. *Galenism: Rise and Decline of Medical Philosophy*. Ithaca: Cornell University Press, 1973.

van der Eijk, Philip. "*Medicine in Early and Classical Greece*." In *The Cambridge History of Science*. Edited by Alexander Jones and Liba Taub, 293–315. Cambridge: Cambridge University Press, 2018.

2

Greek and Latin Word Elements in Medical Terminology

CHAPTER LEARNING OBJECTIVES

1) You will gain a basic understanding of Hippocratic *Aphorism* 1.1.
2) You will have a working knowledge of the etymological approach to medical terminology, which is fundamental to understanding the literal meanings of medical terms.
3) You will learn the principles of analysis and synthesis of compound medical terms.
4) You will learn the classical plural forms of medical terms and the principles of alternate spellings of medical terms.
5) You will learn phonetic spellings and the principles of pronouncing medical terms correctly.
6) You will gain a working knowledge of the vast majority of prefixes and suffixes that you will encounter in medical and scientific terminology.

Lessons from History: *Aphorism* 1.1 and Etymology

Food for Thought as You Read:

To what extant are the language and sentiments expressed in Aphorism 1.1 relevant to modern medicine? What is the etymological approach to medical terminology?

The Greek words in the Rod of Asclepius pictured in Fig. 2.1 are from the famous *Aphorism* 1.1, which is part of a Greek medical text known as the Hippocratic *Aphorisms*. Extending back to the 4ᵗʰ century BC, the *Aphorisms* are a collection of medical aphorisms for the practice of medicine. An aphorism is a short, pithy statement used in wisdom literature to convey some sort of maxim or ideal. The Hippocratic *Aphorisms* are an amalgam of approximately 400 or so sayings derived from different medical texts/authorities. The Hippocratic *Aphorisms* were considered to be an extremely important medical resource, and they were commented upon for centuries by physicians who wanted to gain a "Hippocratic" approach to medicine.

Aphorisms 1.1
Ὁ βίος βραχὺς, ἡ δὲ τέχνη μακρὴ, ὁ δὲ καιρὸς ὀξὺς, ἡ δὲ
πεῖρα σφαλερὴ, ἡ δὲ κρίσις χαλεπή.

Aphorisms 1.1
"Life is short, the art is long, opportunity is fleeting, experiment is
precarious, and judgement is difficult."

The *Aphorisms* begins with the above famous overarching conception of medicine expressed in *Aphorisms* 1.1. The first part of *Aphorisms* 1.1 is translated, "Life is short, the art is long, opportunity is fleeting." By "the art," the author is referring to medicine. Similar to carpentry, shoemaking, and baking, medicine was considered a *techne* (art) in ancient Greek society. The first clause informs the reader that one's life is quite short in comparison to the amount of material one must learn to effectively practice medicine. The last clause warns that when a physician encounters a disease in a patient,

Greek and Latin Roots of Medical and Scientific Terminologies, First Edition. Todd A. Curtis.
© 2025 John Wiley & Sons, Inc. Published 2025 by John Wiley & Sons, Inc.
Companion website: www.wiley.com/go/Curtis

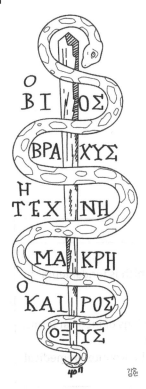

Fig. 2.1 Logo for the Society of Ancient Medicine. *Source:* Chloe Kim.

there will be a brief window of opportunity to make a difference. The latter part of this aphorism, "experiment is precarious, and judgement is difficult," points to the problems of attempting to find the right treatment given the limitations one experiences in the practice of medicine. In many respects, the sentiments of this statement hold true even today; medicine is an art requiring a lifelong commitment to learning and a desire to make the most of every opportunity to heal a patient.

When the Greek words in the aforementioned Aphorism are transliterated into our alphabet (e.g. (βίος) *bios*, (βραχύς) *brachys*, (τέχνη) *techne*, (μακρή) *macre*, (ὀξύς) *oxys*), they become recognizable as common word elements used to form a variety of words. For example, *bios* (life) is evident in terms such as "biology" and "symbiotic"; *brachys* (short) can be seen in "brachypoda" and "brachycephalic"; *techne* (art) is evident in words such as "technology" and "pyrotechnics"; *macre* (long, large) is prevalent in a number of words such as "macroeconomics" and "macrocytosis"; *oxys* (sharp, swift, acid) is apparent in a large collection of words such as "oxygen" and "oxyacusis." It can be discerned that the parts of these Greek words, BIO-, BRACHY-, TECHN-, MACR-, and OXY-, are used as building blocks to construct medico-scientific terms. In this textbook, these building blocks are called **word elements**.

It can also be seen from the Latinized spelling of the Greek word κρίσις (crisis) in the above *Aphorism* that some Greek (and Latin) words have been adopted wholesale into our medical vocabulary as technical terms. In everyday ancient Greek, the word κρίσις could mean "judgment." However, when it was applied to the diagnosis of fevers, ancient Greek physicians used the term κρίσις to "indicate a turning point in a fever." Thus, if a fever broke on the 1st, 2nd, 3rd, or 4th day, they would use this information to determine the patient's prognosis. Today, medicine uses the term "crisis" for a turning point in a disease or the sudden descent of a high temperature. Medical and scientific terminology is replete with Greek and Latin words adopted for technical definitions.

Because Greek and Latin serve as the sources for the vast majority of technical vocabulary in medicine and science, this textbook takes a decidedly etymological approach to learning "medspeak." **Etymology** is the study of the origins and historical meanings of words. An etymological approach to learning medical terminology will involve learning the meanings of word elements and words from Greek and Latin. This is an effective strategy for learning medical terminology because a relatively small amount of Greek and Latin word elements accounts for close to 90% of the technical terms one will encounter in medicine and science. By memorizing the meanings of these word elements, you will be able to recall medical and scientific terms more easily and you will also gain clues as to the potential meanings of unfamiliar medico-scientific terms. The primary focus of this textbook is to help you gain a working vocabulary of these Greek and Latin word elements. We will also be learning the modern usage and meanings of Greek and Latin words such as "crisis" that have become part of our technical language.

In most medical dictionaries, the etymology of a term is set apart in brackets next to the main entry. The abbreviation **L.** and **Gr.** are used to denote whether the term is from Latin or Greek. As discussed in chapter one, you will also run into **ML.** (Medieval Latin) and **NL.** (New Latin) in etymologies. The etymological entry will contain the transliterated Greek or Latin word and its original meaning:

vasotrophic [L. *vas*, vessel + Gr. *trophe*, nourishment]

Some Suggested Readings

Hippocrates. "*Aphorisms.*" In *Hippocrates Volume IV*, Loeb Classical Library 150, trans. by William H. S. Jones., 97–221 Cambridge: Harvard University Press, 1931.

Nybakken, Oscar. *Greek and Latin in Scientific Terminology*. Ames: Iowa State University Press, 1962.

Scarborough, John. *Medical and Biological Terminologies Classical Origins*. Norman: University of Oklahoma Press, 1992.

Etymological Terms

Eponym

An **eponym** is a term used for anything (animal, disease, organ, and function), which is derived from the name of a particular person. Important figures in the history of medicine are often memorialized for their discoveries through the use of eponyms. Medications that are combinations of herbs and organic material are called **Galenicals** due to the influence and nature of Galen's drug recipes. Alois Alzheimer's name is used for the neurological disorder, **Alzheimer Disease**, because he is associated with its discovery. Eponyms are indicated by your medical dictionary's etymological entries as follows:

Galenical [Galen, Claudius, famous Greek physician and writer 129–c.210 AD]
Alzheimer Disease [Alzheimer, Alois, German neurologist, 1864–1915] (Figs. 2.2 and 2.3)

Greek mythological figures are also a common source of eponyms in medico-scientific terminology. They give meaning to an object by associating a distinguishable characteristic of the object with a mythological figure who shares this attribute. In the *Odyssey*, Proteus was a prophetic sea god who was famous for his ability to change shape. Therefore, because of their changeability in aggregate form, a genus of saprophytic motile bacilli is named **Proteus** (Figs. 2.2 and 2.3):

Proteus [Gr. *Proteus*, a sea god who could change his form]

Loan Word

A **loan word** is a Latin or Greek word that has been adopted into English without any significant changes in spelling. Some familiar examples are apex, genesis, and basis. Loan words appear in the etymological entries of medical dictionaries as follows:

apex [L. *apex*, the top]
basis [Gr. *basis*, a base, a place on which one stands]
genesis [Gr. *genesis*, origin, source, production]

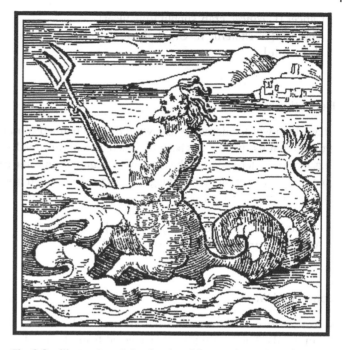

Fig. 2.2 Illustration of the Greek god Proteus by Andrea Alciato from *The Book of Emblems* (1531). *Source:* Jörg Breu the Elder/Wikimedia Commons/Public domain.

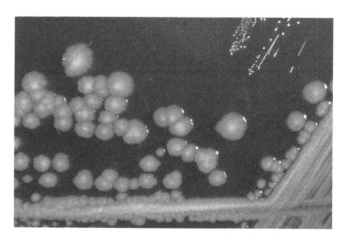

Fig. 2.3 Colonies of *Proteus mirabilis* bacteria. *Source:* U.S. Department of Health & Human Services/Public domain.

It is important to bear in mind that Greek and Latin loan words for diseases, such as **cancer** and **cholera**, often do not reveal their current clinical meanings because the origins of such terms are ensconced within ancient medical concepts of disease. The *chole-* (Gr. *cholē*, bile) in **cholera** reveals the ancient medical belief in disease being the result of humors, such a yellow bile, black bile, blood, and phlegm, becoming peccant. The ancient medical notion of **cancer** being related to ulcerative skin changes has little to do with our modern definition of metastatic cellular diseases. The etymological entries in your medical dictionary provide the original meanings of these loan words.

Cancer [L. *cancer*, crab, suppurating ulcer]

Cholera [L. *cholera*, fr. Gr. *cholera*, a disease affecting humors of the body causing vomiting and diarrhea, fr. *cholē*, bile]

Derivative

Like a loan word, a derivative is a word that is obtained from another language. However, a derivative differs from a loan word in that its spelling has been modified. Often, this involves dropping the inflectional ending of a Greek or Latin word (e.g. **ocular** is derived from the Latin word *ocularis*). In some cases, the deleted inflectional ending is replaced with a suffix common to the vernacular language (e.g. **artery** is derived from the Greek word *artēria*). These changes are quite apparent in their etymological entries:

Ocular [L. *ocularis*, pertaining to the eye]

Artery [Gr. *artēria*, a blood vessel, airway]

Compound Word

Compound words are terms that are created by joining together word elements taken from different Greek and/or Latin words. These terms are constructed from three different types of **word elements**: prefixes, roots, and suffixes. Many of these terms are neologisms. A **neologism** is a new word that is not found in the parent language(s) from which the word is derived. Etymological entries in medical dictionaries reveal that most medical terms are compound words:

Macrocephaly [Gr. *makros*, long, large + Gr. *kephalē*, head]

Semisulcus [L. *semis*, half + L. *sulcus*, a furrow, ditch, groove]

Ceratomandibular [Gr. *keras, keratos*, horn, horn-like + L. *mandibula*, jaw, bone of the lower jaw, fr. L. *mandere* to chew]

Inflection

Greek and Latin are inflected languages. **Inflection** is the modification of a word by adding different endings to the word in order to change the grammatical function of the word. Observe how the changes to the endings of the Latin noun *digitus* (finger or toe) affect the translation of this word in the following anatomical Latin terms:

1) *Digitus secundus.* = 2nd **finger (toe)**
2) *Digiti* = **Fingers (toes)**
3) *Extensor digitorum longus* = Long extender **of the fingers (of the toes)**

By simply changing the endings of *digitus*, one is able to indicate in Latin whether the *digitus* should be translated as a singular or plural (examples 1 and 2), and whether the noun should be translated as a possessive by adding "of the" (example 3).

Because inflectional endings do not change the core meaning of Greek or Latin words, only the grammatical usages, their removal reveals the roots of words:

L. *digitus* – inflectional ending **–us** = Root DIGIT-, finger or toe

Gr. *soma, somatos* – inflectional ending **–os** = Root SOMAT-, body

Because of inflection, Greek and Latin loan words in medical and scientific English will have different nominative plural forms:

Vena (1st declension Latin nominative singular) → Venae (plural)

Trachoma (3rd declension Greek nominative singular) → Trachomata (plural)

Review	Answers
A Greek or Latin word which has been adopted into medical English without any change to its spelling is called a _____.	**loan word**
A medical term that is derived from the name of a person or legendary figure is called an _____.	**eponym**
_____ are words obtained from other languages by modifying the spelling of the original word.	**Derivatives**
_____ are medical terms formed by adding multiple Greek or Latin word elements (i.e. prefix, root, and suffix) together.	**Compound words**
Based on its etymological entry [*Prometheus*, a Titan in Greek mythology who is associated with creating humans], "Promethium" is an _____.	**eponym**
Based on its etymological entry [L. *saeptum*, a wall, barrier + Gr. *plassein*, to form], "Septoplasty" is a _____.	**compound word**
Based on its etymological entry [L. *rostrum*, snout, beak, prow of a ship, a speaker's platform], "Rostrum" is a _____.	**loan word**
Based on its etymological entry [Gr. *konos*, pine cone], "Cone" is a _____.	**derivative**
Because _____ _____ do not change the core meaning of Greek or Latin words, only the grammatical usages, their removal reveals the roots of words. Gr. *soma, somatos* – inflectional ending **-os** = Root SOMAT-, body	**inflectional endings**

Root

While in linguistics, the terms "root," "base," and "stem" have different meanings, for the sake of clarity and as a matter of convention, this textbook does not make a distinction between "root," "base," and "stem." A **root** is the fundamental part of a Greek or Latin word that expresses the basic meaning of the Greek or Latin word. The root is separable from its inflectional endings. Thus, a root often can be recognized in a Greek or Latin word. It is derived by removing the last vowel and any consonant that follows. Roots are primarily derived from Latin and Greek nouns, adjectives, and verbs. In this text, a root will be indicated by the hyphen following the root:

ARTHR-	Gr. *arthron*, joint	**arthr**algia, osteo**arthr**itis
VEN-	L. *vena*, vein	**ven**ectomy, intra**ven**ous

Some roots are not recognizable in the form of the Greek or Latin word provided in the etymological entries in medical dictionaries because these dictionaries only provide the nominative case of a noun (e.g. CORPOR- [L. *corpus*, body]), but for some nouns, particularly Greek and Latin nouns of the 3rd declension, the root is only recognized in the genitive case of the noun (e.g. CORPOR- [L. *corpus*, *corporis*, body]). For such nouns, your textbook will provide both the nominative and the genitive singular form of the Greek or Latin word:

CORPOR-	L. *corpus*, **corpor**is, body	**corpor**eal, bi**corpor**ate
HEPAT-	Gr. *hepar*, **hepat**os, liver	**hepat**itis, **hepat**algia

It is important to bear in mind that more than one root can be derived from a single Greek or Latin word:

FER-, LAT-	L. *ferre*, *latus*, to bear, carry	semini**fer**ous, sub**lat**ion
SOM-, SOMAT-	Gr. *soma*, *somat*os, body	**som**esthetic, **somat**ogenic

A Greek or Latin word can used as the source of a root and be a loan word in medico-scientific terminology. When used as a loan word, the meaning/usage of the word is usually specific to the scientific field in which it occurs. For example, the 23rd Edition of Taber's Medical Dictionary Online provides the following definitions for **soma:** (i) the body as distinct from the mind; (ii) all of the body cells except the germ cells; and (iii) the body of a cell, which contains the nucleus.

Root	Etymology	Loan word
SOM-, SOMAT-	Gr. *soma*, somatos, body	**Soma**
CORPOR-	L. *corpus*, corporis, body	**Corpus**
HEPAT-	Gr. *hepar*, hepatos, liver	**Hepar**
DERM-, DERMAT-	Gr. *derma*, dermatos, skin, hide	**Derma**

Prefix

A **prefix** is a one- or two-syllable word element attached to the beginning of a term, which modifies the meaning of a word. Prefixes are derived from Greek or Latin adverbs and prepositions. Prefixes generally convey concepts such as time, quantity, quality, position, and direction. A prefix will be indicated by the prefix followed by a hyphen (e.g. EU-). Since there is a limited number of prefixes, you can distinguish them from roots by memorizing the list of prefixes provided in the vocabulary at the end of this chapter.

Prefix	Meaning	Examples
EU-	Normal	**eu**pnea (normal breathing)
DYS-	Difficult	**dys**pnea (difficult breathing)
INTRA-	Within	**intra**cystic (pertaining to within a bladder)
EXTRA-	Outside	**extra**cystic (pertaining to outside a bladder)

It is important to bear in mind that not every compound term begins with a prefix, and therefore, one should not assume that the word element in a compound term is a prefix:

Hepatology HEPAT- (root) + LOG- (root) + -Y (suffix)

Suffix

A **suffix** is a one- or two-syllable word element appended to the end of a medical term in order to modify its meaning. The majority of suffixes in medical English are derived from traditional Latin or Greek suffixes. Many of these suffixes have acquired special meanings in medical and scientific terminology that they did not have in antiquity. A suffix will be indicated by a hyphen appearing before the word element:

Suffix	Etymology	Current meanings	Examples
-OMA	Gr. *-oma*	tumor, swelling	derma**toma** (skin tumor)
-ITIS	Gr. *-itis*	inflammation	derma**titis** (inflammation of the skin)
-OSIS	Gr. *-osis*	condition (typically pathological)	derma**tosis** (pathological condition of the skin)

Suffixes also indicate whether a medical term is a noun, adjective, verb, or adverb (i.e. its part of speech). The vast majority of these suffixes indicate the word is a noun or adjective.

Suffix	Part of speech	Meaning	Examples
-IC	Adjective	Pertaining to	phob**ic** (pertaining to fear)
-IA	Noun	Condition	hemipleg**ia** (condition of paralysis of half the body)
-ATE	Verb	To apply, perform	lig**ate** (to apply a ligature)
-AD	Adverb	Toward	cephal**ad** (toward the head)

Certain combinations of suffixes and roots occur so frequently together that they are treated as suffixes in medical terminology (e.g. –LOGY = LOG- + -Y; -SOME = SOM- + -E). For such **compound suffixes**, this book will provide the suffix form with the corresponding root. You should learn the common usage of these compound suffixes, and the individual meanings of the roots and suffixes used to form them.

Root and suffix	Meanings	Etymologies	Example
SOM-, SOMAT-	A body	Gr. *soma, somatos*, body	somesthetic
-SOME	**A body**		chromo**some**
LOG-	Word, speech	Gr. *logos*, word, speech	logorrhea
-LOGY	**The study of**		hepato**logy**

Some Latin and Greek nouns, verbs, and adjectives are also treated as suffixes in medical terminology. You should recognize that these Greek and Latin words are also used as roots in compound terms:

Root and suffix	Meanings	Etymologies	Example
SOM-, SOMAT-	A body	Gr. ***soma***, *somatos*, body	somesthetic
-SOME, **-SOMA**	A body		hypoano**soma**
-PTOSIS	A downward displacement	Gr. ***ptosis***, a falling	blepharo**ptosis**

Combining Vowel and Combing Form

A **combining vowel** is used to join a root to another root or to a suffix. The vowels most commonly used are "o" and "i"; vowels such as "a," "y," and "u" are also used, albeit far less often. There is no uniform rule as to which combining vowel should be added to a particular root. Depending on the term, the same root may use a different combining vowel to join it to another word element. A combining vowel does not add any meaning to the word; it is added simply for the sake of euphony:

HYDR- (root) + **O** (combining vowel) + PHOB- (root) + IA (suffix) = hydr**o**phobia
CEREBELL- (root) + **I** (combining vowel) + PET (root) + AL (suffix) = cerebell**i**petal

A root with a combining vowel is referred to as a **combining form**. The combining forms in the above examples are HYDR/O and CEREBELL/I. Again, the meaning of the root is unchanged by adding a combining vowel.

Usage of Combining Vowels

The following are some general principles for deciding when to add a combining vowel:

1) **A combining vowel is used to combine a root to a root.**
   HEPAT- (root) + **O** (combining vowel) + MEGAL- (root) + Y (suffix) = hepat**o**megaly
   HEPAT- (root) + **O** (combining vowel) + ENTER- (root) + -ITIS (suffix) = hepat**o**enteritis
2) **A combining vowel is used to join a root to a suffix only if the suffix begins with a consonant.**
   HEPAT- (root) + **O** (combining vowel) + -LOGY (suffix) = hepat**o**logy
   HEPAT- (root) + **O** (combining vowel) + -PTOSIS (suffix) = hepat**o**ptosis
3) **If the suffix begins with a vowel, the combining vowel is typically omitted.**
   HEPAT- (root) + -OMA (suffix) = hepatoma
   HEPAT- (root) + -ITIS (suffix) = hepatitis

Elision

Elision is the omission of a letter from a word element in order to make the word easier to pronounce. Elision is common, but not universal, in the following situations:

1) **If a prefix ends with a vowel and the following root or suffix begins with a vowel, the final vowel of the prefix is typically omitted.**
   END**O**– (prefix) + **A**RTERI- (root) + AL (suffix) = endarterial
   MES**O**– (prefix) + **E**NTER- (root) + ON (suffix) = mesenteron

2) **If a root ends with the same vowel that the following root or suffix begins with, the final vowel of the root is usually omitted.**
PERI- (prefix) + CARDI- (root) + ITIS (suffix) = pericarditis
CORE- (root) + ECTASIA (suffix) = corectasia

Assimilation

Certain prefixes may be hard to recognize because their final letter is sometimes changed in response to the first letter of the roots they are attached to. This change is called **assimilation**. Assimilation of prefixes occurs in one of two ways:

1) **The last consonant of a prefix is changed to the same consonant as the following root.**
dis + fusate = diffusate
con + rugator = corrugator
2) **The last consonant is changed to another consonant which allows the combination to be pronounced more easily.**
in + perfect = imperfect
syn + pathy = sympathy

Vowel Gradation (Ablaut)

Vowel gradation is an internal vowel change that occurs to make new words. This can be observed in the alterations of the English word sing, sang, sung, song. With Greek and Latin word elements this also occurs, and these changes are present in medical and scientific terminology.

L. *annus* (year); *perennis* (perennial) = annual, perennial
Gr. *pherein* (to carry); *phoros* (a carrying) = pheresis, dysphoria

Review	Answers
The three types of word elements are _____, _____, and _____.	**prefixes, roots, suffixes**
The fundamental part of a Greek or Latin word which expresses the basic meaning of the Greek or Latin word is called the _____. This type of word element is derived from Greek and Latin _____, _____, and _____.	**root** **nouns, adjectives, verbs**
A _____ is added to the beginning of a compound term. It modifies the term conveying concepts such as _____, _____, _____, _____, and _____.	**prefix** **time, quantity, quality, position, direction**
A _____ is a word element added to the end of a term to modify its meaning. In addition to adding meaning to root, it reveals a medical term is to be used as a _____, _____, _____, or an _____.	**suffix** **noun, adjective, verb, adverb**
Certain combinations of root and suffix which frequently occur together, such as –MEGALY, are called _____ _____.	**compound suffixes**
–STASIS is an example of a Greek word being used as a _____.	**suffix**
A _____ _____ is used to join a root to another root or to a suffix.	**combining vowel**
A root plus a combining vowel is called a _____ _____.	**combining form**
A combining vowel is used to join a root to another _____, as well as a root to a _____ if it begins with a consonant.	**root, suffix**
A combining vowel is not used to join a root to a suffix if the suffix begins with a _____.	**vowel**
The most common combining vowels are _____ and _____. Less common combining vowels are _____, _____, and _____.	**o, i** **a, y, u**

In the following review questions, join the roots and suffixes by adding the combining vowel when needed according the aforementioned principles.

Examples:
ANGI- (root) + ECTOMY (suffix) = **angiectomy**
OSTE- (root) + MEGALY (suffix) = **osteomegal**
VEN- (root) + ARTERI- (root) + OMA (suffix) = **venoarterioma**

Review	Answers
HEMAT- (root) + POIESIS (suffix) = _____	**Hematopoiesis**
VAS- (root) + ECTOMY (suffix) = _____	**Vasectomy**
GASTR- (root) + ENTER- (root) + -CELE (suffix) = _____	**Gastroenterocele**
VEN- (root) + VEN- (root) + -STOMY (suffix) = _____	**Venovenostomy**
ANGI- (root) + ECTASIS (suffix) = _____	**Angiectasis**

In respect to the concepts of elision, assimilation, and vowel gradation answer the following:

Review	Answers
The process of _____ explains why the final vowel of a root or prefix may not be present in a medical term.	**elision**
If a root ends with the _____ _____ that the following root or suffix begins with, the final vowel of the root is usually omitted.	**same vowel**
If a prefix ends with a _____ and the following root or suffix begins with a _____, the final vowel of the prefix is typically omitted.	**vowel, vowel**
The process of _____ explains why a prefix may change its terminal consonant.	**assimilation**
Internal vowel changes which occur to make new words are called _____ _____.	**vowel gradation (ablaut)**

Identify what type of modification has been made to the following word elements:

Example:
CARDI (root) + ITIS (suffix) = Carditis **Elision of the vowel "i" from the root CARDI-**

Review	Answers
PARA- (prefix) + ENTER- (root) + AL (suffix) = parenteral _____	**Elision of the vowel "a" from the prefix PARA-**
OSTE- (root) + ECTOMY (suffix) = ostectomy _____	**Elision of the vowel "e" from the root OSTE-**
CON- (prefix) + LIG (root) + ATE (suffix) = colligate_____	**Assimilation of the consonant "N" to "L" with the prefix CON-**
EPI- (prefix) + ARTERI- (root) + AL (suffix) = eparterial _____	**Elision of the vowel "i" from the prefix EPI-**
SYN- (prefix) + BI- (root) + OSIS (suffix) = symbiosis _____	**Assimilation of the consonant "N" to "M" with the prefix SYN-**

Semantics

Etymology and Semantics

As noted, **etymology** is the study of the history of a word or word element. For the purpose of learning medico-technical jargon, we are focusing on ancient Greek and Latin words and their historical meanings. It is understood that one can trace some Greek and Latin words and word elements beyond these parent languages. For instance, the term *Natrium* is a New Latin termed coined by Jöns Jacob Berzelius in 1814 for the element Sodium (Na). Prior to this, it was called *Natronium* by Ludwig Wilhelm Gilber (1809). The term *Natron* was used by the French in the 17th century. Writing in the 16th century, the famous alchemist and physician Paracelsus used the term *Anatron*, which was derived from the combination of the medieval Arabic term *Natrūn* and its article. The Classical Latin term for sodium *Nitrum* used by ancient Romans is derived from a Greek word *Nitron* (νίτρον), which is a Greek word that etymologists believe has Semitic influence. Ultimately, etymologists trace our Latin term *Natrium* back to the Egyptian *ntrj*. Thus, while the basic etymology of the term Natrium is Latin, its origins go far beyond Latin, and it was not coined directly from a Latin term used for sodium in the Roman world.

Semantics is the study of the meanings of words and parts of words. Tracing a word back to its origins, like *Natrium* to *ntrj*, does not reveal "the true meaning" of a word. The meanings of words change over time and geographical location, as well as in the context in which they are used. For instance, the ancient Egyptian word *ntrj* seems to be derived from a stem for the word "holy or divine," which perhaps is why the Greek historian Herodotus (5th century BC) used the term *Nitron* (νίτρον) when describing the material used by Egyptians for their religious practice of mummification. Semantics reveals that words and word elements can move from abstract to concrete, general to specific, and locative to temporal in their meanings. In regard to scientific jargon, Greek and Latin roots often take on very specific technical meanings. Despite having the same word origin, Natrium (Na), the 11th element on the periodical table, is technically not the same as Natron, which is the naturally occurring sodium carbonate decahydrate believed to have been used in Egyptian mummification. That said, the original meanings of Greek and Latin words are very helpful in recognizing the meanings of compound terms via word analysis.

Meaning via Word Analysis

It is best to think of a compound term as a sentence that needs to be translated. By breaking a compound term down into its word elements and then arranging these parts in a meaningful way, one will arrive at the literal meaning of a word. The following principles are useful in arriving at the literal meaning of a medico-scientific term:

1) As a rule of thumb, when formulating a definition from a term's word elements, the suffix of a term should be translated first followed by the prefix, and then the root or roots. For example:

perineuritis

peri/neur/itis

peri- (prefix, around)/neur- (root, nerve)/-itis (suffix, inflammation)

perineuritis = inflammation around the nerve

2) You need to distinguish between an adjective and a noun in your definition. This can be done by looking at the suffix of the term. Although some adjectival suffixes (e.g. -ic, -al, -ac, -ar, -ous) have special meanings, most can be simply translated as "pertaining to..." or "concerning...."

cardiac

cardi (root) heart/-ac (suffix) pertaining to

cardiac = pertaining to the heart

3) Suffixes, such as –cle, -il, -ole, and –ule, which indicate "smallness" are called "diminutives." They are best translated with the adjective "little" or "small."

arteriole

arteri- (root) artery/-ole (suffix) little

arteriole = small artery

4) Often compound terms have more than one root. The order of the roots typically has no effect on the literal meaning of the term:

psychosomatic

psych- (root) mind/somat- (root) body/-ic (suffix) pertaining to

psychosomatic = pertaining to body and mind

5) Not every compound medical term begins with a prefix:

laterocervical

later- (root) side/cervic- (root) neck/-al (suffix) pertaining to

laterocervical = pertaining to the side of the neck

6) In some instances, a compound term may have more than one prefix. This is particularly true when a prefix is an integral part of an anatomical term (e.g. ENDOCARDI- = *endocardium*). When this occurs, it is best to preserve the anatomical term in your definition:

subendocardial

sub- (prefix) under/endo- (prefix) within + cardi (root) heart + al (suffix) pertaining to

subendocardial = pertaining to under the endocardium

7) Although it is good practice to be able to know the meanings of the roots and suffixes that make up compound suffixes, it is best to give the common usage of the compound suffix in your definition:

hepatomegaly

hepat- (root) liver/megal- (root) large/-y (suffix) state or condition of

hepatomegaly = enlargement of the liver

Word Elements with Multiple Meanings

It is important to remember that a word element can have multiple meanings. The word element **OXY**-, which is derived from the Greek adjective *oxys*, carries with it the ancient Greek meanings of "sharp," "keen," "quick," "pungent," and "acid." Some word elements have acquired new meanings not associated with their original usage in Greek or Latin. **OXY**- has acquired the meaning "oxygen," thanks to the French chemist Antoine-Laurent Lavoisier coining the term "*oxygène*" in 1777 when he mistakenly believed that this gaseous chemical element was the essential component in the formation of acids, hence **OXY**- (acid) + **–GEN** (that which creates). You should learn all the definitions for a given word element so that you will be able to recognize its potential meanings in medicine and science. Your textbook will provide both the ancient and modern definitions, setting the modern meanings off with a semicolon:

OXY-sharp, keen, quick, pungent, acid; oxygen

When faced with a word element having more than one potential meaning, determining the literal definition of a term is often a matter of common sense and context. For instance, the root **PHREN**- can mean "mind" or "diaphragm." If you were reading a text on respiratory diseases and you came across the term phrenoptosis, common sense dictates that "downward displacement of the ...." should be supplied with the term "diaphragm" rather than "mind." But if you were reading about psychological research and you ran across the term bradyphrenia, you should suspect that it refers to the "slowness of the mind."

Synonyms

Synonyms are two different words that refer to the same thing. As was noted in chapter one, medical English makes use of both Greek and Latin words which have similar meanings. The word elements METR- [Gr. *metra*, womb], HYSTER- [Gr. *hystera*, womb], and UTER- [L. *uterus*, womb] are all used today as word elements referring to the "uterus." Other than common usage, there is no reason for the preference of one synonym over another.

Homographs

The etymologies of word elements will also help you to recognize homographs. **Homographs** are words or word elements that have similar spellings but different meanings. The word element PED- in "pediatrics" means "child," but in the word "pedal," it means "foot." The word element PED- in pediatrics is derived from the Greek word "child" [Gr. *pais, paidos*], but in pedal, it is from the Latin word for "foot" [L. *pes, pedis*].

Literal Meaning Versus Technical Definition

The focus of this textbook is on arriving at the literal meanings of medico-scientific terms. It is important to bear in mind that the literal meaning of a term may not encapsulate all the information found in your medical dictionary's definition. The literal meaning of **melanoma**, "black tumor," does not inform you that the tumor is malignant, and it must be inferred that the root **MELAN-** refers to **melanocytes**. Like any language, medical terminology contains idiomatic usages of words. When faced with the term **bradyphrenia**, you could surmise that it refers to either a "condition in which the diaphragm moves slowly," or "a condition in which there is slowness of thought." While the former is a possible literal meaning, the latter is how it is actually used in med-speak. If the meaning of a term is unclear based on your word analysis, consulting a medical dictionary will clarify the term's current usage.

Review	Answers
As a general rule of thumb when arriving at a definition of a term through word analysis, the _____ should be translated 1st, followed by the _____, and then the _____ or _____.	suffix, prefix, root, roots
The roots **PHREN-** and **OXY-** are examples of word elements which have more than one _____.	meaning
The _____ _____ of a compound term is derived through word analysis. This meaning is not always the same as the definition in the dictionary.	literal meaning
PED- is derived from two different words with completely different meanings, which makes it a _____.	homograph

Spelling

The Greek Alphabet

The term "alphabet" is derived from the 1st two letters of classical Greek script, *alpha + beta*. One of the earliest accounts of the origin of the Greek alphabet comes from the 5th century BC historian Herodotus (*Histories* V.58). Using the myth of Cadmus' founding of Thebes, Herodotus describes how Cadmus and his followers brought the letters of the Phoenicians to Greece, which the Greeks later adapted to make their alphabet. Although Herodotus' account has mythological elements to it, his belief that the Greeks acquired their alphabet from the Phoenicians is historically correct. During the 8th century BC, the Greeks adapted the Phoenician alphabet for the purpose of writing their own language. They made numerous changes to the Phoenician script, such as adding letters to represent vowel sounds, ultimately resulting in the 24 letters known as the classical Greek alphabet.

The 24 letters of the classical Greek alphabet overlap with, but differ from, the 26 letters of the English alphabet. The Greek letter, its name, and its English letter equivalents are provided in the following table:

Name of letter	Upper and lower case	English equivalents
Alpha	A α	A a
Beta	B β	B b
Gamma	Γ γ	G g (or N n)
Delta	Δ δ	D d
Epsilon	E ε	E e
Zeta	Z ζ	Z z

Name of letter	Upper and lower case	English equivalents
Eta	H η	E e long
Theta	Θ θ	Th th (or T t)
Iota	I ι	I i
Kappa	K κ	K k (or C c)
Lambda	Λ λ	L l
Mu	M μ	M m
Nu	N ν	N n
Xi	Ξ ξ	X x
Omicron	O ο	O o
Pi	Π π	P p
*Rho	P ρ	R r (or Rh rh)
Sigma	Σ σ or ς	S s
Tau	T τ	T t
Upsilon	Y υ	Y y (or U u)
Phi	Φ φ	Ph ph (or F f)
Chi	X χ	Ch ch
Psi	Ψ ψ	Ps ps
Omega	Ω ω	O o long

Transliteration

Transliteration is the process of representing one writing system in another. The Greek words that appear in the etymological entries in medical dictionaries have been transliterated into English.

One of the obvious ways Greek words are transliterated into English is by replacing the Greek letters with corresponding letters in the Latin (English) alphabet.

ἧπαρ is transliterated into English **hepar** [Gr. *hepar*, liver]

When a Greek word is transliterated into anatomical or biological Latin, its Greek inflectional endings will be changed into Latin inflectional endings. For example, ἧπαρ, ἥπατος is transliterated into anatomical Latin *hepar, hepatis* by removing the Greek inflectional ending for the genitive case (**-os**) and replacing it with the Latin inflectional ending for the genitive case (**-is**). Thus, many of our loan words from anatomical and biological Latin are transliterated Greek words, and these words are declined according to Latin grammar.

Gr. ἀμοιβή, ἀμοιβῆς > biological Latin *amoeba, amoebae* [Gr. *amoibe*, change]
Gr. ἧπαρ, ἥπατος > anatomical Latin *hepar, hepatis* [Gr. *hepar*, liver]

Alternate Spellings of Greek Words

In respect to spelling and the transliteration of Greek words, the following deserves special attention:

1) Greek inflectional endings are often changed into corresponding Latin inflectional endings. This accounts for why Greek words with the terminal ending *–on* will be changed to the Latin *–um*, and likewise, the Greek *-os* will be often rendered as a Latin *–us*.

pericardium [Gr. *perikardion*, around the heart]
strabismus [Gr. *strabismos*, squinting]

2) The inflectional endings of some Greek loan words are simply dropped because English grammar does not require such endings. In other cases, the Greek ending may be changed to a silent "e," or a voiced "y" may be added.

> **stomach** [Gr. *stomachos*, throat, opening, stomach]
> **syringe** [Gr. *syrinx*, pipe]
> **artery** [Gr. *arteria*, windpipe, artery]

3) Some words have alternate spellings because the Greek letter *kappa* may be rendered as a "k" or "c."

> **leukemia** and **leucine** [Gr. *leukos*, white]

4) Some word elements may have alternate spellings because the Greek *upsilon* may be rendered "y" or "u."

> **glucose** and **glycogen** [Gr. *glukus*, sweet]

5) The rough breathing mark ('), which appears over a letter at the beginning of a Greek word is transliterated as an "h."

> **hepar** [Gr. *hēpar*/ἡπαρ, liver]

At the beginning of a Greek word, a *rho* had a rough breathing mark (ῥ) to indicate it was pronounced with an "h" sound. In such cases, it is transliterated "rh."

> **rhinitis** [Gr. *rhis, rhinos*/ῥις ῥινος, nose + -itis, inflammation]

When a *rho* occurs in the middle of a term, it typically has a smooth breathing, and therefore it is transliterated "r."

> **derma** [Gr. *derma*, skin]

Notable exceptions to this rule are the following common suffixes: **-rrhaphy** (suture), **-rrhea** (discharge), **-rrhage** (bursting forth, profuse fluid discharge), and **-rrhexis** (rupture).

6) The Greek diphthong ου (*ou*) is often rendered "u," but it may also appear as "ou."

> **micropus** [Gr. *mikros*, small + *pous*, foot]
> **xanthopous** [Gr. *xanthos*, yellow + *pous*, foot]

7) The Greek diphthong ει is rendered either "i" or "ei."

> **cheirognostic** [Gr. *cheiros*, hand + *gnostikos*, knowing]
> **chiromegaly** [Gr. *cheiros*, hand + *megas*, large]

8) In American English, the Greek diphthongs αι (*ai*) and οι (*oi*) are usually transliterated "e." In British English and scientific Latin, αι (*ai*) and οι (*oi*) are transliterated "ae" and "oe."

> ***anemia*** (American) versus ***anaemia*** (British) [Gr. *anaimia*, want of blood]
> ***diarrhea*** (American) versus ***diarrhoea*** (British) [Gr. *diarrhoia*, a flowing through]

Alternate Spellings of Latin Words

Because English letters are derived from the Latin alphabet, only minor changes in spelling are sometimes observed when Latin words are translated into English. The following should be considered:

1) The Latin diphthongs *ae* and *oe* become *e* in American English words; in British English, these diphthongs are typically retained.

> **septum** [L. *saeptum*, barrier, wall]

2) In English, there is a tendency to drop the inflectional endings of Latin words. That said, the exact Latin spelling will be retained with anatomical and biological terms written in scientific Latin.

> **fibril** [L. *fibrilla*, small fiber]
> **cecal** [L. *caecalis*, pertaining to the cecum]

Review	Answers
The Greek letter φ is transliterated into English as the letters _____.	**PH**
The Greek letter χ is transliterated into English as the letters _____.	**CH**
The Latin diphthongs *ae* and *oe* are often transliterated as the letter _____ in American English.	**E**
The Latin *i* is sometimes transliterated as a letter _____ in Latin words such as *major*.	**J**
With derivatives in English, there is a tendency to drop the _____ _____ of Latin words.	**inflectional endings**
The Greek *kappa*, when transliterated into English, appears either as a letter _____ or as a letter _____.	**K, C**
The Greek diphthongs "ei," "ou," "ai," and "oi" are often rendered as the letters_____, _____, _____, and _____ in American English.	**I, U, E, E**
The Greek *rho* is transliterated as the letter combination ____ at the beginning of a word and as the letter _____ in the middle of a word. Notable exceptions to this rule are the suffixes _____, _____, _____, and _____.	**RH, R, -rrhaphy, -rrhea, -rrhage, -rrhexis**
The Greek *upsilon* is transliterated to the English letter _____ or the letter _____.	**U, Y**
The inflectional endings of some Greek loan words are simply dropped because English grammar does not require such endings. In other cases, the Greek ending may be changed to a silent _____, or a voiced _____ may be added.	**E, Y**
In scientific Latin and English, Greek inflectional endings are often changed into _____ inflectional endings, for example, "os" becoming "us."	**Latin**

Transliterate the following Greek words:

Example: ἀρθρῖτις = arthritis

Review	Answers
γλωττα = _____	glotta
θωραξ = _____	thorax
χολερα = _____	cholera
ψυχη = _____	psyche
ἐκζεμα = _____	eczema

Pluralization

The Greek and Latin loan words, as well as the numerous compound words and Latin phrases used in scientific taxonomies, follow the grammatical rules of their parent languages. Unlike English, Latin and Greek are highly inflected languages. Because of inflection, Greek and Latin loan words in medical and scientific English will have different nominative plural forms.

Vena (1st declension Latin nominative singular) → Venae (plural)
Trachoma (3rd declension Greek nominative singular) → Trachomata (plural)

Common Classical Plural Forms in Medico-Scientific English

Most scientific and medical publications will require the use of classical plural forms. For a small collection of terms, pluralization by adding an "s" or "es" is acceptable and even preferred (e.g. **colons, cancers, hematomas, sinuses, viruses, meatuses, plexuses, and fetuses**). The following table contains the Greek and Latin singular endings commonly found in medical English and their corresponding plural forms:

Singular ending	Plural ending	Singular	Plural
-a	-ae	vertebra	vertebrae
-ax (-ex, -ix)	-aces, (-ices)	thorax (apex, fornix)	thoraces (apices, fornices)
-en	-ina	foramen	foramina
-is	-es	diagnosis	diagnoses
-itis	-itides	arthritis	arthritides
-ons (-ens, -ans)	-ontes (-entes, -antes)	pons (dens, albicans)	pontes (dentes, albicantes)
-oma	-omata	neuroma	neuromata
-on	-a	phenomenon	phenomena
-um	-a	brachium	brachia
-us	-i	fungus	fungi

Provide the plural endings for the following:

For example: coccus = cocci

Review	Answers
blastoma = _____	blastomata
papilla = _____	papillae
lumen = _____	lumina
enteritis = _____	enteritides
endocardium = _____	endocardia
satyriasis = _____	satyriases
encephalon = _____	encephala
cortex = _____	cortices
nevus = _____	nevi
intussuscipiens = _____	intussuscipientes

Pronunciation

The pronunciation of medico-scientific terms is a source of great anxiety for students. This is particularly true of Latin biological and anatomical names, such as *Amphioctopus marginatus* and *flexor digitorum superficialis*. Greek and Latin words in medical and scientific English conform to the principles for the pronunciation of English words. For example, when the Greek word ψυχή (mind) is transliterated into English as "psyche," it loses its Greek pronunciation psu-khē′ and is instead pronounced sī′kē. Likewise, the pronunciation of scientific terms written in Latin differs from the way Latin is believed to have been spoken in antiquity. Today, the term biceps is commonly pronounced bī′sĕps, but in the Latin of ancient Rome, it would have sounded like bī′keps. Although the ancient pronunciation of Latin, often termed the **classical pronunciation**, is still used today in the reading of Latin literature, for the sake of effective communication and uniformity, it is best to use the English principles of pronunciation outlined in this chapter.

Phonetic Spelling

To help with pronunciation, most medical dictionaries provide the **phonetic spellings** of terms. For example, if you were to look up the term omphalopagus, you would find (ŏm″fă-lŏp′ă-gŭs) in Taber's Cyclopedic Medical Dictionary. Phonetic spellings use letters and symbols to indicate how words sound in English. To aid in the pronunciation of vowels and syllables, a phonetic spelling contains diacritical marks called **macron** (‾), **breve** (˘), and **stress mark** (′). Long vowels have a macron (‾) placed over them. Short vowels are indicated by a breve (˘). Syllables are separated by either an accent mark or a hyphen. The stress mark (′) is used to indicated which syllable is given greater emphasis when spoken.

Vowels can be considered long (‾) or short (˘). Long vowels are as follows:

Long a (ā) sound as in *rate*
Long e (ē) sound as in *bee*
Long i (ī) sound as in *eye*
Long o (ō) sound as in *over*
Long u (ū) sound as in *you*

The sounds for short vowels are:

Short a (ă) sound as in *alone*
Short e (ĕ) sound as in *elm*
Short i (ĭ) sound as in *it*
Short o (ŏ) sound as in *ton*
Short u (ŭ) sound as in *cut*

A vowel which does not have a diacritical mark will have a flat sound:

a sound as in *banana*
e sound as in *open*
i sound as in *animal*
o sound as in *got*
u sound as in *put*

Guidelines for the Pronunciation of Medico-Scientific Terms

The English pronunciation of medico-scientific terms has never been fully standardized, and therefore, it may vary from region to region. Because of this, there is not one invariably "correct pronunciation." The phonetic spellings listed in your textbook are, for the most part, consistent with those provided in the 23rd edition of Taber's Cyclopedic Medical Dictionary. The following are general principles to help you produce a reasonable pronunciation when faced with an unfamiliar medico-scientific term in English or Latin.

Vowels

The pronunciation of vowels follows the rules of English. The greatest inconsistency in modern pronunciation of classical words appears to be determining which vowel is long and which is short. For example, when the letter y substitutes for the Greek letter upsilon, it is generally pronounced with a long e (ē) sound, as in **bradycardia** (brăd-ē-kard′ē-ă). However, in some cases, it retains a short i sound (ĭ) as in **symbiotic** (sĭm-bī-ŏt′ĭk). When in doubt about whether and vowel is long or short, consult your dictionary. That said, the following should be taken into consideration with respect to vowels and diphthongs:

Final Vowel

Unlike most English words, the final vowel is almost always voiced in terms derived from Latin and Greek:

Final vowel	Example
a = "ah" sound	amoeba (ă-mē′bă)
i = "eye" sound	fung**i** (fŭn′jī)
e = "ee" sound as in **heel**	syncop**e** (sĭn′kō-pē)
es = "ease" sound	phalang**es** (fă-lăn′jēz)

There are exceptions to this rule with certain word elements in English. Examples of this would be the suffix form -cele (sēl) and the suffix -ode (ōd). There are no exceptions to this rule with anatomical and scientific Latin.

Diphthongs

The combination of two vowels to make a single sound is termed a diphthong. Special attention should be given to the following:

Diphthong	**Example**
au as in "taught"	caudal (kawd′ăl)
eu as in "neuter"	aneurysm (ăn′ū-rĭzm)
oi as in "boy"	koilonychia (koy-lō-nĭk′ē-ă)
ae and oe as in "heel"	paederus (pēd′ĕr-ŭs), coelom (sē′lŏm)
ei as in "eye"	leiomyoma (lī-ō-mī-ō′mă)
ui as in "quick"	equine (ē′kwīn)

In Latin, the vowel combination of *ie* is a diphthong. With words derived from Latin, *ie* is pronounced as two separate vowels. For example, **paries** is pronounced pā′rē-ēz, and **facies** is pronounced fā′shē-ēz. The vowel combination *oi* is not a diphthong in Latin, which explains why in some words derived from Latin the vowels are pronounced separately, as in introitus (ĭn-trō′ĭ-tŭs). That said, by convention, *oi* is typically pronounced "oy" for most words derived from Greek and Latin.

Consonants

Consonants pose problems for students because they are often unsure which sound should be used. The following is a list of English rules for how consonants in words derived from Greek and Latin are pronounced.

Consonant	**Examples**
c before a, o, or u = k	cavus (kā′vŭs)
c before ae, oe, e, i, or y = s	coelom (sē′lŏm)
cc before e, i, or y = ks	cocci (kŏk′sī)
ch = k	chiroplasty (kī-rō-plăs′tē)
g before a, o, or u = g	gonad (gō′năd)
g before ae, oe, e, i, or y = j	angina (ăn-jī′nă)
ph = f	tenophyte (tĕn′ō-fīt)
rh or rrh = r	angiorrhexis (ăn-jē-or-ĕk′sĭs)
s + i before another vowel = zhă as in leisure or zēă	aphasia (ă-fā′zhă) polyphrasia (pŏl-ē-frā′zē-ă)
sc + i or e before another vowel = s	misce (mĭs′ē)
th = th	thenal (thē′năl)
t + i before another vowel = sh	aproctia (ă-prŏk′shē-ă)
x as the 1st consonant of word = z	xerosis (zē-rō′sĭs)
x in the middle of a word = ks	taxis (tăk′sĭs)

Consonant Clusters

At the beginning of a word, the first consonants of the following cluster of consonants are often silent:

Consonant cluster and sound	Examples
chth = th	chthonic (thon′ik)
ct = t	ctenocephalides (tĕn-ō-sĕf-ăl′ĭ-dēz)
gn = n	gnathic (năth′ĭk)
mn = n	mnemic (nē′mĭk)
phth = th	phthisis (thĭ′sĭs)
pn = n	pneumonia (nū-mō′nē-ă)
ps = s	psoriasis (sō-rī′ă-sĭs)
pt = t	pterygoid (tĕr′ĭ-goyd)

When these consonant combinations occur in the middle of a term, the first consonant is typically pronounced, as in **apnea** (ăp-nē′ă), **hemoptysis** (hē-mŏp′tĭ-sĭs), and **amnesia** (ăm-nē′zē-ă).

Syllables

A Latin or Greek word has as many syllables as it has vowel sounds or diphthongs. Every syllable is pronounced. The following are guidelines for the recognition and pronunciation of syllables:

1) A single consonant between two vowels or diphthongs generally goes with the second one.

   meatus (mē-ā′tŭs)

   The exception is the letter *x* because it is treated as two consonants, *ks*, and generally is attached to the previous vowel.

   epistaxis (ĕp-ĭ-stăk′sĭs)

2) Two adjacent consonants between two vowels or diphthongs are generally split.

   verruca (vĕr-roo′kă)

   The following double consonants are treated as single consonants:

   cr, br, dr, gr, kr, pr, tr   **sacrum** (sā′krŭm); **nigra** (nī′gră)
   ch, ph, rh, rrh, th   **gnathus** (nā′thŭs); **trichoma** (trĭk-ō′mă)
   bl, cl, dl, gl, kl, ll, pl, tl   **neuroclonic** (nū-rō-klŏn′ĭk); **neuroglioma** (nū-rō-glī- ō′mă)

3) A syllable is considered long if it contains a long vowel. It is short if it contains a short vowel.

Stress

Stress (or Accent) is the syllable in a multisyllabic word that should be emphasized in pronunciation. In phonetic spellings, the syllable that receives the stress will be indicated by a **stress mark** (′). In general, medico-scientific terms follow the patterns of stress that are found in Latin.

1) In words of two syllables, the stress is placed on the 1st syllable.

   gnathic (năth′ĭk)
   mnemic (nē′mĭk)

2) In words of more than two syllables, the accent is placed on the penult (the next to last) if the last syllable is long.

   chiroplasty (kī-rō-plăs′tē)
   phalanges (fă-lăn′jēz)

3) In words of more than two syllables, the accent is placed on the antepenult (the 2nd from the last) if the syllable is short.

> polyphrasia (pŏl-ē-frā′zē-ă)
> psoriasis (sō-rī′ă-sĭs)

While these are useful rules of thumb, one can find numerous examples of exceptions to these rules:

> ctenocephalides (tĕn-ō-sĕf-ăl′ĭ-dēz)
> angiorrhexis (ăn-jē-or-ĕk′sĭs)

Pronunciation of Word Elements

As noted, many medical terms do not follow the above principles so the best principle is to focus on learning the pronunciation of the word elements because this will get you close to the pronunciation used in the fields of medicine or science. Therefore, this textbook includes the phonetic spelling of the word elements listed in the vocabularies. When learning the meanings of the word elements, you should take the time to learn how to pronounce them.

Word Element	Phonetic Spelling	Etymology
NEUR/O	(nūr-ō)	Gr. *neuron*, nerve
ANTI-	(ant-i)	Gr. *anti-*, against, opposed to
ANTE-	(ant-ē)	L. *ante-*, before, forward
-CELE	(sēl)	Gr. *kele*, tumor, swelling, hernia

Review	Answers
The *pt* in **pterygium** makes a/an _____ sound.	t
The *mn* in **mnemonic** makes a/an _____ sound.	n
The *ch* in **chirality** makes a/an _____ sound.	k
The *g* in **phagic** makes a/an _____ sound.	j
The *es* in **stapes** makes a/an _____ sound.	ēz
The *ei* in **meibomian** makes a/an _____ sound.	ī
The *c* in **caecum** makes a/an _____ sound.	s
The *x* in **xeroderma** makes a/an _____ sound.	z
The *sia* in **polychromasia** makes a/an _____ or a _____ sound.	zhă, zēă
The *pn* in **orthopnea** makes a/an _____ sound.	pn
The *ae* in **paederus** makes a/an _____ sound.	ē
The *chth* in **chthonic** makes a/an _____ sound.	th
The *x* is **taxis** makes a/an _____ sound.	ks
The *t* in **aproctia** makes a/an _____ sound	sh
The *oi* in **koilonychia** makes a/an _____ sound.	oy
The *oe* in **coelom** makes a/an _____ sound.	ē

Vocabulary

Prefixes

Students often struggle with distinguishing between a root and a prefix. The following table contains the Greek and Latin prefixes used in medical terminology. It is imperative that you commit this list to memory. Some prefixes will have more than one meaning, and therefore, it is necessary to adapt the meaning to the particular context or use of a word. The force of the prefix's meaning may vary. In some cases, it is best to interpret it literally (e.g. **pericardium** – tissue which is *around* the heart), and in other cases, it should be understood as conveying a more abstract meaning (e.g. **perinatal** – *around* the time of birth). The changes in the spellings of certain prefixes due to assimilation are provided.

Greek Prefixes

Prefix	Meaning	Example
A- (a-) **AN-** (an-) before a vowel	Not, without	**a**chromatic **an**algesic
AMPHI- (am-fī) **AMPHO-** (am-fō)	Around about, both, both sides, in two ways	**amphi**bious **ampho**diplopia
ANA- (an-ă) **ANO-** (an-ō)	Upward, back, against, again	**ana**phoria **ano**tropia
ANTI- (ant-i)	Against, opposed to	**anti**coagulant
APO- (ap-ŏ)	Away/apart from, derived from	**apo**enzyme
DI- (dī)	Twice, double, two	**di**cephalous
DIA- (dī-ă)	Through, across	**dia**lysis
DICHO- (dī-kō)	In two, twofold	**dicho**tomy
DYS- (dis)	Difficult, painful, faulty	**dys**trophy
EC- (ek) **EK-** (ek) **EX-** (eks)	Out of, outside	**ec**topia **ek**phorize **ex**ophthalmus
ECTO- (ĕk-tō)	On the outside	**ecto**derm
EN- (en) **EM-** (em) before *b*, *m*, and *p*	In, within	**en**cephalon **em**pyesis
ENDO- (en-dō) **ENTO-** (ĕn-tō)	Within	**endo**cardium **ento**blast
EPI- (ep'ĭ-) **EPH-** (ĕf-) before *h*	Upon, on	**epi**dermal **eph**emeral
ESO- (es-ŏ)	Inward, within	**eso**tropia
EU- (ū)	Well, normal, good	**eu**pnea
EXO- (ek-sō)	Outside of, outward	**exo**gamy
HEMI- (hĕm-ē)	Half, partly	**hemi**paralysis
HYPER- (hī-pĕr)	Above, beyond, excessive	**hyper**tonic
HYPO- (hī-pō)	Under, below, deficient	**hypo**tonic
KATA- (kăt-ă)	Down, downward, against, complete, (intensive)	**kata**thermometer
CATA- (kăt-ă) **CAT-** (kăt) before *h*		**cata**tonic **cat**hode
META- (met-ă) **MET-** (met) before a vowel	After, beyond, change	**meta**stasis **met**encephalon
OPISTHO- (ŏ-pis-thŏ)	Behind, backward	**opistho**tonos
PALI- (păl-ĭ) **PALIN-** (păl-ĭn)	Again, once more, backward	**pali**graphia **palin**mnesia
PARA- (par-ă)	Alongside, beyond, opposite; abnormal	**para**noia

Prefix	Meaning	Example
PERI- (per-ĭ)	Around	**peri**osteum
PRO- (prō)	Before, in front of, forward	**pro**enzyme
PROS- (pros)	Toward, in addition, near	**pros**thesis
PROSO- (pros-ŏ)	Forward, before	**proso**plasia
SYN- (sin) **SYM-** (sim) before *b* or *p*	Together, with	**syn**dactyly **sym**biology

Latin Prefixes

Prefix	Meaning	Example
A- (a-) **AB-** (ab)	Away/apart from	**a**vulsion **ab**duct
AD- (ăd) **AF-** (ăf) before *f*	Toward, to, near	**ad**duct **af**ferent
AMBI- (am-bi)	Around, on both sides, both, twofold	**ambi**opia
ANTE- (ant-ē)	Before	**ante**partum
BI- (bĭ) **BIN-** (bĭ-n) before vowels	Twice, two, double, twofold	**bi**ped **bin**aural
CIRCUM- (sĭr″kŭm)	Around	**circum**duct
CON- (kŏn) **COL-** (kŏl) before *l* **COM-** (kŏm) before *b, m, p* **CO-** (kŏ) before *h* **COR-** (kŏr) before *r*	With, together, complete	**con**genital **col**ligate **com**plication **co**hesion **cor**rugator
CONTRA- (kon-tră)	Against, opposite	**contra**lateral
DE- (dē)	Down from, from, not	**de**lactation
DEMI- (dĕm-ĭ-)	Half, part	**demi**facet
DIS- (dĭs) **DIF-** (dĭf) before *f*	Apart from, separate	**dis**tract **dif**ference
E- (ē) **EX-** (eks) **EF-** (ef) before *f*	Out of, off	**e**vagination **ex**tend **ef**ferent
EXTRA- (ĕks-tră) **EXTRO-** (eks-trŏ)	Outside, beyond	**extra**pulmonary **extro**vert
IN- (ĭn) **IM-** (ĭm) before *b, m, p* **IL-** (ĭl) before *l* **IR-** (ĭr) before *r*	Into, in, against, not	**in**duction **im**perfect **il**literate **ir**radiate
INFRA- (in-fră)	Below, lower	**infra**orbital
INTER- (int-er)	Between	**inter**costal
INTRA- (ĭn-tră)	Within, during	**intra**dermal
INTRO- (ĭn-trŏ)	Within, inward	**intro**vert
INTUS- (ĭn-tŭs)	Within	**intus**susception

Prefix	Meaning	Example
JUXTA- (jŭks-tă)	Beside, near to	**juxta**pyloric
NON- (non)	Not, without	**non**occlusion
OB- (ŏb) **OC-** (ŏk) before *c* **OP-** (ŏp) before *p*	Against, in the way, facing	**ob**struction **oc**clusion **op**position
PER- (pĕr)	Through, throughout, (intensive)	**per**cutaneous
POST- (pōst)	After, behind	**post**operative
PRAE- or **PRE-** (prē)	Before, in front of	**pre**cordium
PRO- (prō)	Before, in front of, forth	**pro**tuberance
RE- (rē)	Again, back, (intensive)	**re**nascent
RETRO- (rĕt-rō)	Backward, behind	**retro**flexed
SE- (sĕ)	Aside, apart from	**se**gregate
SEMI- (sem-ē)	Half	**semi**permeable
SUB- (sŭb) **SUC-** (sŭk) before c **SUF-** (sŭf) before *f* **SUG-** (sŭg) before *g* **SUP-** (sŭp) before *p* **SUR-** (sŭr) before *r*	Under, below, less than normal	**sub**cutaneous **suc**cession **suf**fuse **sug**gestible **sup**puration **sur**rogate
SUPER- (soo-pĕr)	Over, above, excessive	**super**numerary
SUPRA- (soo-pră)	Above, upon	**supra**spinatous
TRANS- (trăns)	Across, through	**trans**carpal
ULTRA- (ŭl-tră)	Beyond, excessive	**ultra**sonic

In the following review, identify the prefix and its possible meanings.

Example: Prosencephalon = <u>Proso- forward, before</u>

Review	Answers
Juxtapyloric = _____	**Juxta- beside, near to**
Demifacet = _____	**Demi- half, part**
Symbiotic = _____	**Sym- together, with**
Agnosia = _____	**A- not, without**
Dissection = _____	**Dis- apart from, separate**
Postpartum = _____	**Post- after, behind**
Transurethral = _____	**Trans- across, through**
Analeptic = _____	**Ana- up, back, against, again**
Palilalia = _____	**Pali- again, once more, backward**
Metastasis = _____	**Meta- after, beyond, change**
Catatonic = _____	**Cata- down, downward, against, complete, (intensive)**
Hypertonic = _____	**Hyper- above, beyond, excessive**

Review	Answers
Ambidextrous = _____	**Ambi- around, on both sides, both**
Abduction = _____	**Ab- away from**
Apochromatic = _____	**Apo- away from, derived from**
Occlusion = _____	**Oc- against, in the way, facing**
Contrafissura = _____	**Contra- against, opposite**
Anticoagulant = _____	**Anti- against, opposed to**
Insect = _____	**In- into, in, against, not**
Afferent = _____	**Af- toward, to, near**

In the following review, give the possible prefix that will complete the meaning of each term.

Example: Around the nose = <u>PERI- (or CIRCUM-)</u> nasal

Review	Answers
Alongside the nose = _____nasal	**PARA-**
Below the nose = _____nasal	**INFRA- (or SUB-, HYPO-)**
Above the nose = _____nasal	**SUPRA- (or SUPER-, HYPER-)**
Through the nose = _____nasal	**TRANS- (or DIA-, PER-)**
Half a nose = _____nasal	**SEMI- (or HEMI-, DEMI-)**
Within the nose = _____nasal	**INTRA- (or INTRO-, ENDO-, EN-, INTUS-)**
Near the nose = _____nasal	**JUXTA- (or AD-, PROS-)**
Without a nose = _____nasal	**A-**
Together with the nose = _____nasal	**CON- (or SYN-)**
Upon the nose = _____nasal	**EPI- (or SUPRA-)**
Two nosed = _____nasal	**BI- (or DI-)**
Before or in front of the nose = _____nasal	**PRAE- (or PRO-, PROSO-)**
Behind the nose = _____nasal	**RETRO- (or POST-, OPISTHO-)**
Excessive nosed = _____nasal	**HYPER- (or ULTRA-, SUPER-)**
Apart from the nose = _____nasal	**AB- (or DIS-, SE-, APO-)**
A faulty or painful nose = _____nasal	**DYS-**
A good or normal nose = _____nasal	**EU-**

Suffixes

The suffixes are essential to understanding compound medical terms, and therefore, they should be committed to memory. The following table contains the traditional Greek and Latin suffixes used in medical terminology. The parts of speech (e.g. noun, adjective, and verb) are indicated in the list of meanings. Suffixes having similar meanings have been grouped together.

Greek Suffixes

Suffix	Meaning	Example
ADJECTIVAL SUFFIX		
-AC (ak)	Pertaining to	ili**ac**
-IC (ĭk)		gast**ric**
-TIC (tik)		cathar**tic**
VERB		
-IZE (īz)	To do; to become; to use; to engage in	euthan**ize**
NOUN SUFFIX		
-A (ă)	State or condition of	dyspn**ea**
-ESIS (ē-sĭs)		sudor**esis**
-IA (ē-ă)		man**ia**
-IASIS (ĭ-ă-sĭs)		psor**iasis**
-ISM (ĭzm)		embol**ism**
-OSIS (ō-sĭs)		symb**iosis**
-SIA (shă, sē-ă)		dyspep**sia**
-IAC (ē-ăk)	One who is afflicted with	hemophil**iac**
-ID (ĭd)	(Forms a noun or adjective) like, resembling, in the form of	lip**id**
-OID (oyd)		delt**oid**
-ODE (ōd)		nemat**ode**
-IDES (ĭ-dēz)	Descended from;	Ctenocephal**ides**
-IDAE (ĭ-dē)	**-ides** zoologic "genus"	Musc**idae**
-IDA (ĭ-dă)	**-idae** zoologic "family"	Arachn**ida**
	-ida zoologic "order" and "class"	
-IN (ĭn)	Substance, typically a chemical or hormone	chromat**in**
-INE (ēn) or (ĭn)		chlor**ine**, adrenal**ine**
-IST (-ĭst)	Person interested in; a practitioner who specializes in	herbal**ist**
-ITE (īt)	Belonging to, the nature of	som**ite**
-ITIS (īt-ĭs)	Inflammation	arth**ritis**
-IUM (ē-ŭm)	Tissue or part of the body	endocard**ium**
-OMA (ō-mă)	Tumor	neur**oma**
-Y (ē)	State or condition of, the act of	empa**thy**
		appendectom**y**

Latin Suffixes

The medico-scientific suffixes in the following table are derived from classical Latin suffixes. Most of them have been formed by removing the Latin inflectional endings (e.g. *-alis* = -AL). In some cases, vowels have been added to their original Latin spellings (e.g. *-eus* = -EOUS).

Suffix	Meaning	Example
ADJECTIVAL SUFFIXES		
-ACEOUS (ā-shŭs)	Made of, having the quality of, full of	alli**aceous**
-ANEOUS (ā-nē-ŭs)		succed**aneous**
-EOUS (ē-ŭs)		aur**eous**
-AL (ăl)	Pertaining to	semin**al**
-AR (ăr)		ocul**ar**
-EAL (ē-ăl)		lact**eal**
-ILE (ĭl)		sen**ile**

Suffix	Meaning	Example
-ANS (ăns)/-ANT (ănt) -ENS (ĕns) / -ENT (ĕnt) -IENS (ē-ĕns) / -IENT (ē-ĕnt)	Translated –*ing* added to the verb	devi**ant** abduc**ent** absorbefac**ient**
*SC + ANT, IENT, ENT	*Becoming added to verb + ing	rube**scent**
-BLE (bl) -ILE (ĭl)	Ability to	aud**ible** frag**ile**
-ID (ĭd)	In a state or condition of	frig**id**
-LENT (lĕnt) -OSE (ōs)	Full of	puru**lent** adip**ose**
-ARY (ā-rē) -ORY (ŏr-ē)	Pertaining to; (also forms a noun) place of	mortu**ary** depilat**ory**
ADVERBIAL SUFFIX		
-AD (ăd)	Indicates direction toward a part of the body	cephal**ad**
VERBAL SUFFIX		
-ATE (āt)	To make, to cause, to act upon; (also forms an adjective) having the form of, possessing	decapit**ate** penn**ate**
NOUN SUFFIX		
-TIA (shē-ă) -CE (s) -ITY (ĭ-tē) -TUDE (tood)	State or condition of	demen**tia** sequen**ce** san**ity** alti**tude**
-CLE (k-l) -IL (ĭl) -OLE (ōl) -ULE (ūl) -UNCLE (ŭng-kĕl)	Diminutive (little)	cuti**cle** fibr**il** arteri**ole** ven**ule** carb**uncle**
-IAN (ē-ăn)	Thing or person performing an action; practitioner of	pediatric**ian**
-ION (shŏn) -MENT (mĕnt) -URE (ŭr)	action; condition resulting from an action	liga**tion** liga**ment** fiss**ure**
-OR (or)	Something (usually a muscle) that performs an action; quality of condition	flex**or** pall**or**

In the following review, choose the best suffix to complete the literal meaning of the term.

Example: Inflammation of the heart = cardi-_____.

-itis   -oma   -ia   -esis

Review	Answers
Tissue inside of the heart = endocardi-_____. -oid -ist -ium -ism	**-IUM**
Of the nature of a body = som-_____. -ize -ite -or -ile	**-ITE**

Review	Answers
Pertaining to the liver = hepat-_____. -ic -ist -y -ian	**-IC**
Toward the stomach = gastr-_____. -ose -ion -ad -iac	**-AD**
Tumor of the head = cephal-_____. -ose -oma -ium -ite	**-OMA**
Resembling a nose = rhin-_____. -oid -ium -oma -ole	**-OID**
Full of glands = aden_____. -esis -ose -ac -id	**-OSE**
State or condition causing an abnormally small head = microcephal_____. -ia -iac -ile -ida	**-IA**
A small foot = ped_____. -ole -osus -aceous -alis	**-OLE**
A liberating hormone = liber_____. -osis -id -ode -in	**-IN**
The act of cutting into the heart = cardiotom_____. -y -ist -orium -ode	**-Y**
A muscle that extends a part of the body = extens_____. -or -ium -ida -ule	**-OR**
A biological family of dog-like carnivores = Can_____. -oid -idae -ian -orium	**-IDAE**
A practitioner who cuts into veins to draw blood = phlebotom_____. -y -ist -ate. -ize	**-IST**

3

Anatomical Terminology

CHAPTER LEARNING OBJECTIVES
1) You will learn about the ancient Alexandrian origins of human dissection and the rise of anatomical Latin.
2) You will gain a basic understanding of the grammar of anatomical Latin for medical English.
3) You will learn the Greek and Latin word elements for general parts of the body.

Lessons from History: Alexandrian Origins of Human Dissection and the Rise of Anatomical Latin

Food for Thought as You Read:

> *What role has society played in human dissection?*
> *When did systematic human dissection begin? By whom? What language did they speak and write in? When did it stop?*
> *When and where was human dissection resumed?*
> *Who is Vesalius? Why is he important to human dissection?*
> *Why are anatomical terms written in Latin today?*

The term **anatomy** is derived from the Greek word *anatome* [Gr. *ana*, up + *tome*, cut], which means "the act of dissection." Thanks to its longstanding usage in medical education, when one speaks of "human anatomy" today, one is generally referring to the "structures of the human body" or "the study of the structures of the human body." The dissection of human corpses in medical education can be traced back to the 14th century AD, when annual anatomies became part of the curricula of the Italian universities of Padua and Bologna. That said, long before any medieval anatomist ever touched a scalpel to a human cadaver, the famous Greek physicians, Herophilus of Chalcedon (c. 330–260 BC) and his contemporary Erasistratus of Ceos (c. 315–240 BC) had systematically dissected human cadavers. These physician-anatomists are also infamous figures in the history of medicine largely because they are said to have performed vivisections on condemned criminals to reveal the nature of the hidden parts of the human body (Fig. 3.1).

As Heinrich von Staden has pointed out, the discoveries of Herophilus and Erasistratus were quite remarkable considering that even for modern anatomists, the "thisness" of anatomical structures is far from self-evident amidst the mass of tubules, sinew, and fatty tissue. Without the aid of modern anatomical instruments and cadaveric atlases, Herophilus was able to meticulously differentiate such obscure structures as membranes of the eye, 7 of the 12 pairs of cranial nerves, and the choroid plexus in the ventricles of the brain. Herophilus was the first to make a distinction between motor and sensory nerves, and his discovering of the epididymis and the seminal vessels helped to dispel Aristotle's concept of the testicles functioning as "loom-weights." Many of his Greek anatomical terms live on in Latin. He called the first part of the small intestine the *dodekadaktylos* (12 fingers) because it was 12 fingers long, and the next part of the small intestine the *nestis* (fasting) because it is always found to be deprived of food. His terminology is preserved in the Latin words *duodenum* (12) and *jejunum* (empty) used in modern medical terminology. Herophilus likened the inferior portion of the floor of the 4th ventricle of the brain to a reed pen (Gr. *kalamos*), which today is known as the *Calamus scriptorius* (L. *scribal reed*).

Greek and Latin Roots of Medical and Scientific Terminologies, First Edition. Todd A. Curtis.
© 2025 John Wiley & Sons, Inc. Published 2025 by John Wiley & Sons, Inc.
Companion website: www.wiley.com/go/Curtis

The modern eponym Torcular Herophili also preserves his contribution to human anatomy. The Torcular Herophili is a confluence of cranial venous sinuses that was likened to a "wine vat" (Gr. *lēnos* = L. *torcular*) by Herophilus when he discovered it during his dissections. Erasistratus' discoveries were equally impressive. For example, his portrayal of the heart as a mechanical pump and his theory of junctions (Gr. *sunanastomoses*) between arteries (Gr. *arteriai*) and veins (Gr. *phlebes*) had him flirting ever so closely with recognizing the circulation of blood, a discovery made only much later by William Harvey in the 17th century.

Prior to Herophilus and Erasistratus, direct knowledge of the internal anatomy of the human body was gleaned primarily from the serendipity of a decomposing corpse or from a wound revealing the internal parts of a human being. Aristotle's (384–322 BC) biological studies were an important step toward the act of human dissection.

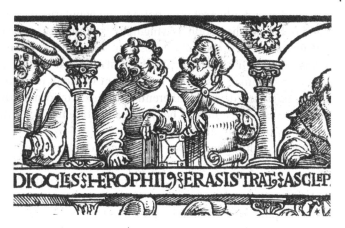

Fig. 3.1 Detail of a 16th century woodcut depicting Herophilus and Erasistratus. It was common for Medieval and Renaissance artists to depict ancient Greek physicians as contemporaries. *Source:* Wellcome Collection/Public domain.

Aristotle's systematic dissections of animals led him to believe that the function and structures of animals reveal a hierarchical relationship between all living things, with mankind being at the apex. For Aristotle, as well as his medical contemporaries, Praxagoras and Diocles of Carystus, animal dissections provided observable information from which to draw conclusions about the human body.

Although a movement from animal to human dissection would seem to be a logical progression to most moderns, Greek sociocultural taboos made it difficult to gain access to a human cadaver, let alone dissect it. Firstly, access to a cadaver would have been limited to those bodies deemed "unworthy" of burial because Greek culture placed great emphasis on the proper funerary treatment of the body, often linking the ceremony to the deceased's journey to the afterlife. Secondly, Greek literature, as well as laws concerning the disposal of bodies, convey a belief that human cadavers were viewed as pollutants to the sacred and the living.

Heinrich von Staden argues that a number of sociocultural factors found in Hellenistic Alexandria, Egypt, not only allowed but also induced Herophilus and Erasistratus to violate the aforementioned social taboos. The early Ptolemies' ambition to establish Alexandria as the center of learning in the Greek world led them to creating the famous museum (Temple of the Muses). Equipped with its own library, the Museum became a place of literary and scientific inquiry attracting the best minds through the lure of Ptolemaic patronage. Greek scientists' such as the Greek mathematician Euclid, whose *Elements* provided the basis for the geometric proofs used today; the inventor Ctesibius, who wrote the first treatise on compressed air and its uses in pumps; and the astronomer Aristarchus of Samos, who is famous for placing the sun at the center of the universe, were all drawn to Alexandria. The culture of intellectual competition and discovery created by the confluence of scientists, philosophers, and physicians in Alexandria may have spurred Herophilus and Erasistratus to take such an original approach to the study of human anatomy. Insulated by the philosophical and scientific culture of Alexandria, their human dissections would have been viewed in quite a different context than in mainstream Greek society. Through the eyes of philosophers living in Alexandria, Herophilus and Erasistratus' human dissections were probably understood as being in-step with Aristotle's biological inquiries. Many of these philosophers' materialistic explanations of the relationship between the *psyche* (soul) and *soma* (body) left the human body both "secularized" and "demystified," and therefore, the human body would have been seen as a suitable subject for dissection. Furthermore, the longstanding Egyptian practice of the religious embalming of corpses may have also provided a sociocultural precedent for these two Greek anatomists to legitimize their human dissections. Lastly and perhaps most importantly, Ptolemaic patronage provided Herophilus and Erasistratus with the means to procure human bodies necessary for their program of dissection.

Curiously, after Herophilus' and Erasistratus' anatomical investigations, neither their followers nor any other ancient Greek anatomists involved themselves in the practice of human dissection. While the aforementioned sociocultural taboos serve as an adequate explanation for the cessation of human dissection among later physicians, it does not fully explain why the students of Herophilus and Erasistratus did not continue their teachers' anatomical investigations.

Von Staden and other scholars point to the popularity of a rival school of medicine as one explanation for the abandonment of human dissection. During mid-3rd century BC, physicians who called themselves "Empiricists" [Gr. *empeirikoi*] put forward a new theoretical position, which held that medical knowledge and practice should be based solely on "experience" [Gr. *empeiria*]. The kind of *empeiria* they sought was limited to observable clinical results. Empiricists considered human dissection impertinent to the practice of medicine. Their argument was that an understanding of human anatomy does not inherently lend itself to formulating cures for disease; and furthermore, death, as well as the act of laying open a human body, alters the true nature of the internal parts, therefore rendering what one observes as irrelevant to human physiology.

After Herophilus and Erasistratus, comparative anatomy based on animal dissections regained its popularity in the 1st and 2nd century AD. Galen of Pergamum became the foremost anatomist during this period. His writings predominated for centuries, becoming the primary source of information for medieval anatomists. Operating under the false belief that Galen had dissected humans, medieval medical schools began to dissect one male and, if possible, one female cadaver per year. The purpose of these dissections was for instructing students on the preexisting physiological theories and anatomical descriptions, which were primarily derived from the writings of Galen. During the 16th century, Andreas Vesalius (1514–1562 AD) took a more investigative approach to dissection. He revealed that many of the errors in Galen's anatomical descriptions could be attributed to Galen's use of animals rather than human cadavers. Vesalius' *De humani corporis fabrica* (*On the Material of the Human Body*, 1543) broke holes in Galenic anatomy, thereby opening the way to a flood of anatomical discoveries made in the following centuries (Fig. 3.2).

Although many of the Greek terms Erasistratus, Herophilus, and Galen used to describe the body are still in play to this day, the language of anatomy is decidedly Latin because Vesalius and the vast majority of subsequent anatomists wrote about their findings in Latin. The modern movement toward international standardization of terminology serves as another explanation for Latin being the language of anatomy. Up until the 19th century, there were no regulations or guidelines for naming the parts of the human body, and therefore, anatomical terminology was fraught with redundancies and inconsistencies caused by a wide variety of different Greek, Latin, and vernacular names being used for the same anatomical structures. To make this terminology logically consistent, intelligible, and concise in form, a committee of anatomists gathered together in Basle, Switzerland during the late 19th century. The result of their efforts was the first international anatomical system, which was published as the *Nomina anatomica* in 1895. The *Nomina anatomica* effectively reduced the number of human anatomical names from over 50,000–5,528 terms, and it dictated that these terms be written in Latin. Following this precedent, the international nomenclatures for human anatomy (*Terminologia anatomica*), tissues (*Terminologia histologia*), embryology (*Terminologia embryologica*) and veterinary anatomy (*Nomina anatomica veterinaria*) all dictated that their terms be written in grammatically correct Latin.

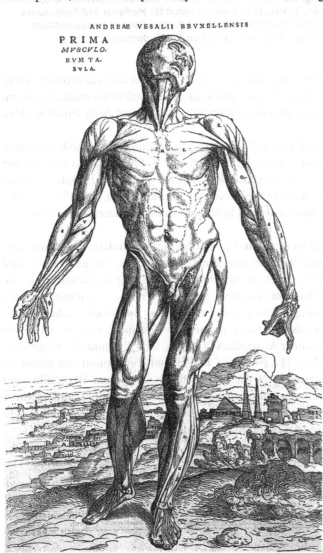

ANDREAE VESALII BRVXELLENSIS

PRIMA MVSCVLO. RVM TA. BVLA.

Fig. 3.2 First of a series of images on the muscles in A. Vesalius, *De humani corporis fabrica*. The letters on the muscles are Vesalius' innovation of labeling individual muscles in anatomical drawings. *Source:* Wellcome Collection/Public domain.

Some Suggested Readings

Duffin, Jacalyn. "*The Fabricated Body: History of Anatomy.*" In *History of Medicine: A Scandalously Short Introduction*, Third Edition, 9–38. Toronto: University of Toronto Press, 2021.

Federative Committee on Anatomical Terminology. *Terminologia Anatomica: International Anatomical Terminology.* New York: Thieme, 1998.

Rocca, Julius. "*Anatomy and Physiology.*" In *A Companion to Science, Technology, and Medicine in Ancient Greece and Rome*, Edited by Georgia L. Irby, 343–359. Hoboken, John Wiley & Sons, 2016.

von Staden, Heinrich. "The Discovery of the Body: Human Dissection and Its Cultural Contexts in Ancient Greece." *Yale Journal of Biology and Medicine* 65 (1992): 223–241.

von Staden, Heinrich. *Herophilus: The Art of Medicine in Early Alexandria.* Cambridge: Cambridge University Press, 1989.

Latin Anatomical Nouns

The following is an introduction to the grammar of anatomical Latin. The grammatical information is restricted to a brief summary of what is relevant to anatomical Latin terms in medical English.

Inflection

Greek and Latin are inflected languages. **Inflection** is the modification of a word by adding endings to it in order to change the grammatical function of the word. Observe the changes to the endings of the noun *digitus* (finger or toe) in the following anatomical terms:

1) *Digit̲u̲s̲ secundus.* = second finger
2) *Digit̲i̲* = Fingers
3) *Extensor digit̲o̲r̲u̲m̲ longus* = Long extender of the fingers

   Note that the meaning of the root *digit-* (finger) is unchanged. By simply changing the endings of *digitus*, one is able to indicate in Latin whether the *digitus* should be translated as a singular or plural (examples 1 and 2), and whether the noun should be translated as a possessive by adding "of the" (example 3). The inflectional ending will indicate both the **case** and the **number** of a noun.

Case

Latin nouns receive inflectional endings to signify the different grammatical usages of a given noun in a phrase or sentence. The different grammatical usages are called **cases**. Latin nouns have five main cases: **nominative, genitive, accusative, dative,** and **ablative**.

   Anatomical and biological taxonomies use only two cases of nouns, the **nominative** and **genitive**.

Nominative Case

The first word of an anatomical term is invariably a noun in the nominative case. The inflectional ending of the first term will indicate whether it should be translated as a nominative singular or plural nominative. This is often done by adding an –s or –es in English.

ven̲a̲ basilica = basilic v̲e̲i̲n̲
(nominative, singular noun)
ven̲a̲e̲ vesicales = vesical v̲e̲i̲n̲s̲
(nominative, plural noun)

N.B.: The nominative singular is also the form listed in the etymological entries in medical dictionaries.

Taber's Cyclopedic Medical Dictionary 23rd Edition:
Venesection [L. *vena*, vein + *sectio*, a cutting]

Genitive Case

In an anatomical term, the genitive case generally, but not necessarily, appears right after the noun it modifies. The inflectional endings will indicate if a noun is a genitive singular or plural. The genitive case is generally translated "of the x."

> *arteria <u>nervi</u>* = artery <u>of the nerve</u>
> (genitive, singular noun)
> *vasa <u>nervorum</u>* = vessels <u>of the nerves</u>
> (genitive, plural noun)

N.B. When you run into a binomial or trinomial Latin term (e.g. *cavitas nasi*), the first word is invariably a noun in the nominative case. Any noun subsequent to the first word is in the genitive case.

> *Cavitas* (nominative, singular) *nasi* (genitive singular)

Number

Number is the grammatical term used to indicate if a noun is singular or plural. A noun that refers to one thing is called **singular**, and a noun that refers to more than one thing is called **plural**. In English, plurals are formed by adding an "s" or "es" to nouns (e.g. dog-dogs, kiss-kisses), or by changing the spelling of the noun (e.g. goose-geese). Latin uses a greater number of endings than English to indicate whether a noun is singular or plural. The plural endings used for Latin words are dependent on the declension a noun belongs to.

The inflectional ending of a noun reveals whether the noun should be translated as a singular or plural. The following are some of the common plural formations. You should already be familiar with most of these Latin endings from Chapter 2.

Nouns of the 1st declension that end in -*a* change to -*ae*	*vena → venae* = vein → veins
Nouns of the 2nd declension that end in -*us* change to –*i*	*nervus → nervi* = nerve → nerves
Nouns of the 2nd declension that end in -*um* change to –*a*	*brachium → brachia* = arm → arms
Nouns of the 3rd declension that end in -*ix* and -*ex* change to –*ices*	*radix → radices* = root → roots *cortex → cortices* = rind/cortex → rinds/"cortices"
Nouns of the 3rd declension that end in -*is* change to –*es*	*febris → fibres* = fever → fevers
Nouns of the 3rd declension that end in -*ns* change to –*ntes*	*dens → dentes* = tooth → teeth *pons → pontes* = bridge → bridges
Nouns of the 3rd declension that end in -*en* change to -*ina*	*foramen → foramina* = opening → openings

Using the inflectional ending changes listed above, write the plural form of the following Latin nouns:

Example: Arteria = **Arteriae**

Review	Answers
cortex	**cortices**
fibula	**fibulae**
lens	**lentes**
labium	**labia**
limen	**limina**
naris	**nares**
nasus	**nasi**
semen	**semina**
frons	**frontes**
coxa	**coxae**

N.B. The Latin singular and plural forms for the 4th and 5th declension nouns are the same. In medical English, loan words of the 4th declension are pluralized by adding the English **-es** (e.g. plexuses, sinuses, and fetuses). Loan words from the 5th declension are rarely pluralized in medical English.

Gender

Every Latin noun has a specific gender associated with it. In grammar, the **gender** of a noun designates whether it is **masculine**, **feminine**, or **neuter**. A neuter is a noun which is neither masculine nor feminine. The gender of a Latin noun often cannot be explained by biological sex. For example, a muscle is neither inherently male nor female, but the Latin word *musculus* (muscle) has a grammatical gender of "masculine" assigned to it.

In Latin dictionaries, the gender of a noun is indicated by m. (masculine), f. (feminine), and n. (neuter).

musculus, -i, **m.** a muscle
vena, -ae, **f.** a vein
brachium, -i, **n.** upper arm

In anatomical Latin, the 1st declension has only feminine nouns; the 2nd declension has masculine and neuter nouns; the 3rd declension has masculine, feminine and neuter nouns; the 4th declension has masculine, feminine and neuter nouns; and the 5th declension has feminine nouns. The neuter variations for these declensions (2nd, 3rd, and 5th declensions) affect the nominative singular and plural endings for these nouns.

Declensions

Latin nouns are divided into groups called declensions. A **declension** is a collection of nouns which follow a similar pattern of endings to indicate their case and number. Observe the different inflectional endings that the 1st declension noun *vena* uses in respect to the 2nd declension noun *musculus*.

Case	1st declension singular	2nd declension singular
Nominative	*Vena*	*Musculus*
Genitive	*Venae*	*Musculi*
Accusative	*Venam*	*Musculum*
Dative	*Venae*	*Musculo*
Ablative	*Vena*	*Musculo*

Latin has five declensions called the **1st declension**, the **2nd declension**, the **3rd declension**, the **4th declension**, and the **5th declension**. A noun will fall into one of these five declensions. The inflectional endings for these five declensions are in the following chart:

	nom. sing.	gen. sing.	nom. plural	gen. plural
1st Declension (feminine)	-a	-ae	-ae	-arum
2nd Declension (masculine)	-us	-i	-i	-orum
2nd Declension (neuter)	-um	-i	-a	-orum
3rd Declension (masculine and feminine)	various	-is	-es	-um (-ium)
3rd Declension (neuter)	various	-is	-a (-ia)	-um (-ium)
4th Declension (masculine and feminine)	-us	-us	-us	-uum
4th Declension (neuter)	-u	-us	-ua	-uum
5th Declension (feminine)	-es	-ei	-es	-erum

Examples of the noun from each declension with their inflectional endings:

	nom. sing.	gen. sing.	nom. plural	gen. plural
1st Declension (feminine)	*Vena* (vein)	*Venae* (of the vein)	*Venae* (veins)	*venarum* (of the veins)
2nd Declension (masculine)	*Musculus* (muscle)	*Musculi* (of the muscle)	*Musculi* (muscles)	*Musculorum* (of the muscles)
2nd Declension (neuter)	*Brachium* (arm)	*Brachii* (of the arm)	*Brachia* (arms)	*Brachiorum* (of the arms)
3rd Declension (masculine and feminine)	*Cavitas* (cavity)	*Cavitatis* (of the cavity)	*Cavitates* (cavities)	*Cavitatum* (of the cavities)
3rd Declension (neuter)	*Os* (bone)	*Ossis* (of the bone)	*Ossa* (bones)	*Ossium* (of the bones)
4th Declension (masculine and feminine)	*Manus* (hand)	*Manus* (of the hand)	*Manus* (hands)	*Manuum* (of the hands)
4th Declension (neuter)	*Genu* (knee)	*Genus* (of the knee)	*Genua* (knees)	*Genuum* (of the knees)
5th Declension (feminine)	*Facies* (face)	*Faciei* (of the face)	*Facies* (faces)	*Facierum* (of the faces)

Note how the genitive singular ending and nominative plural are the same for the 1st declension (*-ae*) and the 2nd declension (*-i*). With binomial and trinomial anatomical terms, the **1st word** is a **noun** in the **nominative case**. Therefore, if the 1st word ends with *–ae* or *-i*, it is a nominative plural, all subsequent nouns ending with *–ae* or *-i* are likely to be a genitive singular. For example:

> *arteriae* cervicis (nominative plural) = arteries of the neck
> corpus *arteriae* (genitive singular) = body of the artery
> *musculi* cervicis (nominative plural) = muscles of the neck
> corpus *musculi* (genitive singular) = body of the muscle

If the noun appears by itself with an *–ae* or *-i* ending, it is a nominative plural.

> *arteriae* (nominative plural) = arteries
> *musculi* (nominative plural) = muscles

Anatomical Latin uses a limited number of 4th and 5th declension nouns. That said, the 4th declension nouns ***manus*** (hand) and ***genu*** (knee), as well as the 5th declension ***facies*** (face) are commonly used in anatomical terms.

Using Latin Dictionaries

The most common declensions in anatomical and scientific Latin are the 1st, 2nd, and 3rd declensions. A noun can only take the pattern of endings of its declension. The **genitive singular** indicates which declension a noun belongs to.

Declension	Genitive singular	Nominative singular	Genitive singular
1st	**-ae**	*vena* (vein)	*venae*
2nd	**-i**	*musculus* (muscle)	*musculi*
3rd	**-is**	*cavitas* (cavity)	*cavitatis*
4th	**-us**	*manus* (hand)	*manus*
5th	**-ei**	*facies* (face)	*faciei*

Latin dictionaries will indicate the declension by providing the genitive singular ending for the noun.

> *vena, -ae*, f., vein

For each entry, the first word (**vena**) is the nominative singular of the noun. The second part, **-ae**, reveals the genitive singular ending of the noun. The **f.** indicates the gender of the noun, and the last word is its English equivalent. It is important to bear in mind that the English equivalent presented in a Latin dictionary may differ from the way the term is used in medicine. The following are examples of the dictionary entries for the five declensions:

Declension	Latin dictionary ending
1st	*vena, -ae*, f. vein
2nd	*musculus, -i*, m. muscle
3rd	*abdomen, abdominis*, n. abdomen
4th	*manus, -us*, m. hand
5th	*facies, -ei*, f. face

Based on this information you can change the endings of a noun, which in grammatical terms is called declining a noun:

1) First, identify which declension a noun belongs to by looking at the second form listed in the Latin dictionary.
   For example, with the above entry for **vena**, the singular genitive, **-ae**, indicates that this noun is of the 1st declension, and therefore this noun will follow the 1st declension's pattern of endings.
2) The root is found by dropping the inflectional ending from the noun.

> *vena, -ae*, f. vein
> *vena* (**a** is nominative singular inflection ending for the 1st declension) = *ven-* (is the root)

For many 3rd declension nouns, the nominative singular does not reveal the root of the noun. The root is observed in the genitive singular form. A Latin dictionary will indicate the root by showing the full genitive singular form, for example:

> *corpus, corporis*, n. body
> *corporis* (**-is** is the genitive ending for the 3rd declension) = *corpor-* (root)
> *cervix, cervicis*, f. neck
> *cervicis* (**-is** is the genitive ending for the 3rd declension) = *cervic-* (root)

3) To change a noun from nominative to genitive case, you add endings according to the declension a noun belongs to. For example, because *vena* is a 1st declension noun, the nominative and genitive endings will be as follows:

Case	Singular	Example	Plural	Example
Nom.	**-a**	*vena*	**-ae**	*venae*
Gen.	**-ae**	*venae*	**-arum**	*venarum*

If the noun is a 3rd declension whose root differs from its nominative singular form like *cervix*, the 3rd declension endings are added to the root:

Case	Singular	Example	Plural	Example
Nom.	**various forms**	*cervix*	**-es**	*cervices*
Gen.	**-is**	*cervicis*	**-um**	*cervicum*

N.B. A single inflectional ending will indicate both the case and the number of a noun. To understand anatomical Latin, you need to be able to recognize the singular and plural forms for the nominative and genitive cases for each declension.

Based on the dictionary entry, give the root and indicate which declensions the following nouns belong to:

Example: *Os, ossis,* n. bone = **OSS-, 3rd declension**

Review	Answers
Os, oris, n. mouth = _____	OR-, 3rd declension
Nasus, -i, m. nose = _____	NAS-, 2nd declension
Coxa, -ae, f. hip = _____	COX-, 1st declension
Cubitus, -i, m. elbow = _____	CUBIT-, 2nd declension
Brachium, -i n. arm = _____	BRACHI-, 2nd declension
Axilla, -ae, f. armpit = _____	AXILL-, 1st declension
Genu, -us, n. knee = _____	GEN-, 4th declension
Femur, femoris, n. thigh = _____	FEMOR-, 3rd declension
Pectus, pectoris, n. chest = _____	PECTOR-, 3rd declension
Auris, auris, f. ear = _____	AUR-, 3rd declension
Facies, -ei, f. face = _____	FACI-, 5th declension

Provide the nominative plural form for the following Latin anatomical nouns:

artereia, -ae, f. artery = **arteriae**
os, oris, n. mouth = **ora**
cavitas, cavitatis, f. cavity = **cavitates**

Review	Answers
cervix, cervicis, f. neck _____	cervices
vena, -ae, f. vein _____	venae
genu, -us, n. knee _____	genua
brachium, -i, n., upper arm _____	brachia
corpus, corporis, n. body _____	corpora
organum, -i, n. organ _____	organa
nasus, -i, m. nose _____	nasi
sinus, -us, m. sinus _____	sinus
frons, frontis, f. forehead _____	frontes
pes, pedis m. foot _____	pedes

Provide a translation for the following underlined nominative and genitive terms.

Example:
corpusculum <u>renis</u> (genitive singular, kidney) = corpuscle **of the kidney**
<u>arteriae</u> (nominative plural, artery) *rectae* = straight **arteries**

Review	Answers
cavitas <u>nasi</u> (genitive singular, nose) = cavity _____	of the nose
<u>musculi</u> fascei (nominative plural, muscle) = _____ of the face	muscles

Review	Answers
extensor <u>digitorum</u> longus (genitive plural, toe/finger) = long extender _____	**of the fingers/toes**
sulcus <u>costae</u> (genitive singular, rib) = groove _____	**of the rib**
<u>vena</u> profunda (nominative singular, vein) = deep _____	**vein**
arteria <u>brachii</u> anterior (genitive singular, upper arm) = anterior artery _____	**of the upper arm**
<u>arteriae</u> cerebelli (nominative plural, artery) = _____ of the cerebellum	**arteries**
tinea <u>barbae</u> (genitive singular, beard) = ringworm _____	**of the beard**
Pediculus humanus <u>corporis</u> (genitive singular, body) = human louse _____	**of the body**
<u>pars</u> sacralis (nominative singular, part) = sacral _____	**part**

Latin Nouns for General Parts of the Human Body

The following are the Latin nouns for the parts of the human body in the *Terminologia Anatomica*. The etymologies present the nominative and genitive singular forms for each Latin noun. The plural forms for the loan words can be found in the examples (e.g. **Corpus**, body, pl. **Corpora**, bodies) (Fig. 3.3).

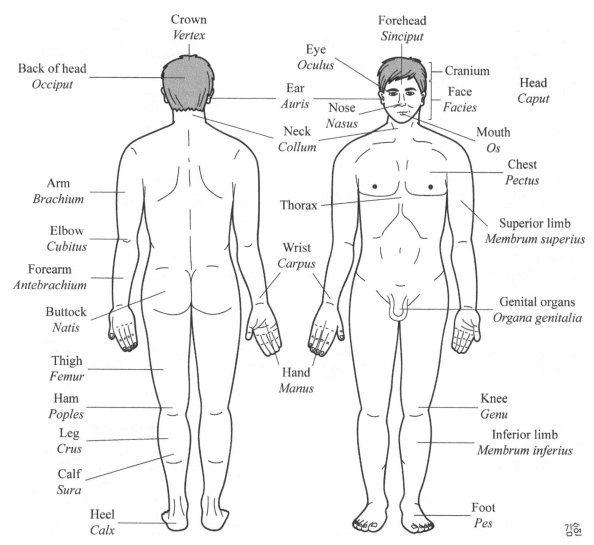

Fig. 3.3 Latin names for the parts of the human body. *Source:* Drawing by Chloe Kim.

Latin word element	Current usage	Etymology	Examples
CORPOR/O (kor-pŏ-rō)	Body	L. *corpus, corporis,* n. body	**Bicorpor**ate, extra**corpor**eal Loan word: **Corpus** (kor′pŭs) pl. **Corpora** (kor′pŏ-ră)
PART/O (par-tō)	Part	L. *pars, partis,* f. part	**Part**ial, **part**icle Loan word: **Pars** (pars) pl. **Partes** (par′tēz)
CAVIT/O (kăv-ĭ-tō)	Cavity	L. *cavitas, cavitatis,* f. cavity, hollow	**Cavit**ation, **cavit**ary Loan word: **Cavitas** (kăv′ĭ-tăs) pl. **Cavitates** (kă-vĭ-tă′tēz)
ORGAN/O (or-gă-nō)	Organ	L. *organum, -i,* n. organ fr. Gr. *organon,* tool, instrument	**Organ**omegaly, **organ**opathy Loan word: **Organum** (or′gă-nŭm) pl. **Organa** (or′gă-nă)
ENCEPHAL/O (ĕn-sef-ă-lō) -ENCEPHALON (en-sef-ă-lŏn)	Brain	L. *encephalon, -i,* n. encephalon, brain fr. Gr. *enkephalos,* brain	**Encephal**omeningitis, Tel**encephal**on, Amyel**encephal**y Loan word: **Encephalon** (en-sef′ă-lŏn) pl. **Encephala** (en-sef′ă-lă)
CORD/O (kor-dō)	Heart	L. *cor, cordis,* n. heart	**Cord**ate, intra**cord**al Loan word: **Cor** (kor) pl. **Corda** (kor′dă)
PULM/O (pŭl-mō) PULMON/O (pŭl-mō-nō)	Lung	L. *pulmo, pulmonis,* m. lung	**Pulm**oaortic, **pulmon**ologist Loan word: **Pulmo** (pŭl′mō) pl. **Pulmones** (pŭl′mō-nēz″)
HEPAT/O (hĕp-ă-tō) HEPAR/O (hep-ă-rō)	Liver	L. *hepar, hepatis,* n. liver fr. Gr. *hepar, hepatos,* liver	**Hepat**itis, **Hepar**in, **hepat**algia Loan word: **Hepar** (hē′par″) pl. **Hepatia** (hē-pat′ē-a)
GASTR/O (gas-trō) -GASTER (găs-tĕr)	Stomach, belly	L. *gaster, gastris,* f. stomach fr. Gr. *gaster, gastros,* belly, stomach	**Gastr**ectasis, proto**gaster**, **gastr**ocele Loan word: **Gaster** (gas′tĕr) pl. **Gastres** (gas′trēz″)
INTESTIN/O (in-tes-tĭn-ō)	Intestine	L. *intestinum, -i,* n. internal, intestine	Gastro**intestin**al, **intestin**iform Loan word: **Intestinum** (in″tĕs-tī′nŭm) pl. **Intestina** (in″tĕs-tī′nă)
VESIC/O (vĕs-ĭ-kō)	Bladder, sac, vesicle	L. *vesica, -ae,* f. bladder, sac	Cervico**vesic**al, **vesic**oclysis, **vesic**ocele Loan word: **Vesica** (vĕ-sī′kă) pl. **Vesicae** (vĕ-sī′kē″)

Latin word element	Current usage	Etymology	Examples
REN/O (rē-nō)	Kidney	L. *ren, renis*, m. kidney	**Ren**ogastric, adre**nal**, supra**ren**al Loan word: **Ren** (rĕn) pl. **Renes** (rĕn′ēz″)
CUT/O (kū-tō) **CUTANE/O** (kū-tā-nē-ō)	Skin	L. *cutis, -is*, f. skin, hide	**Cut**icle, trans**cutane**ous Loan word: **Cutis** (kūt′ĭs) pl. **Cutes** (kūt′ēz″)
GLANDUL/O (glan-jŭ-lō)	Glandule, gland	L. *glandula, -ae*, f. little acorn; gland fr. L. *glans, glandis*, f. acorn; gland	**Glandul**ose, **glandul**ar Loan word: **Glandula** (glan′jŭ-lă) pl. **Glandulae** (glan′jŭ-lē″)
ARTERI/O (ar-tĕr-ē-ō)	Artery	L. *arteria, -ae*, f. artery fr. Gr. *arteria*, windpipe, artery	**Arteri**otomy, intr**arteri**al Loan word: **Arteria** (ar-tĕr′ē-ă) pl. **Arteriae** (ar-tĕr′ē-ē)
VEN/O (vē-nō)	Vein	L. *vena, -ae*, f. vein	**Ven**ectomy, intra**ven**ous Loan word: **Vena** (vē′nă) pl. **Venae** (vē′nē)
VAS/O (vă-zō) **VASCUL/O** (vas-kyŭ-ō)	Vessel (carrying fluids)	L. *vas, vasis*, n. vessel L. *vasculum, i*, n. a small vessel	**Vas**omotor, extra**vas**ate, **vascul**ar Loan word: **Vas** (vas) pl. **Vasa** (va′să)
OSS/O (os-ō)	Bone	L. *os, ossis*, n. bone	**Oss**ific, **oss**eous Loan word: **Os** (ŏs) pl. **Ossa** (os′ă)
MUSCUL/O (mŭs-kyŭ-lō)	Muscle; mouse	L. *musculus, -i*, m. muscle, mouse	**Muscul**ophrenic, intra**muscul**ar Loan word: **Musculus** (mŭs′kyŭ-lŭs) pl. **Musculi** (mŭs′kyŭ-lī)
NERV/O (nĕr-vō)	Nerve	L. *nervus, -i*, m. sinew; nerve	**Nerv**ous, **nerv**imotor Loan word: **Nervus** (nĕr′vŭs) pl. **Nervi** (nĕr′vī)
CAPIT/O (kap-ĭ-tō) **CIPIT/O** (sip-ĭ-tō) **-CIPUT** (sĭp-ŭt) **-CEPS** (seps)	Head	L. *caput, capitis*, n. head	**Capit**ate, bi**cipit**al, sin**ciput**, bi**ceps** Loan word: **Caput** (kap′ŭt) pl. **Capita** (kap′ĭt-ă)

Latin word element	Current usage	Etymology	Examples
CRANI/O (krā-nē-ō)	Cranium, skull	L. *cranium*, *-i*, n. cranium fr. Gr. *kranion*, skull, cranium	**Crani**ocele, intra**crani**al Loan word: **Cranium** (krā′nē-ŭm) pl. **Crania** (krā′nē-ă)
FACI/O (fā-shē-ō)	Face, surface	L. *facies*, *-ei*, f. face	**Faci**oplasty, **faci**al Loan word: **Facies** (fā′shē-ēz) pl. **Facies** (fā′shē-ēz)
OCUL/O (ŏk-ū-lō)	Eye	L. *oculus*, *-i*, m. eye	Bin**ocul**ar, intra**ocul**ar Loan word: **Oculus** (ŏk′ū-lŭs) pl. **Oculi** (ŏk′ū-lī)
*AUR/O (or-lō)	Ear	L. *auris*, *auris*, f. ear	**Aur**iform, **aur**al Loan word: **Auris** (or′is) pl. **Aures** (or′ēz)
NAS/O (nā-zō)	Nose	L. *nasus*, *-i*, m. nose	**Nas**ion, **nas**al Loan word: **Nasus** (nā′sŭs) pl. **Nasi** (nā′sī)
OR/O (ō-rō)	Mouth	L. *os*, *oris*, n. mouth	Ab**or**ad, **or**al Loan word: **Os** (ōs) pl. **Ora** (ō′ră)
BUCC/O (bŭk-ō)	Cheek	L. *bucca*, *-ae*, f. cheek	**Bucc**inator, retro**bucc**al Loan word: **Bucca** (bŭk′ă) pl. **Buccae** (bŭk′ē)
*MENT/O (men-tō)	Chin	L. *mentum*, *-i*, n. chin	Sub**ment**al, **ment**oplasty Loan word: **Mentum** (ment′ŭm) pl. **Menta** (ment′ă)
OCCIPIT/O (ŏk-sĭp-ĭ-tō)	Back of cranium, occiput	L. *occiput*, *occipitis*, n. back of head	Sub**occipit**al, **occipit**ofacial Loan word: **Occiput** (ok′sĭ-pŭt) pl. **Occipita** (ok-sĭp′ĭ-tă)
SINCIPIT/O (sĭn-sĭp-ĭ-tō)	Front of cranium, sinciput	L. *sinciput*, *sincipitis*, n. forehead	**Sincipit**al Loan word: **Sinciput** (sĭn′sĭp-ŭt) pl. **Sincipita** (sĭn-sĭp′ĭ-tă)
VERTIC/O (vĕr-tĭ-kō)	Crown of the cranium, summit	L. *vertex*, *verticis*, m. summit	**Vertic**al, **vertic**omental Loan word: **Vertex** (vĕr′tĕks) pl. **Vertices** (vĕr-tĭ′sēz)

Latin word element	Current usage	Etymology	Examples
FRONT/O (frŏn-tō)	Forehead, front	L. *frons, frontis*, f. forehead	**Front**omalar, naso**front**al Loan word: **Frons** (fronz) pl. **Frontes** (fron'tēz)
COLL/O (kŏl-lō)	Neck	L. *collum, -i*, n. neck	**Coll**ar, **coll**iform Loan word: **Collum** (kŏl'lŭm) pl. **Colla** (kŏl'lă)
CERVIC/O (sĕr-vĭ-kō) **-CERVIX** (sĕr-viks)	Neck	L. *cervix, cervicis*, f. neck	**Cervic**itis, endo**cervix** Loan word: **Cervix** (sĕr'viks) pl. **Cervices** (sĕr'vĭ-sēz)
TRUNC/O (trŭn-kō)	Trunk, cut off	L. *truncus, -i*, m. trunk of a tree, lopped off part fr. L. *truncare*, to cut off	**Trunc**al, **trunc**ate Loan word: **Truncus** (trŭng'kŭs) pl. **Trunci** (trŭng'kī)
THORAC/O (thō-ră-kō) **-THORAX** (thŏr-aks)	Thorax	L. *thorax, thoracis*, m. thorax fr. Gr. *thorax, tharakos*, breastplate, chest	**Thoraco**centesis, **thorac**ic Loan word: **Thorax** (thŏr'aks) pl. **Thoraces** (thŏr'ă-sēz)
PECTOR/O (pek-tŏ-rō)	Chest	L. *pectus, pectoris*, n. chest	Ex**pector**ant, medio**pector**al Loan word: **Pectus** (pek'tŭs) pl. **Pectora** (pek'tŏ-ră)
DORS/O (dor-sō)	Back	L. *dorsum, -i*, n. back	**Dors**ad, **dors**al Loan word: **Dorsum** (dor'sŭm) pl. **Dorsa** (dor'să)
ABDOMIN/O (ab-dom-ĭ-nō)	Abdomen	L. *abdomen, abdominis*, n. paunch, belly	Sub**abdomin**al, intra**abdomin**al Loan word: **Abdomen** (ab-dō'mĕn) pl. **Abdomina** (ab-dom'ĭ-nă)
INGUIN/O (ing-gwĭ-nō)	Groin	L. *inguen, inguinis*, n. groin	**Inguin**al, ex**inguin**al Loan word: **Inguen** (ing'gwĕn) pl. **Inguina** (ing'gwĕ-nă)
PELV/O (pel-vō)	Pelvis	L. *pelvis, -is*, f. a basin, basin shaped cavity	Intra**pelv**ic, **pelv**irectal Loan word: **Pelvis** (pel'vĭs) pl. **Pelves** (pel'vēz)
CINGUL/O (sing-gyŭ-lō)	Girdle	L. *cingulum, -i*, n. belt, girdle	**Cingul**otomy, **cingul**ate Loan word: **Cingulum** (sing'gyŭ-lŭm) pl. **Cingula** (sing'gyŭ-lă)

Latin word element	Current usage	Etymology	Examples
MEMBR/O (mem-brō)	Limb	L. *membrum, -i*, n. limb	Loan word: **Membrum** (mem′brŭm) pl. **Membra** (mem′bră)
AXILL/O (ak-sil-ō)	Armpit, axilla	L. *axilla, -ae*, f. armpit	Sub**axill**ary, **axill**ar Loan word: **Axilla** (ak-sil′ă) pl. **Axillae** (ak-sil′ē)
BRACHI/O (brăk-ē-ō)	Upper arm, brachium, arm-like process	L. *brachium, -i*, n. upper arm fr. Gr. *brachion*, arm	**Brachi**oplasty, **bachi**ocephalic Loan word: **Brachium** (brā′kē-ŭm) pl. **Brachia** (brā′kē-ă)
CUBIT/O (kū-bĭ-tō)	Elbow	L. *cubitus, -i*, m. elbow fr. L. *cubitum, -i*, n. elbow	Sub**cubit**al, **cubit**ocarpal Loan word: **Cubitus** (kū′bĭ-tŭs) pl. **Cubiti** (kū′bĭ-tī)
ANTEBRACHI/O (ant-ē-brăk-ē-ō)	Forearm	L. *antebrachium, -i*, n. forearm fr. Gr. *brachion*, arm	**Antebrachi**al Loan word: **Antebrachium** (ant-ē-brā′kē-ŭm) pl. **Antebrachia** (ant-ē-brā′kē-ă)
MAN/O (mă-nō)	Hand	L. *manus, -us*, f. hand	Bi**man**ual, dextro**man**ual Loan word: **Manus** (mă′nŭs) pl. **Manus** (mă′nŭs) or **Manuses** (mă′nŭs-es)
***CARP/O** (kăr-pō)	Wrist	L. *carpus, -i*, m. wrist fr. Gr. *karpos*, wrist	**Carp**optosis, **carp**ometacarpal Loan word: **Carpus** (kăr′pŭs) pl. **Carpi** (kăr′pī)
METACARP/O (met-ă-kar-pō)	Metacarpus	L. *metacarpus, -i*, m. metacarpus fr. Gr. *karpos*, wrist	**Metecarp**ectomy, carpo**metacarp**al Loan word: **Metacarpus** (met-ă-kar′pŭs) pl. **Metacarpi** (met-ă-kar′pī)
PALM/O (pal-mō)	Palm of the hand	L. *palma, -ae*, f. palm	**Palm**oplantar, **palm**ar Loan word: **Palma** (păl′mă) pl. **Palmae** (păl′mē)
VOL/O (vō-lō)	Palm of the hand	L. *vola, -ae*, f. palm	**Vol**ar Loan word: **Vola** (vō′lă) pl. **Volae** (vō′lē)
DIGIT/O (dij-ĭt-ō)	Finger, toe	L. *digitus, -i*, m. finger of toe	**Digit**iform, **digit**al Loan word: **Digitus** (dij′ĭt-ŭs) pl. **Digiti** (dij′ĭt-ī)

Latin word element	Current usage	Etymology	Examples
POLLIC/O (pŏl-ĭk-ō)	Thumb	L. *pollex, pollicis*, m. thumb	**Pollic**ization, **poll**ical Loan word: **Pollex** (pŏl'ĕks) pl. **Pollices** (pŏl'i-sēz″)
*NAT/O (nă-tō)	Buttocks, nates	L. *nates, -ium*, f. buttocks	**Nat**al Loan word: **Nates** (nă'tēz)
CLUN/O (klŭ-nō)	Buttocks, clunes	L. *clunes, -ium*, f. buttocks	**Clun**eal Loan word: **Clunes** (klŭ'nēz)
COX/O (kŏk-sō)	Hip	L. *coxa, -ae*, f. hip	**Cox**odynia, **cox**ofemoral Loan word: **Coxa** (kok'să) pl. **Coxae** (kok'sē)
FEMOR/O (fem-ŏ-rō)	Thigh, femur bone	L. *femur, femoris*, n. thigh	**Femor**otibial, inter**femor**al Loan word: **Femur** (fē'mŭr) pl. **Femora** (fem'ŏ-ră)
*GEN/O (jĕn-ō)	Knee	L. *genu, -us*, n. knee	**Gen**ucubital, super**gen**ual Loan word: **Genu** (jē'nū) pl. **Genua** (jen'ū-ă)
POPLIT/O (pop-li-tō)	Hollow of the knee, poples	L. *poples, poplitis*, m. posterior thigh, hamstring	**Poplit**eus, **poplit**eal Loan word: **Poples** (pŏp'lēz) pl. **Poplites** (pŏp-lit'ēz)
CRUR/O (kroo-rō)	Leg, leg-like part	L. *crus, cruris*, n. leg	**Crur**al, inguino**crur**al Loan word: **Crus** (kroos) pl. **Crura** (kroor'ă)
SUR/O (sū'rō)	Calf	L. *sura, surae*, f. calf	**Sur**al Loan word: **Sura** (sū'ră) pl. **Surae** (sū'rē)
*PED/O (ped-ō)	Foot	L. *pes, pedis*, m. foot	**Ped**icle, carpo**ped**al Loan word: **Pes** (pĕs) pl. **Pedes** (pe'dēz)
TARS/O (tar-sō)	Ankle, flat of the foot, edge of the eyelid	L. *tarsus, -i*, m. ankle fr. Gr. *tarsos*, flat of foot	**Tars**algia, **tars**omegaly Loan word: **Tarsus** (tar'sŭs) pl. **Tarsi** (tar'sī)

Latin word element	Current usage	Etymology	Examples
*CALC/O (kăl-kō)	Heel	L. *calx, calcis*, f. heel	**Calc**aneous Loan word: **Calx** (kălks) pl. **Calces** (kal′sēz)
METATARS/O (met-ă-tar-sō)	Metatarsus	L. *metatarsus, -i*, m. metatarsus fr. Gr. *tarsos*, flat of foot	**Metatars**algia, **metatar**sal Loan word: **Metatarsus** (met-ă-tar′sŭs) pl. **Metatarsi** (met-ă-tar′sī)
HALLIC/O (hal-ĭk-ō) **HALLUC/O** (hal-ŭk-ō)	Big toe	L. *hallux, hallucis*, or *hallex*, *hallicis*, m. big toe	**Hallic**al, **halluc**al Loan word: **Hallux** (hal′ŭs) pl. **Halluces** (hal′ŭ-sēz″)
PLANT/O (plan-tō)	Sole (of foot), sprout or cutting, plant	L. *planta, -ae*, f. sole (of foot) fr. L. *planta*, a sprout, seedling	**Plant**ar, **planti**grade Loan word: **Planta** (plănt′ă) pl. **Plantae** (plăn′tē)

N.B. To avoid confusion, be aware of the following homographs:

AUR/O: Ear [L. *auris*, ear]; Gold, golden [L. *aurum*, gold]
CARP/O: Wrist [L. *carpus*, wrist]; Fruit [Gr. *karpos*, fruit]
CALC/O: Heel [L. *calx, calcis,* heel]; Calcium, limestone, stone [L. *calx, calcis*, a stone]
PED/O: Foot (L. *pes, pedis*, foot) Child (Gr. *pais, paidos*, child)
GEN/O: Knee (L. *genu*, knee); Cheek (L. *gena*, cheek); Become, born, produced, race (Gr. *genos*, race, kind)
NAT/O: Buttocks (L. *nates*, buttocks); Born (L. *nasci, natus*, to be born)
MENT/O: Chin (L. *mentum*, chin); Mind (L. *mens, mentis*, mind, reason)

Review	Answers
The combining form in vasotomy indicates that this is a surgical incision into a _____.	**vessel**
The Latin anatomical term for a vein is _____.	**vena**
The combining form in ossification indicates that the _____ is affected.	**bone**
The Latin anatomical term for chin is _____.	**mentum**
The Latin anatomical term for the upper arm is _____, and the anatomical term for the forearm is _____.	**brachium, antebrachium**
The combining forms for buttocks are _____ and _____.	**CLUN/O, NAT/O**
The plural form for the Latin anatomical term for calf is _____.	**surae**
The adjective crural in crural ligament indicated that this ligament is located in the _____.	**leg**
The translation of *Cervix organi* is _____.	**neck of the organ**
The axillary nerve is located in the _____, and the inguinal artery is located in the _____.	**armpit, groin**
Coxalgia is pain in the _____.	**hip**
Genu valgum affects the _____.	**knee**
The anatomical Latin terms for the palm are _____ and _____.	**vola, palma**

Review	Answers
The *Cingulum pectorale* is the pectoral _____. The Latin adjective "*pectorale*" is formed from the Latin noun meaning _____.	**girdle, chest**
The Latin combining forms for eye, nose, and ear are _____, _____, and _____.	**ocul/o, nas/o, aur/o**
Digiti pedis is best translated _____ of the foot, and *Digiti manus* is best translated _____ of the hand.	**toes, fingers**
The cubital fossa is located at the _____, and the carpal tunnel is located at the _____.	**elbow, wrist**
The combining form BUCC/O in buccocervical means _____.	**cheek**
The translation of *Pars arteriae* is _____.	**part of the artery**
The translation of *Cavitas thoracis* is _____.	**cavity of the thorax**
The plural form for the Latin anatomical term meaning thigh is _____.	**femora**
The back of the cranium is called the _____; the top of the cranium is called the _____; and the front of the cranium is called the _____.	**occiput, vertex, sinciput**
Orofacial apraxia affects the _____ and the _____.	**mouth, face**
The translation of *Nervi musculi* is _____.	**nerves of the muscles**
The popliteal artery is located at the _____ of the knee.	**back**
Encephalitis is a condition that effects the _____.	**brain**
The anatomical Latin word *cor* means _____, and its corresponding root is _____.	**heart, CORD-**
Hepatalgia affects the _____.	**liver**
The anatomical Latin word cutis means _____, and its corresponding roots are _____ and _____.	**skin, CUT-, CUTANE-**
The combining form for stomach is _____.	**GASTR/O**
The adjective renal refers to the _____.	**kidneys**
The Latin combining form for intestine is _____.	**INTESTIN/O**
The anatomical Latin word for "bladder" is _____.	**vesica**
The anatomical Latin word for "lung" is _____, and its corresponding roots are _____ and _____.	**pulmo, PULM-, PULMON-**

Greek Anatomical Nouns

Declensions

Greek has three declensions. The following are examples of the different Greek inflectional endings for these three declensions with transliterations of the Greek.

Case	1st Declension		
Nominative	κεφαλή *kephale* (head)	κοιλία *coelia* (cavity)	
Genitive	κεφαλῆς *kephales*	κοιλίας *coelias*	

	2nd Declension		
Nominative	ὀστέον *osteon* (bone)	τράχηλος trachelos (neck)	
Genitive	ὀστέου *osteou*	τραχήλου *trachelou*	

	3rd Declension		
Nominative	σῶμα *soma* (body)	ῥίς *rhis* (nose)	θώραξ thorax (thorax)
Genitive	σώματος *somatos*	ῥινός *rhinos*	θώρακος thorakos

With the 1st and 2nd declension nouns, the roots can be found by removing the inflectional endings from the nouns: *-os, -on, -e,* and *-a.* However, as in Latin, the 3rd declension nouns reveal their common root in the genitive singular. The etymological entries in the textbook's vocabulary provide the genitive singular for these 3rd declension nouns [Gr. *soma, somatos*). For the Greek loan words in English, the plural form is provided in the vocabulary (e.g. **Soma**, body, pl. **Somata** bodies).

Greek Nouns in Anatomical Latin

Most of the anatomical terms derived from Greek words have been Latinized, and therefore they appear with Latin declension endings.

Greek nouns ending with *–os* (-ος) become *–us* and are declined according to the pattern of Latin 2nd declension masculine nouns.

Gr. καρπός *karpos* > L. *carpus*

Greek nouns with *–e* (-η) or *–a* (-α) become *–a* and are declined with 1st declension feminine endings.

Gr. ἀρτηρία *arteria* > L. arteria

Greek nouns ending with *–on* (-ον) become *–um* and are declined according to 2nd declension neuters.

Gr. βραχίων *brachion* > L. *brachium*

Greek nouns from the 3rd declension are transliterated into Latin and declined as 3rd declension Latin nouns.

Gr. θώραξ, θώρακος thorax, thorakos > L. thorax, thoracis

There are two Greek inflectional endings that are sometimes retained in anatomical Latin:

1) The Greek neuter ending *–on* is sometimes retained in the nominative singular. However, it is declined as if it was a 2nd declension.

Case	Singular	Plural
Nominative	*ganglion* (knot; mass of nerve cells)	*ganglia*
Genitive	*ganglii*	*gangliorum*

2) The Greek ending *–ma* is a neuter singular ending. Its plural form is *–mata.* Both nominative singular and plural forms are occasionally used in anatomical Latin.

Case	Singular	Plural
Nominative	*bregma* (intersection of the coronal and sagittal sutures of skull)	*bregmata*

Greek word element	Current usage	Etymology	Examples
SOMAT/O (sō-măt-ō)	Body	Gr. *soma, somatos*, body	**Somat**ogenic, di**som**us, chromo**some**
SOM/O (sō-mō)			Loan word: **Soma** (sō'mă) pl. **Somata** (sō'măt-ă)
-SOME (sōm)			

Greek word element	Current usage	Etymology	Examples
*MER/O (mĕr-ō) **-MER** (mĕr) **-MERE** (mēr)	Part, partial	Gr. *meros, mereos*, part	**Mero**tomy, iso**mer**, sarco**mere**
COEL/O (sē-lō) ***CEL/O** (sē-lō) **CELI/O** (sē-lē-ō) **-COELE** (sēl) ***-CELE** (sēl)	Cavity, abdomen	Gr. *koilia*, cavity	**Coel**enterate, **cel**oschisis, **celi**ac syringo**coele**, syringo**cele**
CARDI/O (kard-ē-ō)	Heart	Gr. *kardia*, the heart	**Cardi**ology, endo**cardi**tis
PNEUM/O (nū-mō) **PNEUMON/O** (noo-mŏ-nō)	lung	Gr. *pneumon, pneumonos*, lung	**Pneum**ocentesis, **pneumon**ectasis
ENTER/O (ent-ĕ-rō)	Intestine (usually the small intestine)	Gr. *enteron*, that within, intestine	Gastro**enter**itis, my**enter**on, **enter**olith Loan word: **Enteron** (ĕn′tĕr-ŏn)
NEPHR/O (nef-rō)	Kidney	Gr. *nephros*, kidney	**Nephr**itis, **nephr**oabdominal, **nephr**oblastoma Loan word: **Nephros** (nĕf′rŏs)
CYST/O (sis-tō)	Bladder, sac, cyst	Gr. *kystis*, bladder	**Cyst**ocele, **cyst**ocentesis, **cyst**algia
ADEN/O (ad-ĕn-ō)	Gland	Gr. *aden, adenos*, gland	Thyro**aden**itis, **aden**opathy, lymph**aden**itis
DERM/O (dĕr-mō) **DERMAT/O** (dĕr-mă-tō) **-DERM** (dĕrm)	Skin	L. *dermis, -is*, f. dermis fr. Gr. *derma, dermatos*, skin	Ecto**derm**, **dermat**ocele Loan word: **Dermis** (dĕr′mĭs) pl. **Dermes** (dĕr′mēz″)
MY/O (mī-ō) **MYOS/O** (mī-ō-sō) **MYS/O** (mī-sō)	Muscle, mouse	Gr. *mys, myos*, muscle, mouse	**Myo**mere, endo**mys**ium

Greek word element	Current usage	Etymology	Examples
OSTE/O (os-tē-ō)	Bone	Gr. *osteon*, bone	**Oste**oclast, **oste**osis Loan word: **Osteon** (os′tē-on) pl. **Ostea** (os′tē-a)
NEUR/O (noor-ō)	Nerve	Gr. *neuron*, nerve, tendon, sinew	**Neur**algia, **neur**al Loan word: **Neuron** (noor′on) pl. **Neura** (noor′a)
PHLEB/O (flĕ-bō)	Vein	Gr. *phleps, phlebos*, vein	**Phleb**otomy, **phleb**itis
ANGI/O (an-jē-ō)	Vessel	Gr. *angeion*, vessel	**Angi**oma, eu**angi**otic
CEPHAL/O (sĕf-ă-lō)	Head	Gr. *kephale*, head	Clino**cephal**y, **cephal**ad
METOP/O (me-top-ō)	Forehead	Gr. *metopon*, forehead	**Metop**ic, **metop**ism
PROSOP/O (prō-sō-pō)	Face	Gr. *prosopon*, face	Macro**prosop**ia, **prosop**algia
RHIN/O (rī-nō) **-RHINE** (rīn)	Nose	Gr. *rhis, rhinos*, nose	**Rhin**orrhea, lepto**rhine**
OPHTHALM/O (of-thal-mō) **-OPHTHALMUS** (ŏf-thăl-mŭs)	Eye	Gr. *ophthalmos*, eye	Xer**ophthalm**ia, crypt**ophthalmus**
OT/O (ō-tō)	Ear	Gr. *ous, otos*, ear	An**ot**ia, **ot**ic
STOMAT/O (stō-măt-ō) **STOM/O** (stō-mō)	Mouth, outlet, opening	Gr. *stoma, stomatos*, mouth	**Stomat**ocyte, macro**stom**ia Loan word: **Stoma** (stō′mă) pl. **Stomata** (stō′măt-ă)
*MEL/O (mĕl-ō)	Cheek	Gr. *melon*, cheek	**Mel**itis, **mel**oncus
GENI/O (jē-nē-ō)	Chin	Gr. *geneion*, chin	**Geni**oplasty, micro**geni**a
TRACHEL/O (trak-ĕ-lō)	Neck, cervix	Gr. *trachelos*, neck, throat	**Trachel**odynia, **trachel**itis
*MEL/O (mĕl-ō)	Limb	Gr. *melos, meleos*, limb	A**mel**us, macro**mel**ia
MASCHAL/O (măs-kāl-ō)	Armpit	Gr. *maschale*, armpit	Trago**maschal**ia, **maschal**oncus

Greek word element	Current usage	Etymology	Examples
OLECRAN/O (ō-lek-ră-nō)	Elbow	Gr. *olekranon*, elbow	**Olecran**oid, **olecran**arthritis Loan word: **Olecranon** (ō-lek′ră-non) pl. **Olecrana** (ō-lek′ră-na)
ANCON/O (ang-kō-nō)	Elbow	Gr. *ankon*, elbow	**Ancon**ad, **ancon**itis
CHEIR/O (kī-rō) CHIR/O (kī-rō)	Hand	Gr. *cheir, cheiros*, hand	A**cheir**ia, **chir**opractic
DACTYL/O (dak-tĭ-lō) -DACTYL (dak-tĭl)	Finger or toe	Gr. *daktylos*, finger or toe	Syn**dactyl**ism, iso**dactyl**ism Loan word: **Dactyl** (dak′tĭl)
LAPAR/O (lap-ă-rō)	Abdomen	Gr. *lapara*, loin, flank, abdomen	**Lapar**otomy, **lapar**oscopy
PYG/O (pī-gō)	Buttocks	Gr. *pyge*, buttocks	**Pyg**algia, **pyg**omelus
GLUT/O (gloo-tō)	Buttock	Gr. *gloutos*, buttock	**Glut**itis, **glut**oid
ISCHI/O (ĭs-kē-ō)	Hip, ischium bone	Gr. *ischion*, hip	**Ischi**algia, **ischi**al
*MER/O (mĕr-ō)	Thigh	Gr. *meros, merou*, thigh	**Mer**ocele, **mer**oparesthesia
GONY/O (gŏn-ĭ-ō) GONAT/O (gŏn-ăt-ō)	Knee	Gr. *gony, gonatos*, knee	**Gony**campsis, **gonat**ocele
KNEM/O (nē-mō) CNEM/O (nē-mō)	Lower leg	Gr. *kneme*, lower leg, shin	**Knem**ometry, a**cnem**ia
PTERN/O (tĕr-nō)	Heel	Gr. *pterna*, heel	**Ptern**algia
POD/O (pŏ-dō) -PUS (pŭs) -POD (pod)	Foot, foot-like structure, stalk	Gr. *pous, podos*, foot	**Pod**agra, poly**pus**, arthro**pod**

N.B. To avoid confusion, be aware of the following homographs:

MER/O: Thigh [Gr. *meros, merou*, thigh]; Part [Gr. *meros, mereos*, part]
MEL/O: Limb [Gr. *melos, meleos*, limb]; Cheek [Gr. *mela*, cheek]
-CELE: Cavity, abdomen [Gr. *koilia*, cavity]; Hernia, tumor [Gr. *kele*, tumor]

Review	Answers
The suffix in gastropod means _____.	foot
The combining form in knemometry means _____.	lower leg
Aconad is in the direction of the _____.	elbow
A laparoscopic surgery involves looking in the _____.	abdomen
The combining form MER/O can mean _____ or _____ because it is a homograph.	part, thigh
The combining form CHIR/O in chiropractor indicates that this practitioner works with his or her _____.	hands
The plural form of Olecranon is _____.	Olecrana
The Greek synonym for MUSCUL/O is _____.	my/o
Trachelocele is a protrusion at the _____.	neck
The plural form of stoma is _____.	stomata
Otitis is an inflammation of the _____.	ear
A genioplasty is a surgical reconstruction of the _____.	chin
The compound suffix "-some" in chromosome means _____.	body
Tragomaschalia is a condition of foul odor from the _____.	armpit
Pternalgia is a pain in the _____.	heel
The Greek synonym for the Latin combing form NAS/O is _____.	RHIN/O
Prosoponeuralgia is nerve pain affecting the _____.	face
A phlebitis is an inflammation of a _____.	vein
The Greek synonym for the Latin combining from VAS/O is _____.	ANGI/O
The combining form MEL/O can mean _____ or _____ because it is a homograph.	limb, cheek
Xerophthalmia affects the _____.	eye
The celiocentesis is a surgical puncture and aspiration of the _____.	abdomen
The Greek combining form for the Latin anatomical term *frons* is _____.	METOP/O
Dactyledema is swelling in the _____ or _____.	fingers, toes
Gonycampsis is an abnormal curvature of the _____.	knee
The roots DERM- and DEMAT- mean _____.	skin
The root in adenitis means _____.	gland
Pneumoconiosis affects the _____.	lungs
The combining form NEPHR/O means _____.	kidney
The Greek combining form for the Latin anatomical term *vesica* is _____.	CYST/O
The Greek root for the heart is _____.	CARDI-
The Greek combining form for the intestines is _____.	ENTER/O

Latin Anatomical Adjectives

Types of Latin Adjectives

An **adjective** is a word that describes or modifies a noun. Adjectives are an important part of anatomical Latin. Adjectives distinguish an anatomical structure by revealing its defining characteristic (e.g. *ligamentum flavum*, the **yellow** ligament) or its physical location (e.g. *musculus temporalis*, the **temple** muscle). The latter can also be translated using "of the" (e.g. *musculus temporalis*, the muscle **of the temple**).

A Latin adjective always agrees with the noun it modifies, that is to say, the ending of the adjective reflects the **number**, **case**, and **gender** of the noun it modifies.

Number: If the noun is a singular, then its adjective must be singular. If the noun is a plural, then its adjective must be plural.

> singular: *os long**um*** (long bone)
> plural: *ossa long**a*** (long bones)

Case: If the noun is in the nominative case, then its adjective is in the nominative case. If the noun is in the genitive case, then its adjective is in the genitive case.

> nominative: *os long**um*** (long bone)
> gentive: *nervus ossis long**i*** (nerve of the long bone)

Gender: If the noun is a feminine (masculine, neuter), then the adjective will take a feminine (masculine, neuter) form.

> masculine: *musculus long**us*** (long muscle)
> feminine: *arteria long**a*** (long artery)
> neuter: *os long**um*** (long bone)

Latin adjectives typically appear after the nouns they modify. However, in some instances, an adjective will appear disjointed from the noun it modifies. For example, in the term *musculus flexor digitorum profundus* (the deep flexing muscle of the fingers), the adjective *profundus* (deep) modifies the noun *musculus* rather than *digitorum* (of the fingers). The noun it modifies is made evident by the fact that the grammatical ending of *profundus* agrees with the number, case, and gender of *musculus* rather than the number, case, and gender of *digitorum*. If there were such a thing as "the flexing muscle of the deep fingers," it would be *musculus flexor digitorum profundorum*.

There are two types of adjectives: (i) adjectives which follow the 1st and 2nd declension endings and (ii) adjectives which follow 3rd declension endings.

1st and 2nd Declension-Type Adjectives

These types of adjectives follow the patterns of the 1st declension or the 2nd declension nouns to agree with the gender, case, and number of the nouns they are modifying.

First declension endings *–a* are used to agree with nouns whose gender is feminine. Second declension endings *–us* are used to agree with masculine nouns. Second declension neuter endings *–um* are used to agree with neuter nouns.

	Singular			**Plural**		
	2nd (masc.)	1st (fem.)	2nd (neut.)	2nd (masc.)	1st (fem.)	2nd (neut.)
Nom.	*intern**us*** (internal)	*intern**a***	*intern**um***	*intern**i***	*intern**ae***	*intern**a***
Gen.	*intern**i***	*intern**ae***	*intern**i***	*intern**orum***	*intern**arum***	*intern**orum***

There are several of these adjectives which follow this pattern whose nominative ends in *–er*. Whether these nouns drop the *–e* or keep it is apparent in the feminine and neuter forms of these adjectives.

	Singular			**Plural**		
	2nd (masc.)	1st (fem.)	2nd (neut.)	2nd (masc.)	1st (fem.)	2nd (neut.)
Nom.	*dext**er*** (right)	*dextr**a***	*dextr**um***	*dextr**i***	*dextr**ae***	*dextr**a***
Gen.	*dextr**i***	*dextr**ae***	*dextr**i***	*dextr**orum***	*dextr**arum***	*dextr**orum***

	Singular			Plural		
	2ⁿᵈ (masc.)	1ˢᵗ (fem.)	2ⁿᵈ (neut.)	2ⁿᵈ (masc.)	1ˢᵗ (fem.)	2ⁿᵈ (neut.)
Nom.	*liber* (free)	*libera*	*liberum*	*liberi*	*liberae*	*libera*
Gen.	*liberi*	*liberae*	*liberi*	*liberorum*	*liberarum*	*liberorum*

The dictionary entry for these types of adjectives provides the nominative singular endings for masculine, feminine, and neuter:

internus, -a, -um, internal
dexter, -tra, -trum, right

Third Declension-Type Adjectives

Most of the 3ʳᵈ adjectives used in anatomical Latin use two terminations for the three grammatical genders. Thus, one ending is used for both masculine and feminine nouns, and another is used for the neuter nouns.

	Singular		Plural	
	masc. and fem.	neut.	masc. and fem.	neut.
Nom.	*-is*	*-e*	*-es*	*-ia*
Gen.	*-is*	*-is*	*-ium*	*-ium*
Nom.	*medialis* (medial)	*mediale*	*mediales*	*medialia*
Gen.	*medialis*	*medialis*	*medialium*	*medialium*

The dictionary entry for these adjectives provides the nominative singular for the masculine/feminine and the neuter endings:

brevis, -e, short
dorsalis, -e, dorsal

Comparative Adjectives

When Latin adjectives are used to compare the characteristics of nouns, a comparative adjective is used. **Comparative adjectives are usually translated by adding an –er to the adjective (e.g. great → greater, low → lower, small → smaller).** In Latin, comparative adjectives are often recognized by the *–ior* ending, and sometimes with the *–or* ending. Comparative adjectives follow the pattern for 3ʳᵈ declension nouns.

	Singular		Plural	
	masc. and fem.	neut.	masc. and fem.	neut.
Nom.	*-ior (-or)*	*-us*	*-es*	*-a*
Gen.	*-is*	*-is*	*-um*	*-um*
Nom.	*inferior* (lower)	*inferius*	*inferiores*	*inferiora*
Gen.	*inferioris*	*inferioris*	*inferiorum*	*inferiorum*
Nom.	*major* (greater)	*majus*	*majores*	*majora*
Gen.	*majoris*	*majoris*	*majorum*	*majorum*

The dictionary entries for comparatives provide the nominative singular for the masculine/feminine and neuter:

Anterior, anterius, anterior
Minor, minus, lesser, minor

Creation of Latin Anatomical Adjectives

Anatomical Latin adjectives are often created by adding the 3rd declension endings *–alis* or *–aris* to the root of an anatomical Latin noun.

>*cranium*, cranium + *-alis* →*cranialis, -e*, cranial
>*frons*, *frontis*, forehead + *-alis* →*frontalis, -e*, frontal
>*palma*, palm + *-aris* →*palmaris, -e*, palmar
>*vola*, palm + *-aris* →*volaris, -e*, volar

Anatomical Latin adjectives are also created by adding the 1st and 2nd declension endings to the root of the anatomical Latin noun.

>*poples*, *poplitis*, m. hollow of the posterior knee → *popliteus, a, um* pertaining to the posterior knee, popliteal

Roots can be combined to form compound anatomical adjectives.

>*anter-* + *o* + *medialis* = *anteromedialis, -e*, anteromedial
>*pont-* + *o* + *cerebell-* + *aris* →*pontocerebellaris, -e*, pontocerebellar

Latin Adjectives for Positions and Planes of the Body

Fig. 3.4 Planes, positions, and directions of human and quadruped animals. *Source;* Drawing by Chloe Kim.

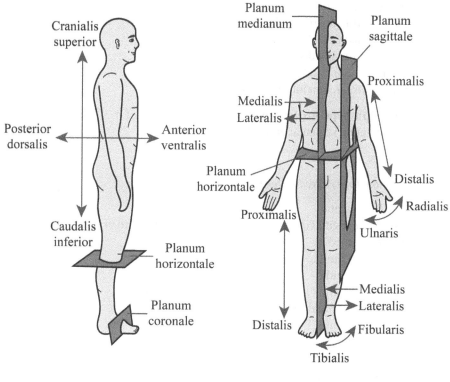

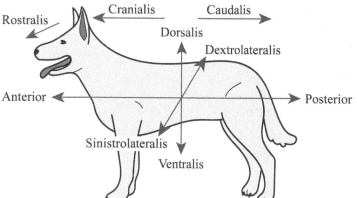

The **anatomical position** is a term used for the purpose of describing the body (Fig. 3.4). For humans, the anatomical position is standing, feet flat and together, arms to the side with palms facing forward. For quadruped animals the anatomical position is standing on all fours, and therefore some anatomical terms are not synonymous with human anatomical terms of position (e.g. anterior of a dog is his face and the ventral part is his belly). Human anatomists divide the body into planes which in English are termed the **coronal plane** (or **frontal plane**), **sagittal plane** (or **medial plane**), and **transverse plane**. The **coronal plane** (or **frontal plane**) is a vertical line which divides the body into **anterior** (**ventral**) and **posterior** (**dorsal**). The **sagittal plane** (or **medial plane**) is a vertical plane dividing the body into left and right. The **transverse plane** is horizontal division separating the upper and lower body. These planes help to determine positions such as **lateral**, **medial**, **distal**, **proximal**, **anterior**, **posterior**, **ventral**, and **dorsal**.

1ˢᵗ and 2ⁿᵈ Declension-Type Adjectives: The dictionary entries for the 1ˢᵗ and 2ⁿᵈ declension-type adjectives show the nominative singular endings (masculine, feminine, and neuter) of the adjective in the following way:

> *externus, -a, -um,* external
>
> *sinister, -tra, -trum,* left

1ˢᵗ and 2ⁿᵈ Declension-Type Adjectives for Planes and Positions:

> *internus, -a, -um* internal
> *externus, -a, -um* external
> *transversus, -a, -um* transverse
> *dexter, dextra, dextrum* right
> *sinister, sinistra, sinistrum* left
> *profundus, -a, -um* deep;
> *medius, -a, -um* middle
> *intermedius, -a, -um* intermediate

3ʳᵈ Declension-Type Adjectives: The dictionary entries for 3ʳᵈ declension adjectives are the nominative (masculine/feminine, and neuter) singular endings for these adjectives:

> *medialis, -e,* medial

3ʳᵈ Declension-Type Adjectives for Planes and Positions:

> *lateralis, -e* lateral
> *sagittalis, -e* sagittal (*on or parallel to the sagittal suture of the skull)
> *medialis, -e* medial
> *cranialis, -e* cranial
> *caudalis, -e* caudal
> *rostralis, -e* rostral
> *coronalis, -e* coronal (*on the coronal suture of the skull)
> *frontalis, -e* frontal
> *dorsalis, -e* dorsal
> *ventralis, -e* ventral
> *superficialis, -e* superficial
> *longitudinalis, -e* longitudinal
> *transversalis, -e* transverse
> *proximalis, -e* proximal
> *distalis, -e* distal
> *palmaris, -e,* palmar
> *volaris, -e,* volar
> *plantaris, -e,* plantar

Comparative Adjectives: The dictionary entries for a comparative adjective are as follows:

inferior, -ius, inferior
major, -us, greater

Planes and Positions:

anterior, -ius anterior
posterior, -ius posterior
superior, -ius superior
inferior, -ius inferior

Latin word element	Current usage	Etymology	Examples
SINISTR/O (sĭn-ĭs-trō)	Left	L. *sinister, -tra, -trum,* left	**Sinistr**ad, **sinistr**aural Loan word: **Sinister** (sĭn-ĭs′tĕr)
***LEV/O** (lē-vō)	Left	L. *laevus, -a, -um,* left	**Lev**ocardia, **lev**oscoliosis
DEXTR/O (deks-trō)	Right	L. *dexter, -tra, -trum* right	**Dextr**ad, **dextr**ocular Loan word: **Dexter** (dĕks′tĕr)
LATER/O (la-ĕ-rō)	Side	L. *lateralis, -e,* pertaining to the side, lateral fr. L. *latus, lateris,* n. side	Bi**later**al, infero**later**al Loan word: **Latus** (lat′ŭs) **Lateralis** (lăt-ĕr-ā′lĭs)
MEDI/O (mēd-ē-ō)	Middle	L. *medius, -a, -um,* middle	**Medi**an, **medi**olateral Loan word: **Medius** (mēd′ē-ŭs)
EXTER/O (eks-tĕ-rō) **EXTERNAL/O** (ĕks-tĕr-nā-lō) **EXTREM/O** (ĕks-trēm-ō)	Outside, outermost	L. *exter,* outward L. *externalis, -e,* outside L. *extremus, -a, -um,* outermost	**Exter**oceptive, **external**ia **extrem**ophile
INTERN/O (ĭn-tĕr-nō)	Within, inside	L. *internus, -a, -um,* within, inside	**Intern**ist, **internal**
DORS/O (dor-sō)	Back	L. *dorsalis, -e,* dorsal, pertaining to the back fr. L. *dorsum, -i,* n. back	**Dors**ad, **dors**al Loan word: **Dorsum** (dor′sŭm) pl. **Dorsa** (dor′sa)
VENTR/O (ven-trō)	Belly, abdomen, cavity	L. *ventralis, -e,* pertaining to the belly, ventral fr. L. *venter, ventris,* m. belly	**Ventr**al, **ventr**ad Loan word: **Venter** (vent′ĕr) **Ventralis** (ven-tra′lĭs)

Latin word element	Current usage	Etymology	Examples
ROSTR/O (rŏs-trō)	Snout, beak	L. *rostralis, -e*, pertaining to the snout or beak, rostral fr. L. *rostrum, -i*, n. snout, beak	**Rostr**iform, **rostr**al Loan word: **Rostrum** (rŏs'trŭm) pl. **Rostra** (rŏs'tra)
CAUD/O (kowd-ō)	Tail, tail-like	L. *caudalis, -e*, pertaining to the tail, caudal L. *cauda, -ae*, f. tail	**Caud**al, **caud**ad Loan word: **Cauda** (kowd'ă) pl. **Caudae** (kowd'ē)
PROXIM/O (prok-sĭm-ō)	Nearest (to a given part or center of body)	L. *proximalis, -e*, proximal *proximus, -a, -um*, nearest, closest *superlative from L. *propior*, nearer	**Proxim**ad, **proxim**al
DIST/O (dĭs-tō)	Farthest (from a given part of the center of the body)	L. *distalis, -e*, apart from, distal	**Dist**olabial, **dist**al
CORON/O (kor-ō-nō)	On the coronal suture of the skull, crown, circular, coronary arteries	L. *coronalis, -e*, coronal; the coronal suture fr. L. *corona, -ae*, f. crown, garland	**Coron**avirus, **coron**al Loan word: **Corona** (kŏ-rō'nă) pl. **Coronae** (kŏ-rō'nē)
SAGITT/O (să-jĭ-tō)	On or parallel to the sagittal suture of the skull, arrow	L. *sagittalis, -e*, pert. to an arrow; the sagittal suture fr. L. *sagitta, -ae*, f. arrow	**Sagitt**ocyst, **sagitt**al
ANTER/O (ant-ĕ-rō)	Front, anterior	L. *anterior, -ius*, more forward, anterior	**Anter**ograde, **anter**ograde Loan word: **Anterior** (an-tēr'ē-ŏr)
POSTER/O (pŏs-tĕr-ō)	Behind, posterior	L. *posterior, -ius*, more behind, posterior	**Poster**oinferior, **poster**oanterior Loan word: **Posterior** (pŏs-tē'rē-or)
SUPER/O (soo-pĕr-ō)	Above, superior	L. *superior, -ius*, more above, superior	**Super**olateral Loan word: **Superior** (soo-pē'rē-or)
INFER/O (in-fĕr-ō)	Below, inferior	L. *inferior, -ius*, more below, inferior	**Infer**olateral Loan word: **Inferior** (in-fēr'ē-ŏr)

Review	Answers
The dextrolateral side of animals is to its _____ side.	**right**
A caudal direction is literally toward the _____.	**tail**
A levoscoliotic curve is bent to the _____.	**left**
A rostrifom structure is in the shape of a _____.	**snout, beak**
Arteria lateralis is translated _____.	**lateral artery**
A ventral direction is literally toward the _____.	**belly, abdomen**
Venae internae is translated _____.	**internal veins**

Review	Answers
The _____ plane separates the anterior and posterior part of the bodies.	**coronal**
The _____ plane separates the body into left and right.	**sagittal**
For bipedal animals, ventral is the same as _____ and dorsal is the same as _____.	**anterior, posterior**
The opposite of distal is _____.	**proximal**
The opposite of ventral is _____.	**dorsal**
Sinistrad is toward the _____.	**left**
The anatomical Latin noun for "crown" is _____.	**corona**
The anatomical noun for "tail" is _____.	**cauda**

4

Diagnostic and Therapeutic Terminology

CHAPTER LEARNING OBJECTIVES
1) You will learn about Celsus' account of Greek medicine in *De medicina*.
2) You will learn about the patient case histories in the Hippocratic *Epidemics*.
3) You will learn the word elements used in diagnostic and therapeutic terms.
4) You will learn the abbreviations and format of modern progress notes.

Lessons from History: Celsus' Description of Greek Medicine

Food for Thought as You Read:

How is Celsus' conception of medicine different from our own? How is it similar?
How would a Roman recognize who is and who is not a "medicus"? How do we recognize who and who is not a physician?

> Just as the art of agriculture promises food for healthy bodies, likewise the art of medicine promises health for sick bodies ... truly it has been cultivated considerably more among the Greeks than in the other nations, and it was not among them from the beginning, but within a few generations before us.
>
> Celsus, *De medicina*, Proemium I.1, Loeb, pp. 2–3.

The above Latin passage is part of the proemium (prefatory remarks) to Book I of Aulus Cornelius Celsus' *De medicina* (*On Medicine*), Fig. 4.1. Celsus was a 1st-century-AD Roman author who wrote encyclopedias on the arts of agriculture, medicine, rhetoric, philosophy, law, and military practices. Of these works, only *De medicina* has been preserved. The proemium to Book I provides a detailed account of the history of ancient Greek medicine. This historical account is followed by eight books on the practice of medicine. Book I addresses dietetics and the preservation of health; Book II addresses the signs and symptoms of disease; Book III is on the treatment of specific diseases affecting the whole body; Book IV deals with the treatment of diseases affecting specific parts of the body; Book V discusses drugs for diseases of the whole body; Book VI is on drugs for diseases affecting specific parts; and Books VII and VIII describe different types of surgeries. Unlike most medical texts in the Greco-Roman world, *De medicina* was written in Latin rather than Greek. This made *De medicina* more accessible to a Roman audience, and it also helped to make it an important text for the development of Latin medical terminology during the Renaissance. Similar to agriculture, Celsus sees Greek medicine as art (L. *ars*, Gr. *techne*) worthy for Romans to study. Medicine promises the restoration of health (L. *sanitas*), which was termed *hygieia* in Greek. The fact that Celsus' encyclopedia of medicine is decidedly Greek reveals how influential ancient Greek medicine had become in the Roman world (Fig. 4.2).

Greek and Latin Roots of Medical and Scientific Terminologies, First Edition. Todd A. Curtis.
© 2025 John Wiley & Sons, Inc. Published 2025 by John Wiley & Sons, Inc.
Companion website: www.wiley.com/go/Curtis

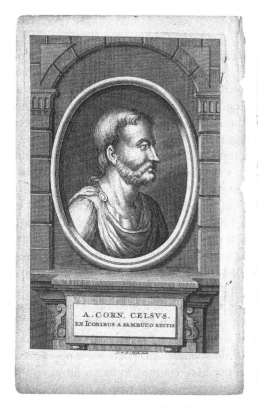

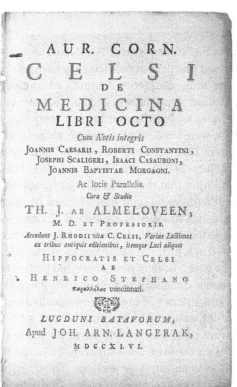

Fig. 4.1 Artist depiction Aulus Cornelius Celsus and the title page of a 1746 edition of *De medicina*. Celsus and the medical Latin of *De medicina* were highly regarded during the Renaissance. The text depicted here is one of 45 different editions of *De medicina* that were published during the period of 300 years (1478–1785). *Source:* Wellcome Collection/Wikimedia Commons/CC BY 4.0.

Fig. 4.2 Anonymous woodcut of the "Symphony of Plato" (1516). The image is of Plato, Aristotle, Hippocrates and Galen playing in a string quartet suggesting the harmonization of these two philosophers and two physicians. The attempt to harmonize the views of ancient philosophers and physicians can be observed in ancient Greek and Roman authors as well. For instance, Galen, the famous 2nd-century-AD physician, suggests that Plato's approach to the natural philosophy is consistent with Hippocrates' understanding of the human body in Galen's treatise *On the Opinions of Hippocrates and Plato*. *Source:* Unknown Source/Wikimedia Commons/Public domain.

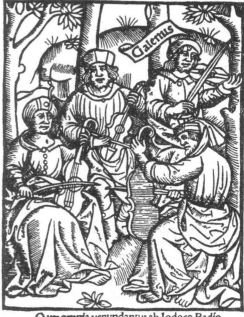

What defines Greek medicine in the Roman world? For Celsus and other Romans, Greek medicine is a collection of empirically and theoretically derived practices of medicine that are commonly associated with the Hippocratic Corpus (5th–4th century BC). One of the most distinctive features of ancient Greek medicine is its reliance on natural explanations for the causes of disease. Another recognizable feature is its tendency toward theoretical explanations that relied on overarching principles to describe the unseen workings of the human body. In many respects, these theoretical explanations of disease were similar to the various reductionist arguments that were used by ancient Greek philosophers, such as Parmenides of Elea (c. late 6th or early 5th century BC), Empedocles (c. 494–434 BC), Democritus of Abdera (c.460–370 BC), Plato (429–347 BC), and Aristotle (384–322 BC), to explain the origin and nature of the cosmos. It is important to bear in mind that there was a lack of consensus among medical authors as to what exactly caused the disease. Some medical authors thought that diseases resulted from residues; others attributed diseases to imbalances in fluids of the body called humors; some linked diseases to the restriction of the movement of a breath called pneuma; and still others saw disease as a failure of the body to function properly. By late antiquity, the theoretical explanation that the body consisted of four fluids identified as blood, bile, black bile, and phlegm (i.e. the four humors) became the predominate theory by which human physiology and pathophysiology were understood, and this theoretical model continued to have an influence on medicine well into the early modern period of western civilization.

In the Greco-Roman world, a practitioner of medicine was called an *iatros* in Greek and a *medicus* in Latin. Both titles indicated what the person did, meaning quite literally "one who heals," rather than his education or status in society. The *iatros* and *medicus* were viewed as practitioners of a *techne* (i.e. an "art"), much like architects, cooks, and poets. The criteria for becoming a doctor were quite different from the modern-day physician. There were no medical degrees or licensing to qualify one as an *iatros* or *medicus*. Thus, anyone could have claimed to be an *iatros* in the Greco-Roman world. What separated the educated physician from other practitioners of medicine was his knowledge of the most important medical writings, the names of the practitioners under whom he studied, and most importantly, his ability to cure patients. Today, the word-elements **IATR-** and **MEDIC-** are used in medical terminology for "medicine," "healing," or "physician" (e.g. iatrology, iatrogenic, medicine, and medicated) (Fig. 4.3).

The terms "doctor" and "physician" used today have their origins with the rise of medical universities in the 12th century AD. These terms were used to distinguish university trained doctors from a litany of other practitioners of medicine existing in the Medieval and Renaissance societies. Medical education in Medieval and Renaissance universities primarily involved studying a collection of treatises attributed to Hippocrates and Galen under the guidance of a *doctor*, which meant "teacher" or "scholar." By the 14th century, it began to mean "a holder of the highest degree in a university." The term "physician," as well as "physicist," comes from the Latinized Greek term for the study of nature, *physica*. The ancient Greek philosophers who focused on studying nature (Gr. *physis*) were termed "natural philosophers" (Gr. *physiologoi* or *physikoi*), and in many respects, their theoretical explanations of nature represented ancient Greek science. In Medieval universities, *physica* encompassed a wide variety of studies of the natural world, ranging from Aristotle's (384–322 BC) systematic approach to motion and causality to the medical theories of Galen. Later, *physica* came to be used extensively for the art of medicine. This connection can be seen in Chaucer's *Canterbury Tales* (1387–1400) when the character of a learned medical practitioner, who has studied the writings of a long list of ancient Greek and Islamic doctors, is identified as a "*Doctour of Phisyk* (Fig. 4.4)."

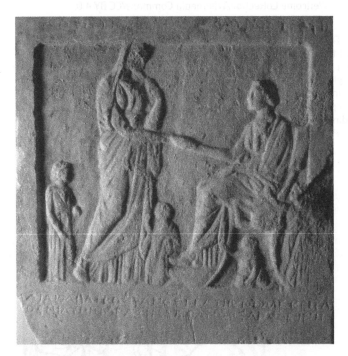

Fig. 4.3 Although ancient Greek medicine was predominately practiced by men, there is evidence that some women were recognized as having practiced medicine. The above image is of Phanostrate (seated), who was Greek-Athenian midwife and doctor practicing in the 4th century BC. Her epitaph reads: μαῖα καὶ ἰατρὸς Φανοστράτη ἐνθάδε κεῖται, οὐθενὶ λυπηρά, πᾶσιν δὲ θανοῦσα ποθεινή = "Midwife (*maia*) and doctor (*iatros*), Phanostrate lies here, who caused pain to no one, and having died, is missed by all." *Source:* Courtesy of National Archaeological Museum of Athens.

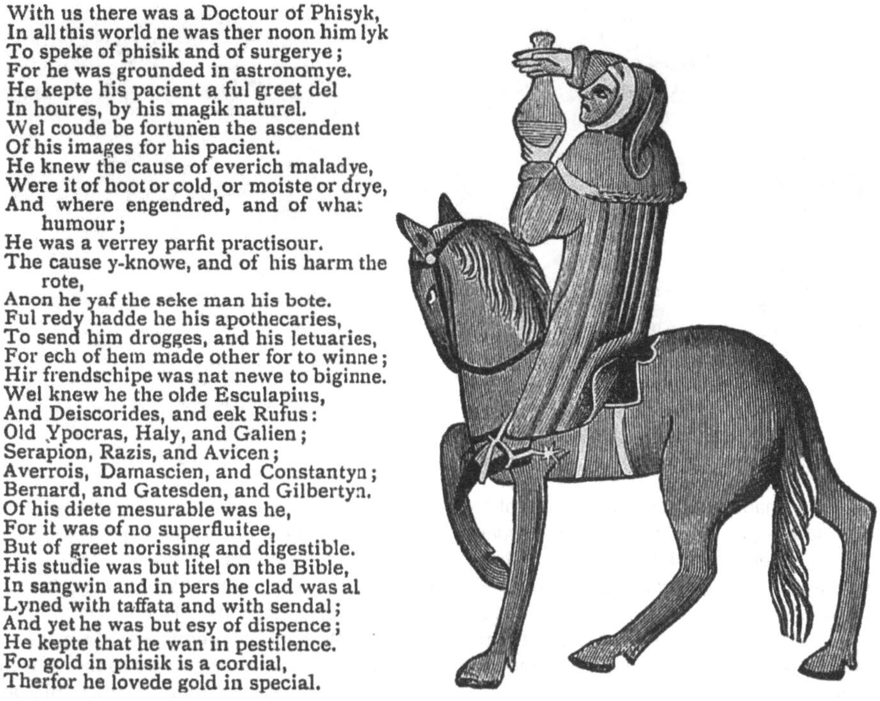

Fig. 4.4 Image of Chaucer's "Doctour of Phisyk," who is holding a matula (a glass jar) of urine for the purpose of medical uroscopy. *Source:* Colin Waters/Alamy Stock Photo.

With us there was a Doctour of Phisyk,
In all this world ne was ther noon him lyk
To speke of phisik and of surgerye ;
For he was grounded in astronomye.
He kepte his pacient a ful greet del
In houres, by his magik naturel.
Wel coude be fortunen the ascendent
Of his images for his pacient.
He knew the cause of everich maladye,
Were it of hoot or cold, or moiste or drye,
And where engendred, and of wha:
    humour ;
He was a verrey parfit practisour.
The cause y-knowe, and of his harm the
    rote,
Anon he yaf the seke man his bote.
Ful redy hadde he his apothecaries,
To send him drogges, and his letuaries,
For ech of hem made other for to winne ;
Hir frendschipe was nat newe to biginne.
Wel knew he the olde Esculapius,
And Deiscorides, and eek Rufus :
Old Ypocras, Haly, and Galien ;
Serapion, Razis, and Avicen ;
Averrois, Damascien, and Constantyn ;
Bernard, and Gatesden, and Gilbertyn.
Of his diete mesurable was he,
For it was of no superfluitee,
But of greet norissing and digestible.
His studie was but litel on the Bible,
In sangwin and in pers he clad was al
Lyned with taffata and with sendal ;
And yet he was but esy of dispence ;
He kepte that he wan in pestilence.
For gold in phisik is a cordial,
Therfor he lovede gold in special.

According to Celsus, Greek medicine was divided into three parts: regimen (Gr. *diatetike*), drugs (Gr. *pharmakeutike*), and surgery (Gr. *cheirourgia*). The Greek words for these parts form the roots **DIET-**, **PHARMAC-**, and **CHIRURGIC-** used in modern medical terminology for "diet," "drugs/medicines," and "surgery." Regimen involved mostly what one ate or drank. However, regimen also involved prescribing a way of life to prevent or to treat disease. Bathing, diet, exercise, sleep, and sexual activity were all parts of the art of regimen, and therefore, almost every aspect of a person's life could fall under the physician's direction. For example, whether one bathed in hot or cold water, how long he bathed, as well as what time he bathed were believed to have different effects on the body, making it soft, hard, dry, or moist. With this in mind, ancient physicians often based their remedies on the principle of "opposites cure opposites." For instance, if they believed a disease was engendered by a wet and cold humor, then a regimen with a drying and heating effect would be used. Likewise, Greek medicine's use of drugs was based upon the theory that materials have properties which affect the body. Therefore, depending on their ingredients, some drugs dry the body, others make it moist, some cause a cooling effect, others heat, some are diuretic, others laxative.

The Greek term for "surgery," comes from the Greek words *cheir* "hand" + *ergon* "work," and it quite literally meant "the art of working with one's hands." In the Greco-Roman medicine, *cheiriourgia* was defined as the use of one's hands on the patient's body to produce a desired effect, and it was considered one of the three divisions of medicine. A wide variety of treatments (e.g. trepanation, bloodletting, wound care, resetting of broken bones, and the removal of kidney stones) fell under the Greek category of *cheiriourgia*. Surgeons have not always been as highly esteemed as they are today. Medieval society made distinction between medicine and surgery. A "surgeon" was often viewed as merely a "practitioner of a handicraft," and therefore his method of healing was deemed beneath the more "cerebral" practices of regimen and drugs used by academically trained physicians. Medieval surgeries were often performed by nonacademics, such as barbers and bonesetters. During the Renaissance, surgery gradually took on a greater role in academic medicine. The distinction between medicine and surgery is nevertheless still evident in British and commonwealth countries where the degrees of Bachelor of Medicine (*Medicinae Baccalaureus*) and Bachelor of Surgery (*Baccalaureus Chirurgiae*) are simultaneously awarded upon graduation from medical school, which is abbreviated MB ChB, MB BCh, or MBBS (Fig. 4.5).

At the time Celsus was writing, medicine was quite sectarian. Greek physicians divided themselves along the lines of which famous teacher they followed (e.g. Herophileans, Erasistrateans, and Hippocratics), or by what causal theories they used to explain diseases (e.g. Humoralists and Pneumatists), or along the epistemic methods by which they derived their cures (e.g. Empiricists, Rationalists, and Methodists). Celsus spends much of his history of medicine describing the

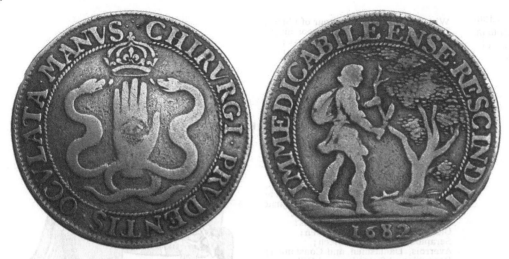

Fig. 4.5 Image of 1682 Jeton (token) of a corporation of surgeons. The front has a hand with an eye and two Aesculapian snakes. The Latin phrase (*oculta manus chirurgic prudentis*) is translated "the hand with an eye of the experienced surgeon." The back has a man pruning a tree with a knife. The Latin phrase (*immedicabile ense rescindit*) is translated "he cuts away with the scalpel the incurable." The corporation was an economic and regulatory movement that joined barber surgeons and medical-school surgeons, which were two distinct groups who practiced surgery, into one body of practitioners. Due to their abilities with razors, barbers were called upon to practice surgery since the Medieval period. The medical-school surgeons would separate themselves from the barber surgeons in the 18th century. The barber pole's characteristic red and white stripes are said to derive from the barber's surgeon's practice of bloodletting; the red representing bandages soaked in blood. The continued relationship between barbers and surgery can also be observed in the different versions of the Sweeney Todd story, in which Sweeney Todd is commonly identified as a barber-surgeon. *Source:* CGB/Wikimedia Commons/CC BY-SA 3.0.

differences between the Empiricists, the Rationalists, and the Methodists. Empiricists derived their cures through individual and collective *empeiria* (experience), without the use of theoretical explanations for the unseen causes of disease. As noted in Chapter 3, they also did not value human dissection as the means of discovering cures for their patients. Rationalists, on the other hand, held it was important to know the hidden causes of disease in order to arrive at a cure. Thus, they made use of evident causes and what they thought were the natural actions of the body. Because they considered the nature of the internal parts of the body as being necessary to know in order to find cures for disease, they were proponents for anatomical dissections. The Methodists were physicians who rejected being classed as relying solely on theoretical reasons such as the Rationalists, and they also believed one cannot find cures from experience alone. Instead, they developed a "method of inquiry," in Greek *methodos* (*meta-* + *hodos,* a road, path), to find cures for diseases. This "method" involved seeing commonalities in diseases, which could be expressed in three broad categories: diseases of flux, diseases of constriction, and diseases that manifest a combination of both. In some respects, the epistemological questions raised by these sects still exist in medicine when we consider to what extent experience versus theory comes into our making decisions when treating patients.

Some Suggested Readings

Celsus. *On Medicine, Volume I: Books 1-4.* Translated by Walter G. Spencer. Loeb Classical Library 292. Cambridge, MA: Harvard University Press, 1971.
Cruse, Audrey. *Roman Medicine.* Stroud: The History Press, 2004.
Jones-Lewis, Molly. "*Physicians and 'Schools'.*" In *A Companion to Science, Technology, and Medicine in Ancient Greece and Rome,* Edited by Georgia L. Irby, 386–401. Hoboken, John Wiley & Sons, 2016.
Jackson, Ralph. *Doctors and Diseases in the Roman Empire.* London: British Museum, 1988.
Scarborough, John. *Roman Medicine.* London: Thames and Hudson, 1969.

Vocabulary

Greek or Latin word element	Current usage	Etymology	Examples
IATR/O (ī-a-trō)	Medicine, physician	Gr. *iatros*, physician, healer	**Iatr**ogenic, psych**iatry**
-IATRY (ī-ă-trē)	medical treatment	*iatreia*, medicine, healing	
MEDIC/O (měd-ĭ-kō)	Medicine, medical treatment	L. *medicus, -i*, m. physician; medicine, healer	**Medic**ochirurgical, **medic**ation
THERAP/O (thěr-ă-pō) **THERAPEUT/O** (thěr-ă-pū-tō) **-THERAPY** (ther-ă-pē)	Treatment	Gr. *therapeuein*, to take care of, to heal, to treat Gr. *therapeutike*, treatment -therapy, treatment	**Therap**ist, **therap**eutic, aroma**therapy**
PHARMAC/O (făr-mă-kō) **PHARMACEUTIC/O** (făr-mă-sū-tĭ-kō)	Drugs, medicine	Gr. *pharmakon*, a drug, poison Gr. *pharmakeutikos*, by means of a drug or poisons	**Pharmac**ochemistry, **pharmaceut**ical
DIET/O (dī-ě-tō)	Food	Gr. *diaita*, way of living/ regimen; diet	**Diet**itian
CHIRURGIC/O (kĭ-rŭr-jĭ-kō)	Surgery	Gr. *chirurgia*, surgery	Odonto**chirurgic**al
LOG/O (log-ō) **-LOGY** (lŏ-jē)	Word, speech The study of	Gr. *logos*, word, speech, reason, thought of	**Log**orrhea, arthro**logy**
NOM/O (nŏ-mō) **-NOMY** (nŏ-mē)	Law, custom Knowledge/laws of	Gr. *nomos*, law, custom	Ergo**nom**ics, taxo**nomy**
PHYSI/O (fĭz-ē-ō) **PHYSIC/O** (fĭz-ĭ-kō-kō)	Nature, growth, function Physical, natural	Gr. *physis*, nature, growth, function Gr. *physikos*, of nature	**Physi**ognomy, **physic**ochemical
TECHN/O (tek-nō)	Art, skill	Gr. *techne*, art, skill, craft	**Techn**ology, **techn**ophobic
ERG/O (ěr-gō) **-ERGASIA** (ěr-gā-sē-ă)	Work, function	Gr. *ergon*, work	Syn**erg**ic, hyper**ergasia**

Review	Answers
Physiology is the study of the functions of living organisms. The word is formed from root _____, which means _____, _____, and _____, and the compound suffix _____, which literally means _____.	**PHYSI-, nature, growth, function -LOGY, the study of**
Hypoergasia is defined as decreased functional activity. It is formed from the prefix HYPO- and the compound suffix _____, which means _____ and _____.	**-ERGASIA, work, function**
Ergophobia is a fear of _____.	**work**
Any injury or illness that occurs because of medical care is termed "iatrogenic." The root IATR- means _____ and _____.	**medicine, physician**
Based on its word elements the adjective "medicochirurgical" pertains to _____ and _____.	**medicine, surgery**
Technetium was the first element to be produced artificially. It is named after the Greek word *technetos*, which means "artificial." One can see that the Greek word *technetos* is derived from the Greek word *techne*, which means _____, _____, and _____.	**art, skill, craft**
Ergonomics is the science of fitting a workplace to the user's needs and health. The root NOM- in this word can mean _____, _____, and _____.	**laws, customs, knowledge of**
The branch of medicine that provides medical treatment for mental illnesses is called psych_____.	**-iatry**
The term "pharmacotherapy" is composed of two word elements: PHARMAC-, which means _____ or _____, and -THERAPY, which means _____.	**drugs, medicine treatment**

Lessons from History: Celsus on the Preservation of Health

Food for Thought as You Read:

How is Celsus' understanding of health different from our own? How is it similar?

Celsus was not the first to discuss the preservation of health. The preservation of health has been a topic of Greek medicine since the 5th century BC. Likewise, the Greek goddess of health, Hygeia, whose name is related to our word elements for health **HYGIEN-** and **HYGIEI-**, was always associated with Asclepius, the Greek god of medicine (Fig. 4.6). In Book I of *De medicina*, Celsus makes a distinction between the healthy regimen of the *homo sanus* (healthy human) and the *homo imbecillus* (weak human). As would be expected with other Greek medical works devoted to the preservation of health, the healthy regimen involves the knowledge of salubrious eating, drinking, exercise, sleep, living quarters, copulation, bathing, ointments, purging, and venesection. However, there is no universal healthy regimen, because each person has his or her unique needs. Celsus states that one should take into consideration the individual's kind of body (*genus corporis*), sex (*sexus*), age (*aetas*), and the time of the year (*tempus ani*) when considering the precepts of a healthy regimen. For example, in respect to the kind of body, the principle of opposites is applied: a thin body should be thickened; a thick body should be thinned; a cold body should be warmed; a hot body should be cooled; a soft body should be hardened; and a hard body should be softened. He informs the reader that a body can be thickened (*implere*, to fill in) by moderate exercise, frequent rest, by contraction of the bowels, by anointing, by bathing after a meal, by adequate sleep, by a soft couch, by a tranquil spirit, by winter cold in moderation, by sweet and fatty food, and by – not surprisingly – frequent meals.

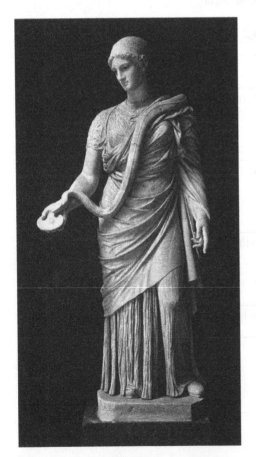

Fig. 4.6 Image of Pentelic marble statue of the Greek goddess of health, Hygeia. Found in 1797 at Ostia. Hygeia is commonly depicted with a snake or with Asclepius himself. *Source:* Wellcome Collection/CC BY 4.0.

In respect to age, there are also different needs to maintain health. For example, he recommends that wine should be diluted for children (*pueri*) and undiluted for the old (*senes*). This recommendation has nothing to do with the effects of alcohol; it is derived from a belief that the nature and temperament of human bodies changes over time. This belief is also evident in ancient Greek concepts of male versus female bodies, which are often described as having somewhat antithetical qualities (e.g. females are moist and males are dry). As to the time of the year, one should change their regimen to combat or lessen the effects of the excessive qualities (e.g. hot, cold, wet, and dry) of the seasons. Regimens should also be tailored to individual weaknesses: for a lax and painful colon due to flatulence (*inflatio*, swollen, and puffed up), a person should promote the movement of the gas by reading aloud, by taking hot baths, by eating hot food and drink, and by avoiding the cold.

He also includes a detailed regimen for how to preserve one's health if one is unable to leave an area during *pestilentia* (plague, unhealthy condition), and he argues one should follow this same regimen when visiting harsh places (*graves regiones*) or traveling during a harsh season (*grave tempus*). The precepts or rational behind his advice amounts to avoiding extremes in one's regimen when one is exposed to an unhealthy environment. Celsus' account of the preservation of health during *pestilentia* preserves the Greek distinction between disease that arises in an individual and disease that arises in a group of peoples due to external factors, which was generally called an *epidemia*. The Greek term *epidemia*, from which we get our term "epidemic," appears to be derived from the combination *epi-* "upon" and *demos* "people." Although similar to our modern definition of an epidemic – "a disease affecting a high percentage of people in a community or large area at one time" – Greek medicine did not recognize that epidemics could be caused by infectious diseases. Although the Latin word *contagium* (fr. L. *contingere*, to touch) was associated with defilement and disease by some authors, the phenomenon of passing a disease by touch was not recognized by Greek physicians as an explanation for epidemics. An *epidemia* was generally believed to be caused by people breathing in an unhealthy emanation in the air (Fig. 4.7). Similarly, any severe climatic change could be seen as the cause for groups of people experiencing a similar malady.

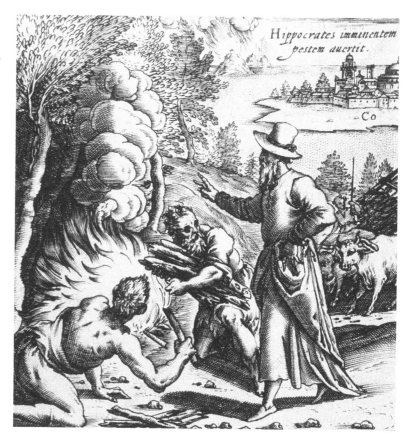

Fig. 4.7 Image of Hippocrates averting an impending plague (*Hippocrates imminentem pestem avertit*) from the frontispiece of *Hippocratis Coi Opera: Quae Extant Graece Et Latine Veterum Codicum Collatione Restituta, Nouo Ordine in Quattuor Classes Digesta, Interpretationis Latinae Emendatione & Scholijs Illustrata a Heiron Mercurali Forloiviensi*, 1588. The image is of Hippocrates averting miasma (peccant air) from entering a setting creating a bonfire. This speaks to a Hellenistic legendary account of Hippocrates being so great of a physician that he could help against a plague, which is something ancient Greek physicians would not realistically claim to be able to do. The image also preserves the link between pestilence and miasma that was quite evident in the medical attempts to avert the Black Death by fumigation and aromatic substances. *Source:* Wellcome Collection/Public domain.

Some Suggested Readings

Celsus. *On Medicine, Volume I: Books 1-4*. Translated by Walter G. Spencer. Loeb Classical Library 292. Cambridge, MA: Harvard University Press, 1971.

Jouanna, Jacques, and Neil Allies. "*Dietetics in Hippocratic Medicine: Definition, Main Problems, Discussion.*" In *Greek Medicine from Hippocrates to Galen: Selected Papers*, Edited by Philip van der Eijk, 137–154. Leiden: Brill, 2012.

König, Jason. "*Regimen and Athletic Training.*" In *A Companion to Science, Technology, and Medicine in Ancient Greece and Rome*, Edited by Georgia L. Irby, 450–464. Hoboken: John Wiley & Sons, 2016.

Tountas, Yannis. "The Historical Origins of the Basic Concepts of Health Promotion and Education: The Role of Ancient Greek Philosophy and Medicine." *Health Promotion International* 24, no. 2 (2009): 185–192.

Vocabulary

Greek or Latin word element	Current usage	Etymology	Examples
SAN/O (să-nō) **SANIT/O** (san-ĭ-tō)	Health	L. *sanus, -a, -um*, healthy L. *sanitas, sanitatis*, f. health	**Sane**, **insan**ity
HYGIEN/O (hī-jēn-ō) **HYGIEI/O** (hī-jē-ō)	Health	Gr. *hygieine*, healthful Gr. *hygieia*, health	**Hygien**ist, **hygiei**ology Loan Word: **Hygiene** (hī′jēn″)
ANTHROP/O (an-thrŏ-pō)	Human	Gr. *anthropos*, a human being	**Anthrop**oid, **anthrop**ology
***HOM/O** (ho-mō) **HOMIN/O** (hŏm-ĭn-ō)	Human	L. *homo, hominis*, m. a human being	**Hom**icidal, **homin**id Loan word: **Homo** (hō′mō)
IDI/O (ĭd-ē-ō)	Individual, distinct	Gr. *idios*, private, personal, peculiar	**Idi**opathic, **idi**oglossia
DEM/O (de-mō)	People	Gr. *demos*, people of a country or land	Epi**dem**ic, **dem**ographics
ETHN/O (ĕth-nō)	Race, culture	Gr. *ethnos*, race, nation	**Ethn**ography, **ethn**ocentric
***GEN/O** (jē′nō)	Race, kind, hereditary, gene	Gr. *genos*, kind, race, descent; *genea*, stock, descent L. *genus, -eris*, n. family	**Gen**odermatosis, **gen**ogram Loan word: **Genus** (jē′nŭs, jen′ŭs)
ANDR/O (an-drō)	Male, masculine, stamen of a flower	Gr. *aner, andros*, man; stamen of flower	**Andr**ogen, **andr**oid
VIRIL/O (vĭr-ĭl-ō)	Male, masculine	L. *virilis, -e*, male fr. L. *vir, viri*, m. man, male	**Viril**ism, **viril**e
GYN/O (jin-ō) or (gĭn-ō) **GYNEC/O** (jin-ĕkō) or (gĭn-ĕkō)	Female, feminine, pistil of a flower (gynoecium)	Gr. *gyne, gynaikos*, woman	Andro**gyn**ous, **gynec**oid
FEMIN/O (fem-ĭn-ō)	Female, feminine	L. *femina, -ae*, f. woman, female	**Femin**ine, **femin**ism

Greek or Latin word element	Current usage	Etymology	Examples
*PED/O (pē-dō)	Child	Gr. *pais, paidos*, child	**Ped**iatric, **ped**odontics
PUERIL/O (pū-ĕ-rĭ-lō)	Child	L. *puerilis, -e* child-like fr. L. *puer, -i,* m. child	**Pueril**e, **pueril**ism
GER/O (jer-ō) GERONT/O (jer-ŏn-tō)	Elderly, Old age	Gr. *geron, gerontos*, old person	**Ger**iatrics, **geront**ology
PRESBY/O (prez-bĭ-ō)	Elderly, old age	Gr. *prespys, presbytes*, elder, old person	**Presby**acusia, **presby**iatrics
SEN/O (sĕ-nō) SENIL/O (sē-nĭ-lō)	Elderly, old age	L. *senex, senis,* n. old, old person L. *senilis, -e,* old	**Sen**escence, **senil**ity

N.B.

GEN/O is a homograph see **GEN/O** (Gr. *gignomai,* to come into being) = To become, be produced.
GER/O is a homograph see **GER/O** (L. *gerere,* to carry, bear) = To carry, bear.
HOM/O is a homograph see **HOM/O** (Gr. *homos,* same) = Same.
PED/O is a homograph see **PED/O** (L. *pes, pedis,* foot) = Foot.

Review	Answers
The use of measures to promote conditions favorable to health is termed "sanitation." The Latin root SANIT- means _____. The Greek roots that have the same meaning are _____ and _____.	**health HYGIEN-, HYGIEI-**
Senility and senile share a common root that means _____ or _____. The process of growing old is called senescence. The root in this word that means "old age" is _____.	**elderly, old age SEN-**
The branch of health care concerned with the care of the aged is termed geriatrics. The root in this word that means "old age" is _____. Gerontology is the study of the processes and effects of aging and of age-related diseases on humans. The combining form in this word that means "old age" is _____.	**GER- GERONT/O**
Gynecology is a branch of medicine that focuses on women's health, particularly reproduction and reproductive organs. The combining form in gynecology means _____ or _____. The Latin combining form for "female" is _____. In botany, _____ is used for the ovary of the plant.	**female, feminine FEMIN/O GYN/O**
Pediatrics is the field of medicine concerned with the maintenance of children's health and the treatment of their diseases. The root in the pediatrics that means "child" is _____.	**PED-**
An androgen is a substance that stimulates _____ or _____ characteristics in a person. The combining form for the stamen of a plant is _____.	**male, masculine ANDR/O**
Based on the Greek root for human, "something that resembles a human" is termed an _____oid. Based on the Latin root, the family of primates that includes humans is termed _____idae. The Greek combining form HOM/O, which means "same," should not be confused with the Latin loan word Homo, which means _____.	**anthrop homin human**
A disease that typically occurs in a given population is said to be endemic to that group. An epidemic is disease that has become exceptionally high in a given population. A pandemic is defined as an exceptionally widespread disease, affecting a high percentage of people. Epidemic, pandemic, and endemic all share the root DEM-, which means _____.	**people**

Review	Answers
Virile is an adjective that means _____ or _____. The root in virile is _____. It should not be mistaken for the adjective viral, which means "virus." The root for virus is VIR-.	**male, masculine** **VIRIL-**
Ethnogerontology studies the effects of aging in different cultures and races. The combining form in ethnogerontology that means "race" and "culture" is _____.	**ETHN/O**
The loss of hearing associated with old age is termed presbyacusia. The root in this word that means "old age" is _____.	**PRESBY-**
Childishness is termed puerilism. The root that means "child" in puerilism is _____.	**PUERIL-**
Illnesses that have an uncertain or undetermined cause are termed idiopathic. The combining form IDI/O in this term literally means _____ or _____.	**individual, distinct**
Genotype is the genetic constitution present in an organism. This word contains the combining form GEN/O, which can mean _____, _____, _____, and _____.	**race, kind, hereditary, gene**

Lessons from History: Celsus and the Diagnosis of Disease

Food for Thought as You Read:

How is Celsus' understanding of disease different from our own? How is it similar?

> Now there are many signs for an impending ill health. In these interpretations, I will not hesitate to use the authority of ancient men, particularly Hippocrates, since recent physicians, as much as they have made changes to the curing of certain diseases, however they admit that those men best prognosticated these things.
>
> Celsus, *De medicina,* Proemium II.1, Loeb, pp. 84–85

Book II of *De medicina* addresses the signs of disease for the purpose of prognosis (L. *praesagire,* to foretell, to say beforehand). Greek medicine placed great value on making a correct prognosis. Unlike modern medicine, which makes a distinction between prognosis (Gr. *prognosis,* foreknowledge) and diagnosis (Gr. *diagnosis,* discernment), the former being the "prediction of the future course of a disease" and the latter being "the identification of a disease by its signs and symptoms," ancient Greek prognosis could involve recognizing the past, present, and the future nature of a disease based on the current signs and symptoms of a patient. That said, in general, medical prognosis was the art of recognizing and correctly interpreting the preceding signs of disease, and thus, it was often compared and contrasted with religious prophecy. Celsus notes that certain diseases can be anticipated based on the season, the weather, age and the type of body of the patient. Prognostic signs were useful because they allowed an ancient physician to "see" the hidden pathophysiology of the body. Celsus states, "if blood (*sanguis*) and heat (*calor*) are abundant, it follows that there may be a hemorrhage (*profluvium sanguinis*) from some part"; and elsewhere he posits, "those who cough out bloody sputum, there is a defect (*vitium*) in the lung." As is the case with Hippocratic works on prognosis, *De medicine* contains lists of signs that indicate a deadly disease. "Red and thin urine is usual in severe indigestion (*cruditas*) ... and so when such urine persists for a long time, it indicates that there is a danger of death." In other cases, the location of the disease is important: "A disease of the small intestine, unless it dissipates, kills within seven days." Greek physicians generally would not treat a patient who had the signs of imminent death because short-term palliative care for the terminally ill was not a part of Greek medicine, and because one's reputation as a *medicus* or *iatros* was dependent on restoring a patient to health. Celsus acknowledges that these signs of approaching death were sometimes misunderstood. He tells how the famous physician, Asclepiades, when he met up with a funeral procession, recognized that a man who was being carried was not dead. The point of the story is that one should not ascribe blame to the art of medicine because it was the first prognosticator's inability to correctly interpret the signs that led to this mistake.

At the beginning of Book III of *De medicina,* Celsus explains the classifications of disease (L. *genera morborum*) and their treatment. Similar to modern medicine, Greek medicine divided disease into two species: acute (Gr. *oxys,* sharp, swift) and chronic (Gr. *chronos,* time, long time). According to Celsus, acute diseases are known by their quick onset, severe pain without intermission, and rapid mortality. Chronic diseases were considered long-lasting diseases that were difficult to fully eradicate once they became deep-seated. Interestingly, Celsus adds two more classes of disease. The third class is said to be at one time acute and at another time chronic. He notes that some fevers are this type of disease. The fourth class is neither acute, because it is not fatal, nor is it chronic, because the patient is easily restored to health.

In addition to classifying diseases as being acute or chronic, Celsus also divides the diseases of the whole body (L. *totum corpus*) from diseases that affect a specific part of the body (L. *pars corporis*). Book III addresses diseases of the whole body, while Book IV addresses diseases arising from and affecting a specific part of the body. In some respects, this is similar to modern medicine's distinction between local and systemic diseases. Today, a local disease is understood as being limited to one place or part, and a systemic disease is a general disease affecting multiple parts or the whole body.

In Books III and IV, one finds numerous similarities and differences between modern and ancient Greek terminologies and concepts of disease. In Book III, Celsus notes that the Greeks identified different types of chronic and dangerous wasting diseases. One of these diseases was termed *atrophia* (fr. Gr. *a-* lack of + *trophe*, nourishment), and it was described as a wasting of the body due to the patient's dread of food. The modern meaning of the derivative "atrophy" is "an abnormal decrease in the size of cell, organ, or tissue. (Fig. 4.8)" Celsus uses the term *cachexia* (fr. Gr. *kakos*, bad + *hexis*, habit of body) for another type of wasting. He explains that this wasting disease causes digested food to be corrupted due to the bad habit of the body. This bad habit of the body could be due to prolonged illness, bad medications, or unserviceable food having been consumed. "Cachexia" is a loan word used today for a state of ill health, malnutrition, loss of weight, and wasting of muscle. The last form of wasting he notes is called *phthisis* (perishing, decaying) by the Greeks. This disease is said to start as drainage from the head into the lungs causing ulceration, periodic fevers, frequent cough, and pus being excreted. Today the term "phthisis" is used primarily for tuberculosis, but it is sometimes used for wasting of a part not due to tuberculosis (e.g. phthisis bulbi). Celsus uses the general term *tabes* for wasting or

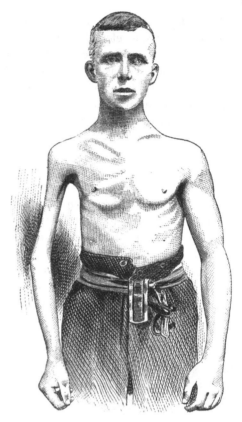

Fig. 4.8 Image of a boy with atrophy of his right arm due to acute anterior polymyelitis. Image found in *An American Textbook of the Diseases of Children*, 1895. *Source:* Internet Archive Book Images/Flickr/CC0.

malnutrition due to pestilence, disease, or want of food. This term is still used today for "a gradual wasting/emaciation due to a chronic disease." Tabes comes from the Latin verb *tabere*, which means "to waste away, be consumed."

Celsus places a collection of diseases that have adverse effects on behavior and mental faculties under the category of *insania* (madness, unsound mind). Today, the term "mental illness" or "mental disorder" are used for any disorder affecting behavior or mood, and the term insane is defined as "mentally deranged and therefore legally incompetent." The diseases Celsus places in the category of *insania*, such as *phrenesis* and *melancholia*, are not strictly "mental illnesses" because they have somatic etiologies. Melancholia (Gr. *melas*, black + *chole*, bile), which was associated with a wide variety of mental illnesses, particularly depression, was thought be caused by the presence of black bile in the body. And *phrenesis* is said to be a delirious state associated with attacks of fever. "Melancholy" is used today as a non-technical term for depression, and *phrenesis'* influence on our vocabulary can be seen in the term "phrenetic," which is defined as "a maniacal or frantic behavior."

Celsus states that the signs of inflammation are four: *rubor* (redness), *tumor* (swelling), *calor* (heat), and *dolor* (pain). These Latin terms are still considered the four cardinal signs of inflammation. In the 19th century, Rudolph Virchow added a fifth sign of inflammation, *functio laesa*, loss of function, to the Celsus' tetrad. Celsus notes that the Greek term for inflammation is *phlegmone*. Today this word can be seen in the compound term "phlegmasia" (an inflammation) and the derivative "phlegmon" (an acute pyogenic inflammation of soft tissue). The terms *inflammatio*, which is derived from *inflammare* (to set on fire), and *phlegmone*, which comes from the verb *phlegein* (to burn) emphasize heat being an important sign of this disease. Ancient humoral theories of inflammation generally attribute the swelling and heat to the effects of superfluous blood flowing into an area. Today, inflammation is described as a complex cascade of biological processes that occurs primarily at the cellular level.

In Book III, Celsus informs his reader that *febris* (fever) is another class of disease that is common and affects the whole body. Following the Greek manner of classifying fevers, which are termed *pyretoi* (fevers) in Greek, he divides them according to their reoccurrences. Quartan fevers reoccur on the 4th day; tertian fevers reoccur on the 3rd day; and quotidian fevers reoccur daily. These patterns of sudden attacks of fever are evident in the different types of malaria, which is why they today are termed "quartan malaria," "tertian malaria," and "quotidian malaria." A sudden, periodic attack of fever, as well as other diseases, is referred to today as a "paroxysm," thanks to the Greek word *paroxysmos* (irritation). Ancient Greek medical authors, such as the Hippocratic text *On the Nature of Man*, viewed these *pyretoi* as diseases which had specific humoral causes, such as too much bile in the body. However, for modern medicine, fever is merely a sign of another disease. The term malaria appears to have been coined in the 17th century via the Italian word mal'aria, from L. *mala aer*, which literally means "bad air." The belief that peccant air could cause a wide spread disease in a given population extends back to the ancient Greek world, and such a cause of disease was sometimes termed a *miasma* (Gr. defilement, pollution). Interestingly, Rome's susceptibility to malaria due to its marshy landscape may account for why they had three sanctuaries to a goddess of fevers, named Febris.

In Book V, among Celsus' discussions of the different types of skin lesions, one will find a description of a "*carcinoma*." Here, as in other places, Celsus is using a word that has been transliterated from a Greek medical term, *karkinoma*. The use of terms *karkinoma* and *karkinos* dates back to the 5th century BC, where they were used interchangeably for ulcerative lesions in the Hippocratic Corpus. Similar to the literal meaning of *cancer* in Latin, *karkinos* is a Greek word for "crab." That said, Celsus appears to make a distinction between a *carcinoma* and *cancer*. Both are placed under the category of *ulcus* (ulceration), which is a term used for a wide variety of skin lesions. Celsus points out that there are different species of *cancer*. Whatever its species, a *cancer* corrupts not only the part it occupies but it also "creeps" (L. *serpere* to creep, crawl) to other areas. *Cancer* in some cases can be a red and painful ulceration above the inflammation; in other cases, *cancer* is a black ulceration with foul odor and putrefaction of the flesh. What makes these lesions forms of *cancer* is that like a crab, they spread out devouring nearby flesh. A *carcinoma*, according to Celsus, is a *vitium* (defect, blemish) typically found in the upper parts of the body: face, nose, ears, lips, and the breasts of women. In some cases, the part becomes harder or softer, often without ulceration. This type of *carcinoma* is only dangerous if it is irritated by impudent surgical treatment. The other type of *carcinoma* is the worst, and Celsus tells his reader that the Greeks call this type *cacoethes* (fr. Gr. *kakoetheia* malignant, bad disposition). He notes how this carcinoma has stages: first, it is without ulceration; then it ulcerates; and lastly, it forms a warty excrescence (*thymium*). He states that this type of *carcinoma* must be removed immediately, because its other stages do not allow for medical intervention and often lead to death. In some respects, Celsus' description of the *cacoethes carcinoma* resembles the stages of cancer, particularly breast cancer, and his use of *cacoethes*, is similar to when we identify a cancerous tumor as being "malignant" (L. *malignus*, bad-natured) and a noncancerous tumor as being "benign" (L. *benignus*, good-natured) (Fig. 4.9). For modern medicine, the term "cancer" is used for a large collection of malignant neoplasia that is recognized by their uncontrolled formation of cells, and a cancer that arises from epithelial tissue is called a "carcinoma."

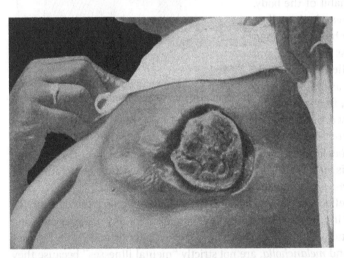

Fig. 4.9 Picture of an observable carcinoma of patient's breast. The patient had been treated with arsenic paste, which was often used in the early 1900s for cancer. *The Breast: Its Anomalies, Its Diseases, and Their Treatment*, 1917. *Source:* Internet Archive Book Images/Flickr/CC0.

Some Suggested Readings

Celsus. *On Medicine, Volume I: Books 1-4.* Translated by Walter G. Spencer. Loeb Classical Library 292. Cambridge, MA: Harvard University Press, 1971.

Celsus. *On Medicine, Volume II: Books 5-6.* Translated by Walter G. Spencer. Loeb Classical Library 292. Cambridge, MA: Harvard University Press, 1961.

Langslow, David. "The Formation and Development of Latin Medical Vocabulary." PhD thesis, University of Oxford, 1991.

Nikita, Efthymia, Anna Lagia, and Sevi Triantaphyllou. "*Epidemiology and Pathology*." In *A Companion to Science, Technology, and Medicine in Ancient Greece and Rome*, Edited by Georgia L. Irby, 465–482. Hoboken: John Wiley & Sons, 2016.

Pagel, Walter. "Prognosis and Diagnosis: A Comparison of Ancient and Modern Medicine." *Journal of the Warburg Institute* 2, no. 4 (1939): 382–398.

Rosenthal, Thomas. "Aulus Cornelius Celsus – His Contributions to Dermatology." *Archives of Dermatology* 84, no. 4 (1961): 613–618.

Vocabulary

Greek or Latin word element	Current usage	Etymology	Examples
GNOS/O (nō-sō) GNOST/O (nos-tō) -GNOSIA (gnō-sē-ă) -GNOSIS (gnō-sĭs) -GNOMY (gnō-mē)	Knowledge, knowing; -GNOMY = a means of knowing	Gr. *gnosis*, knowledge Gr. *gnomon*, judge, a means of knowing	**Agnos**ia, pro**gnos**is, **agnost**ic, physio**gnomy**
ETI/O (ēt-ē-ō) *AETI/O (ēt-ē-ō)	Cause	Gr. *aitia*, cause	**Eti**ology, **eti**otropic
ESTHESI/O (ĕs-thē-zē-ō) -ESTHESIA (es-thē-zh(ē-)ă)	Sensation, feeling	Gr. *aesthesis*, feeling, sensation	**Esthesi**ology, an**esthesia**
MORB/O (mor-bō)	Disease	L. *morbus, -i*, m. disease	**Morb**ific, pre**morb**id
NOS/O (nō-sō) -NOSIS (*nō-sĭs*)	Disease	Gr. *nosos*, disease	**Nos**ology, hemato**nosis**
PATH/O (path-ō) -PATHY (pă-thē) -PATH (path)	Disease, feeling, suffering; -PATH = one affect by a disease, one who treats a disease	Gr. *pathos*, feeling, suffering, disease	**Path**ogen, sym**pathy**, osteo**path**
MORT/O (mor-tō)	Death	L. *mors, mortis*, f. death	**Mort**ality, pre**mort**al
THANAT/O (thă-nă-tō) -THANASIA (thă-nă-zē-ă)	Death	Gr. *thanatos*, death	**Thanat**omania, eu**thanasia**
NECR/O (nĕk-rō)	Dead body, dead	Gr. *nekros*, dead body; dead	**Necr**osis, **necr**opsy
FEBR/O (fē-brō)	Fever	L. *febris, -is*, f. fever	Post**febr**ile, a**febr**ile
PYR/O (pī-rō) PYRET/O (pī-rĕ-tō)	Fever, fire; PYRET- = fever	Gr. *pyr*, fever, fire, heat; Gr. *pyretos*, fire, fever	**Pyr**ogen, anti**pyret**ic

Greek or Latin word element	Current usage	Etymology	Examples
HEM/O (hē-mō) **HEMAT/O** (hĕm-ă-tō) **-EMIA** (ĕm-ē-ă) **-HEMIA** (hĕm-ē-ă)	Blood; -EMIA = condition of blood	Gr. *haima, haimatos,* blood	**Hem**olytic, **hemat**ology, isch**emia**
POLY- (pŏl-ē)	Many	Gr. *polys,* much, many	**Poly**pnea, **poly**uria
MULT/I (mŭl-tē)	Many	L. *multus, a, um,* many	**Multi**-infection, **mult**ifid
CAL/O (kă-lō) **CALOR/O** (kă-lo-rō)	Heat, calorie	L. *calor, -is,* m. heat; fr. *calere* to heat	**Cal**efacient, **calor**ic Loan word: **Calor** (kă′lor)
RUBR/O (roo-brō)	Red, redness	L. *ruber, rubra, rubrum,* red; *rubor, ruboris,* m. redness	**Rubr**ospinal, **rubr**othalamic Loan word: **Rubrum** (roo′brŭm) **Rubor** (roo′bor)
ERYTHR/O (ĕ-rĭth-rō)	Red, redness (red blood cells)	Gr. *erythros,* red	**Erythr**openia, **erythr**ocyte
TUM/O (tū-mō)	Swelling, tumor, abnormal mass	L. *tumor, tumoris,* m. swelling, mass	**Tum**efacient, **tum**escence Loan word: **Tumor** (too′mŏr)
ONC/O (ong-kō) **-ONCUS** (ong-kus)	Swelling, tumor, abnormal mass	Gr. *onkos,* mass, tumor	**Onc**ocyte, blephar**oncus**
EDEMAT/O (ĕ-dĕ-mă-tō) **-EDEMA** (ĕ-dĕ-mă)	Swelling	Gr. *oidema, oidematos,* swelling	**Edemat**ous, cephal**edema** Loan word: **Edema** (ĕ-dĕ′mă)
TROPH/O (trŏ-fō) **-TROPHY** (trŏ-fĕ)	Nourishment, growth	Gr. *trophe,* nourishment	**Troph**ectoderm, hyper**troph**y
TABET/O (tă-be-tō)	Wasting	L. *tabes, -is,* f. wasting away, decay	**Tabet**ic Loan word: **Tabes** (tă′bēz″)
***CEL/O** (sē-lō) **KEL/O** (kĕ-lō) **-CELE** (sēl)	Hernia, protrusion	Gr. *kele,* tumor, hernia	**Cel**osomia, **kel**oid, entero**cele**
CYT/O (sĭ-tō)	Cell	Gr. *kytos,* a hollow receptacle	**Cyt**ogenesis, **cyt**otoxin

Greek or Latin word element	Current usage	Etymology	Examples
CELL/O (se-lŏ) **CELLUL/O** (sĕl-ŭ-lŏ)	Cell	L. *cella, ae*, f. room, chamber L. *cellula, -ae*, f. little room, chamber	**Cell**ucidal Bi**cellul**ar Loan word: **Cellula** (sĕl'ŭ-lă) pl. **Cellulae** (sĕl'ŭ-lē)
CANCER/O (kan-ser-ŏ)	Cancer, crab	L. *cancer, cancri*, m. crab	Pre**cancer**ous, **cancer**ology Loan word: **Cancer** (kan'sĕr)
CARCIN/O (kar-sĭ-nŏ)	Cancer, crab	Gr. *karkinos*, crab, creeping ulcer; cancer	**Carcin**ogen, **carcin**omata
MAL/O (măl-ŏ) **MALIGN/O** (mă-lĭg-nŏ)	Bad, faulty; MALIGN- = Cancerous, becoming worse	L. *malus, -a, -um*, bad L. *malignus, -a, -um*, ill-disposed, wicked	**Mal**occlusion, **malign**ant
KAK/O (ka-kŏ) **CAC/O** (ka-kŏ)	Bad, faulty	Gr. *kakos*, bad	**Kak**idrosis, **cac**ogeusia
PHLOG/O (flŏ-gŏ)	Inflammation	Gr. *phlogosis*, inflammation Gr. *phlegmone*, inflammation Gr. *phlegmasia*, inflammation, heat	**Phlog**ogenic, anti**phlog**istic Loan words: **Phlegmon** (flĕg'mŏn) **Phlegmasia** (fleg-mā'zhă)
DOLOR/O (dŏ-lŏ-rŏ)	Pain	L. *dolor, doloris*, m. pain	**Dolor**imeter, **dolor**ific Loan word: **Dolor** (dŏ'lor) pl. **Dolores** (dŏ-lo'rēz")
NOC/O (nŏ-kŏ) **NOXI/O** (nŏk-shŏ)	Pain	L. *nocere*, to harm, hurt L. *noxius, -a, -um*, hurtful	**Noc**iceptive, **noxi**ous
ALG/O (al-gŏ) **-ALGIA** (al-j(ē-)ă) **-ALGESIA** (al-jē'zē-ă)	Pain; -ALGIA = Painful condition; -ALGESIA = Sense of pain	Gr. *algos*, pain;	**Alg**ophobia, arthr**algia**, hyper**algesia**
ODYN/O (ŏ-dĭn-ŏ) **-ODYNIA** (ŏ-dĭn-ē-ă)	Pain; -ODYNIA = Painful condition	Gr. *odyne*, pain	An**odyn**e, enter**odynia**
ACU/O (ă-kū-ŏ) **ACUT/O** (ă-kū-tŏ)	Needle, sharpness, pointed	L. *acus, -us*, f. needle, sharp L. *acutus, -a, -um*, sharp, pointed	**Acu**puncture, **acut**e Loan word: **Acute** (ă-kūt')

Greek or Latin word element	Current usage	Etymology	Examples
OXY/O (ŏk-sē-ō) -OXIA (ok-sē-ă)	Sharpness, quick, acid, oxygen; -OXIA = Oxygen condition	Gr. *oxys*, sharp, swift, sour, acid; oxygen	**Oxy**esthesia, an**oxia**
CHRON/O (kro-nō)	Time (prolonged)	Gr. *chronos*, time	**Chron**ic, **chron**ology
PUR/O (pŭ-rō) PURUL/O (pŭr-yŭ-lō)	Pus	L. *pus, puris,* n. pus L. *purulentia, -ae,* f. collection of pus	**Pur**ohepatitis, **purul**ent
PY/O (pī-ō)	Pus	Gr. *pyon*, pus	**Py**uria, nephro**py**osis
RHE/O (rē-ō) -RRHEA (rē-ă)	Flow; -RRHEA = A discharge (of a fluid)	Gr. *rheein*, to flow;	**Rhe**ology, pyo**rrhea**
-(R)RHEXIS (rek-sĭs)	A rupture	Gr. *rhexis*, burst, rupture	Myo**rrhexis**, amnio**rrhexis** Loan word: **Rhexis** (rĕk'sĭs)
-RRHAGIA (rā-jē-ă) -RRHAGE (răj)	Rupture with profuse discharge of a fluid (typically blood)	Gr. *rhegnynai*, to break, burst forth	Gastro**rrhagia**, hemo**rrhage**
RHAGAD/O (răg-ă-dō)	Tear, fissure, cleft	Gr. *rhagas, rhagados,* cleft, fissure	**Rhagad**iform, **rhagad**es
-PENIA (pē-nē-ă)	Decrease, deficiency	Gr. *penia*, poverty;	Cyto**penia**, osteo**penia**
MEGA- (mĕg-ă) MEGAL/O (meg-ă-lō) -MEGALY (meg-ă-lē)	Enlargement, large	Gr. *megas, megalou,* large	**Mega**dose, **megal**encephaly, cardio**megaly**
MICR/O (mī-krō)	Small	Gr. *mikros*, small	**Micr**obe, **micr**ocephalic
MACR/O (mak-rō)	Large, long	Gr. *makros*, long, large	**Macr**ocyte, **macr**oscopic
LYS/O (lī-sō) -LYSIS (lī-sĭs)	Breakdown, dissolving	Gr. *lysis,* a loosening, setting free	**Lys**ogen, anti**lysis** Loan word: **Lysis** (lī'sĭs) pl. **Lyses** (lī'sēz)
MALAC/O (mal-ă-kō) -MALACIA (mă-lā-shē-ă)	Soft, abnormal softening	Gr. *malakos*, soft	**Malac**osarcosis, myelo**malacia**

Greek or Latin word element	Current usage	Etymology	Examples
-PTOSIS (ptō-sĭs)	Downward displacement, prolapse	Gr. *ptosis*, a dropping, falling	Pseudo**ptosis**, nephro**ptosis**
			Loan word: **Ptosis** (tō′sĭs) pl. **Ptoses** (tō′sēz)
-ECTASIS (ek-tă-sĭs)	Dilation, expansion	Gr. *ektasis*, stretching out	Gast**rectasis**, angio**ectasia**
-ECTASIA (ek-tā-zhē-ă)			Loan word: **Ectasis** (ek′tă-sĭs) pl. **Ectases** (ek-tă′sēz)
SCHIZ/O (skĭ-zō)	A splitting, a cleft	Gr. *schizein*, to split, cleave	**Schiz**ocyte, rhachi**schisis**
-SCHISIS (skĭ-sĭs)			
STAS/O (stă-sō) **STAT/O** (stă-tō) **-STASIS** (stă-sĭs) **-STAT** (stăt)	A standing, stoppage, cause to stand; -STAT = A device for stopping, ceasing something	Gr. *stasis*, standing, stoppage	**Stas**iphobia, **stat**oacoustic, meta**stasis**, hemo**stat** Loan word: **Stasis** (stă′sĭs) pl. **Stases** (stă′sēz)
POIET/O (poy-ĕ-tō) **-POIESIS** (poy-ē-sĭs)	To make, produce	Gr. *poieein*, to make, produce	Angio**poiet**in, angio**poiesis**
PLAST/O (pla-stō) **-PLAST** (plast) **-PLASIA** (plă-zē-ă)	formed, molded; -PLAST = Forming cell or organelle; -PLASIA = Condition of formation, growth	Gr. *plastos*, formed, molded	**Plast**id, chloro**plast**, neo**plasia**
FAC/O (fak-ō) **FIC/O** (fĭk-ō) **FACT/O** (fak-tō) **FECT/O** (fek-tō)	To make, cause	L. *facere*, *factum*, to make, do	Rubi**fac**ient, calci**fic**ation, putre**fact**ion, af**fect**
GEN/O (jē′nō) **-GEN** (jĕn)	To become, be produced	Gr. *gignomai*, to come into being	Pyro**gen**, psycho**gen**ic

Greek or Latin word element	Current usage	Etymology	Examples
GRAPH/O (gra-fŏ) **-GRAPH** (graf) **-GRAPHY** (gră-fē)	Writing; -GRAPH = A device for an image or written record, or the record itself; -GRAPHY = Process of recording, writing	Gr. *graphein*, to write, inscribe	**Graph**eme, radio**graph**, angio**graphy**
GRAMMAT/O (gra-mă-tŏ) **-GRAM** (gram)	Something written or drawn; -GRAM = A record or image of something	Gr. *gramma, grammatos*, something written or drawn	Para**grammat**ism, angio**gram**
*METR/O (mĕ-trŏ) **-METER** (mĕt-ĕr) **-METRY** (mĕ-trē)	Measure, measurement; -METER = Measuring instrument; -METRY = The process of measuring something	Gr. *metron*, a measure	A**metr**opia Dolori**meter** Hystero**metry**

N.B.

CEL/O is a homograph see **CEL/O** (Gr. *koilos*, hollow, cavity) Hollow, cavity.
METR/O is a homograph see **METR/O** (Gr. *metra*, womb) Uterus.
ETI/O is commonly spelled **AETI/O** outside the United States.

Review	Answers
The study of the causes of diseases is termed _____ology.	**eti- or aeti**
Necrotic tissue is said to be _____ tissue.	**dead**
The process of measuring cells is termed cyto_____. An instrument for measuring angles of joints is called gonio_____. Hypometria is a decreased range of measurable movement. The root in hypometria means _____ or _____.	**metry** **meter** **measure, measurement**
The formation of blood vessels is termed angiopoiesis. The suffix meaning "make" or "produce" is _____. Similarly, synthetic erythropoietin is used for the _____ of red blood cells.	**-POIESIS** **production (making)**
Pathology is the study of the nature and cause of diseases. The combining form PATH/O can mean _____, _____, and _____.	**disease, suffering, feeling**
Nosology is the study of the description or classification of _____.	**disease (diseases)**
A high mortality rate is a high number of _____ in a population. A high morbidity in a population means there is a high number of _____ in a population.	**deaths** **diseases**
A patient is said to be afebrile if he or she does not have a _____.	**fever**
An antipyretic drug is used against _____.	**fevers**
A rupture with a profuse discharge of blood is called a hemo_____. A discharge of pus is called pyo_____. A rupture of an artery is called arterio_____.	**rrhage** **rrhea** **rrhexis**
Atrophy is the decreased size of tissue or organ. Hypertrophy is the increased size of a tissue or organ. The root that they share is TROPH-, which means _____.	**nourishment**

Review	Answers
Cachexia is a loan word that is used as "a state of ill health, malnutrition, loss of weight, and wasting of muscle." "Cachexia," "kakidrosis," and "cacogeusia" are derived from the Greek word *kakos*, which means _____.	**bad**
Ectasis is a loan word that means _____ or _____. Its root commonly shows up in the compound suffix _____.	**dilation, expansion -ECTASIA**
A prolapse or downward displacement of spleen would be a spleno_____.	**ptosis**
A phlogogenic substance creates an _____. Likewise, an acute pyrogenic inflammation of subcutaneous connective tissue is called a phlegmon. And a painful white inflammation due to a deep venous thrombosis is called phlegmasia alba dolens.	**inflammation**
A hernia of an organ is a splanchno_____.	**cele**
The combining forms used for "cell" are _____, _____, and _____. The loan word cellula is used for "a minute cell' or "a small compartment."	**CELL/O, CELLUL/O CYT/O**
Softening of a vessel is termed angio_____. Malacotic tissue is _____ tissue.	**malacia soft**
Lysis is the gradual decline of a fever or disease; it is the opposite of crisis. Lysin is a substance that dissolves or destroys a substance, particularly cells. Lysol is a disinfectant. The common root in these words is LYS-, which means _____ and _____.	**breakdown, dissolving**
Enlargement of an organ is called splanchno_____.	**megaly**
The Latin word element for "many" is _____ and the Greek word element for "many" is _____. These Greek and Latin adjectives are treated as prefixes in compound medical terms.	**MULTI-, POLY-**
The four cardinal signs of inflammation are "tumor," "rubor," "dolor," and "calor," which mean _____, _____, _____, and _____.	**swelling, redness, pain, heat**
The Greek combining form for "small" is _____. The Greek combining form MACR/O can mean _____ and _____.	**MICR/O large, long**
The combining form for "heat" is _____.	**CAL/O**
The combing forms for "redness" are _____ and _____. The term for "reddening of the skin" is erythema.	**RUBR/O, ERYTHR/O**
The combining forms for pain are _____, _____, _____, _____, and _____.	**ALG/O, ODYN/O, NOC/O, NOXI/O DOL/O**
The combining forms for swelling are _____, _____, and _____. A tumor can refer to a swelling as well as a mass. The common suffix used for tumor is -OMA.	**TUM/O, ONC/O, EDEMAT/O**
A neoplasia is the formation of new tissue or tumors. The compound suffix meaning a condition of formation or growth is _____. Plastic surgery repairs or restores missing structures through the transfer of tissue or the use of synthetic materials. The root in "plastic" means _____ and _____. An osteoplast (more commonly known as a osteoblast) is a term used for a bone-_____ cell.	**-PLASIA formed, molded forming**
A cancerous tumor that arises from the epithelial cells is called a _____oma. Both a malignant neoplasia and the sign of the Zodiac that looks like a crab are called _____.	**carcin cancer**
A decrease or deficiency of glucose in the blood is termed glyco_____.	**penia**
The roots FIC-, FAC-, FACT-, and FECT- are all derived from a Latin verb that means to _____ or _____.	**make, cause**
Tabes is a loan word used for _____ due to a chronic disease. The combining form for tabes is _____.	**wasting TABET/O**
The movement of bacteria or cancer cells from one part to another is called "metastasis." The adjective for this is "metastatic." The suffix and root in these words are derived from a Greek word meaning _____ and _____. Likewise, a device that stops blood from flowing is a hemo_____.	**standing, stoppage stat**
An instrument for recording vessels is called an angio_____. An image of a vessel is called an angio_____.	**graph gram**
The combining forms _____ and _____ can refer to something that has a "cleft" in it.	**SCHIZ/O, RHAGAD/O**
Pyorrhea would be a discharge of _____. The other combining form meaning for "pus" is _____.	**pus, PUR/O**

Review	Answers
A chronic disease is a progressive, long-lasting disease. The root in chronic means _____. An acute disease is a rapid onset, severe, and short-coursed disease. The root in acute means _____ and _____.	**time** **sharp, pointed**
The suffix -ONCUS, as in blepharoncus, means _____. The suffix -EDEMA, as in lymphedema, means _____.	**tumor** **swelling**
A benign disease is defined as a nonreoccurring and nonprogressive disease. A malignant disease is defined as a cancerous or extremely harmful disease. The words malignant, malocclusion, and malformation share the root MAL-, which means _____ or _____.	**bad, faulty**
An exacerbation or sudden recurrent attack of a disease is referred to as a _____. The derivative paroxysm shares a root with terms such as oxylalia, oxycephalous, and oxytocic. The root OXY- can mean _____, _____, _____, and _____. When -OXIA is used as a suffix, it typically refers to an _____ condition.	**paroxysm** **sharp, quick, acid, oxygen** **oxygen**
Thanatology is the study of _____. In Greek mythology, the god of death was called Thanatos. His brother, Hypnos, was the god of sleep. Today we use the term eu_____ for the deliberate ending of a life due to an incurable illness or unbearable suffering. Originally, it meant an "easy or happy death." Around the mid-nineteenth century it took on its current meaning.	**death** **thanasia**
Placebo effect is the phenomenon in which some people experience a benefit after the administration of an inactive substance or treatment. Placebo comes from the Latin verb meaning "I will please." Nocebo effect is the opposite phenomenon; it is when you are given an inactive substance, and being told that it produces negative effects, you experience these symptoms. Nocebo means "I will _____."	**harm (cause pain)**
The suffix -GEN means to _____ and to be _____. It will often be made into an adjective by adding -IC or -OUS to it (e.g. iatrogenic and enterogenous).	**become, produced**
A paresthesia is an abnormal or painful sensation that is often a result of damage to a nerve or nerves. The prefix in this word PARA- means abnormal, and the suffix _____ means sensation. An esthesiometer is a devise used for tactile _____.	**-ESTHESIA** **sensation**
The Greek combining forms commonly used for "blood" are _____ and _____. The suffixes _____ and _____ are commonly used for pathological conditions associated with blood.	**HEM/O, HEMAT/O** **-EMIA, -HEMIA**

Lessons from History: Celsus and Ancient Greek Surgery

Food for Thought as You Read:

How is Celsus' understanding of surgery different from our own? How is it similar?

> The third part of medicine, which cures by the hand, is commonly recognized and has been put forth by me. It does not lay aside the use of medicaments and method of regimen, but performs most by hand, and its effect is the most visible among all the parts of medicine.
>
> Celsus, *De medicina*, Proemium VII.1, Loeb pp. 294–295.

In Books VII and VIII of *De medicina*, Celsus, provides a detailed account of ancient surgeries. In his prefatory remarks to Book VII, he claims that surgery was practiced more by Hippocrates than all his predecessors. Over time, it began to have its own *professores* (L. *professor*, an expert, a public teacher). Alexandria, Egypt, was an important center for the teaching of surgery. Celsus notes how "in Egypt surgery grew greatly by the author Philoxenus, who very accurately put together this part of medicine from many volumes of writings. Gorgias and also Sostratus and Heron and the two Apollonii and Ammonius, the Alexandrians, and many other famous men, each found out something." He then describes the characteristics of an ideal surgeon: he should be a steady-handed, ambidextrous young man with good vision. He also claims that a surgeon should have pity, so that he wishes to cure his patient, but he should not be overly moved by his patient's cries that he cuts too fast. This statement, as well as the numerous descriptions of how the surgical attendants were used to restrain the patient from moving, point to the fact that ancient Greek surgeries were performed without the benefit of anesthesia.

Based on Celsus' descriptions of ancient Greek surgeries, we can recognize that ancient Greek surgery encompassed performing surgical reconstructions, incisions, excisions of body parts, surgical punctures for aspiration, creating an orifice in the body, suturing wounds, and surgical fixations/suspension of body parts. Thus, the scope of their surgeries covers the corresponding surgical suffixes used today: -**PLASTY, -TOMY, -ECTOMY, -CENTESIS, -STOMY, -RRHAPHY, -PEXY**. Ancient Greek surgeons practiced some forms of eye surgeries (couching cataracts) and cosmetic surgeries (e.g. restoration of foreskin). However, when compared to modern surgical procedures, ancient Greek surgeries could be quite dangerous in terms of infections, and the lack of anesthesia limited how invasive the procedures could be. For example, a modern lithotomy (Gr. *lithos*, stone + *tome*, cut), a surgical incision to remove a stone from the urinary tract, is a somewhat routine surgery with a very good success rate, thanks to antiseptic technique and the ability to anesthetize a patient. However, in ancient Greek medicine, this surgery was quite dangerous due to postsurgical infections and because it was performed without any painkillers.

Some surgeries which we might consider quite dangerous were commonly and "successfully" performed. The act of drilling into cranium is called trepanation or trephination (Fig. 4.10). Skeletal records reveal that this practice was widespread and predated ancient Greek medicine. The long cylindrical surgical device used in this surgery is called a trephine or a trepan (Gr. *trypanon*, a borer, auger). Celsus' description of trepanation reveals that it was used to excise black or decaying bone from the cranium. He describes two sizes of trepans, which he calls in Latin *terebrae* (borers). The larger of the two trepans was used for large areas of bone decay. In his description of trepanation of the cranium, Celsus describes how surgeons used bone dust to determine the depth of the cut, and they protected the dura mater of the brain from damage by using a bronze plate called a *meningophylax* (guardian of the membrane). The edges of the bone are then filed smooth, and, next, medicaments are placed in the exposed part and covered with wool dressing soaked in oil and vinegar. As Celsus correctly notes, the flesh will eventually fill the hole. Making burr holes in the cranium is still practiced today, albeit for different reasons. It can be used to treat pooling of blood under the dura mater of the brain, called a subdural hematoma. However, if a modern surgeon makes a hole in a skull, he or she will typically replace the bone and patch it up.

In addition to the trepan, ancient Greek physicians made use of a wide variety of tools that modern surgeons would recognize: *katheter* (catheter), *psalis* (surgical scissor), *agkistran* (hook), *kauterion* (cautery iron), *mochliskos* (lever) *spathumele* (spatula probe), *cyathiscomele* (probe), and different types of *macharia* (scalpels). Much like modern physicians, Greek physicians also made use of devices for looking into the body such as the *hedrodiastoleus* (Fig. 4.11), which is a type of anal speculum used for looking for anal fistulae, and the vaginal *dioptra*, which was a speculum used in ancient gynecology. In modern medical terminology, the suffix used for a

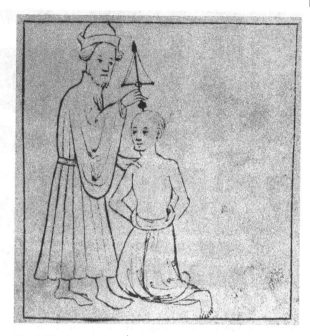

Fig. 4.10 Image of 13th century trepanation. *Source:* Wellcome Collection/CC BY 4.0.

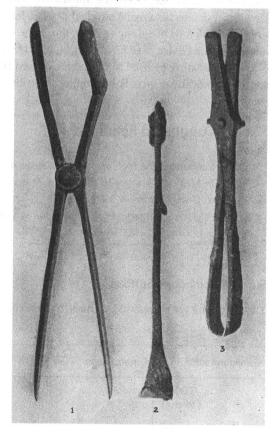

Fig. 4.11 1. *Hedrodiastoleus* (rectal speculum), 2. *lithoulkos* (stone scoop), 3. *litholobos* (stone forceps), Plate XLVI in John S. Milne. Surgical Instruments in Greek and Roman Times. Oxford, England: Clarendon Press, 1907. *Source:* Wellcome Collection/Wikimedia Commons/CC BY 4.0.

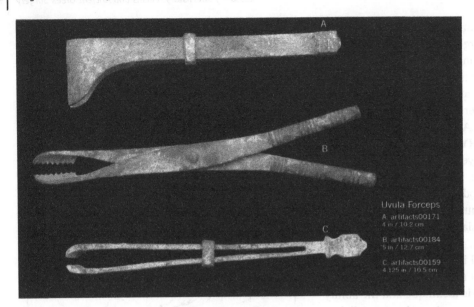

Fig. 4.12 *Staphylagra* (uvula forceps) from a collection of surgical instruments found at Pompey after the eruption of Mount Vesuvius (79 AD). *Source:* Courtesy of Claude Moore Health Sciences Library, University of Virginia.

devise for looking into a specific body part is -**SCOPE**, which is derived from the Greek word *skopeein*, "to look at." Likewise, there are devices whose names reveal they were for specific surgeries. For example, the devices called the *litholobos* (stone forceps) and the *lithoulkos* (stone scoop) reveal that they were designed to be used in a lithotomy. Ancient Greek physicians also made surgical devices for specific body parts. A *staphylagra* (*staphyle*, uvula + *agra*, a catching, hunting) was a device designed to remove the uvula (Fig. 4.12). An *osteotome* (*osteon*, bone + *tome*, a cutting) was an ancient Greek device used for cutting bones to help with reducing fractures. We still use the term "osteotome" for an array of chisel-like devices used to cut bones. Today, the surgical suffix -**TOME** is added to a combining form to denote the specific use of the device. For example, an atriotome is a device used for cutting into the atria of the heart.

Some Suggested Readings

Bliquez, Lawrence. *The Tools of Asclepius: Surgical Instruments in Greek and Roman Times.* Leiden: Brill, 2014.

Celsus. *On Medicine, Volume III: Books 7-8.* Translated by Walter G. Spencer. Loeb Classical Library 336. Cambridge, MA: Harvard University Press, 1979.

Le Blay, Frédéric. "Surgery." In *A Companion to Science, Technology, and Medicine in Ancient Greece and Rome*, Edited by Georgia L. Irby, 371–385. Hoboken: John Wiley & Sons, 2016.

Surgical Compound Suffixes

The following are compound suffixes that are commonly used to describe surgeries.

Compound suffix	Current usage	Etymology	Examples
-**TOMY** (tŏ-mē)	Incision	Gr. *tome*, a cutting; Gr. *ek* out + *tome*, a cutting	Cardio**tomy**, gastr**ectomy**, procto**tome**
-**ECTOMY** (ek-tŏ-mē)	Excision		
-**TOME** (tōm)	Device for making an incision		
-**STOMY** (stŏ-mē)	Surgical creation of an opening (stoma)	Gr. *stoma, stomatos*, mouth, opening	Colo**stomy**, venoveno**stomy**

Compound suffix	Current usage	Etymology	Examples
-PLASTY (plas-tē)	Surgical reconstruction	Gr. *plastos*, formed, molded	Rhino**plasty**, cheilo**plasty**
-RRHAPHY (ră-fē)	Surgical suturing	Gr. *rhaptein*, to sew, stitch	Arterio**rrhaphy**, myo**rrhaphy**
-PEXY (pĕk-sē)	Surgical fixation	Gr. *pexis*, a fixing together of something	Organo**pexy**, nephro**pexy**
-TRIPSY (trip-sē)	Crushing	Gr. *tripsis*, a rubbing, friction	Neuro**tripsy**, litho**tripsy**
-SCOPY (skŏ-pē) **-SCOPE** (skōp)	Examination, esp. with a device; -SCOPE = A device for looking into a body part	Gr. *skopeein*, to look at, view	Cranio**scopy**, naso**scope**
-DESIS (dē-sĭs)	Surgical binding, fusion	Gr. *deein*, to bind	Syn**desis**, arthro**desis** Loan word: **Desis** (dē′sĭs)
-CENTESIS (sen-tē-sĭs)	Surgical puncture for aspiration	Gr. *kenteein*, to goad, prick	Abdomino**centesis**, thoraco**centesis** Loan word: **Centesis** (sen-tē′sĭs) pl. **Centeses** (sen-tē′sēz)
-SECTION (sek-shŏn)	A cutting	L. *secare, sectum*, to cut	Re**section**, pro**section**
-CLASTY (klas-tē)	A surgical breaking	Gr. *klastos, broken*	Litho**clasty**
-TRYPESIS (trĭ-pē-sĭs)	A surgical boring	Gr. *trype*, a piercing, a hole	Sterno**trypesis**, cranio**trypesis**

Review	Answers
A device for cutting into a joint is termed an arthro _____.	**tome**
An excision of part of a joint is termed an arthr _____.	**ectomy**
A surgical reconstruction of a joint is called an arthro _____.	**plasty**
A surgical crushing or breaking down of a stone in the body is a litho _____.	**tripsy**
A suturing of joint is termed an arthro _____.	**rrhaphy**
A fusion or binding of a joint is an arthro _____.	**desis**
The visual examination of a joint with a surgical device is an arthro_____.	**scopy**
The making of a surgical opening in a joint is an arthro _____.	**stomy**
An incision into a joint is an arthro _____.	**tomy**
A device for looking inside a joint is an arthro _____.	**scope**
A surgical puncture for aspiration of a joint is an arthro _____.	**centesis**
A cutting of anatomical structure into two parts is called bi _____.	**section**
A surgical fixation of an organ is an organo _____.	**pexy**
A surgical boring or perforation of the skull is a cranio_____.	**trypesis**

Surgical Word Elements

The word elements that form the aforementioned surgical compound suffixes are important to recognize because they are present in medical and scientific terms.

Greek or Latin word element	Current usage	Etymology	Examples
TOM/O (tŏ-mō)	Cut, a section	Gr. *tomos*, cutting	**Tom**ography, hylo**tomous**
STOM/O (stō-mō) **STOMAT/O** (stō-mă-tō)	A mouth, an opening	Gr. *stoma*, *stomatos*, a mouth; opening	Xero**stom**ia, **stomat**odynia Loan word: **Stoma** (stō′mă) pl. **stomata** (stō′măt-ă)
PEX/O (pĕ-ksō) **-PEXIS** (pĕk-sĭs)	Fixation, binding	Gr. *pexis*, a fixation, binding	Colo**pex**ostomy, hemato**pexis** Loan word: **Pexis** (pek′sĭs) pl. **pexes** (pek′sēz)
RHAPH/O (rā-fō) **R(H)APHID/O** (rā-fĭ-dō)	Seam, suture; R(H)APHID/O = Needle, needle-like	Gr. *raphe*, a suture, seam Gr. *rhaphis*, *rhaphidos*, needle	**Raphid**es Loan word: **Rhaphe** (or **raphe**) (rā′fē) pl. **rhaphes** (rā′fēz)
CLAST/O (klăs-tō) **-CLAST** (klăst) **-CLASIS** (klă-sĭs) **-CLASIA** (klă-zē-ă)	Broken, breaking; -CLAST = A breaker of things; -CLASIS and -CLASIA = A breaking of something	Gr. *klastos*, broken	Glyco**clast**ic, osteo**clast**, auto**clasis**
SCOP/O (skō-pō)	To view	Gr. *skopeein*, to look at, view	**Scop**ophilia, micro**scop**ic
SECT/O (sĕk-tō) **SEC/O** (sē-kō)	Cut, a section	L. *secare*, *sectum*, to cut	Bi**sect**ion, **sec**odont
CIS/O (sī-sō) **-CIDE** (sĭd)	Kill, cut	L. *caedere*, *caesum*, to cut, kill	In**cis**ion, vermi**cide**
TRIPT/O (trip-tō)	crushing, grinding	Gr. *tripsis*, a rubbing, friction, massage	Litho**tript**er Loan word: **Tripsis** (trip′sĭs) pl. **Tripses** (trip′sēz)
TREPAN/O (trĕ-păn-ō) **TREPHIN/O** (trĕ-fĭ-nō) **TRYPAN/O** (trĭ-pă-nō)	Borer, drilling; TRYPAN- = Borer; a genus of parasitic protozoa called trypanosomes	L. *trepanum*, *-i*, fr Gr. *trypanon*, a borer	**Trepan**ation, **trephin**e **trypan**ocide

Review	Answers
CT stands for computed tomography, which is a computerized x-ray scanning system that creates a sectional anatomic image. The combining form in "tomography" means _____ or _____.	**cut, section**
The genus of parasitic protozoa is called the Trepanosoma. The name is derived from the Greek *trypanon*, which means _____ and *soma*, which means _____.	**borer, body**
Inflammation of the mouth is called _____itis. A stoma literally means an _____ or a _____. "Stoma" is also a term used for a surgically created opening or passageway.	**stomat** **opening, mouth**
A cell that breaks down bone is termed an osteo_____. The breaking down of bone is termed osteo_____ or osteo_____.	**clast** **clasis, clasia**
Something that is sectile is capable of being _____.	**cut**
An anatomical rhaphe is a structure that looks like a _____ or _____. However, the combining form RHAPHID/O means _____ or _____.	**suture, seam** **needle, needle-like**
Scopophobia is an abnormal fear of being _____.	**viewed (seen)**
A colopexostomy is the creation of a colostomy by connecting the colon to the abdominal wall. The combining form PEX/O in this term means _____ or _____.	**fixation, binding**
Tripsis is a loan word that means _____ or _____.	**crushing, rubbing**
Incision literally means the _____ into something. The word suicide is formed from the Latin reflexive possessive *suus, -a, -um*, which means "his, her, its," and the suffix -cide, which means to _____.	**cutting** **kill**

Lessons from History: Hippocratic Epidemics and Progress Notes

Food for Thought as You Read:

How are the case studies in the Hippocratic Epidemics similar to modern progress notes? How are they different?

Our earliest example of a Greek physician recording the progression of a patient's disease can be found in the 5th and 4th century BC texts known as the Hippocratic *Epidemics I–VII*. The seven books of the *Epidemics* are not collective work of a single author. Scholars see them as three groups of treatises with different authors. The authors appear to be itinerant Greek physicians who are moving through foreign lands, such as Thasos. The title is slightly misleading in that these works do not pertain to the modern connotation of epidemics. It is possible that the Greek title of these works (*epidemiai*) speaks to the rise of diseases in communities due to changes in weather and seasons. These accounts of the types of diseases that befall a people are commonly referred to as "constitutions" by modern scholars on account of the abrupt changes in the weather causing changes in the constitutions of people in the area. However, these works also include chronological accounts of the signs and symptoms of individual patients. The accounts of individuals are referred to as "case studies" by modern scholars. The following is one example of the detailed observation of a patient captured in very succinct language. The following account of a patient named Philiscus is identified as Case I in Book I of the *Epidemics*:

Philiscus lived by the wall; he took to his bed.

First day. Acute fever and sweating; night uncomfortable.

Second day. General exacerbation; later a small clyster moved the bowels well. Restful night.

Third day. Early and until midday he appeared to be without fever; but toward evening acute fever with sweating; thirst; dry tongue; he passed dark urine; uncomfortable night, without sleep; completely out of his mind.

Fourth day. All symptoms exacerbated; urines dark; more comfortable night; urines of a better color.

Fifth day. About midday slight epistaxis of unmixed blood; urines varied, with scattered, round particles suspended in them, resembling semen; they did not settle. On the application of a suppository the patient passed, with flatulence, a little excreta. A distressing night, spells of sleep, talking; wandering of the mind; extremities everywhere cold, and difficult to warm back up; he passed dark urine; spells of sleep toward dawn; speechless; cold sweat; extremities livid.

Sixth day, around noon the patient died.

The breathing throughout was as though the patient was recollecting to do it: rare and large. Spleen raised in a round swelling; cold sweats all the time. The exacerbations on even days.

Hippocrates. *Epidemics I* translated by Paul Potter. Loeb Classical Library 147:192–195.

From this case history, one can observe the level of detailed observations that an ancient Greek physician would record when treating a patient, and one can also observe by the recording of days that the physician recognized that the chronology is imperative when recording signs and symptoms. While this recording of a patient's signs and symptoms is reminiscent of modern progress notes and case studies, the above account of Philiscus' disease, as well as the other cases in the *Epidemics*, differs in a number of important ways from modern medical records. Aside from the obvious lack of patient confidentiality, the most striking element in these histories is the number of patients who are recorded as having died. Thus, the emphasis of these accounts is not to demonstrate successful outcomes. While treatment of the patient is mentioned ("small clyster moved the bowels well"), the focus of this case, as well as the majority of cases in the *Epidemics*, is not on the patient's response to the treatment. Instead, the recording of the days in which there were dramatic changes in signs and symptoms appears to be what these ancient physicians are trying to record (e.g. "the exacerbations on even days"). Another interesting feature of these case studies is that the authors often do not provide a name of the disease the patient is suffering from. This raises the question: how was this information of any use to an ancient physician? It seems that these case histories reveal a belief that diseases, named or not named, can be recognized by the chronicity of the signs and symptoms. Therefore, if physicians were to recognize the pattern of critical days of a disease, they would be better able to anticipate changes in the patient's condition and recognize the window of opportunity for treatment.

Today, a progress note is a very common medical record that is used by healthcare professionals to document a patient's health and response to treatment during the course of care. Unlike the case studies in the *Epidemics*, diagnosis and treatment of the patient is imperative to these medical records. While the date of the note is important, providing a chronological account of the patient's signs and symptoms is not the formatting structure of these notes.

Some Suggested Readings

Galen. *Commentary on Hippocrates' Epidemics Book I, Parts I-III*. Translated by Uwelator Vagelpohl. Berlin: De Gruyter Akademie Forschung, 2014.

Hippocrates. *Ancient Medicine. Airs, Waters, Places. Epidemics 1 and 3. The Oath. Precepts. Nutriment*. Edited and translated by Paul Potter. Loeb Classical Library 147. Cambridge, MA: Harvard University Press, 2022.

Langholf, Volker. *Medical Theories in Hippocrates: Early Texts and the 'Epidemics'*. Berlin, Boston: De Gruyter, 1992.

SOAP Notes

Progress notes are typically written in a SOAP format. SOAP is an acronym for the parts this type of progress note:

S-subjective	**Patient's experiences, personal views, or feelings.**
O-objective	**Observable signs and the results of tests that the clinician has performed.**
A-assessment	**Evaluation of the patient's signs/symptoms and progress**
P-plan	**Determination of how to proceed or alter the plan of care**

Some common abbreviations in these notes are as follows:

pt – **Patient**
CC – **Chief complaint**
y.o. – **Year old**
c/o – **Complains of**
WDWN – **Well-developed and well-nourished**
CP – **Chest pain**

WNL – Within normal limits

Hx – history

s/p – status post

Sx – symptoms

R/O – Rule out *meaning that this needs to be determined

D/C – Discharge, discontinue

SOB – Shortness of breath

RRR – Regular rate and rhythm

T – Temperature

UE – Upper extremity

LE – Lower extremity

R – Respiration

BP – Blood pressure

P – Pulse

ETOH – Alcohol

NKDA – No known drug allergies

RTC – Return to the clinic

RTO – Return to the office

Read the following progress note and answer the questions:

CC: 25 y.o. WDWN female, s/p arthrocentesis of right knee, who c/o swelling and pain in bilateral LE.

S: Denies Hx of LE trauma, carcinoma, SOB, or dorsalgia. Pt acknowledges regular consumption of ETOH. She is currently not taking any medications, and she has NKDA.

O: Pt is afebrile, T 98.6, BP 130/80, P 60, R 15, lungs are clear, heart RRR, LE strength WNL without any notable atrophy. No apparent organomegaly or hematomata with palpation, strong pedal pulses; moderate pitting crural edema noted in bilateral LE.

A: Idiopathic pitting edema, R/O acute kidney failure and angiopathy

P: Referral for urinalysis, lower extremity angiography; DC ETOH, RTC next week.

Review	Answers
True or False, based on the chief complaint, the patient has pain and swelling in both lower extremities.	**True (bilateral LE)**
True or False, based on the chief complaint, the patient recently had a surgical aspiration of her right knee.	**True (arthrocentesis of right knee)**
True or False, based on the subjective, the patient has a history of back pain and cancer.	**True (dorsalgia, carcinoma)**
True or False, based on the subjective, the patient is allergic to certain medications.	**False (NKDA)**
True or False, based on the objective, the patient regularly drinks alcohol.	**True (ETOH)**
True or False, based on the objective, the physician observed swelling in both of the patient's lower legs.	**True (crural/bilateral)**
True or False, based on the objective, the physician took the pulse at the patient's feet.	**True (pedal)**
True or False, based on the objective, the physician did not feel (palpation) any enlargements of the organs or a tumor of blood.	**True (no organopathy and hematomata)**
True or False, based on the assessment, the physician does not know the etiology of the patient's edema, and the physician wants to rule out a disease of the blood vessels and kidney failure.	**True (idiopathic pitting edema, R/O...)**
True or False, based on the plan, the physician wants to run diagnostic imaging of the blood vessels, and the physician has asked the patient to stop drinking alcohol.	**True (angiography, DC ETOH)**

5

Chemical and Pharmacological Terminology

CHAPTER LEARNING OBJECTIVES

1) In this chapter, we will look at the letters, numbers, signs, abbreviations, and word elements that are commonly used in chemistry and pharmaceutical terms.
2) You will also learn the history of the Greek alphabet and Roman numbers, the elements in ancient Greek science, the origins of chemistry and chemical terms, and ancient Greek drugs.

Lessons from History: The Greek Alphabet and Modern Scientific Notation

Food for Thought as You Read:

What does isopsephy reveal about the relationship between letters and numbers?

Ancient Greeks used the letters of their alphabet as symbols for numbers. Each Greek letter was assigned a specific number value. This numerical system required the use of 27 letters, which is three more letters than the 24 found in the classical Greek alphabet. To account for this, the Greeks used three archaic letters for the missing numbers of 6, 90, and 900. An example of how this numbering system works can be seen in the following table:

Arabic number	1	2	3	4	5	6	7	8	9
Greek number	α	β	γ	δ	ε	Ϝ	ζ	η	θ
Greek name	Alpha	Beta	Gamma	Delta	Epsilon	Digamma	Zeta	Eta	Theta
Arabic number	10	20	30	40	50	60	70	80	90
Greek number	ι	κ	λ	μ	ν	ξ	ο	π	ϙ
Greek name	Iota	Kappa	Lambda	Mu	Nu	Xi	Omicron	Pi	Koppa
Arabic number	100	200	300	400	500	600	700	800	900
Greek number	ρ	σ	τ	υ	φ	χ	ψ	ω	ϡ
Greek name	Rho	Sigma	Tau	Upsilon	Phi	Chi	Psi	Omega	Sampi

Using letters as numbers led to the practice of **isopsephy** (Gr. *isos* = equal and *psephos* = pebble). The etymology of isopsephy indicates that it comes from the ancient Greek practice of arranging pebbles into patterns to learn arithmetic and geometry. However, the term is also used for the ancient practice of adding up the numerical value of letters in a word or words to form a single number. For example, in the *Lives of the Twelve Caesars*, the Roman historian Suetonius (AD 69–122) relates how the Roman Emperor Nero's nefarious deed of killing his own mother was linked to the numerical value of Nero's

Greek and Latin Roots of Medical and Scientific Terminologies, First Edition. Todd A. Curtis.
© 2025 John Wiley & Sons, Inc. Published 2025 by John Wiley & Sons, Inc.
Companion website: www.wiley.com/go/Curtis

name in Greek (Fig. 5.1). Suetonius cites a slogan going around Rome, which states, "count the numerical values of the letters in Nero's name, and in 'murdered his own mother' and you will find their sum is the same." The numerical value of the Greek letters in Nero's name comes to 1005 (Νερων = 50 + 5 + 100 + 800 + 50). Likewise, the Greek phrase "murdered his own mother" (ιδιαν μητερα απεκτεινε = [10 + 4 + 10 + 1 + 50] + [40 + 8 + 300 + 5 + 100 + 1] + [1 + 80 + 5 + 20 + 300 + 5 + 10 + 50 + 5]) comes to 1005.

The most famous example of isopsephy in the modern world is the so-called "Number of the Beast" found in the book of *Revelation* (also known as the *Apocalypse of John*) in the Bible. When writing about an anti-Christ figure known as the Beast, the author of *Revelation* informed his audience that with "wisdom" and "insight" they would be able to "calculate the number of the beast, for it is man's number. His number is 666" (*Revelation* 13 : 18). Thanks to its association with the Beast, the number 666 appears in a number of modern horror films that evoke modern conceptions of the Devil (also known as Satan and Lucifer). There is still no scholarly consensus as to the identity of the name associated with this number. At the beginning of the 20th century, it was pointed out that the Greek spelling of "Nero Caesar," when transliterated into Hebrew and then calculated via numbers associated with Hebrew letters, equals 666. Interestingly, in some ancient manuscripts of *Revelation*, the number is written 616, rather than 666. This variant 616 seems to add credence to the belief that Nero was the intended name because the Hebrew transliteration of the Latin spelling of "Nero Caesar" totals 616. Of the Roman Emperors in the 1st-century AD, Nero is the only Emperor's name that can account for both 666 and 616, which is perhaps the most compelling argument that Nero was the intended referent (Fig. 5.2). Furthermore, for these numbers to have any significance for a reader of the late 1st-century AD, which is the traditional period of the composition of Revelation, it would seem likely that these numbers should refer to a contemporary historical figure, particularly one who persecuted Christians, something for which Nero is quite infamous. However, some scholars have argued that since Greek is the language of the New Testament, it stands to reason that this would be the numerical letters that would have been intended for the Number of the Beast, and consequently, the various Greek numerical values for Nero's name and title would not add up to 616 or 666. In his *contr. Haer.* (5.29–30), Irenaeus (c. AD 130–202), the first Christian author to address the number of the Beast in *Revelation*, claims that 666 is the actual number of the Beast. Irenaeus does not even consider Nero as a potential candidate for this number, and instead, he lists a number of Greek names that potentially could fit this numerical number. Irenaeus uses this list of potential names to illustrate that it is impossible to know for certain whom the number refers to since the name has not been revealed by God to mankind.

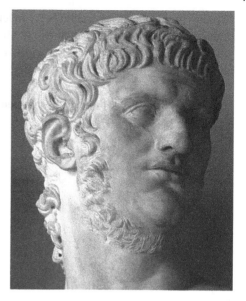

Fig. 5.1 Bust of Nero, c. 1st-century AD, Capitoline Museum. *Source:* Unknown Source/ Wikimedia Commons/CC BY-SA 3.0.

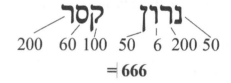

Nero Caesar (Latin)

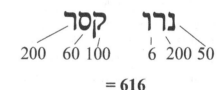

Fig. 5.2 The Latin and Greek spellings of the Nero's name and their respective calculations. *Source:* Courtesy of Tim Hegg, Torah Resource, https://torahresource.com/ number-666-revelation-1318/last accessed 19 January 2024.

Some Suggested Readings

Ast, Rodney, and Julia Lougovaya. "*The Art of Isopsephism in the Greco-Roman World.*" In *Ägytische Magie und ihre Umwelt.* Edited by Andrea Jördens, 82–98. Wiesbaden: Harrassowitz, 2015.

Cole, Zachary. *Numerals in Early Greek New Testament Manuscripts: Text-Critical, Scribal, and Theological Studies.* Leiden: Brill, 2017.

Today, the classical Greek alphabet is widely used to denote various constants and values within the fields of mathematics, science, engineering, and medicine (e.g. δ indicates declination in astronomy and σ is used in mechanics for stress). These letters commonly appear in the names of various medications, and therefore, it is useful to memorize the following Greek letters and their names.

Name of letter	Upper and lower cases	Name of letter	Upper and lower cases
Alpha	A α	Nu	N ν
Beta	B β	Xi	Ξ ξ
Gamma	Γ γ	Omicron	O o
Delta	Δ δ	Pi	Π π
Epsilon	E ε	*Rho	P ρ
Zeta	Z ζ	Sigma	Σ σ or ς
Eta	H η	Tau	T τ
Theta	Θ θ	Upsilon	Y υ
Iota	I ι	Phi	Φ φ
Kappa	K κ	Chi	X χ
Lambda	Λ λ	Psi	Ψ ψ
Mu	M μ	Omega	Ω ω

Using the above table of classical Greek letters and their English equivalents, answer the following:

Review	Answers
The SI unit of measure of electric resistance, Ω = ohm, is designated by the Greek letter which is called an _____. Likewise, ω-3 fatty acid is called _____-3 fatty acid.	**Omega** **Omega**
The sign for curvature is κ, which is the Greek letter _____.	**Kappa**
The coefficient of friction in physics, μ, is designated by the lowercase Greek letter which is called a _____.	**Mu**
β-reduction in lambda calculus = _____-reduction in lambda calculus.	**Beta**
θ (lowercase) represents a plane angle in geometry. The name of this Greek letter is _____.	**Theta**
Λ (capital) represents the cosmological constant. The name of this Greek letter is _____.	**Lambda**
"I don't care one ι" = "I don't care one _____."	**Iota**
The symbol for torque is τ, which is the Greek letter _____.	**Tau**
The symbol for damping ratio is ζ, which is the Greek letter _____.	**Zeta**
The symbol for emissivity is ε, which is the Greek letter _____.	**Epsilon**
A finite difference is represented by a capital delta, which is written_____.	Δ
The symbol for gamma rays is a lowercase Greek "gamma," which is written _____.	γ
The potential energy of water is represented by an upper-case Greek "psi," which is written _____.	Ψ
A universal set in logic is represented with the lowercase "chi," which is written _____.	χ
Stress in mechanics is denoted with a lowercase "sigma," which is written _____.	σ
The kinematic viscosity of liquids is denoted with a lowercase "nu," which is written _____.	ν
The ratio of a circle's circumference to its diameter is denoted with a lowercase "pi," which is written _____. This constant is also named after the 3rd-century-BC Greek mathematician from Syracuse, Archimedes.	π
Resistivity is represented by a lowercase "rho," which is written _____.	ρ
The symbol for an eta-meson is the lowercase letter "eta," which is written _____.	η
The symbol for an alpha-particle is a lowercase "alpha," which is written _____.	α

For Fun: Transliterate your name into Greek and provide its numerical value.

Example: Todd Curtis = τοδδκυρτις = (300 + 70 + 4 + 4) + (20 + 400 + 100 + 300 + 10 + 200) = 1404

Roman Numerals

Roman numerals have not been used in mathematics since Leonardo of Pisa (c. 1180–1250) published his famous book *Liber abaci*, which popularized the Hindu-Arabic number system in the Latin-speaking West. However, Roman numerals have continued to be used for clock faces, dates, ornate enumerations, and in particular, with the dosages in pharmaceutical prescriptions. The Roman numerals used today are derived from the actual number system of the Roman Empire. These basic numbers can be expressed in capital or lowercase letters as follows:

Roman numeral and their Arabic number equivalent
I or i = 1
V or v = 5
X or x = 10
L or l = 50
C or c = 100
D or d = 500
M or m = 1000

To form larger numbers, the Roman numeric symbols are combined, with the larger unit preceding the smaller. The actual number is found by adding all the numeric symbols together. For example, VII represents 7, CCLXVI represents 266, and MDCCCCXXVI is 1926. Likewise, on prescriptions, one will find lowercase Roman numerals, such as iii tab. represents 3 tablets, vi gtt represents 6 drops, and xvi tab. represents 16 tablets.

To shorten the length of certain numbers, a subtraction notation was sometimes employed by the Romans, and it is still used to this day. The **subtraction notation** places the smaller unit before the larger to indicate that the actual number is derived from the smaller numerical value being subtracted from the larger. The subtraction notation is only used for the following six numbers:

IV = 4, **IX** = 9, **XL** = 40, **XC** = 90, **CD** = 400, **CM** = 900

The subtraction rule is useful because it allows for large numbers to be reduced to a smaller notation.

1949 = MDCCCCXXXXVIIII = MCMXLIX

Give the Hindu-Arabic number for the following:

Review	Answers
The prescription "iv tab." is equal to _____ tablets.	4
The date MCDXXV is equal to _____.	1425
The prescription xi suppositories is equal to _____ suppositories.	11
XL Olympiad is equal to _____ th Olympiad.	40
The date MMXVII is equal to _____.	2017

Word Elements for Greek and Latin Numbers

In addition to Greek and Roman numerical symbols, the word elements derived from Greek and Latin numbers are commonly used in scientific terminology. This is particularly true with chemical compositions.

Greek Cardinal Numbers

The following are the most commonly used Greek cardinal numbers. Cardinal numbers denote quantity and are equivalent to 1, 2, 3, 4, etc. The numeral word elements mon/o, tri/o, tetr/a, pent/a, hex/a, and oct/a are commonly used in the naming of chemical compounds and complexes, such as tetrachlorodibenzo-p-dioxin, carbon monoxide, and octadecatrienoic acid. Interestingly, the word elements di- and non-, which come from Latin, are used for chemical compounds instead of their corresponding Greek numbers. Chemical compound numbers from 11–19 will have deka/deca attached to the ordinal number (18-octadeca-, 15-pentadeca-, 12-dodeca-, etc.). Unlike many other roots, the most common combining vowels for some of these numbers is not O, and therefore, the following word elements reflect differing combining vowels for each root.

Greek word element	Current usage	Etymology	Examples
HEN/O (hen-ō)	One	Gr. *hen*, one	**Hen**otic, **hen**ogeneis
MON/O (mŏn-ō)	One, alone	Gr. *monos*, alone, single	**Mon**oblepsia, **mon**androus
DY/O (dī-ō)	Two, a pair	Gr. *dyo*, two	**Dy**ad, **dy**aster
TRI/O (trī-ō)	Three	Gr. *treis*, three	**Tri**gastric, **tri**actinal
TETR/A (tĕt-ră)	Four	Gr. *tetra*, four	**Tetr**ablastic, **tetr**ad
PENT/A (pen-tă)	Five	Gr. *pente*, five	**Pent**abasic, **pent**adactyl
HEX/A (heks-ă)	Six	Gr. *hex*, six	**Hex**apoda, **hex**ahedron
HEPT/A (hĕp-tă)	Seven	Gr. *hepta*, seven	**Hept**achromic, **hept**agynous
OKT/A (ŏk-tă) **OCT/A** (ŏk-tă)	Eight	Gr. *okto*, eight	**Oct**aploid, **oct**opus
ENNE/A (en-nē-ă)	Nine	Gr. *ennea*, nine	**Enne**agon, **enne**aphylla
DEC/A (dek-ă)	Ten	Gr. *deka*, ten	**Dec**agram, **dec**apod
HENDEC/A (hen-dek-ă)	Eleven	Gr. *hendeka*, eleven	**Hendec**ahedron, **hendec**agon
DODEC/A (dō-dek-ă)	Twelve	Gr. *dodeka*, twelve	**Dodec**ahedron, **dodek**agynus
HECAT/O (hĕk-ă-tō) **HECT/O** (hĕk-tō)	One hundred	Gr. *hekaton*, one hundred	**Hecat**omeric, **hect**ogram
CHILI/O (kil-i-ō) **KIL/O** (kil-ō)	One thousand	Gr. *chilioi*, one thousand	**Chili**ad, **kil**ometer
MYRI/O (mĭr-ē-ō)	Ten thousand, innumerable	Gr. *myrioi* ten thousand, innumerable	**Myri**apoda, **myri**ad

Review	Answers
Literally and numerically, the subphylum myriapoda have _____ feet. In actuality, the number of feet/legs of the species in this subphylum ranges from less than 10–750. The root MYRI/A could also mean _____.	**10 000** **Innumerable**
A hecatophyllus plant literally means that this plant has _____ leaves (Gr. *phyllon*, leaf).	**100**
In the chemical term tetraaquadichlorochromium, the word element TETR/A means _____.	**4**
Octadecatrienoic acid is listed by its lipid number (octadeca) _____: (tri)_____.	**18 : 3**
Carbon monoxide has _____ oxygen atom. The word element MON- can also mean _____ in other contexts. Another Greek combining form for "one" is _____.	**1** **alone** **HEN/O**
Hendecagon literally has _____ angles/corners (Gr. *gonia*, angle).	**11**
An enneagynous flower has _____ pistils, which are the female reproductive parts of the flower.	**9**
Hexachlorophene is an antibacterial compound that has _____ chlorine atoms.	**6**
A pentandrous flower has _____ stamens, which are the male reproductive parts of the flower.	**5**
The heptathlon has _____ events.	**7**
A dyad is a _____ of chromosomes formed by meiosis of a tetrad.	**pair**
A Chilianthus arboreus is a plant whose name means _____ flowers (Gr. *anthos*, flower).	**1000**

Greek Ordinal Numbers

The following are commonly used Greek ordinal numbers. **Ordinal numbers** tell the position/order of something. They are commonly used in chemistry, and like other Greek numbers, they are also used in the physical sciences. It is important to bear in mind that they are sometimes translated as cardinal numbers (i.e. one, two, three, and four) rather than as ordinal numbers (i.e. 1st, 2nd, 3rd, and 4th).

Greek word element	Current usage	Etymology	Examples
PROT/O (prō-tō)	1st	Gr. *protos*, 1st	**Prot**otype, **prot**ogyny
DEUTER/O (dū-tĕr-ō)	2nd	Gr. *deuteros*, 2nd	**Deuter**oplasm, **deuter**opathy
TRIT/O (trīt-ō)	3rd	Gr. *tritos*, 3rd	**Trit**anopia, **trit**ocone
TETART/O (te-tar-tō)	4th, one-fourth	Gr. *tetartos*, 4th	**Tetart**anopia, **tetart**ohedral

Adverbs and Numbers

In Chemistry, Greek and Latin adverbs are used as prefixes to indicate the number of coordinating groups or ligands within a molecule. They are also a part of the Latin used in pharmaceutical prescriptions (e.g. Twice a day = BID = *bis in die*; Three times a day = TID = *ter in die*).

Greek and Latin word element	Current usage	Etymology	Examples
BIS- (bis)	Two times, two	L. *bis*, two times	**Bis**acromial, bisaxillary
TRIS- (tris)	Three times, three	Gr. *tris*, three times	**Tris**-(ethylenediamine) cobalt (III)
TER- (tĕr)		L. *ter*, three times	**Ter**tian

Greek and Latin word element	Current usage	Etymology	Examples
TETRAKIS- (tĕ-tră-kis)	Four times, four	Gr. *tetatrakis*, four times	**Tetrakis**(triphenylphosphine)-palladium(0)
QUATER- (kwŏ-tĕr)		L. *quater*, four times	**Quater**nary

Review	Answers
A tetartoanopia is a loss of _____ of one's visual field.	**one fourth**
Protobiology is the study of viruses. The combining form PROT/O means _____.	**1st**
Deuterostomes differ from protostomes because their _____ opening becomes the mouth.	**2nd**
Tritolyl contains _____ tolyl radicals in the molecule.	**three**
Bisiliac pertains to the _____ iliac crests. BID in prescriptions stands for *bis in die*, which means "_____ in a day."	**two** **twice**
If a molecule has three ligands, the prefix _____ is used. If it has four ligands, the prefix _____ is used.	**TRIS-** **TETRAKIS-**

Latin Cardinal Numbers

Although the naming of chemical compounds and complexes is primarily derived from Greek numbers, Latin numerals and ordinals are occasionally used. The following roots are from commonly used Latin ordinal numbers. Unlike many other roots, the common combining vowels for these numbers is not O, and therefore, the following word elements reflect differing combining vowels for each root.

Latin word element	Current usage	Etymology	Examples
UN/I (ŭ-ni)	One	L. *unus*, one	**Uni**lateral, **uni**fied
DU/O (dū-ŏ)	Two	L. *dou*, two	**Duo**genarian, **du**plex
TRI- (trĭ)	Three	L. *tres, tria*, three	**Tri**ceps, **tri**dent
QUADR/I (kwŏd-rĭ)	Four	L. *quattuor*, four	**Quadr**uped, **quadr**angle
QUINQU/E (kwĭn-kwē)	Five	L. *quinque*, five	**Quinqu**evalent, **quinqu**efoliolate
SEX/A (sĕks-ă)	Six	L. *sex*, six	**Sex**agenarian, **sex**ipara
SEPT/I (sĕp-tĭ)	Seven	L. *septem*, seven	**Sept**ivalent, **sept**ennial
OCT/O (ŏk-tŏ)	Eight	L. *octo*, eight	**Oct**aploidy, **oct**ipara
NOV/I (nŏ-vĭ)	Nine	L. *novem*, nine	**Nov**ember, **nov**ennial
DEC/A (dek-ă)	Ten	L. *decem*, ten	**Dec**ember, **dec**imal
CENT/O (sĕn-tŏ)	One hundred	L. *centum*, one hundred	**Cent**imeter, **cent**enary
MILL/I (mĭl-ĭ)	One thousand	L. *mille*, one thousand	**Mill**ipede, **mill**imeter

Latin Ordinal Numbers

The following roots are from the most commonly used Latin ordinals. Unlike many other roots, the most common combining vowels for these numbers is not O, and therefore, the following word elements reflect differing combining vowels for each root:

Latin word element	Current usage	Etymology	Examples
PRIM/I (prĭ-mĭ)	1st, one	L. *primus*, 1st	**Prim**ate, **prim**ordial
SECUND/I (sĕ-kŭn-dĭ)	2nd, two	L. *secundus*, 2nd	**Secund**igravida, **secund**iflorus
TERTI/A (tĕr-shē-a)	3rd, three	L. *tertius*, 3rd	**Terti**ary, **tert**ian
QUART/A (kwor-tă)	4th, four	L. *quartus*, 4th	**Quart**an, **quart**ile
QUINT/A (kwĭn-tă)	5th, five	L. *quintus*, 5th	**Quint**uplet, **quint**isternal
SEXT/I (sĕks-tĭ)	6th, six	L. *sextus*, 6th	**Sext**ipara, **sext**uplet
SEPTIM/A (sĕp-tĭ-mă)	7th, seven	L. *septimus*, 7th	**Septim**al, **sept**uplet
OCTAV/A (ŏk-tă-vă)	8th, eight	L. *octavus*, 8th	**Octav**e, **octav**o
NON/A (nŏn-ă)	9th, nine	L. *nonus*, 9th	**Non**agenarian, **non**agon
DECIM/O (dĕs-ĭ-mŏ)	10th, 10	L. *decimus*, 10th	Hexa**decim**al, **decim**ate

Review	Answers
Possessing the power of combining or replacing one atom of hydrogen is called _____-valent.	**uni**
A woman's _____ pregnancy is called primigravida. A woman in her _____ pregnancy is called secundigravida.	**1st 2nd**
Tertiary syphilis is the _____ stage of syphilis.	**3rd**
Quaternary substances are composed of _____ elements.	**4**
A nonane has _____ carbon atoms.	**9**
Literally, a centipede has _____ feet. Despite the name, centipedes have varying amount of legs, with some species having up to 354 legs.	**100**
Our term "mile" comes from the Roman unit of measure *mille passuum*, which is _____ paces, as measured by every other step in a march.	**1000**
A quartan fever associated with malaria occurs every _____ day.	**4th**
Having _____ pregnancies that produce viable infants is termed sextipara. That said, a woman who gives birth to_____ children from a single pregnancy is said to have had septuplets.	**6 7**
The Calendar of Romulus, which was named after the legendary founder of Rome, Romulus, had 10 months. This calendar began with the month of March. In the Calendar of Romulus, September, October, November, and December correspond to the _____th, _____th, _____, th, and _____th months. The Roman Republic Calendar moved the 1st month to January and added two more months to the 10 months of the legendary Calendar of Romulus.	**7, 8, 9, 10**
The biceps muscle has _____ "heads" or "origins," and the triceps muscle has _____ "heads" or "origins."	**2, 3**
A quadriplegic is a term that denotes the number of paralyzed limbs of a person, which is _____. QID stands for "quattuor in die" which means "_____ times in a day."	**4 4**
Parthenocissus quinquefolia comes from the Greek *parthenos* "virgin" and the Latinized *cissus* meaning "ivy." The species is called *quinquefolia* because it has _____ leaves.	**5**

Lessons from History: The Four Classical Elements and the Elements of Chemistry

Food for Thought as You Read:

Is reductionism scientific? What makes it appear scientific?

From its early beginnings, Greek philosophers attempted to explain the origin and nature of the universe via naturalistic explanations that relied on some universal principle or cause. Their reductionist approach to explaining the physical universe is evident in the ancient Greek medical theories.

One of their approaches was to reduce the universe into a number of physical forces (e.g. binding, loosening, heat, cold, wet, dry, etc.), which were later referred to as physical *dynameis* (singular *dynamis*). The Greek word *dynameis* is often translated as "powers," but in natural philosophy, it seems to refer to the sum total of a thing's characteristics or qualities. The early theories typically spoke of opposing forces being at work in the formation of the universe. For example, the Greek philosopher Empedocles spoke in metaphorical terms about the opposing physical forces of "attraction" and "repulsion" as "love" and "strife." Such theoretical approaches to the physical universe were also applied to the medical concepts of health and disease. For example, writing in the 5th century BC, Alcmaeon of Croton (S. Italy) opined that "what preserves health is the equal distribution (*isonomian*) of its forces (*dynameis*) – moist, cold, hot, bitter, sweet, and so on – and the dominion (*monarchian*) of any one of them creates disease (D. 442)." While Alcmaeon's conception of health as being an equality (*isonomia*) and disease being a monarchy (*monarchia*) has political undertones, his theory is similar to other philosophers and physicians who conceived of health as being a balance or equilibrium and disease being a disruption of this balance of powers.

A number of Greek philosophers and physicians delimited the physical forces of the universe to four: heat (*thermos*), cold (*psychros*), wet (*hygros*), and dry (*xeros*). Their choice of these four can be partially explained by their understanding of the predominate qualities of the four seasons. The Hippocratic work entitled *On the Nature of Man* (*Nat. Hom.*) links each season to a predominate quality that corresponds to the weather of each season (i.e. Winter is cold, Spring is wet, Summer is hot, and Fall is dry). The author of *Nat. Hom.* argues that these four qualities can be linked to a predominance of a specific humor (i.e. blood, phlegm, bile, black bile) because the season and the humor share a predominate quality. Phlegm is more prevalent in man during the winter; blood becomes dominant during the Spring; bile is dominant in the Summer; and black bile is more prevalent in the Fall. The link between the four seasons and the four humors is part of *Nat. Hom.*'s explanation as to why certain diseases are more prevalent at different times of the year, which this author attributes to an unhealthy predominance of a single humor that was engendered in the human body by the season's corresponding quality. Although we no longer consider these qualities to be the primary forces that formed the universe, their combining forms, **THERM/O (heat, temperature), PSYCHR/O (cold), HYGR/O (wet)**, and **XER/O (dry)**, are commonly used in medicine and science due to their corresponding qualities. Likewise, the combining form **DYNAM/O** is commonly used in compound terms to indicate "power, force" (e.g. dynamometer and isodynamic).

Another line of inquiry taken by natural philosophers was to consider what is the fundamental material of the universe (Fig. 5.3). For some philosophers, such as Democritus of Abdera (c. 450 BC), the universe was composed of an infinite number of uncuttable forms of matter and the void around them. This "uncuttable" form of matter was often referred to as an *atomon*, from which we get our word "atoms." Another approach was to reduce the material of the universe into a limited number of observable "elements," particularly *ge* (**earth**), *hydor* (**water**), *pyr* (**fire**), and *aer* (**air**). These elements were often referred to as *stoicheia*, which is a Greek word used for the rudimentary parts of a whole, such as the letters of the Greek alphabet. However, there was no consensus as to their number and nature. Some philosophers were monists: Thales of Miletus (c. 600 BC) considered *hydor* (**water**) to be the element of the universe; Anaximenes (c. 550 BC) argued that *aer* (**air**) was the fundamental principle; and Heraclitus (500 BC) believed it to be *pyr* (**fire**). Other philosophers were dualists: Parmenides of Elea (c. 475 BC) thought the universe was composed of *ge* (**earth**) and *pyr* (**fire**), while Hippon (c. 450 BC) believed them to be *pyr* (**fire**) and *hydor* (**water**). In his Metaphysics (985a31-3), Aristotle (385–322 BC) credits the 5th-century-BC philosopher, Empedocles, with being the first to propose that there were four elements that made up the universe: *ge* (**earth**), *hydor* (**water**), *pyr* (**fire**), and *aer* (**air**). These four elements were commonly referred to as "the four elements"; today, we refer to them as the "classical elements." Although what constitutes an element is much different in modern science, we continue to use the ancient Greek word *stoicheia* via our combining form **STOICHI/O** for "**element**." The Greek words for the four classical elements are preserved in the combining forms **GE/O** (earth), **HYDR/O** (water), **PYR/O** (fire, fever), and **AER/O** (air).

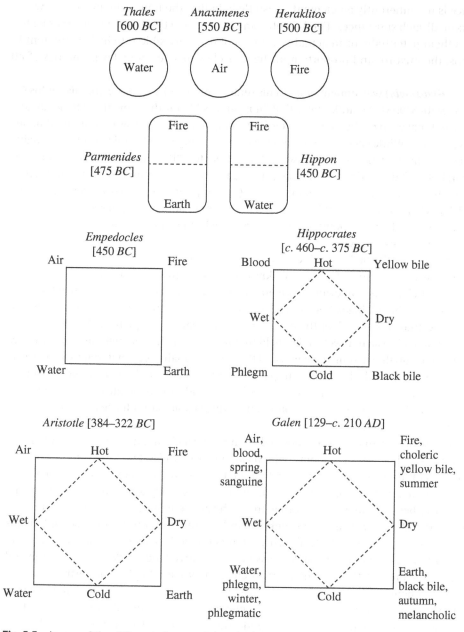

Fig. 5.3 Image of the different elemental theories in philosophy and medicine. As can be seen, Galen mated and medicalized the Aristotelian model by adding and associating the four humors to the four elements. Galen also mated the four humors to the four temperaments, which was a theory of personality and characteristics of individuals born with a predominate humoral mixture (i.e. melancholic, choleric, sanguine, and phlegmatic). *Source:* Drawing by Chloe Kim.

While Empedocles may have been the first philosopher to speak to four elements making up the universe, it is Aristotle's systematic approach to the four elements that had a profound effect on philosophy and medicine for centuries. Similar to modern chemistry, Aristotle focused on the nature of physical substances and the forces involved in their alterations and compositions. Aristotle recognized that some material things were composed of multiple substances. For example, something made of rock and wood can be clearly seen as having been composed of multiple substances. Therefore, he called these compounds *heterogenous* (Gr. *heteros*, other, another, different + *genos*, kind). He also recognized that some things were uniform in substance (e.g. wood, bone, and stone), which he called *homoeomerous* (Gr. *homoios*, similar, like + *meros*, part, portion). The key criteria for a substance to be *homoeomerous* material was that each and every part of such a substance must be the same as the whole. Thus, heterogenous compounds can be broken down into homoeomerous substances. For example, a body can be broken down into bones, tendons, muscle, skin, etc.

That said, a homoeomerous substance is not inherently an element. Aristotle held that the four elements (earth, water, fire, and air) were the building blocks of all such substances. For Aristotle, an element "is a body into which other bodies may be analyzed, which is present in them potentially or in actuality, and is not itself divisible into bodies different in form (*De caelo*, III.3, 302a15ff)." Thus, the mixture and proportion of the four elements accounts for properties of all substances.

Aristotle's belief in the four qualities (*dynameis*) was fundamental to his understanding of the four elements. In his *On Generation and Corruption* (*DG* II.3, 330a30–330b5), Aristotle states that "it is impossible for the same thing to be hot and cold, or moist and dry." Aristotle theorized that each of the four qualities (hot, cold, dry, and wet) was predominant in one of the four elements (earth, water, fire, and air). While each element embodied one primary quality and a secondary quality that was not in opposition to its primary quality (e.g. hot-dry or hot-wet). Aristotle states, "It is evident that the 'couplings' of the elementary qualities will be four: hot with dry and hot with moist, and again cold with dry and cold with moist. And these four couples have attached themselves to the apparently 'simple' bodies (fire, air, water, and earth) in a manner consonant with theory. For fire is hot and dry, whereas air is hot and moist (air being a sort of aqueous vapor); and water is cold and moist, while earth is cold and dry." Because the four qualities are forces by which substances are formed, the four elements are potentially or actually evident in all substances.

Humoralism, the belief that the certain fluids in the body explained disease and health, became one of the more common medical theories among the philosophically inclined sect of physicians known as Rationalists. Writing in the 2nd-century AD, Galen argued that the theory of the four elements is relevant to the practice of medicine because it explained the quality and nature of the four humors (i.e. phlegm, blood, black bile, and yellow bile), which in turn, explained the origins of health and disease. Following Aristotle, he argued that each of the four elements is a pairing of qualities. Earth was cold/dry; fire was hot/dry; water was cold/wet; and air was hot/wet. Galen held that nature, which he sometimes characterizes as a Demiurge (Craftsman), used the hot/cold qualities as instruments and the dry/wet qualities as material to form everything in the universe. Galen's systematic approach to linking the four qualities and elements to the four humors, coupled with his claim that his theory accurately reflected the true approach to medicine found in Hippocrates' *On the Nature of Man*, led to the four quality/element/humor theory becoming the dominant medical explanation for health, disease, and medical treatments in Medieval and Renaissance medicine.

Our modern understanding of what constitutes an element is derived from modern chemistry. The origins of chemistry are historically linked to the practices and beliefs of alchemy, which extends back to Hellenistic Egypt. Steeped in mysticism, and pulling from the art of metallurgy, alchemy was based on the belief that base metals, such as lead and copper, could be transmuted into purer metals such as gold and silver by a legendary substance known as the Philosopher's Stone. Medieval alchemists believed metals and other inert physical elements were formed from the same original substance in varying degrees of purity. They also sought to find a universal cure for disease and means to prolong life, which was known as "the Elixir of Life." While alchemy often operated in secrecy and at the periphery of science, over time, quite a number of famous scientists of the Renaissance and Early Modern Period drew from and dabbled in alchemy, such as Sir Isaac Newton and the famous English chemist, Robert Boyle. The term chemistry comes from the medieval Latin word for alchemy (*alkimia*), which is derived from the Arabic *al-kimiya*, which appears to be from the Greek *chemeia*. As to the origins of this Greek word, some argue that it is from an old name for the "black earth of Egypt," an area with strong ties to the practice of alchemy, and others argue that it is from a Greek word meaning "to pour."

The use of chemical elements in medicine is often tied to the famous 16th-century physician and alchemist, Paracelsus. Breaking from the Galenist of the 16th century, Paracelsus argued that the four-element and humor model was an erroneous model for health and disease. Among Paracelsus' five different sources of disease, he put forward that there are three principles that are inherent in all matter and essential to life: the fiery, volatile principle was associated with sulfur, the solid and inert principle was said to be salt, and the fluid and changeable element was mercury. Paracelsus' cures for disease relied much more heavily on being mineral and metal-based than the Galenists, and in keeping with the practices of alchemy, he attempted to distill and transform such material to remove impurities, thereby making them more therapeutic. His reliance on empirical evidence versus scholastic medical theories led him to the discovery of a number of revolutionary ideas and treatments, most notably the use of mercury in the treatment of syphilis. Although Paracelsus is thought of as the first medical chemist, he is an alchemist whose writings are full of astrology and religious mysticism, and his explanations of chemical preparations were often rife with magico-spiritual conceptions of the elements. That said, the practices of his followers led to the chemical approach of deriving medications that came to its fruition in western medicine.

Some Suggested Readings

Aristotle. "*On Generation and Corruption.*" In *The Complete Works of Aristotle* Volume 1, Edited by Jonathan Barnes, 512–554. Princeton: Princeton University Press, 1984.

Aristotle, "*On the Heavens,*" In *The Complete Works of Aristotle* Volume 1, Edited by Jonathan Barnes, 447–511. Princeton: Princeton University Press, 1984.

Loyson, Peter. "Influences of Ancient Greek on Chemical Terminology." *Journal of Chemical Education* 86, no. 10 (2009): 1195–1199.

Loyson, Peter. "Influences from Latin on Chemical Terminology." *Journal of Chemical Education* 87, no. 12 (2010): 1303–1307.

Pagel, Walter. *Paracelsus: An Introduction to Philosophical Medicine in the Era of the Renaissance.* Basel: Karger Medical and Scientific Publishers, 1982.

Weisberg, Michael, Paul Needham, and Robin Hendry. "*Philosophy of Chemistry.*" In *The Stanford Encyclopedia of Philosophy* (Spring 2019 Edition). Edited by Edward, N. Zalta: Springer, 2019. https://plato.stanford.edu/archives/spr2019/entries/chemistry/.

Etymological Explanations: Chemical Elements

Etymologies of Chemical Elements Derived from Greek

Today, chemical elements are defined as what constitutes the ordinary matter of the universe. They are recognized by their atomic number, and currently, 118 elements have been identified. They are commonly linked to their chemical properties and health effects (Fig. 5.4).

The chemical elements of the periodic table reveal that most of these symbols and terms are derived from Greek and Latin word elements commonly used in the natural sciences and medical terminology. The following is a list of etymologies of some of the Greek combining forms for elements in chemistry:

Greek combining form	Current meaning	Etymology	Symbol and rationale for chemical element
HYDR/O (hĭ-drŏ)	Water, liquid, hydrogen	Gr. *hydros*, water	H Hydrogen Named "water creator" because it forms water.
HELI/O (hē-lē-ŏ)	Sun, helium	Gr. *helios*, sun	He Helium It was discovered in the spectrum of the sun.
LITH/O (lĭth-ŏ)	Stone, lithium	Gr. *lithos*, stone	Li Lithium It was discovered in minerals.
NITR/O (nĭ-trŏ)	Nitrogenous	Gr. *nitron*, sodium bicarbonate; niter	N Nitrogen Named "niter creator" because this gas was found through the analysis of niter.
OX/O	Oxygen	Gr. *oxys*, acid, sharp, keen	O Oxygen Named "Acid creator" because it was thought to be the element which formed acids.
NEON/O (nĕ-on-ŏ)	Neon	Gr. *neos*, new, recent, young	Ne Neon New discovery found in air residues.
NE/O (nĕ-ŏ)	New, recent		

Greek combining form	Current meaning	Etymology	Symbol and rationale for chemical element
PHOSPH/O (fŏs-fō-rō)	Phosphorus	*Gr. phosophoros*, light bringer, morning star	P Phosphorus Named "light bearer" because phosphorus emits light.
CHLOR/O (klō-rō)	Green, Chlorine	*Gr. chloros*, green	Cl Chlorine Named after the color of the gas.
CHROMI/O (krō-mē-ō)	Chromium	*Gr. chroma, chromatos*, color	Cr Chromium Chromium compounds have different colors.
CHROM/O (krō-mō)	Color		
CHROMAT/O (krō-mă-tō)			
SELENI/O sĕ-lĕ-nē-ō)	Selenium	*Gr. selene*, moon	Se Selenium Named "moon" because it was confused with tellurium, which meant "earth."
SELEN/O (sĕ-lē-nō)	Moon, crescent-shaped		
BROM/O (brō-mō)	Foul-smelling, bromine	*Gr. bromos*, foul-smelling	Br Bromine Named because the element has a foul smell.
CRYPT/O (krip-tō)	Hidden, covered, krypton	*Gr. kryptos*, covered, hidden	Kr Krypton Named for the difficulty in discovering it.
KRYPT/O (krip-tō)			
RHOD/O (rō-dō)	Rose, red, rhodium	*Gr. rhodon*, rose, rose-colored	Rh Rhodium Named for the color of solutions containing it.
XEN/O (zen-ō)	Foreign, strange, xenon	*Gr. xenon*, foreign, strange	Xe Xenon Last of a series of gases to be discovered.
BAR/O (bar-ō)	Weight, pressure	*Gr. baros*, weight, pressure	Ba Barium Named such because it was present in the mineral barytes "heavy spar".
BARY/O (bar-ĭ-ō)	Heavy, dull	*Gr. barys*, heavy	
OSM/O (oz-mō)	Odor, smell, osmium	*Gr. osme*, smell, scent odor	Os Osmium Named for the strong smell of its oxide.
THALL/O (thăl-lō)	Young branch, shoot, simple plants (i.e. fungi, lichens, algae) thallium	*Gr. thallos*, young shoot or branch	Tl Thallium Named for the green line visible in its spectrum.
AKTIN/O (ak-ti-nō)	Ray, ray-like, radiation, actinium	*Gr. aktinos*, ray	Ac Actinium Actinium is radioactive.
ACTIN/O (ak-ti-nō)			

Periodic table of elements:

#	Symbol	Name	Atomic mass
1	H	Hydrogen	1.008
2	He	Helium	4.003
3	Li	Lithium	6.94
4	Be	Beryllium	9.012
5	B	Boron	10.81
6	C	Carbon	12.011
7	N	Nitrogen	14.007
8	O	Oxygen	15.999
9	F	Fluorine	18.998
10	Ne	Neon	20.180
11	Na	Sodium	22.990
12	Mg	Magnesium	24.305
13	Al	Aluminium	26.982
14	Si	Silicon	28.085
15	P	Phosphorus	30.974
16	S	Sulfur	32.06
17	Cl	Chlorine	35.45
18	Ar	Argon	39.948
19	K	Potassium	39.098
20	Ca	Calcium	40.078
21	Sc	Scandium	44.956
22	Ti	Titanium	47.867
23	V	Vanadium	50.942
24	Cr	Chromium	51.996
25	Mn	Manganese	54.938
26	Fe	Iron	55.845
27	Co	Cobalt	58.933
28	Ni	Nickel	58.693
29	Cu	Copper	63.546
30	Zn	Zinc	65.38
31	Ga	Gallium	69.723
32	Ge	Germanium	72.630
33	As	Arsenic	74.922
34	Se	Selenium	78.97
35	Br	Bromine	79.904
36	Kr	Krypton	83.798
37	Rb	Rubidium	85.468
38	Sr	Strontium	87.62
39	Y	Yttrium	88.906
40	Zr	Zirconium	91.224
41	Nb	Niobium	92.906
42	Mo	Molybdenum	95.95
43	Tc	Technetium	[97]
44	Ru	Ruthenium	101.07
45	Rh	Rhodium	102.906
46	Pd	Palladium	106.42
47	Ag	Silver	107.868
48	Cd	Cadmium	112.414
49	In	Indium	114.818
50	Sn	Tin	118.710
51	Sb	Antimony	121.760
52	Te	Tellurium	127.60
53	I	Iodine	126.904
54	Xe	Xenon	131.298
55	Cs	Caesium	132.905
56	Ba	Barium	137.327
57 – 70	*	(Lanthanide series)	
71	Lu	Lutetium	174.967
72	Hf	Hafnium	178.49
73	Ta	Tantalum	180.948
74	W	Tungsten	183.84
75	Re	Rhenium	186.207
76	Os	Osmium	190.23
77	Ir	Iridium	192.212
78	Pt	Platinum	195.084
79	Au	Gold	196.992
80	Hg	Mercury	200.592
81	Tl	Thallium	204.38
82	Pb	Lead	207.2
83	Bi	Bismuth	208.980
84	Po	Polonium	[209]
85	At	Astatine	[210]
86	Rn	Radon	[222]
87	Fr	Francium	[223]
88	Ra	Radium	[226]
89 – 102	**	(Actinide series)	
103	Lr	Lawrencium	[262]
104	Rf	Rutherfordium	[267]
105	Db	Dubnium	[270]
106	Sg	Seaborgium	[269]
107	Bh	Bohrium	[270]
108	Hs	Hassium	[270]
109	Mt	Meitnerium	[278]
110	Ds	Darmstadtium	[281]
111	Rg	Roentgenium	[281]
112	Cn	Copernicium	[285]
113	Nh	Nihonium	[286]
114	Fl	Flerovium	[289]
115	Mc	Moscovium	[289]
116	Lv	Livermorium	[293]
117	Ts	Tennessine	[293]
118	Og	Oganesson	[294]

*Lanthanide series

#	Symbol	Name	Atomic mass
57	La	Lanthanum	138.905
58	Ce	Cerium	140.116
59	Pr	Praseodymium	140.908
60	Nd	Neodymium	144.242
61	Pm	Promethium	[145]
62	Sm	Samarium	150.36
63	Eu	Europium	151.964
64	Gd	Gadolinium	157.25
65	Tb	Terbium	158.925
66	Dy	Dysprosium	162.500
67	Ho	Holmium	164.930
68	Er	Erbium	167.259
69	Tm	Thulium	168.934
70	Yb	Ytterbium	173.045

**Actinide series

#	Symbol	Name	Atomic mass
89	Ac	Actinium	[227]
90	Th	Thorium	232.038
91	Pa	Protactinium	231.036
92	U	Uranium	238.029
93	Np	Neptunium	[237]
94	Pu	Plutonium	[244]
95	Am	Americium	[243]
96	Cm	Curium	[247]
97	Bk	Berkelium	[247]
98	Cf	Californium	[251]
99	Es	Einsteinium	[252]
100	Fm	Fermium	[257]
101	Md	Mendelevium	[258]
102	No	Nobelium	[259]

Fig. 5.4 Periodic table of elements as of 2016. *Source:* https://commons.wikimedia.org/wiki/File:Periodic_Table_Of_Elements_Black_And_White.svg.

Etymologies of Chemical Elements Derived from Latin

The following is a list of etymologies of some of the Latin combining forms for elements in chemistry:

Latin combining form	Current meaning	Etymology	Symbol and rationale for chemical element
CARB/O (kar-bō)	Carbon, carbon dioxide	L. *carbo, carbonis*, coal, charcoal	C Carbon Found in graphite and charcoal
NATRI/O (nā-trē-ō) NATR/O (nā-trŏ)	Sodium	L. *natrium*, salt	Na Sodium Latin name for carbonate salt found in Egypt
SILIC/O (sĭl-ĭ-kō)	Silica, silicon	L. *silex, silicis*, flint; silica	Si Silicon Found in flint
KALI/O (kal-ē-ō) KAL/O (ka-lō)	Potassium	L. *kalium*, potash	K Potassium Later Latin derived from Arabic al-qaliy "burnt ashes", alkali
*CALC/O (kal-kō)	Calcium, lime	L. *calx, calcis*, limestone, lime concretion	Ca Calcium Same
FERR/O (fĕr-ō)	Iron	L. *ferrum*, iron	Fe Iron Same
ARGENT/O (ar-jent-ō)	Silver	L. *argentum*, silver	Ag Silver Same
CUPR/O (kū-prŏ)	Copper	L. *cuprum*, copper	Cu Copper Named for of the island of Cyprus, where copper was mined by the Romans
STANN/O (stan-ō)	Tin	L. *stannum*, tin	Sn Tin Same
*AUR/O (or-ō)	Gold	L. *aurum*, gold	Au Gold Same
HYDRARGYR/O (hī-dror-jĭ-rō)	Mercury	L. *hydrargyrum*, mercury, liquid silver	Hg Mercury Latinized Greek for "silver" (argyr/o) and "water" (hydr/o)

N.B.
The roots **CALC-** and **AUR-** are homographs whose Latin roots also mean "heel" and "ear" respectively. **CALC-** will usually use the combining vowel **I** when it refers to "calcium."

Greek Mythological Characters and the Etymology of Modern Elements

The elements Titanium, Tantalum, Promethium, and Mercury are all eponyms for famous Greek mythological figures. Martin Heinrich Klaproth, a German chemist, named the element **Titanium (Ti)** because he discovered it after **Uranium**. Titanium is derived from the Greek term for the children of the Greek god Ouranos (Uranus). Ouranos, whose name means "Sky" or "Heavens," was the consort of Gaia (Earth). Via Gaia, Ouranos became the father of the Titans. Cronus, the youngest of the Titans, overthrew his father by castrating him (Fig. 5.5). Hesiod's *Theogony* suggests that Titan's name is derived from the verb *titainein* "to stretch." Ouranos calls them the Titans because they "over-reached" their position as gods when they castrated their father with the help of their mother, Gaia. Today, the combining form **TITAN/O** is used for Titanium or for "an object/person of enormous size".

Promethium (Pm) is a radioactive metallic element that was discovered in the fusion products of uranium while working on the Atomic bomb. The element Promethium (Pm) is named after the Titan, Prometheus. In Greek mythology,

Prometheus stole the fire that Zeus had withheld from mankind, and after he gave it to mortals, Zeus punished Prometheus by having him chained to a mountain and letting an eagle eat Prometheus' liver every day. In later Greco-Roman myths, Prometheus is described as creating mankind and teaching them the arts (Fig. 5.6). The relationship between fire/fusion and danger to the discoverer explains why the name of this Titan was chosen for Promethium. Furthermore, the adjective **promethean** is used for "someone or something that is daringly creative".

The element **Tantalum (Ta)** is named after the Greek mythological figure, Tantalus. According to some Greek myths, Tantalus was punished by the gods because he gave the food of the gods, ambrosia and nectar, to mortals. In other myths, Tantalus is punished because he chopped up his son and attempted to feed him to the gods. Tantalus' eternal punishment

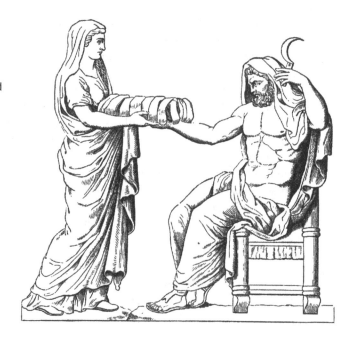

Fig. 5.5 Roman image of Cronus with his iconic sickle being offered a swaddled rock by his wife, Rhea. The image captures how Cronus repeated his father's treachery toward his kids, by swallowing the infants in order to avoid being usurped by one of his sons. As in the case of his father, Cronus is overthrown through the scheming of his wife, who offers Cronus a swaddled stone to swallow instead of her last child, Zeus. Line drawing of Imperial Roman base metope found on the Capitoline Hill. Line drawing found in *Galerie mythologique recueil de monuments pour servir à l'étude de la mythologie, de l'histoire e de l'art, de l'antiquité figurée, et du langage allégorique des anciens*, by A. L. Millin, 1811. *Source:* Numérisation Google/Wikimedia Commons/Public domain.

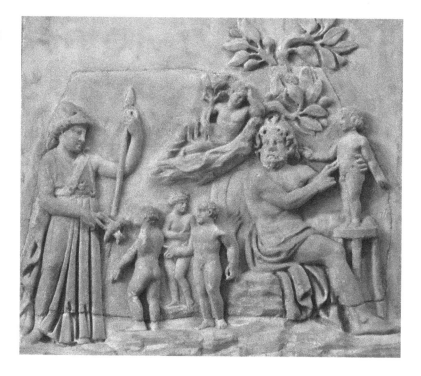

Fig. 5.6 Image of a 3rd-century-AD Roman base relief of Prometheus creating humans with Athena looking on. Louvre Museum. *Source:* Jastrow/ Wikimedia Commons/Public domain.

in the afterlife was to be standing in a pool of water with branches of fruit overhead. Every time he reaches for the fruit, it eludes his grasp, and the water always recedes before he can take a drink. The element was named Tantalum because it was not able to take on water. The word **tantalize** originates from the story of Tantalus. If something is called tantalizing, it's because it is desirable yet always just out of reach.

The element **Mercury** has the chemical symbol **(Hg),** which comes from the Latinized Greek word hydrargyrum (G. *hydor*, water + Gr. *argyros*, silver). This element ultimately derives its name from the Roman god of commerce, travelers, and merchants. The Roman god, Mercury, was commonly linked to the Greek god, Hermes. Due to this connection, Mercury plays the role of herald and ambassador of his father, Jupiter, in Roman literature. This connection with Hermes also explains why the planet is also called Mercury. Greek astronomers called this planet the "star of Hermes," claiming that this "star" should be called Hermes because he was the 1st to determine the order of the heavens (Eratosthenes, *Epitome* 43). Given the planet Mercury's rapid movement and its antegrade and retrograde movements that seem to communicate with the other planets, it is likely that the celerity and messenger qualities of the god Hermes were factors that led to this planet being named after this god. Mercury's connection with Hermes seems to explain why the element is also called Mercury. In the Greco-Roman world, a mystic figure named Hermes Trismegistus (Thrice-Greatest) was associated with a collection of writings related to magic, mysticism, and alchemy, which were called *Hermetica* (Fig. 5.7). Hermes Trismegistus is believed to be a syncretizing of the Greek god Hermes with the Egyptian god Thoth, but for later Christian authors, Hermes Trismegistus was considered a wise pagan prophet. In the late medieval and early Renaissance, the figure of Hermes Trismegistus became popularly associated with mystic religious views of alchemy. The element Mercury was of central importance to alchemists. This element was commonly referred to as *Argent Vive* (living silver), and its mutable nature was believed to hold the key to the chemical transformations that Alchemists sought to understand. At this time period, Alchemists began to refer to *Argent Vive* as "our Mercury" to show their own philosophical understanding of the secrets of this liquid metal. It is likely that Hermes Trismegistus' association with alchemy led to this essential element of the Alchemists being called by the god's Roman name, Mercury. Whether this is the case or not, the connection between alchemy and the name of the element was well understood by authors of the scientific revolution, such as Francis Bacon:

> There bee two Great Families of Things; You may terme them by severall Names; Sulphureous and Mercureall, which are the Chymists Words: (as for their Sal, which is their Third Principle, it is a Compound of the other two;) Inflammable, and Not Inflammable; Mature and Crude; Oily and Watry.
>
> -Francis Bacon, *Experiments Touching Sulphur and Mercury*

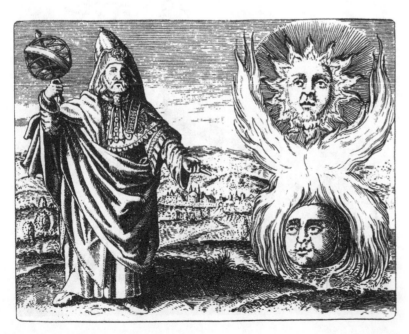

Fig. 5.7 Woodcut image of Hermes (Mercurius) Trismegistus with the alchemical Sun and Moon from Daniel Stolz von Stolzenberg, *Viridarium Chymicum*, 1624. Stolz was a physician and writer of alchemy. *Source:* Unknown Source/Wikimedia Commons/Public domain.

Review	Answers
Heliox is a mixture of the elements _____ and _____. The first root also means _____, which is evident in terms such as heliotropic and heliophobia.	**helium, oxygen sun**
The combining from for Selenium is SELENI/O. It is formed from the Greek root SELEN/O, which is used currently for _____ or _____, as in selenoid and geoselenic.	**moon, crescent-shaped**
The root in bromine literally means _____, which is the meaning used in terms such as bromhidrosis and bromomenorrhea.	**foul-smelling**
Stannosis is a condition associate with the element _____.	**tin**
Aurotherapy uses _____ to treat rheumatoid arthritis. The root is a homomorph, which has the additional meaning of _____ from the Latin word *auris*.	**gold, ear**
The cupric in cupric sulfate reveals that it is associated with _____.	**copper**
The root in ferritin reveals it is associate with _____.	**iron**
A person with hypernatremia has too much _____ in his or her blood.	**sodium**
In addition to referring to the element Krypton, the root in krypton, (usually as CRYPT-) also means _____ or _____.	**hidden, covered**
The combining forms that mean "color" are _____ and _____. CHROMI/O is used for the element _____.	**CHROM/O, CHROMAT/O Chromium**
The root in chlorine is associated with the color _____ and the root in rhodium is associated with color _____.	**green, red (rose)**
Osmiophobic is resistant to a stain with the element _____, osmophobia literally could pertain to a fear of _____.	**osmium, odor (smell)**
In addition to the element Actinium, the combining form means _____, _____, or _____, as in the words actinodermitis and actinomyces.	**ray, ray-like, radiation**
The root in Xenon literally means _____ or _____.	**foreign, strange**
Hyperkalemia is a condition that has too much _____ in the blood.	**Potassium**
The root in lithium means _____, as in the words rhinolith and lithotomy.	**stone**
The element named after the Roman messenger god is _____. The combining form used for this element is _____, which comes from the Latinized Greek word for liquid silver.	**Mercury, HYDRARGYR/O**
The combining form for the element silver is _____, which is formed from the Latin word for silver.	**ARGENT/O**
The root in the element Thallium's name also means_____, _____, or _____, as in heterothallic and merithallos.	**shoot, young branch, simple-plant**
The combining form for Phosphorus is _____; the combining form for Silicon is _____; and the combining form for Carbon is _____, which also means_____.	**PHOSPHOR/O, SILIC/O, CARB/O, carbon dioxide**
The etymology of the element Barium provides two commonly used combining forms BARY/O and BAR/O. The first combining form is used for _____ and _____, as in baryglossia and baryphonia. The second combining form is used for _____ and _____, as in barometer and barotitis.	**heavy, dull pressure, weight**
The combining form OX/O is used for _____. The root OXY- can be used for oxygen, acid, keen, and sharp.	**oxygen**
The combining form for Neon is NEON/O. The root in neon means _____ and _____, and is used in words such as neoplasm and neonatal.	**new, recent**
CALC/O is used for the element _____. It is a homograph, and therefore, it also can mean _____ from another Latin word.	**Calcium, heel**

Commonly Used Greek and Latin Word Elements in Chemical Terminology

In addition to the numbers and elements you have already learned, these word elements are used to explain chemical compounds and complexes, and they also can be found in medical terminology:

Greek or Latin word element	Current usage	Etymology	Examples
HEDR/O (hē-drō)	Side	Gr. *hedra*, side	Poly**hedr**al, dodecahedron
MER/O (mĕr-ō) **-MER** (mĕr) **-MERE** (mĕr)	Part, partial	Gr. *meros*, a part	**Mer**otomy, poly**mer**, blasto**mere**
GONI/O (gō-nē-ō) **GON/O** (go-nō) **-GON** (gon)	Angle	Gr. *gonia*, angle	**Goni**ometer, tri**gon**al, hexa**gon**
ERG/O (ĕr-gō) **-URGY** (ŭr-jē)	Work	Gr. *ergon*, work	Syn**erg**ic, metall**urgy**
PYR/O (pī-rō)	Fire, fever	Gr. *pyr*, fire, fever	**Pyr**ogen, **pyr**omania
HYGR/O (hī-grō)	Moisture, wet, humidity	Gr. *hygros*, wet	**Hygr**ometer, **hygr**ophilous
THERM/O (thĕr-mō) **-THERM** (thĕrm)	Heat, temperature	Gr. *thermos*, heat	**Therm**ometer, ecto**therm**
CALOR/O (kă-lo-rō) **CAL/O** (kă-lō)	Heat, calorie	L. *calor, caloris*, heat	**Calor**ic, trans**cal**ent
STOICHI/O (stoy-kē-ō)	Element	Gr. *stoicheion*, element	**Stoichi**ometry, **stoichi**ometric
PSYCHR/O (sī-krō)	Cold	Gr. *psychros*, cold	**Psychr**oalgia, **psychr**ophilic
XER/O (zer-ō)	Dry	Gr. *xeros*, dry	**Xer**oderma, **xer**ostomia
GE/O (jē-ō)	Earth, land	Gr. *ge*, earth	**Ge**obiology, apo**ge**otropic
AER/O (ĕ-rō)	Air	Gr. *aer*, air	An**aer**obic, **aer**obe
TOP/O (tō-pō) **-TOPE** (tōp)	Place	Gr. *topos*, place	**Top**ognosia, iso**tope**

Greek or Latin word element	Current usage	Etymology	Examples
TROP/O (trŏ-pō) **-TROPE** (trŏp)	Turn, change	Gr. *trope*, turn, change	Allo**trop**ic, somato**trope**
CIS/O (sīz-ō) **-CIDE** (sīd)	Cut, kill	L. *caedere, caesum*, to kill, cut	In**cis**ion, pisci**cide**
TRANS- (trans)	Across, through	L. *trans*, across	**Trans**ient, **trans**calent
CIS- (sĭs)	On this side	L. *cis*, on this side	**Cis**gender, **cis**platin
SESQUI- (sĕs-kwĭ)	One and a half	L. *sesqui*, one and a half	**Sesqui**hora, **sesqui**centennial
IS/O (ī-sō)	Equal	Gr. *isos*, equal	**Is**omer, **iso**tope
HOM/O (hŏm-ō)	Same	Gr. *homos*, like, same	**Hom**ograft, **hom**oblastic
HETER/O (hĕt-ĕr-ō)	Different from, other	Gr. *heteros*, other of two	**Heter**ogeneous, **heter**oalbumose
ENANTI/O (ĕn-ăn-tē-ō)	Opposite	Gr. *enanta*, opposite	**Enanti**omer, **enanti**omorph
ALL/O (al-ō)	Different, other, foreign	Gr. *allos*, other of a group	**All**omerism, **all**oantigen
NEUTR/O (nū-trō)	Neither, neutral	L. *neuter, neutra, neutrum*, neither	**Neutr**on, **neutr**ocytic
ELECTR/O (ĕ-lek-trō)	Electricity	Gr. *elektron*, amber	**Electr**ode, **electr**on
HOD/O (hō-dō) **OD/O** (ōd-ō) **-ODE** (ōd)	Road, path, traveling	Gr. *hodos*, road, path	**Hod**ograph, meth**od**, an**ode**
MOL/O (mōl-ō) **MOLECUL/O** (mŏ-lek-yŭ-lō)	Mass, mole Molecule	L. *moles*, a mass L. *molecula*, little mass	**Mol**ar, **mol**ecular Loan word **Mole** (mōl)
OSM/O (oz-mō)	Impulse, push, osmosis	Gr. *osmos*, impulse, push	**Osm**otic, **osm**osis
VAL/O (va-lō) or (vă-lō)	Strength	L. *valere*, to be strong	Co**val**ence, mono**val**ent
STERE/O (stĕr-ē-ō)	Solid, three-dimensional	Gr. *stereos*, solid	**Stere**oacuity, **stere**otropism

Review	Answers
The roots in proton, neutron, and electron meanings are correspondingly _____, _____, and _____.	**first, neither (neutral), electricity**
Stoichemetry literally means the measurement of _____.	**elements**
The suffix –mer means _____. Quite literally a polymer has _____ parts; an isomer has _____ parts; an enantiomer has _____ parts; an allomer has _____ parts; a homomer has the _____ parts.	**part (partial), many, equal, opposite, different (other), same**
OSM/O is a homomorph. One of the etymological meanings is _____ because it comes from the Greek word *osme*, and the other etymological meaning is _____ because it comes from the Greek word *osmos*.	**odor (smell) push (impulse, osmosis)**
The suffix in cathode and anode means _____, _____ or _____. The combining form is _____.	**road, path, traveling HOD/O**
An isomeric structure with the parts on "this side" would have the prefix _____ attached to the compound, and an isomeric structure with the parts being "across" from each other would use the prefix _____.	**CIS-, TRANS-**
A heterocyclic compound is a cyclic compound that has at least two different elements. The prefix HETERO- means _____, but it can also mean _____.	**different from, other**
According to Taber's, 1 mole of a substance contains as many atoms as exist in 0.012 kg of carbon 12. The original meaning of MOL/O is _____.	**mass**
By definition, a sequioxide is an oxide in which the oxygen is present in the ratio of three atoms to two of another element. The prefix SESQUI- indicates this because it means _____.	**one and a half**
Quite literally, a thermometer measures _____; a hygrometer measures _____; a psychrometer measures _____; and a xerometer measures _____.	**heat, humidity (moisture), cold, dry**
A hexagonic structure has six _____, but a hexaheronic structure has six _____.	**angles, sides**
Literally, a calorie is a unit of _____.	**heat**
The word stereoisomer refers to the spatial arrangement, since STERE/O means _____ or _____.	**solid, three-dimensional**
Based on its combining form and the ancient Greek theory of the four elements, geology is literally the study of _____; pyrology is literally the study of _____; aerology is literally the study of _____; and hydrology is literally the study of _____.	**earth, fire, air, water**
TROP/O and TOP/O are easily confused; TROP/O means _____, and _____. TOP/O means _____. TROP/O is also easily mistaken for TROPH/O, which means _____.	**turn, change place nourishment**
The suffix -URGY in metallurgy and the combining form ERG/O in ergonomics both come from the Greek word *ergon*, which means _____.	**work**
The valence is the property of an atom that allows it to combine in definite proportion with other atoms. The root in valence is _____, which means _____.	**VAL- strength**
The suffix in bactericide and acaricide means _____.	**kill (cut)**

Lessons from History: Ancient Greek Drugs and Modern Pharmaceutical Terminology

Food for Thought as You Read:

What makes something a drug? How do society and science affect what is and what is not considered a drug?

Based on various drugs being mentioned in Homer's *Odyssey*, it is quite clear that the medicinal use of plants and herbs extends as far back as the earliest Greek writings. Thus, Archaic Greek pharmacy appears to be a collection of plant lore derived from empirical evidence, as well as superstition. Beginning in the 5th- and 4th-century BC, philosophical and medical theories of the elements and qualities were used to explain some of the medicinal effects of these plants and herbs. Such medical materials were often referred to as ***pharmaka*** in medical and non-medical texts. Today, the roots from the Greek words *pharmakon* and *pharmakeutikos* are used for the combining forms meaning drug/medication, **PHARMAC-** and **PHARMACEUT-**. That said, what constituted a *pharmaka* (medications, drugs, and poison) in ancient Greek medical writings is quite different from our chemically derived drugs. Often this medical material could be considered both a food and a drug. For example, different wines were recommended as being a part of the person's diet, and these same wines are also found in lists of *materia medica* for their specific medicinal powers.

Furthermore, the term *pharmaka* was also used for toxic material derived from plants and animals. Writing in the 2nd-century BC, Nicander of Colophon composed two medical poems entitled *Theriaca* and *Alexipharmaca*. The former text deals with the poisons from animals. Hence, the title is derived from the Greek word for "wild beast," *therion*. He details the poisons of cobras, wasps, and centipedes. The latter text addresses antidotes to poisons. The work contains information on deadly plants such as aconite, which we recognize as a potent neurotoxin that can be fatal in two to six hours, and hemlock, which causes death via paralysis of respiratory muscles. One can surmise medical knowledge of antidotes and poisons would be highly valued by political figures, who lived in fear of being poisoned by their enemies.

In general, Greek *pharmaka* could be a simple or a compound medication. One of the most famous examples of a collection of simple medications is Dioscorides' *De materia medica*. Written in the 1st-century AD, *De materia medica* contains lists of medicinal properties for slightly more than 1,000 plants, minerals, and animals. These simple medications were organized according to medical material, which was mostly from the plant kingdom, and according to the type of *dynameis* (powers/properties) of the material (e.g. warming, mollifying, binding, drying, cleaning, making thin, cooling, concocting, etc.). For the plants, each entry more or less contains the following information: name of the plant, appearance, properties, medicinal usages, preparation, application, and storage. An example follows:

> Wild lettuce is similar to the cultivated, larger stalk; leaves: whiter, thinner, more rough, and bitter to taste. To some degree its properties are similar to those of opium poppy, thus some people mix its juice with opium. Whence its sap 2 obols [1.14 grams] in weight with sour wine purges away watery humors through the digestive tract; it cleans away abulgo [a white opacity of the cornea], misty eyes. It assists against burning [of the eyes] anointed on with woman's milk. Generally, it is sleep inducing and anodyne. It expels the menses; given in a drink for scorpion and venomous spider bites. The seeds, similar to that of cultivated kind, drunk avert dreams and sexual intercourse. Its juice produces the same things but with a weaker force. The sap extracted in an earth bowl, exposed to sunlight first as it were, and remaining juice stored.
>
> Translation John Riddle in *Dioscorides on Pharmacy and Medicine*. Austin: The University of Texas Press, 1985, 25.

These descriptions are informative but terse, and therefore, they are often lacking the kind of "how to" information necessary for anyone unfamiliar with the preparations of medications. According to Riddle, of the over 4,740 medicinal usages listed in this text, the scientific efficacies of these simple medicines varied from erroneous and purely speculative to uncertain or marginally effective in producing what was claimed. Some medicinal usages appear to be based on the appearance of the medical material. For instance, the hairy appearance of seahorses (hippocampi) appears to be the justification for using an ointment from this animal for alopecia. Some medicinal usages, such as white willow acting as a contraceptive, have been partially supported through modern scientific studies. Dioscorides' information for these medical materials is derived from (i) botanical writings, such as Theophrastus' (c. 371–c. 287 BC) *Enquiry into Plants*, (ii) medical texts, such Nicandor of Colophon's *Theriaca* and *Alexipharmaca*, (iii) the drug lore of "druggists" (*pharmakopolai*), "root cutters" (*rhizotomoi*), "ungent makers" (*myrepohoi*), "mixture sellers" (*migmatopolai*), and (iv) his own personal observations based on his travels.

The use of compound drugs, medicaments with identifiable recipes of ingredients from various *medica materia*, dates back to the Hippocratic Corpus. Most of these recipes can be found in the gynecological treatises of the Hippocratic Corpus and, in this early stage of their development, they are categorized primarily by their usage. An example of this from *Diseases of Women* (L. 8.172) is as follows:

> An agent to accelerate birth: take turpentine and honey, twice this amount of olive oil, and some very pleasant fragrant wine, mix together, warm, and give many times to drink; this will also settle the uterus if it is inflamed.
>
> Hippocrates, *Disease of Women I*, XI Loeb Classical Library, translation Paul Potter, 178–179. Cambridge: Harvard University Press, 2018.

Over time, large collections of recipes were gathered together and placed into written accounts by physicians. The purpose of these tomes of drug recipes may be dual in that they disseminated medical information as well as served as an advertisement of the expertise of the author in such matters. Some of the most influential collections of drug recipes were Galen's writings: *On the Composition of Medications According to Place*; *On the Composition of Medications According to Kind*; *On Antidotes*; and *On Theriac for Pison*. Galen's habit of systematizing previous medical knowledge according to recognizable categories led to his pharmaceutical works being influential on the ever-growing collections of medical recipes. What can be seen from Galen's writings is that many of these recipes became attached to famous physicians and political figures, which probably lent credibility to their readers' belief in these drugs' efficacies. The following recipe for alopecia is listed among those from Cleopatra's *Cosmetics*:

> Another [remedy against alopecia]. The power of this [remedy] is better than that of all the others, as it works also against falling hair and, mixed with oil or perfume, against incipient baldness and baldness of the crown; and it works wonders. One part of burnt domestic mice, one part of burnt remnants of vine, one part of burnt horse teeth, one part of bear fat, one part of deer marrow, one part of reed bark. Pound them dry, then add a sufficient amount of honey until the thickness of the honey is convenient, and then dissolve the fat and the marrow, knead and mix them. Place the remedy in a copper box. Rub the alopecia until new hair grows back. Similarly, falling hair should be anointed every day.
>
> Galen, *Composition of Medicines According to Places* 1.2, K. 12.404, Translation Laurence Totelin, "Cold, Dry, and Bald," *The Recipes Project*, https://recipes.hypotheses.org/.

While its association with a legendary figure in cosmetics would have made this recipe for alopecia attractive, its ingredients are not devoid of qualities that ancients would have found to have effects on hair growth. As Totelin points out, one could go further than the perceived effects of the warm and moistening qualities of the ingredients in this medication to understand its rationale for its use on baldness; it may extend to the notion of the effects on plants due to the qualities of the seasons being associated with similar effects on hair loss and growth (i.e. Fall is cold/dry = leaves falling/grass dying; Spring is warm/wet = leaves and grass growing). Based on Galen's writings, one can observe that the philosophical rationale behind the different ingredients in these recipes may lie in the modification and additions of the specific powers (*dynameis*) of the ingredients. In other words, if one desired the strong emetic effect of one medical material, but not its excessively cold quality, one would add a warm ingredient to diminish the intensity of the cooling ingredient. Likewise, if one wanted to add an antidote quality to this emetic, one would add an ingredient with the appropriate antidote faculty. Today, thanks to Galen's influential writings, medicines composed of herbs and vegetables that are prepared according to an official formula are referred to as **Galenics** or **Galenicals**.

One of the most sought-after compound drugs in the history of medicine is a drug called Mithridatum. Its name had a strong influence on the centuries of belief in its medicinal efficacy. Mithridatum is named after the famous King of Pontus on the Black Sea, Mithridates VI (120–63 BC). Much like Attalus III of Pergamum (ruled 138–133 BC), Mithridates allegedly carried out pharmacological experiments on prisoners to determine the efficacy of various poisons. Through these means and through physician knowledge of *medica materia*, Mithridates was said to have developed a compound drug that contained all known antidotes to all poisons. He would take an almond-sized portion of this antidote on a daily basis to make himself immune to being poisoned. According to Roman legend, Mithridates was so accustomed to taking this antidote that, when he was facing defeat at the hands of the Roman general Pompey, he had to commit suicide by the sword because he unfortunately had made himself immune to poison. Based on this legend, a wide variety of recipes were lauded as the actual ingredients of Mithridates' antidote. In Book V of *De Medicina* (V.23.3), Celsus provides one of the earliest accounts of the ingredients of Mithridatum:

> But the most famous antidote is that of Mithridates, which that king is said to have taken daily and by it to have rendered his body safe against danger from poison. It contains costmary 1.66 grams, sweet flag 20 grams, hypericum, gum, sagapenum, acacia juice, Illyrian iris, cardamon, 8 grams each, anise 12 grams, Gallic nard, gentian root and dried rose-leaves, 16 grams each, poppy-tears and parsley, 17 grams each, casia, saxifrage, darnel, long pepper, 20.66 grams each, storax 21 grams, castoreum, frankincense, hypocistis juice, myrrh and opopanax, 24 grams each, malabathrum leaves 24 grams, flower of round rush, turpentine-resin, galbanum, Cretan carrot seeds, 24.66 grams each, nard and opobalsam, 25 grams each, shepherd's purse 25 grams, rhubarb root 28 grams,

saffron, ginger, cinnamon, 29 grams each. These are pounded and taken up in honey. Against poisoning, a piece the size of an almond is given in wine. In other affections, an amount corresponding in size to an Egyptian bean is sufficient."

Celsus, *De medicina*, II. Loeb Classical Library, translation W. G. Spencer, 56–57. Cambridge: Harvard University Press, 1953.

In addition to having ingredients such as castoreum and opium that have recognizable medicinal effects, the litany of different exotic medical materials in Mithridatum made this an expensive drug, which undoubtedly also added to the belief in its medicinal value. The actual ingredients of Mithridates' antidote varied considerably from author to author. Over time, a wide variety of drug recipes became known as Mithridatum. At first, Mithridatum was considered strictly an antidote for all poisons; over time, it became used as a drug for a wide variety of illnesses, a kind of **panacea** (Gr. *panakes*, pan-all + *akos* cure). Today, immunity to a poison that is acquired by taking it in gradually increasing doses is referred to as **Mithridatism**.

Unlike in antiquity, the names of the drugs today are highly regulated. A medication will have three names: **chemical name**, **generic name**, and a **trade/brand name**. The chemical name is written according to the drug's chemical structure. The generic name is the nonproprietary name of a drug, and it is based on one or more of the chemicals in the drug. The brand name is the drug manufacture's trademarked name for a drug. For example, the three names for Valium are as follows:

Chemical: 7-chloro-1, 3-dihydro-1-methyl-5-phenyl-2H-1,4-benzodiazepin-2-one.
Generic: Diazepam
Brand: Valium

Similar to Mithridatum, the brand name of a modern drug affects the perception of the medication's effectiveness. This is why pharmaceutical companies spend quite a lot of money finding a name that will suggest its usage without jeopardizing the nonpropriety name being approved by the FDA. Surprisingly, Latin or Greek word elements are often used in these names:

Valium: used to treat anxiety disorders (L. *Vale* = Farewell)
Paxil: an antidepressant and antianxiety drug (L. *Pax* = Peace)
Lunesta: a sleeping medication (L. *Luna* = Moon)
Viagra: A medication for erectile dysfunction (L. *Vir* = Man + L. *Agra* = fertile or farmed land in Latin and Greek)

Some Suggested Readings

Dioscorides. *De Materia Medica*. Third Edition. Translated by Lily Beck. New York: Greg Olms Verlag, 2017.

Riddle, John. *Dioscorides on Pharmacy and Medicine*. Austin: The University of Texas Press, 1985.

Scarborough, John. *Pharmacy and Drug Lore in Antiquity: Greece, Rome, Byzantium*. Vermont: Ashgate Publishing, 2010.

Totelin, Laurence. "Mithradates' Antidote: A Pharmacological Ghost." *Early Science and Medicine* 9, no. 1 (2004): 1–19.

Totelin, Laurence. *Hippocratic Recipes: Oral and Written Transmission of Pharmacological Knowledge in Fifth- and Fourth-Century Greece*. Leiden: Brill, 2009.

The Recipes Project, https://recipes.hypotheses.org/.

Etymological Explanations: The Abbreviations and Symbols Used in Prescriptions

Rx is the symbol for the modern **prescription** (Fig. 5.8). The symbol Rx is an abbreviation of the Latin second-person singular imperative *recipe*, which means "take." *Recipe* was once the word written by physicians at the head of medical prescriptions. In the early 1800s, the word "recipe" came to mean "instructions for preparing food." Today, the symbol Rx retains the original medical meaning of *recipe*. The modern medical prescription is a written direction by a physician for dispensing and administering a medication. The prescription will identify the name, strength, and quantity of the drug to be provided to the patient. The **Signa**, or **Sig.**, of the prescription provides specific instructions for the

NAME ___Ima En Pain___ AGE __41__
ADDRESS _____ DATE 11/11/20

DIRECTIONS:

Rx Vicoden 20 mg/40 tbs
     Sig: i tab. p.o. q4h prn mild pain,
     or ii tab. p.o. q4h prn moderate pain

_____
SIGNATURE

Fig. 5.8 Sample of abbreviations used in prescriptions.

administration of the medication. Signa is another second-person singular imperative that comes from the Latin verb *signare*, which means "to indicate."

Most of the contractions and abbreviations that appear in the instructions of modern prescriptions are derived from Latin words and phrases. Many of these go back to the abbreviations used in medieval manuscripts. Medieval scribes would shorten the spelling of common Latin words to save transcription space and work. Symbols such as "-," "~," were added above a letter to indicate it is a shortened word (e.g. ā). By the 18th century, the growing movement for the use of national languages in science greatly reduced the amount of medical material written in Latin. As medico-scientific authors increasingly turned to their respective vernacular to express their ideas, Latin began to function less as a language and more as a code for technical phrases in medicine, such as *nihil per os* (**NPO** = nothing by mouth) and *bis in die* (**BID** = twice a day). Today's medical terminology, particularly for prescriptions of medication, makes frequent use of these Latin phrases via abbreviations and symbols.

In addition to abbreviations, some of the symbols used in medicine have classical origins. The symbol ϴ used today for "none or negative" is derived from the ancient symbol called the *theta nigrum* (black theta) or the *theta infelix* (unfortunate theta), which was a symbol of death in Greek and Latin epigraphy (Fig. 5.9). The use of the Greek letter "theta" signified the Greek word *thanatos* (death), and it is commonly used in images of gladiatorial battles to indicate the outcome of the battle. Likewise, the symbols for female and male, respectively ♀ and ♂, are the astrological symbols for the planets Venus and Mars. The symbol for Venus (♀) is said to represent a hand mirror since Venus is a goddess of physical beauty. The symbol for Mars (♂) represents a shield and spear, owing to its association with the god of war.

The following is a list of some of the common abbreviations used in prescriptions and medical notes:

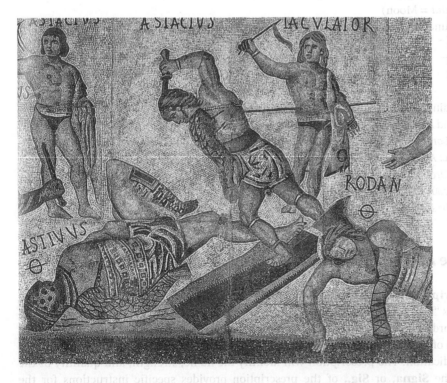

Fig. 5.9 The *theta nigrum* in a 4th-century AD gladiatorial scene from a mosaic in the Villa Borghese. *Source:* Storiaviva Viaggi Tour Operator/Wikimedia Commons/ Public domain.

Abbreviation	Latin	Current Meaning
p.o.	*per os*	Through the mouth; orally
SL	*sub linguam*	Sublingual
PR	*per rectum*	Through the rectum; rectally
PV	*per vaginam*	Through the vagina; vaginally
ID		Intradermal
IM		Intramuscular
IV		Intravenous
SC (Sub-Q)		Subcutaneous
ad	*ad*	To, up to
ad lib.	*ad libitum*	At pleasure (as desired)
alt.h.	*alternis hora*	Every other hour
ā	*ante*	Before
a.c.	*ante cibum*	Before food
a.m.	*ante meridiem*	Before midday (morning)
aq.	*aqua*	Water
aur.; a	*auris*	Ear
a.d.	*auris dextra*	Right ear
a.s.	*auris sinistra*	Left ear
a.u.	*auris utraque*	Each ear
bis	*bis*	Twice
b.i.d.	*bis in die*	Twice a day
c̄	*cum*	With
c.c.	*cum cibo*	With food
d	*dies*	Day
d/c		Discharge, discontinue
Dx	*diagnosis*	Diagnosis
et	*et*	And
h.	*hora*	Hour
h.s.	*hora somni*	Hour of sleep (at bedtime)
noc.	*nocte*	At night
NPO	*nihil per os*	Nothing by mouth
o.d.	*oculus dexter*	Right eye
o.s.	*oculus sinister*	Left eye
o.u.	*oculus uterque*	Each eye (both)
o.m.	*omni mane*	Every morning
o.n.	*omni nocte*	Every night
p̄	*post*	After
per	*per*	Through
p.c.	*post cibum*	After meal
p.m.	*post meridiem*	After midday (i.e. afternoon)
p.r.n.	*pro re nata*	Under the present circumstance (i.e. as needed)
q	*quaque*	Every

Abbreviation	Latin	Current Meaning
q.d. (q.2d., q.3d.)	*quaque die*	Every day (every two days, every three days)
q.h. (q.2h, q.3h.)	*quaque hora*	Every hour (every two hours, every three hours)
q.i.d.	*quarter in die*	Four times a day
R_x	*recipe*	Prescription
s̄	*sine*	Without
s̄s̄	*semis*	One half
S, Sig.	*Signa*	Indicate (on label)
stat.	*statim*	Immediately
t.i.d.	*ter in die*	Three times a day
ut dict.; u.d.	*ut dictum*	As directed

Translate the following prescriptions. Bear in mind the following drug abbreviations: tab. = tablet; cap. = capsule; SUP = suppository; gt = drop (L. *gutta*); gtt = drops (L. *guttae*). Roman numerals are often in the lower case when they appear in scripts. Indication of the duration of days is typically written with X before an Arabic number (e.g. X 5 d = for five days):

Review	Answers
Vicodin, ii tab p.o. q3h prn mild pain	**Vicodin, two tablets by mouth, every three hours, as needed for mild pain**
Ducolax, SUP. iv PR o.m. u.d.	**Ducolax, suppository four through the rectum every morning, as directed**
Lunestra 3 mg p.o. h.s. prn sleep	**Lunestra, 3 mg by mouth, at bedtime, as needed for sleep**
cap. ii STAT, then i q6h	**Two capsules immediately, then one every six hours**
gtt iii a.u. noc. ad lib.	**Three drops each ear, as desired**
V-Go inject SC i qd u.d.	**V-Go subcutaneous injection one daily, as directed**
i SL tid p.c. X 6 d	**One under the tongue, three times a day, after meals, for six days**

Convert the following into the appropriate abbreviations:

Review	Answers
Two suppositories through the vagina at bedtime	ii SUP, PV h.s.
Four drops in the left eye every four hours	iv gtt o.s. q4h
Two capsules by mouth three times a day for seven days	ii cap. p.o. t.i.d. X 7 d
Two by mouth every other hour with food	ii p.o. alt.h. c.c.
One liter intravenous immediately, then 50 ml every six hours	i L IV stat., then 50 ml q6h
Three tablets by mouth two times a day, morning and evening	iii tab. p.o. b.i.d., a.m. and p.m.
Intradermal injection every night without alcohol	ID inject qnoc s̄ ETOH

Unit II

Body Systems

6

Integumentary System

CHAPTER LEARNING OBJECTIVES

3) In this chapter, you will learn the Greek and Latin word elements for the anatomy, physiology, pathologies, and surgical interventions that pertain to the integumentary system.
4) You will also become familiar with the ancient Greek concepts of skin and its role in society, as well as ancient Greek classifications and treatments of skin lesions.

Lessons from History: Ancient and Modern Concepts of Skin and Its Appendages

Food for Thought as You Read:

How are ancient and modern concepts of skin similar? How are they different?

Skin is considered the largest organ in the body. On average, skin weighs about eight pounds, and its area is roughly 20 sq ft. As an organ, the skin serves a number of important functions: it is our 1st defense against infection; it acts as a water barrier; it regulates our body temperature; and it enables our sensations of touch, heat, and cold. Skin (L. *cutis, -is*) is composed of three different layers: the **epidermis** (L. *epidemis, -is*), **dermis** (L. *dermis, -is*), and **hypodermis** (L. *hypodermis, -is*). The lowest part of the epidermis, the *stratum basale*, is where the cells known as **melanocytes** create our skin tones via the production of a pigment known as **melanin**. The **dermis** (L. *dermis, -is*), also known as the **corium** (L. *corium, -i*), contains blood capillaries, nerve endings, hair follicles, and sweat and sebaceous glands. The layer of connective tissue and fat immediately under the dermis is known as the **hypodermis** or the **subcutaneous layer** (*subcutis, -is*). It functions as a place to store fat, as well as the layer that connects the skin to the flesh and bones of the body. Skin is the primary part of the **integumentary system**, the other parts being the **nails** (L. *unguis, -is*), **hair** (L. *pilus, -i*), the **sebaceous glands** (L. *glandula sebacea, glandulae sebaceae*), **sweat glands** (L. *glandula sudorifera, glandulae sudoriferae*), and **fat** (L. *adeps, adipis*).

The term "skin" is derived from an old Norse word for "animal hide." Likewise, the ancient Greek word *derma, dermatos* referred to "human skin, animal hides, and the leather used for shields and bags." It was derived from the Greek verb *derein*, "to skin or flay." The use of *derma* for animal and human skin extends back to Homer's *Iliad* and *Odyssey* (c. 8th–7th century BC). In the Hippocratic Corpus, *derma* continued to be used for "human skin." Similar to the Greek word *derma*, the Latin words *pellis*, *corium*, and *cutis* also referred to "human skin, animal hide, and leather." Among ancient physicians, there was no universally accepted technical distinction between these words, and, therefore, they were used somewhat interchangeably.

As to the nature and origin of skin, some Greek medico-philosophical authors considered skin to have been formed from the element "earth." Of the four classical elements (i.e. earth, water, air, fire), the earth was considered to be dry in nature. In his *On the Generation of Animals* (782a-b), Aristotle had the following to say about the formation of skin:

> In general, the nature of skin (derma) is fundamentally earthy. Being on the surface, skin becomes solid and earthy as the water evaporates from it. Hair (thrix) and its analogs do not arise from flesh (sarx) but from the skin as the water evaporates and exhales in the hair.

Greek and Latin Roots of Medical and Scientific Terminologies, First Edition. Todd A. Curtis.
© 2025 John Wiley & Sons, Inc. Published 2025 by John Wiley & Sons, Inc.
Companion website: www.wiley.com/go/Curtis

Aristotle's distinction between flesh and skin in the above passage seems to be based on the theory that structures of the body are different from each other due to the combination of elemental qualities that formed them. In the case of skin, it is earthier in nature because the element, earth, creates its primary quality of "dryness." As can be observed in the above passage, the Greek word for "skin," *derma, dermatos*, was contrasted with the word for "flesh," *sarx, sarkos*. The same distinction can be seen in Roman authors' usages of the Latin words *cutis, -is* (skin) and *caro, carnis* (flesh).

In his *On the Generation of Animals*, Aristotle went on to explain how hair (*thrix, trichos*) and its analogs were formed from the skin. By "analogs," Aristotle was referring to spines, feathers, and the scales of animals. For Aristotle, hair formation was dependent on the presence of heat and water, and correspondingly, a lack of hair or baldness was associated with cold and dry conditions. The correlation between the nature of skin and the nature of hair is quite evident in many of Aristotle's explanations for the different features of hair. For example, he states that thick hair comes from thick skin, and thin hair comes from thin skin. If the skin should be more porous and thicker, the hairs will be thick because of the abundance of earthy substances and on account of the large size of the pores in the skin. The reverse is true for thin-haired animals and people. Although Aristotle's theory that skin and its analogs are formed from earth has been disproven, modern science does reveal that the outer layer of skin, as well as the appendages of hair, nails, feathers, hooves, and talons, do indeed share a common "substance" in that they are formed by the protein "keratin."

In addition to skin serving as a removable covering over the flesh, ancient Greek philosophers and physicians associated the sense of touch with the skin. This theoretical position can be found in the medical writings of Galen. In his *On Mixtures* (*De temperamentis*, K. 1.563-68), Galen claims that the ideal mixture of elemental qualities that comprise human *derma*, particularly the skin of the palm and fingers of the hand, make this *derma* an organ (Gr. *organon*) perfectly suited for the sense of touch. From Galen onward, skin was considered by physicians as an organ of touch. However, Galen's conception of an *organon* differs from our modern understanding of an organ. Galen was unable to see the different tissues that make up the structure and determine the functions of organs. Today, a bodily **organ** (**ORGAN-**) is defined as "a distinct structure made of several tissues that all contribute to specific functions." By using the Greek word *organon*, Galen was likening skin to a "tool or instrument used for making or doing something." This etymology explains why the ancient musical instrument called the *hydraulis* was also called an *organon*. Created by the Hellenistic engineer Ctesibius of Alexandria (285–222 BC), the *hydraulis* was a musical instrument that is recognized as the ancient origin of our modern church organ (Fig. 6.1).

In Galen's *The Use of the Parts* (*De usu partium* K. III.14–18), which is a text that he wrote to describe the purposes of the parts of the human body, Galen argues that the human fingernail (Gr. *onyx, onychos*) is a part that reveals how the human hand was uniquely designed by Nature for decidedly human activities (e.g. writing, sculpting, etc.). He claims that human fingernails give structure to the softer and more deformable flesh of the fingers. He claims that the combination of soft flesh and hard nails makes the fingers well suited to gripping small, hard objects. Galen goes on to say that the length and shape of human fingernails are important to the function of human prehension, which is why human fingernails should

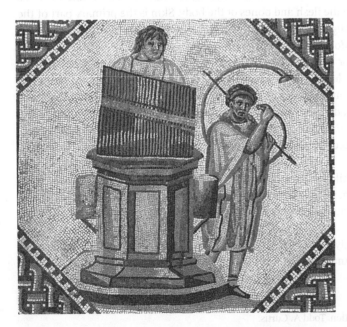

Fig. 6.1 Image of a 3rd century AD Roman mosaic of a hydraulis (Gr. *hydor*, water + *aulos*, pipe instrument) found at Nennig, Germany. *Source:* TimeTravelRome/Wikimedia Commons/CC BY 2.0.

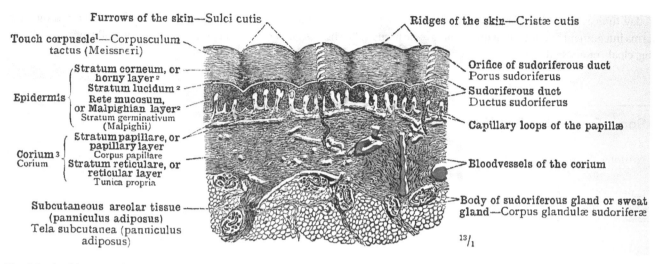

Furrows of the skin—Sulci cutis

Ridges of the skin—Cristæ cutis

Touch corpuscle[1]—Corpusculum tactus (Meissneri)

Epidermis { Stratum corneum, or horny layer[2] / Stratum lucidum[2] / Rete mucosum, or Malpighian layer[2] / Stratum germinativum (Malpighii)

Corium[3] Corium { Stratum papillare, or papillary layer / Corpus papillare / Stratum reticulare, or reticular layer / Tunica propria

Subcutaneous areolar tissue (panniculus adiposus) Tela subcutanea (panniculus adiposus)

Orifice of sudoriferous duct Porus sudoriferus

Sudoriferous duct Ductus sudoriferus

Capillary loops of the papillæ

Bloodvessels of the corium

Body of sudoriferous gland or sweat gland—Corpus glandulæ sudoriferæ

13/1

Fig. 6.2 In this anatomical image of the layers of the skin, note that the corium is associated with bottom two layers of the epidermis. *Source:* Carl Toldt et al. 1919/Rebman Company/Public domain.

not be too long, like the claws or talons of animals. As to the modern understanding of the function of fingernails, scientists consider the broad and flat shape of human fingernails to be a distinct feature of primates that evolved for the purpose of grasping smaller objects. While Galen's understanding of the function of human nails is similar to a modern understanding of their function, Galen's conception of what determined the formation of human fingernails has little to do with the evolutionary theories used in modern biology. Galen describes Nature (*Physis*) in terms of a divine creator, which Galen often likens to a Demiurge (craftsman). Nature created the different features of the animal bodies to meet the unique purposes of their souls. While Galen suggests that humans are a type of animal, Galen believes that the soul of a human is distinct from other animals due to its intelligence and divine nature.

With the discovery of the layers of skin, Greek and Latin words for articles of clothing and woven material came to be commonly used in science and medicine for the naming of new structures of the integumentary system. The recognition that skin is composed of multiple layers began with the advent of the microscope. The famous Italian biologist and physician, Marcello Malpighi (1628–1694), made extensive use of the microscope in his research on human, animal, and plant anatomy. In Malpighi's *De externo tractus organo anatomica observatio* (*Anatomical Observation of the External Organ of Touch*), which was published in 1665, he discovered a layer that gave pigment to the skin. He called this layer the *rete mucosum* (mucous net), which is the layer we currently call *stratum basale* or the "Malpighian layer." By the term *rete*, which is a Latin word for a "net" or "web," Malpighi conceptualized the layer of skin as "woven material." This became the basis for many of the subsequent terms used for layers of skin or tissues (Fig. 6.2). Karl Mayer's *Ueber Histologie und eine neue Eintheilung der Gewebe des menschlichen Koerpers* (*Concerning Histology and a New Classification of the Tissue of Human Bodies*), which was published in 1819, was the first text that used the term "histology" for "the study of tissues." In so doing, Karl drew from the thesaurus of Greek words to find a suitable technical term for this new field of study. He chose the Greek word *histos* because it meant a "web" or "something woven," and therefore, it had a similar meaning to the German word *Gewebe* (fabric, tissue) and the French word *Tissu* (fabric, tissue), which were vernacular words for tissue. The Latin word *tela*, which originally meant "that which is woven," became the anatomical Latin term for "tissue." The Latin word *tunica* was used for a short-sleeved garment often worn under a Roman's toga (Fig. 6.3).

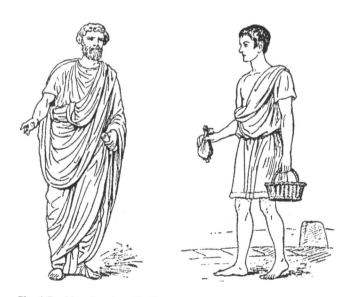

Fig. 6.3 Line drawing of a Roman toga (left) and a tunica (right). *Source:* John Williamson / Wikimedia commons / Public domain.

Today, tunica is used for "a layer or coat of tissue." In the late 1600s, the term *integumentum*, from which we derive our modern terms integument and integumentary, came to be used for "skin." *Integumentum* is a Latin word that originally meant a "covering, cloak, or a disguise".

Some Suggested Readings

Aristotle. *Generation of Animals.* Translated by Arthur L. Peck. Loeb Classical Library 366. Cambridge: Harvard University Press, 1942.

Galen. *Galen and the Usefulness of the Parts of the Body.* Volume 2. Translated by Margaret T. May. Ithaca: Cornell University Press, 1968.

Etymological Explanations: Common Terms and Word Elements for the Anatomy of the Integumentary System

In the following discussion of the anatomical terms associated with the integumentary system (Figs. 6.4 and 6.5), the nominative and genitive singular forms of the anatomical Latin term are provided in parenthesis. The Greek and Latin roots are formatted in all caps and emboldened.

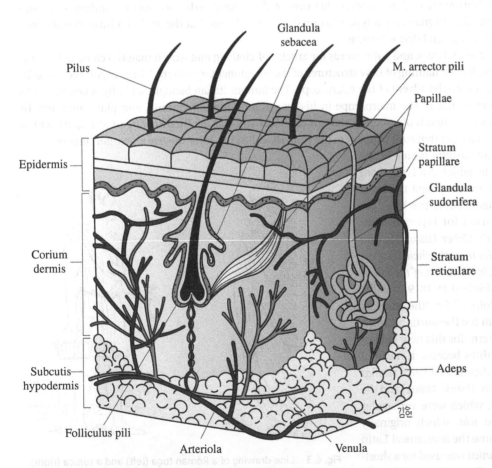

Fig. 6.4 Anatomical Latin terms for skin. *Source:* Chloe Kim.

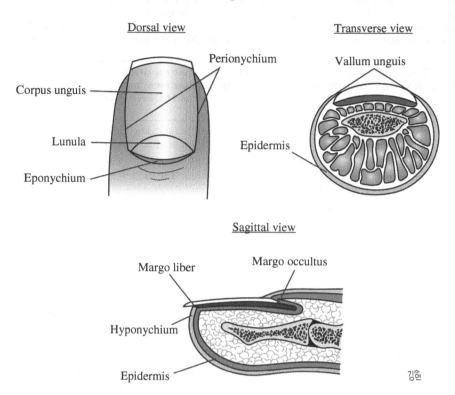

Fig. 6.5 Anatomical Latin terms for the nail (unguis). *Source:* Line drawing by Chloe Kim.

Skin

Skin or Cutis (L. *cutis, -is*) – Skin, also known as the **cutis**, is composed of three different layers: the **epidermis** (L. *epidemis, -is*), **dermis** (L. *dermis, -is*), and **hypodermis** (L. *hypodermis, -is*). The roots **CUT-** and **CUTANE-**, as well as the Latin loan word cutis, refer to "the whole skin, i.e. the dermis and epidermis." The Latin root **PELL-** from *pellis* is also used for "skin" and appears in a collection of medico-scientific terms such as pellagra, apellous, and pellicle. The Greek roots for "skin," **DERM-** and **DERMAT-**, can also refer specifically to the layer of skin called the dermis. Today, as a loan word, **derma** and its anatomical Latin derivative **dermis** refer to the aforementioned layer of the skin.

Epidermis (L. *epidermis, -is*) – The outermost layer of skin is called the epidermis. It derives its name from its position; it sits upon the layer of the "true skin," known as the dermis. The epidermis has five layers, or **strata**, which are from deepest to most superficial, the *stratum basale* (basilar layer), *stratum spinosum* (spiny layer), *stratum granulosum* (granular layer), *stratum lucidum* (clear layer), and *stratum corneum* (horn-like layer). **STRAT-** is the root for "stratum" or "anything that spread out." The lowest part of the epidermis, the *stratum basale*, is where the cells known as melanocytes create our skin tones via the production of a pigment known as **melanin**. In dermatological nomenclature, the root **MELAN-** stands for "melanocyte" or "black."

Dermis (L. *dermis, -is*) or Corium (L. *corium, -i*) – The dermis contains blood capillaries, nerve endings, hair follicles, and sweat and sebaceous glands. Corium originally meant "hide," but it has acquired a technical meaning in modern medicine, specifically referring to "the layer of skin called the dermis." However, the root **CORI-** is also often used nonspecifically for "skin."

Hypodermis (L. *hypodermis, -is*) –The layer of connective tissue and fat immediately under the dermis is known as the hypodermis or the **subcutaneous layer** (L. *tela subcutanea*). It functions as a place to store fat, as well as the layer that connects the skin to the flesh and bones of the body.

Nails (L. *unguis, -is*) – The finger and toe nails are appendages of the skin. The root **ONYCH-** is used for "fingernails, toenails, talons, claws, and hooves." Similarly, its Latin synonym, **UNGU-**, is used today for "fingernails, toenails, talons, claws, and hooves." The anatomical Latin term for the nail is **unguis**. The tissue around the human fingernail is called the **perionychium**. The thickened layer of skin at the base of the nail is called the **eponychium**. The **hyponychium** is the skin just under the free edge of the nail. The crescent-shaped area of nailbed growth is called the **lunula** (L. *lunula, -ae*, little moon). The "body of the nail" is the *corpus unguis*. The free border of the nail is the *margo liber*, and the covered border is the *margo occultus*.

Hair (L. *pilus*, *-i*) – The Greek root **TRICH-** and the loan word **thrix** are used today for "hair" (e.g. thrix, endothrix, and trichosis). The Latin synonym for *thrix* is *pilus*. The Latin root **PIL-** and the loan word **pilus** are also commonly used for "hair" in modern medical and scientific terminology (e.g. pilus incarnates, pilifer, pilomotor). A small sac-like structure containing hair that is located in the dermis is called a **follicle**. Derived from the Latin word for a bag, *follis*, the root **FOLLICUL-** typically refers to a "hair follicle" but it can also mean "little bag."

Keratin – The protein keratin gives hair and nails structural strength. The term "keratin" comes from the Greek word for "horn," *keras, keratos*. The root **KERAT-** (also spelled **CERAT-**) is used in modern medico-scientific language for a "horn," "horn-like substance," or the "cornea." The Latin synonym for *keras* is *cornu*, which explains why the Latin roots **CORNE-/CORN-** are also used today for "horn," "horn-like structure," and the "cornea."

Oil gland or Sebaceous Gland (L. *glandula sebacea*, *glandulae sebaceae*) – The oil glands of the skin are called sebaceous glands, which are located in the dermis. The combining forms used for "sebum," which is the oily substance secreted by the sebaceous glands, are **SEB-**, **STEAT-**, and **STEAR-**.

Sweat gland (L. *glandula sudorifera*, *glandulae sudoriferae*) – Sudor is the loan word for sweat. The sudoriferous glands of the skin are located in the dermis. The combining forms for sweat are **HIDR-**, **SUD-**, and **SUDOR-**.

Fat (L. *adeps, adipis*) – The anatomical Latin term for fat is *adeps*. Based on its root, adipose tissue is full of fat cells. The roots for "fat" are **LIP-**, **ADIP-**, **STEAR-**, and **STEAT-**.

Flesh and tissue

Flesh (L. *caro, carnis*) – The Greek word *sarx*, and the Latin *caro* are synonyms meaning "flesh, muscles, or the inner fleshy part of fruit." The roots from *sarx, sarkos*, and *caro, carnis* (i.e. **SARC-** and **CARN-**) are still used in modern medicine for "flesh" and "muscle" (e.g. carnivore, sarcomere). The roots **CRE-** and **CREAT-**. Today, skin is considered an organ of the integumentary system, and "flesh" is defined as "the soft tissue of the body, particularly the muscles, between the skin and bones."

Tissue (L. *tela, -ae*) – The Greek roots **HIST-** and **HISTI-** are commonly used for "tissue" in modern medicine. The anatomical Latin term for tissue is *tela*, and the loan word for a layer of tissue is **tunica**. Tissue is defined today as "a collection of similar cells and their intercellular substances that perform a specific function."

Epithelium (L. *epithelium, -i*) – One of the most etymologically peculiar terms associated with skin is the word epithelium, which is from the Greek *epi*, which means "on top of," and *thele*, which means "nipple." As to the origin of the term epithelium, Frederick Ruysch introduced the term "epithelium" in his *Thesaurus Anatomicus*, which was published in 1703. Ruysch used the term epithelium to describe a coating, which he discovered in various parts of the body. Because the coating was associated with microscopic nipple-like structures he called it epithelium as well as the *tunica papillosa*. The Latin adjective *papillosa*, is derived from the Latin word for "nipple," *papilla*. Following the influence of Ruysch's terminology, the terms endothelium and mesothelium were later coined. Today, the roots **THEL-** and **PAPILL-** are commonly used for "a nipple or a nipple-like structure," and likewise papilla is used for "nipple," particularly the nipple-like structures of the corium that indent into the epidermis. There are different types of epithelial cells. Epithelium derived from embryonic mesenchymal cells is termed **mesothelium**. It is the serous epithelia that forms the lining of several body cavities: pleura, peritoneum, mediastinum, and pericardium. The squamous epithelium-like tissue that lines the inside of blood and lymphatic vessels, the heart, as well as various other body cavities, is called the **endothelium**. It differs from epithelium in that it is derived from **mesoderm**; epithelium is derived from **ectoderm** and **endoderm**. The terms ectoderm, mesoderm, and endoderm refer to the germ layers of the embryo.

Greek or Latin word element	Current usage	Etymology	Examples
CUT/O (kū-tō)	Skin	L. *cutis, -is*, f. skin, hide	**Cuticle, trans**cutane**ous**
CUTANE/O (kū-tā-nē-ō)			Loan word: **Cutis** (kūt′ĭs) pl. **Cutes** (kūt′ēz″)
DERM/O (dĕr-mō)	Skin	L. *dermis, -is*, f. dermis fr. Gr. *derma, dermatos*, skin	Ecto**derm, derma**tocele
DERMAT/O (dĕr-mă-tō)			Loan word: **Dermis** (dĕr′mĭs) pl. **Dermes** (dĕr′mēz″)
-DERM (dĕrm)			

Greek or Latin word element	Current usage	Etymology	Examples
CORI/O (kŏ-rē-ō)	Skin, dermis	L. *corium*, *-i*, n. hide, skin	Ex**cori**ation, **cori**aceous Loan word: **Corium** (kŏ′rē-ŭm) pl. **Coria** (kŏ′rē-ă)
PELL/O (pĕ-lō)	Skin	L. *pellis*, *-is*, f. hide, skin	**Pell**agroid, **pell**agra
SARC/O (săr-kō)	Flesh, muscle	Gr. *sarx*, *sarkos*, flesh, fleshy pulp of fruit	**Sarc**oadenoma, **sarc**oma
CARN/O (kar-nō)	Flesh	L. *caro*, *carnis*, f. flesh, fleshy pulp of fruit	**Carn**ophobia, **carn**ivore
CRE/O (krē-ō) **CREAT/O** (krē-ăt-ō)	Flesh, muscle	Gr. *kreas*, *kreatos*, flesh, muscle	**Cre**osote, **creat**ine
HISTI/O (hĭs-tē-ō) **HIST/O** (hĭs-tō)	Tissue	Gr. *histion*, web, sail	**Histi**ocyte, **hist**oblast
STRAT/O (stră-tō)	Layer	L. *stratum*, *-i*, n. covering fr. L. *sternere*, to spread out	**Strat**ify, **strat**ification Loan word: **Stratum** (strat′ŭm) pl. **Strata** (strat′ă)
THEL/O (thē-lō) **-THELE** (thē-lē)	Nipple, nipple-like structure	Gr. *thele*, nipple	Epi**thel**ium, neuro**thele**
PAPILL/O (pap-ĭ-lō)	Nipple, nipple-like structure	L. *papilla*, *-ae*, f. nipple	**Papill**oma, **papill**iform Loan word: **Papilla** (pă-pil′ă) pl. **Papillae** (pă-pil′ē″)
KERAT/O (kĕr-ăt-ō) **CERAT/O** (sĕr-ăt-ō)	Horn, hard, horn-like, keratin, cornea	Gr. *keras*, *keratos*, horn	**Kerat**ocele, **cerat**otome
CORNE/O (kor-nē-ō) **CORN/O** (kor-nō)	Horn, hard, horn-like, cornea	L. *cornu*, *-us*, n. horn	**Corne**ous, **corn**ification Loan word: **Cornu** (kor′nū) pl. **Cornua** (kor′nū-a)
PIL/O (pī-lō)	Hair	L. *pilus*, *-i*, m. a hair	**Pil**omotor, de**pil**ate Loan word: **Pilus** (pī′lŭs) pl. **Pili** (pī′lī″)
TRICH/O (trĭk-ō) **-THRIX** (thrĭks)	Hair	Gr. *thrix*, *trichos*, hair	**Trich**oma, endo**thrix** Loan word: **thrix** (thrĭks)

Greek or Latin word element	Current usage	Etymology	Examples
FOLLICUL/O (fŏ-lĭk-yŭ-lō)	Little bag, follicle	L. *folliculus, -i*, n. little bag fr. L. *follis*, bag, purse	**Follicul**ostatin, **follicul**itis Loan word: **Folliculus** (fŏ-lĭk′ū-lŭs) pl. **Folliculi** (fŏ-lĭk′ū-lī″)
UNGU/O (ŭng-gwō, or ŭng-gyō)	Fingernail, toenail, claws, talon, hoof	L. *unguis, -is*, m. fingernail, talon, hoof	**Ungu**late, sub**ungu**al Loan word: **Unguis** (ŭng′gwĭs) pl. **Ungues** (ŭng′gwēz″)
ONYCH/O (ŏn-ĭ-kō)	Fingernail, toenail, claws, talon, hoof	Gr. *onyx, onychos*, fingernail, claw, hoof	**Onych**algia, **onych**orrhexis Loan word: **Onyx** (ŏn′ĭks)
HIDR/O (hi-drō)	Sweat	Gr. *hidros*, sweat	**Hidr**opoiesis, hyper**hidr**osis
SUD/O (sood-ō) **SUDOR/O** (sood-ŏ-rō)	Sweat	L. *sudor, sudoris*, m. sweat	**Sud**omotor, **sudor**esis Loan word: **Sudor** (sood′ŏr)
SEB/O (se-bō, or sē-bō)	Sebum	L. *sebum, -i*, n. tallow, fat; sebum	Anti**seb**orrheic, **seb**aceous Loan word: **Sebum** (sē′bŭm) pl. **Seba** (sē′bă)
STEAR/O (stē-ă-rō) **STEAT/O** (stē-ă-tō)	Sebum, fat	Gr. *stear, steatos*, tallow, fat	**Stear**odermia, **steat**adenoma
LIP/O (lip-ō)	Fat	Gr. *lipos*, fat	**Lip**ocele, **lip**oma
ADIP/O (ad-ĭ-pō)	Fat	L. *adeps, adipis*, m. fat L. *adiposus, -a, -um*, fatty	**Adip**ectomy, **adip**ose Loan word: **Adeps** (a′deps)

Review	Answers
The flesh is composed of the soft tissue of the body, especially muscles. The combining forms for flesh are _____, _____, _____, and _____.	**SARC/O, CARN/O, CRE/O, and CREAT/O**
Skin is an organ of the integumentary system. The combining forms for skin are _____, _____, _____, _____, _____, and _____.	**DERM/O, DERMAT/O, CUT/O, CUTANE/O, CORI/O, PELL/O**
The subdermal layer is also known as the _____ layer. This layer is just below the _____, which is also called the _____. The thin outer layer of skin that lays over the dermis is called the _____.	**subcutaneous dermis, corium epidermis**
Tissue is a collection of particular cells and intercellular substances that have a specific function. The combining forms for "tissue" are _____ and _____. The anatomical Latin term for tissue is _____, and the loan word for a layer of tissue is _____.	**HIST/O, HISTI/O tela, tunica**

Review	Answers
Based on its root, adipose tissue is full of _____ cells. The other roots for "fat" are _____, _____, _____, and _____.	**Fat** **ADIP-, LIP-, STEAT-, STEAR-**
The oil glands of the skin are called sebaceous glands, which are located in the dermis. The combining forms used for "sebum," which is the oily substance secreted by the sebaceous glands, are _____, _____, and _____.	**SEB/O, STEAT/O, STEAR/O**
The cells covering the internal and external surfaces of the human body are called epithelium. The shared root in epithelium, mesothelium, and endothelium means _____ or _____.	**nipple, nipple like**
The papillary layer of the skin has dermal papillae, which look like _____.	**nipples**
Sudor is the loan word for _____. The sudoriferous glands of the skin are located in the dermis. The combining forms for sweat are _____, _____, and _____.	**sweat** **HIDR/O, SUD/O, SUDOR/O**
STRAT/O is the combining form for _____. The corresponding loan word is _____.	**layer** **stratum**
Keratin is the hard protein material found in the epidermis, hair, and nails. The root in keratin means _____, _____, _____, and _____. The Latin synonyms for this root are _____ and _____.	**horn, horn-like, hard, and cornea** **CORN-, CORNE-**
A small sac-like structure containing hair that is located in the dermis is called a _____. The combining forms for hair are _____ and _____.	**Follicle** **PIL/O, TRICH/O**
Nails are outgrowths of the skin composed of keratin. They are analogous to the hooves and talons of animals, and, therefore, the combining forms _____ and _____ can mean hoof, talon, claws, fingernail, and toenail.	**ONYCH/O, UNGU/O**

Lessons from History: Hippocrates' *On Ulcers* and Dermatology

Food for Thought as You Read:

What does the treatise On Ulcers *tell us about Hippocratic treatments of lesions? How is the Greek word helkos used in this text? How does the ancient meaning of a helkos differ from our modern understanding of an ulcer? When and how did the field of dermatology begin?*

Dermatology is a relatively new field of medicine that began in the late 18th and early 19th centuries. The understanding that the *cutis* is an organ that has its own specific diseases is, therefore, a rather modern concept. Anne Charles Lorry's *Treatise on Cutaneous Diseases* (*Tractatus de morbis cutaneis,* 1777), Louis Alibert's *Description de maladies de la peau* (1806), and Robert Willan's *On Cutaneous Diseases* (1808) were three seminal works that helped to create the field of dermatology. The development of this specialized field of medicine was dependent on the invention of the microscope, which allowed physicians to recognize skin as a complex structure.

Prior to the 18th century, due to the influence of ancient Greek medicine, manifest changes to the skin were primarily treated as signs that could be used to determine the unseen pathological condition within the body. That is not to say that ancient Greek medicine did not write about skin diseases. Written in the 5th century BC, the Hippocratic text entitled *On Ulcers* (Greek Περὶ ἑλκέων and in Latin *De ulceribus*) provides an early example of a Greek medical work dedicated to the treatment of lesions of the skin. The English title of this work is somewhat misleading because it does not deal with the specific type of lesions that we refer to as "ulcers." In *On Ulcers*, wounds, burns, and pathological changes to skin fell broadly under the Greek term *helkos*. Modern medicine uses the term "**lesion**" for both wounds (i.e. damage to the skin caused by trauma) and pathological alterations of the skin. Interestingly, today, we use the Greek root **HELC-** or **HELK-** for specific types of lesions, the round and irregular secondary lesions that we define as **ulcers** (Fig. 6.6).

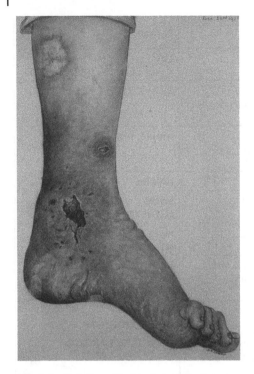

Fig. 6.6 S. A. Sewell's drawing of the lower leg and foot of a female patient showing ulceration, which is part of St. Bartholomew's Hospital Archive and Museum. *Source: Wellcome Collection/CC BY 4.0.*

The technical advice provided in *On Ulcers* makes it clear that ancient Greek physicians took into consideration many of the same factors we use today to identify the nature of a lesion and its corresponding treatment: the color and shape of the lesion, the location on the body, the type of drainage, the presence of swelling, and whether the lesion is new or chronic. Broadly speaking, the advocated treatments for various lesions consisted of the types of therapeutic interventions that are found in modern wound care, such as cleaning, bandaging, applying medications, changing a patient's diet, and surgery when indicated. That said, the lack of understanding of bacterial infection and the reliance on humoral theory also led to recommending erroneous and somewhat deleterious treatment. For instance, the author of *On Ulcers* recommends bleeding old lesions. Most notable was the practice of engendering **suppuration** (formation of pus) in a lesion. The author distinguishes between healthy and bad pus (Gr. *pyon*), which was described as being black and foul smelling. Healthy pus was believed to have been formed from blood that was altered by heat, and it was a good sign of healing. Thus, the author recommends giving rise to pus early so as to avoid swelling. The belief that there is good and bad pus would continue all the way into the 19th century. Although we recognize pus as being produced by an infection, we continue to use the Greek root **PY-** for pus.

The latter part of *On Ulcers* provides a list of recipes for medications that were believed to have specific effects on lesions. Some recipes were for moistening, others for drying, other medications were styptic (i.e. causing bleeding to stop) effects, and some were used for specific types of lesions (e.g. burns, scars). The various geographic provenance of the *materia medica* in these recipes extends to Egypt and as far west as Illyricum. This can be seen in the following recipe:

> For spreading ulcers: Alum, both the baked Egyptian, and the Melian; first rub it off with baked natron and soak it up, and the burnt rock alum; bake until it becomes fiery-red.

> *On Ulcers*, L. 18.1

As to the efficacy of the medications, *materia medica*, such as alum, honey, and wine, may have had some unintended benefits in that these ingredients are mild antiseptics. Others were less beneficial to wound healing; for example copper oxide is a crude antiseptic, but it also kills tissue cells. In other cases, the *materia medica* would have produced effects that were opposite to what was intended. As Majno notes, on the basis that fig-tree latex curdles milk, fig-tree latex was used to reduce bleeding. However, opposite to its effect on milk, fig-tree latex actually prevents the blood from clotting at its normal rate.

Modern dermatology is the branch of medicine for the treatment of skin, hair, and nails and the conditions associated with them. Dermatological conditions are diagnosed by the patient's history, physical examination, and laboratory testing. Most dermatological diseases are managed with medications (topical and systemic). Some require procedures such as surgery, cryotherapy, radiotherapy, or phototherapy. That said, approximately 50% of skin-related consultations are initially assessed by non-dermatologists. A physical assessment of the skin involves identifying types of skin lesions and their characteristics. The location, number, size, color, texture, shape, and distribution of lesions are all part of this assessment. Skin lesions are classified as being primary or secondary. Primary lesions appear as a direct result of a disease. Based on morphology, the following terms are used for different types of primary lesions: macules, vesicles, bullae, chancres, pustules, papules, wheals, plaques, and tumors. Secondary lesions develop from primary lesions (e.g. scales and ulcers) or as a result of external trauma (e.g. scratching). The common terms for these secondary lesions are fissures, crusts, excoriations, scales, scars, ulcers, and changes in pigmentation. It is important to recognize what type of lesion is present because lesions are used as signs that are indicative of different types of disease.

Some Suggested Readings

Hippocrates. *Ulcers*. Translated by Paul Potter. Loeb Classical Library 482. Cambridge: Harvard University Press, 1995.

Santoro, Rosa. "Skin Over the Centuries. A Short History of Dermatology: Physiology, Pathology, and Cosmetics." *Medicina Historica* 1, no. 2 (2017): 94–102.

Etymological Explanations: Lesions

In addition to associating a name to type of lesion (Fig. 6.7), knowing the etymologies of the terms for these lesions is useful to recalling the shape and appearance of a lesion. For instance, the term "plaque" comes from the French word for "a metal

Primary lesions: develop as a direct result of the disease process from previously normal skin

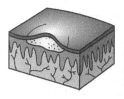

Vesicle
Description: Small, fluid-filled distinct elevation
Example: Blister

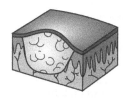

Nodule/Tumor
Description: Solid, palpable, raised mass; nodules have distinct borders; tumors extend deep into the dermis
Example: Wart, large lipoma

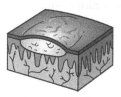

Plaque
Description: Larger, flat, elevated patch with solid surface
Example: Psoriasis

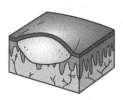

Wheal
Description: Smooth, slightly raised localized area of edema; often irregular and variable in size and color
Example: Hives, insect bites

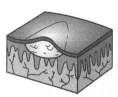

Papule
Description: Small, circular, solid elevations with sharp borders
Example: Mole

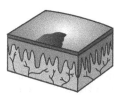

Macule
Description: Flat, discolored spot on skin
Example: Freckles, flat moles

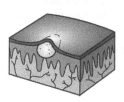

Pustule
Description: Raised lesion vesicle filled with pus
Example: Acne, carbuncles

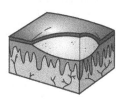

Bulla
Description: Large, fluid-filled elevation
Example: Burn blisters

Secondary lesions: evolve from primary lesions

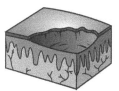

Ulcer
Description: Open sore on skin caused by breaking of necrotic tissue, past the epidermis
Example: Stasis ulcer

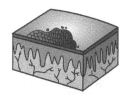

Crust
Description: Hard, dried residue of exudates (either serum, blood or pus or a combination)
Example: Residue of impetigo

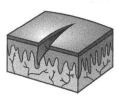

Fissure
Description: Cleft or groove in the skin
Example: Athlete's foot

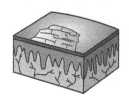

Scale
Description: Flaking of outermost layer of the skin; usually due to excessive dryness
Example: Dandruff

Fig. 6.7 Image of types of primary and secondary lesions. *Source:* Line drawing by Chloe Kim.

plate," which is an accurate description of these types of lesions. The etymologies of lesions also help one to recognize how the root can be used in different contexts.

Some primary and secondary lesions
Macule (L. *macula*, *-ae*) – The term macule comes from the Latin word for "spot" or "stain," *macula*. Therefore, the loan word macula and the root **MACUL-** can be used for macule (e.g. a freckle), as well as any structure that is spotted (e.g. macula lutea, maculated).
Nodule (L. *nodulus*, *-i*) – The term nodule comes from the Latin diminutive *nodulus* (little knot) from the Latin word *nodus* (knot). This word picture helps one to understand that a solid knot-like structure is called a node, nodus, and nodulus. Likewise, the roots **NOD-** and **NODUL-** refer to structures that resemble knots (e.g. lymph nodes).
Vesicle (L. *vesicula*, *-ae*) – The Latin word for a "small bag or bladder" was *vesicula*, which is a diminutive of the Latin word for bladder or bag, *vesica*. This explains why the small, palpable, fluid-filled lesion is called a vesicle and why the root for types of "bladders" (e.g. gall bladder, urinary bladder) is **VESIC-**.
Bulla (L. *bulla*, *-ae*) – Larger, palpable, fluid-filled lesions are called bullae. This term comes from the Latin word for a round swelling, as well as a type of sac-like amulet worn around the necks of Roman boys that they would later lay aside when they took on the white toga of manhood (i.e. *toga virilis*).
Papule (L. *papula*, *-ae*) – The Latin term *papula* means "pimple," and therefore, the root **PAPUL-** refers to lesions and other objects that look like pimples.
Pustule (L. *pustula*, *-ae*) – The Latin word *pustula* was used for an inflamed sore or blister. It is derived from the Latin word *pus*, *puris*, which was used for morbid matter coming from a wound. Today, the roots **PUR-** and **PURUL-** are associated with the fluid that we now call pus. Interestingly, our word "pure" is derived from a related Latin adjective *purus*, *pura*, *purum*, which meant, among other things, "being free from morbid matter."
Fissure (L. *fissura*, *-ae*) – The Latin word *fissura* was used for "a crack" or "the process of splitting." It is derived from the Latin verb *findere*, which means "to split, cleave." Thus, the roots **FISS-** and **FISSUR-** carry with them the meaning of "a crack" or "the process of splitting."

Purpuric lesions and vascular lesions are also categories of lesions. The following are the etymologies of some of these types of lesions.

Some purpuric and vascular lesions
Purpuric lesions (L. *purpura*, *-ae*) – Purpuric lesions are a category of lesions in which blood cells leak into the skin or mucous layers. The Latin word *purpura* meant "purple." Today, the root **PURPUR-** is commonly used for purpuric lesions and for things that resemble the color purple. The smallest of these non-blanching lesions are called **petechia** (from Italian for "specks on the face") and look like small, purplish spots. The larger of these lesions, which is associated with broad bruising, is called **ecchymosis**. This term is derived from ancient Greek medicine for blood or other humors appearing under the surface of the skin (Ge. *ek-* outside + *chymos*, humor).
Vascular lesions (L. *vascula*, *-ae*) – Vascular lesions include acquired diseases of the blood vessels, birthmarks, and vascular malformations. The Latin word *vascula* means "little vessel." **Telangiectasis** (Gr. *telos*, end + *angion*, vessel + *-ectatis*, dialation) is a vascular lesion where there is a dilation of a group of small blood vessels. A **hemangioma** (Gr. *haima*, blood + *angion*, vessel + *-oma*, tumor), which is a benign tumor of encapsulated blood vessels in the skin, is another type of vascular lesion.

In addition to knowing the etymologies of the types of lesions, it is also good to know the common name and its corresponding Latin or Greek word for common skin pathologies.

Common names
Wart (L. *verruca*, *-ae*) – A wart is called a **verruca**, which in Classical Latin meant "a small fault" or "wart."
Mole (L. *nevus*, *-i*) – A mole is called a **nevus**, which in Classical Latin means "birthmark" and "mole."
Hive (L. *urtica*, *-ae*) – A hive is sometimes called **urtica**, which in Classical Latin meant "stinging nettle." **Urticaria** is a common cause of the wheals called hives.
Scar (L. *cicatrix*, *cicatricis*) – A scar is called a **cicatrix**. In Roman literature, a soldier whose scars were on the front of his body (*cicatrices corpore adverso*) indicated bravery in battle because he did not turn and flee from the enemy.
Blackhead/Pimple (L. *comedo*, *comedonis*) – A blackhead/pimple is referred to as a **comedo**, which is a Classical Latin term for "a glutton." It was also formerly used as a term for "worms that devour the body."

Boil (L. *furunculus, -i*) – A boil is called a **furuncle** or **furunculus**, which meant in Classical Latin "a petty thief or pilferer." As noted earlier, **-UNCULUS**, as well as its anglicized **-UNCLE**, is a Latin diminutive suffix that shows up in terms such as carbuncle/ carbunculus (little coal), peduncle/pedunculus (little foot), and homunculus (little human).

Greek or Latin word element	Current usage	Etymology	Examples
HELC/O (hĕl-kō)	Ulcer	Gr. *helkos*, skin lesion	**Helc**oma, **helc**oid
ULCER/O (ŭl-sĕr-ō)	Ulcer	L. *ulcus, ulceris*, n. skin lesion, open sore; ulcer	**Ulcer**ation, **ulcer**ous Loan word: **Ulcer** (ŭl′sĕr) pl. **Ulcera** (ŭl′sĕr-ă)
MACUL/O (mak-yŭ-lō)	Macule, spot	L. *macula, -ae*, f. spot, stain	**Macul**ation, **macul**opathy Loan word: **Macula** (mak′yŭ-lă) pl. **Maculae** (mak′yŭ-lē″)
NEV/O (nē-vō)	Mole	L. *nevus, -i*, m. birthmark, mole	**Nev**olipoma, **nev**oid Loan word: **Nevus** (nē′vŭs) pl. **Nevi** (nē′vī″)
VERRUC/O (vĕr-roo-kō)	Wart	L. *verruca, -ae*, f. wart	**Verruc**iform, **verruc**osis Loan word: **Verruca** (vĕr-roo′kă) pl. **Verrucae** (vĕr-roo′kē″)
CICATRIC/O (sĭk″ă-trĭ-kō)	Scar	L. *cicatrix, cicatricis*, f. scar	**Cicatric**otomy, **cicatric**ose Loan word: **Cicatrix** (sĭ-kā′triks) pl. **Cicatrices** (sik-ă-trī′sēz″)
NOD/O (nō-dō)	Knot-like, node nodule	L. *nodus, -i*, m. a knot	**Nod**ose, **nodul**ar Loan words: **Nodus** (nŏd′ŭs) pl. **Nodi** (nō′dī″)
NODUL/O (nŏd-ū-lō)		L. *nodulus, -i*, m. a little knot	**Nodulus** (nŏd′ū-lŭs) pl. **Noduli** (nŏd′ū-lī″)
PUSTUL/O (pŭs-tū-lō)	Pustule	L. *pustula, -ae*, f. blister, pimple	**Pustul**ant, **pustul**ar Loan word: **Pustula** (pŭs′tū-lă) pl. **Pustulae** (pŭs′tū-lē″)
PAPUL/O (pap-yŭ-lō)	Papule	L. *papula, -ae*, f. pimple, pustule	**Papul**osis, maculo**papul**ar Loan word: **Papule** (păp′yūl)
COMED/O (kŏm-ă-dō)	Pimple, blackhead, whitehead	L. *comedo, comedonis*, m. a glutton; pimple fr. L. *comedere*, to eat up	**Comed**ocarcinoma, **comed**onal Loan word: **Comedo** (kŏm′ă-dō) pl. **Comedones** (kŏm′ă-dō-nēz″)

Greek or Latin word element	Current usage	Etymology	Examples
URTIC/O (ŭrt-i-kō)	Wheal, hive	L. *urtica, -ae*, f. stinging nettle	**Urtic**aria, **urtic**ant Loan word: **Urtica** (ŭrt'i-kă)
FURUNCUL/O (fū-rŭng-kū-lō)	Furuncle, boil	L. *furunculus, -i*, m. boil, a petty thief	**Furuncul**oid, **furuncul**osis Loan word: **Furuncle** (fū'rŭng-k'l)
CYST/O (sĭs-tō)	Cyst, sac, bladder	Gr. *kyste*, sac	**Cyst**oadenoma, **cyst**itis Loan word: **Cyst** (sist)
VESIC/O (vě-sĭ-kō) **VESICUL/O** (vě-sĭk-ū-lō)	Bladder, vesicle, VESICUL = vesicle, small blister	L. *vesica, -ae*, f. bladder *vesicula, -ae*, f. little bladder	**Vesic**ant, **vesic**ular Loan words: **Vesica** (vě-sī'kă) pl. **Vesicae** (vě-sī'sē") **Vesicula** (vě-sĭk'ū-lă) pl. **Vesiculae** (vě-sĭk'ū-ē")
BULL/O (bŭl-ō)	Bulla, large blister	L. *bulla, -ae*, f. round swelling, amulet, water bubble	**Bull**ectomy, **bull**ous Loan word: **Bulla** (bŭl'ă) pl. **Bullae** (bŭl'ē)
PURPUR/O (pŭr-pyŭ-rō)	Purpura, purple	L. *purpura, -ae*, f. purple	**Purpur**ic, **purpur**omycin Loan word: **Purpura** (pŭr'pyŭ-ră) pl. **Purpurae** (pŭr'pyŭ-rē)
ECCHYM/O (ěk-ĭ-mō)	Broad bruising, ecchymosis	Gr. *ecchymosis*, bruise	**Ecchym**otic Loan word: **Ecchymosis** (ěk-ĭ-mō'sĭs) pl. **Ecchymoses** (ěk-ĭ-mō'sēz")
PETECHI/O (pē-tē'kē-ō)	Petechia, red spots	Italian *petecchia*, skin spot	**Petechi**al Loan word: **Petechia** (pē-tē'kē-ă)
TELE- (tel-ĕ)	Distant	Gr. *tele*, distant, far off	**Tele**metry, **tele**phone
TEL/O (těl-ō)	End, complete, purpose	Gr. *telos*, end, fulfillment, purpose	A**tel**ocardia, **tel**angiectasia

Review	Answers
A small fluid-filled lesion, such as a blister, is called a _____. The root for this term means _____ and _____. Latin loan words associated with the root meaning "bladder" and "little bladder" are _____ and _____. The Greek root that is a synonym for the root VESIC- is _____.	**Vesicle, bladder, vesicle** **Vesica, vesicula** **CYST-**
The combining form _____ is used for the purpuric lesion, whose etymology means "little spots (on the face)."	**PETECHI/O**
The loan word ecchymosis is used for the purpuric lesions that exhibit "broad _____."	**bruising**

Review	Answers
The loan word for a "mole" is _____. The loan word for a "wart' is_____. Respectively, the combining forms for these loan words are _____ and _____.	**nevus** **verruca** **NEV/O, VERRUC/O**
The root MACUL- can refer to the lesion called a _____, or it can simply refer to a _____.	**macule, spot**
Urtica is also called a _____ or a_____.	**hive, wheal**
The roots for a "knot-like" structure or lesion of the body are _____ and _____.	**NOD-, NODUL-**
A "boil" is also called a _____. A "scar" is also called a _____. Respectively, the combining forms for these are _____ and _____.	**Furuncle** **Cicatrix** **FURUNCUL/O,** **CICATRIC/O**
The two roots that in general mean "ulcer" are _____ and _____.	**ULCER/O, HELC/O**
A large blister-like lesion is called a _____, which is also the Latin word for a pouch-like type of Roman amulet.	**bulla**
The suffix -UNCULUS and its derivative -UNCLE mean _____ or _____.	**small, little**
The loan word for "pimple/blackhead" that comes from the Latin word for a glutton is _____. The Latin terms *papula* and *pustula* both meant "pimple." Today, a papule is pimple-like lesion that does not have pus, and a pustule is a pimple-like lesion that contain pus. Their respective combining forms are _____ and _____.	**Comedo** **PAPUL/O, PUSTUL/O**
Telangiectasis (or Telangiectasia) is a vascular lesion that causes dilations to small vessels, i.e. the 'ends' of blood vessels. The root TEL- in this word means _____, _____, or _____. It should not be confused with the prefix TELE-, which means _____, or *Tela*, which is the anatomic Latin word used for _____.	**end, complete, purpose** **distant** **tissue**
Purpuric lesions are associated with disorders of coagulation and thrombosis. The root in purpuric means _____ and _____.	**purple, purpura**

Lessons from History: Skin Color in Ancient Greek Medicine and Science

Food for Thought as You Read:

What role does the integumentary system play in ancient Greek racism and colonial racism? How were ancient Greek concepts of humor used in support of these views? What does this say about science and society?

In ancient Greek medicine, skin color was used as a means of determining the presence of disease. For instance, Celsus (V.26.31.A) remarks how one can know that a wound has taken a turn for the worse if it becomes livid: "sometimes the wound becomes the seat of chronic ulceration, and it becomes hardened (*callus*), and the thickened margins become a livid color (*livent*)." In other cases, the name of the disease is based on the color of the skin, as Celsus notes (V.26.31.B), "sometimes a redness (*rubor*), over and above the inflammation, surrounds the wound, and this spreads with pain (the Greeks term is erysipelas). Formed from the Greek words *erythros* (red) and *pella* (skin), **erysipelas** is still used in modern medicine as a term for an infection that causes a bright red rash and swelling. Skin color was also used as a taxonomic sign for distinguishing different species of lesions. This can be observed in Celsus' description of **vitiligo**. Using latinized Greek terms, Celsus (V.28.19) notes that there are three types of vitiligo: *melas* (black), *leuce* (white), and *alphos* (white). Celsus distinguishes *alphos* from *leuce* vitiligo by claiming that *leuke* vitiligo is more whitish (*magis albida*) and deeper. Celsus claims that vitiligo is not dangerous, but it is 'foul' (*foeda*), and it is caused by a 'bad nature of the body' (*malo corporis habitu*). Celsus' vitiligo appears to be a combination of different skin diseases based on our current pathological classifications. Today, vitiligo is a skin disorder that has localized loss of melanocytes causing a patchy loss of skin pigment. In respect to the color terms used by Celsus, **MELAN-**, which is the root derived from the Greek word for 'black' or 'dark,' *melas*, is commonly used in medicine. By extension it is also used for the skin pigment produced by melanocytes, called **melanin**. Likewise, **LEUK-** is commonly used for 'white,' which is its original meaning. *Alphos* is not currently used as a root in modern medicine, but its Latin derivative, *albus*, is used both in scientific Latin and as a root **ALB-** for 'white.' **Albino,** the Portuguese derivative of the Latin *albus*, is used today for 'an individual organism with an inherited partial or total absence of pigment in skin, hair, and eyes.'" Curiously, the term "albino" comes from an 18th-century Portuguese word used for Africans with vitiligo rather than for **albinism**.

In Greek natural philosophy and medicine, skin color was used to biologically justify social perceptions about the sexes and the surrounding peoples. The 3rd century BC Greek treatise *Physiognomonica*, which is attributed to Aristotle but was written by another author, used a variety of different physical appearances (e.g. skin, limbs, nails, hair, nose, lips) as signs of the nature and character of people, as well as animals. For example, he claims (806b) that "a bright complexion is indicative of a hot and sanguine disposition, a whitish-red complexion indicates a good disposition, when it occurs on smooth skin (*leiou chrotos*)." Thus, according to this author, the complexion of a person reveals the character of the person, which is dependent on the heat and humoral mixture of the body. This text contains a famous passage (812a) that is often used in modern discussions about ancient Greek racism: "Those who are too black/dark (*melanes*) are cowards; witness Egyptians, Ethiopians." While this seems to suggest that Greeks held views about Africans similar to those found in colonial racism, the following passage makes such an interpretation somewhat problematic: "those who are too white are cowards as well; witness women. The color that contributes to bravery must necessarily be in the middle of these two." Thus, the author does not see being white-skinned as being indicative of racial superiority, since Greek women are not another race, and the author is not arguing that the white complexion is the antithesis of black. Rather, he appears to be arguing that a sort of mean between these complexions is indicative of a well-balanced inner constitution of the body, which, in turn, determines the character of groups of people. That said, it is quite clear that the complexion of skin is still sexist and racist by modern standards since it is still being used by this author as biological justification for the Greek notions of male and racial superiority.

The connection between skin color and Greek humoral theory was part of colonial racist views in the natural sciences of the 18th and 19th centuries. This is quite evident in Carl Linnaeus' *Systema naturae*, which was a seminal work for our modern taxonomy of genus and species. Carl Linnaeus was the first to classify humans as primates. In his 9th edition of *Systema naturae* (1756), Linnaeus further divided humans into four "species" based on generalizations about their complexions and geographic location (Fig. 6.8): *Homo rufus* (red human) is *Americanus* (American), *Homo albus* (white human) is *Europeus* (European), *Homo luridus* (pale yellow human) is *Asiaticus* (Asian), and *Homo niger* (black human) is *Afer* (African). He then adds that *Homo rufus* is *cholericus* (choleric), *Homo albus* is *sanguineus* (sanguine), *Homo luridus* is *melancholicus* (melancholic), and *Homo niger* is *phlegmaticus* (phlegmatic). The humoral categories of choleric, sanguine, phlegmatic, and melancholic were understood as speaking to the four temperaments. The concept of humoral temperaments goes back to ancient Greek medicine where it was believed that an innate predominance of one of the four humors (i.e. bile, blood, phlegm, and black bile) dictated the type of personality and health of a human being. By creating this humoral link, Linnaeus departs from purely geographical and environmental factors. Not surprisingly, given his time

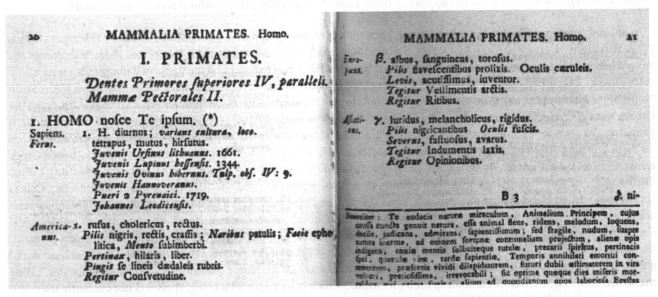

Fig. 6.8 Image of Linnaeus' classification of Homo sapiens. *Caroli Linnaei ... Systema Naturae: Per Regna Tria Naturae, Secundum Classes, Ordines, Genera, Species, Cum Characteribus, Differentiis, Synonymis, Locis.* Holmiae: Salvius, 1758.

period, Linnaeus ascribes moral characteristics to these "races" of peoples, reserving the better of the humoral categories (sanguine) for Europeans. His 10th edition expands upon these four "species" of humans describing their differences in body posture, eye and hair color, facial features, behavior, manner of clothing, and forms of government. In some respects, Linnaeus' approach to categorizing the human species can be traced back to the Hippocratic treatise *Airs, Waters, and Places*, which links the environment of different geographic regions to the appearance, character, and customs of Greek and non-Greek peoples. Therefore, it would appear that medicine and the natural sciences have not been immune to the "disease of racism" that has plagued human thinking for centuries.

Some Suggested Readings

Kennedy, Rebecca, Sydnor Roy, and Max Goldman. *Race and Ethnicity in the Classical World: An Anthology of Primary Sources in Translation*. Indianapolis: Hackett Publishing Company, 2013.

Linnean Society. "Linnaeus and Race." Accessed January 4, 2021. www.linnean.org/learning/who-was-linnaeus/linnaeus-and-race.

Walsh, Lisl. "Blog: What a Difference an ἦ Makes: Hippocrates, Racism, and the Translation of Greco-Roman Thought." *Society of Classical Studies*. Accessed January 4, 2021. www.classicalstudies.org/scs-blog/lisl-walsh/blog-what-difference-ἦ-makes-hippocrates-racism-and-translation-greco-roman.

Vocabulary

Quite a number of roots that we use today to denote color in dermatology come from ancient Greek and Latin, which can be seen in the following list of vocabulary:

Greek or Latin word element	Current usage	Etymology	Examples
MELAN/O (mĕl-ăn-ō)	Black, dark	Gr. *melas, melanos*, black, dark	**Melan**oderma, **melan**oma
NIGR/O (ni-grō)	Black, dark	L. *niger, nigra, nigrum*, black	**Nigr**icans, **nigr**ostriatal
LEUC/O (loo-kō) **LEUK/O** (loo-kō)	White	Gr. *leukos*, white	**Leuk**oderma, **leuc**emia
ALB/O (al-bō) **ALBIN/O** (al-bĭ-nō)	White	L. *albus, alba, album*, white *albino*, Portuguese fr. L. *albus*	**Alb**icans, **albin**uria
PALLID/O	Pale, globus pallidus	L. *pallidus, -a, -um*, pale	**Pallid**ectomy, **pallid**al Loan word: **Pallid** (păl'ĭd)
ERYTHR/O (ĕ-rith-rō)	Red	Gr. *erythros*, red	**Erythr**oderma, **erythr**ocyte
ERYTHEM/O (er-ĭ-thē-mō)	Erythema, a redness of skin	Gr. *erythema*, redness of skin	**Erythem**ogenic, **erythem**atous Loan word: **Erythema** (er"ĭ-thē'mă)
RUBR/O (roo-brō)	Red	L. *ruber, rubra, rubrum*, red	**Rubr**ospinal, **rubr**icyte

Greek or Latin word element	Current usage	Etymology	Examples
XANTH/O (zan-thō)	Yellow	Gr. *xanthos*, yellow	**Xanth**oderma, **xanth**oma
FLAV/O (flā-vō)	Yellow (bright yellow)	L. *flavus, flava, flavum*, yellow	**Flav**obacterium, **flav**in

Review	Answers
Flavism indicates something has a _____ color.	yellow
"A condition of redness of skin" is called _____. Erythroderma is a condition with widespread erythema and scaling of the skin. It is related to the Greek root for "red," which is _____. The corresponding Latin root for "red" is _____.	erythema ERYTHR- RUBR-
Xanthoderma is a condition in which the skin appears _____.	yellow
Melanoderma is a condition in which the skin has _____ or _____ spots of discoloration.	dark, black
The globus pallidus is also called the pallidum. The shared root in these terms means _____.	pale
The root in the participle nigricans means _____ or _____.	dark, black
The loan word for "an individual organism with inherited partial or total absence of pigment in skin, hair, and eyes" is _____. This term ultimately comes from the Latin root for "white," which is _____. The Greek root for "white" is _____.	albino ALB- LEUC- (or LEUK-)

Lessons from History: Terms for Skin Diseases in Ancient Greek and Modern Medicine

Food for Thought as You Read:

What does Celsus' On Medicine reveal about ancient pathological terms for skin disease and their modern definitions?

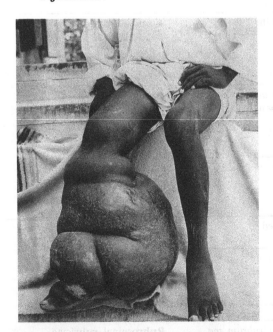

Fig. 6.9 Photograph of a man with elephantiasis in the right leg. *Source:* Wellcome Collection/CC BY 4.0.

Many of our terms for skin diseases can be found in ancient Greek medicine, especially in Celsus' *De medicina*. The use of such terminology testifies to ancient Greek medicine making distinctions between types of skin diseases. That said, while they used similar terms to denote different skin diseases, the corresponding descriptions of these skin diseases varied from author to author. Although terms such as elephantiasis, phagedena, and cancer are still in use, their ancient medical definitions do not correspond to their modern medical meanings. What is lost on the modern user of such pathological terms is that these terms convey that something is attacking either the body or the lesion resembles an animal or the part of an animal. The following is a collection of the ancient terms for skin diseases still used in modern medicine.

Elephantiasis is a condition of large swelling of extremities due to the obstruction of lymphatic vessels. It is caused by filarial parasites and malignancies (Fig. 6.9). This is quite a departure from the original usage in ancient Greek medicine. As Santoro points out, the terms *elephantiasis, elephas morbus,* and *elephantia* (Celsus III.25.1; Scribonius Largus 250) were used to describe a deadly disease characterized by a thickening of the skin similar to an elephant's skin. Celsus describes how this disease affects the whole body, causing spots and swellings, which change to black in color. The skin is thickened and thinned in an irregular way, and when the disease is long-standing, the fingers and toes are sunk under the swelling. He claims it is unknown in Italy, but it is frequently occurring in certain regions. Based on this description, some scholars believe elephantiasis to be what we now call **Hansen Disease**, also known as **leprosy**, which is a chronic infectious disease of the skin and nerves caused by the bacteria *Mycobacterium leprae*. The term leprosy is derived from the Greek word *lepros*, which means "scaly." However, when early ancient Greek authors describe the disease *lepra*, it is quite apparent that they are referring to diseases such as psoriasis that produce scales or plaque-like lesions rather than Hansen Disease. In late antiquity, *lepra* and *elephantiasis* were used synonymously, and, even later, *lepra* became the preferred term of the two.

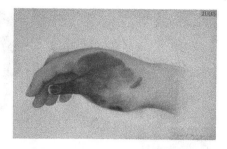

Fig. 6.10 Painting by Thomas Godart of a hand with dry gangrene. St Bartholomew's Hospital Archives & Museum. *Source:* Wellcome Collection/CC BY 4.0.

Gangrene (Gr. *gangraina*, which gnaws away) was an ancient Greek medical term for a lesion that had become black/livid, shriveled, and foul-smelling. Because *gangraina* was believed to be putrefaction caused by corrupt blood, it was treated with bleeding and medications to promote suppurations. Today, the term gangrene is used for necrotic tissue associated with a loss of blood supply to an area (Fig. 6.10).

Phagedena (Gr., which eats or swallows) was a term associated with spreading gangrene. It is derived from the Greek verb *phagein*, which means "to eat, devour." Today, a sloughing ulcer that spreads rapidly is called phagedena (Fig. 6.11).

Impetigo is a contagious bacterial infection of the skin around the mouth and nostrils producing pustules that burst, causing weeping and crusted yellowish lesions (Fig. 6.12). Its name is derived from the Latin verb *impetere*, "to attack." Celsus (V.28.16) claims there are four types of impetigo; these descriptions speak to a sudden onset of some forms of skin disease, similar to what we now call **eczema** (also known as **dermatitis**). In modern medicine, eczema is a general term for an itchy red rash with swollen papules and vesicles that weep serum and may become crusted, thickened, or scaly. Eczema is derived from the Greek verb *ekzein* (to boil out), and it was used in ancient Greek medicine for a variety of skin eruptions.

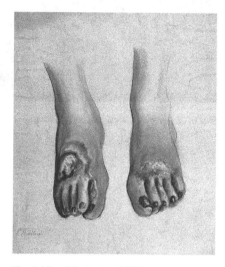

Fig. 6.11 Painting by C. D'Alton of feet of a woman with sloughing phagedena. *Source:* Wellcome Collection/Public domain.

Pediculosis is a term used for a lice infestation of the body (Fig. 6.13). Pediculus (little feet) is the Latin term for a louse.

Cancer is the Latin word for "a crab." The term is used today for a variety of malignant cellular pathologies. Originally, cancer was used to describe a variety of recalcitrant and progressive ulcerations of the skin. This ancient meaning is preserved via the term **cancrum**; a rapidly spreading ulcer is called a cancrum in modern medicine.

Herpes, which comes from the Greek verb *herpein* (to creep, to crawl) and the noun *herpeton* (creeping thing, reptile), was a term used for types of widespread ulcers believed to be caused by yellow bile under the skin. Today, the virus called herpes gets its name from the vesicle eruptions that accompany this virus. The **herpes simplex** (L. *simplex*, simple, unmixed) **type I** causes vesicles around the mouth and nose, while **herpes simplex type II** is sexually transmitted, causing ulcer-like lesions on the genital and anorectal areas. **Herpes zoster** (Gr. *zoster*, a girdle) is a viral disease that causes painful blisters along the pathway of a peripheral nerve, hence creating a girdle-like eruption of vesicles, also known as **shingles** (L. *cingulus*, a girdle) (Fig. 6.14).

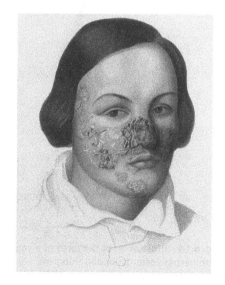

Fig. 6.12 Painting of a woman's face infected with impetigo from *Leçons sur les maladies de la peau, professées à l'École de médecine de Paris. Source:* Wellcome Collection/Public domain.

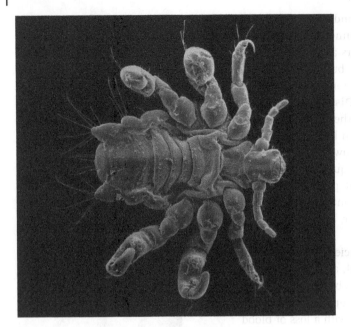

Fig. 6.13 Ventral view of a pubic louse. *Source:* Wellcome Collection/CC BY 4.0.

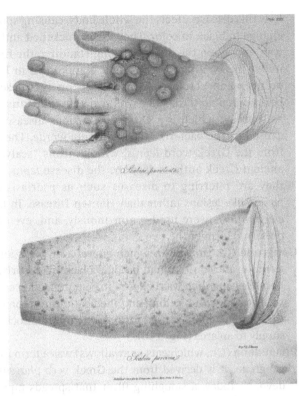

Fig. 6.15 Illustration depicting Scabies purulenta (top) and Scabies porcina (below). *Source:* Wellcome Collection/ Public domain.

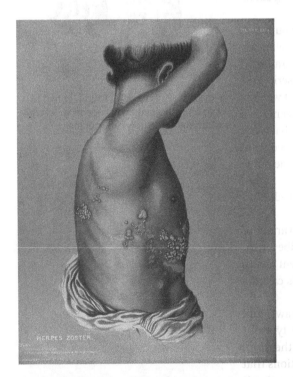

Fig. 6.14 Illustration of the torso of a young man with herpes zoster (common shingles). Chromolithograph by E. Burgess, 1850/1880. *Source:* Wellcome Collection/Public domain.

Scabies: In modern medicine, scabies is a contagious infestation of the skin caused by an itch-mite known as the *Sarcoptes scabiei* (Fig. 6.15). This mite infestation leads to an intense, itching rash of scaly papules and tunnels dug by this parasite. The Latin term scabies is derived from the verb *scabere* (to scratch). Celsus (V.28.15) describes scabies as hardening and redness of the skin with pustules producing persistently itchy ulcers. Its association with roughening and hardening of the skin suggests that it may be quite different from modern scabies, and possibly it was a condition such as modern psoriasis and eczema. That said, Celsus links scabies to the Greek term *agria* (savage).

Psoriasis: Psoriasis is a chronic skin disorder characterized by scaly, silvery plaques covering red papules that commonly occur at the elbows, knees, arms, legs, and scalp (Fig. 6.16). It comes from the Greek verb *psorav* (to itch). What ancient Greek medicine describes as psoriasis seems to correspond loosely to what we term as an itch, mange, and possibly scurvy.

Exanthema: In ancient Greek medicine, an *exanthema* was used for eruptions of the skin. The word is partially derived from the Greek word for "a flower," *anthos*. Today we use exanthema for rashes of the skin, particularly eruptions caused by a viral disease (e.g. **scarlet**

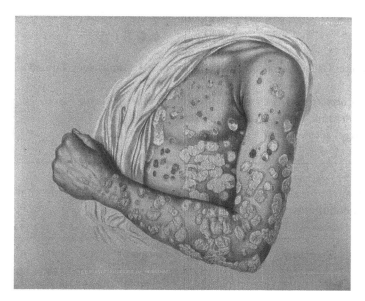

Fig. 6.16 Illustration depicting the torso of a man with psoriasis. *Source:* Wellcome Collection/Public domain.

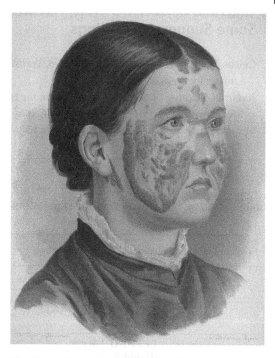

Fig. 6.17 Illustration of lupus erythematosus. *Source:* Wellcome Collection/Public domain.

fever, **rubella = German measles**, **rubeola = measles**, and **varicella = chickenpox**).

Lupus: Our modern term lupus (Fig. 6.17), which is a chronic autoimmune disease characterized by inflammation and ulceration of the body, is derived from the Latin word for "wolf." It first appeared as a medical term in the 14th century, when it was used for types of "devouring" lesions.

Tinea: Tinea is a collection of fungal infections of the skin and its appendages (e.g. **tinea corporis, tinea pedis, tinea barbae, tinea cruris, tinea unguium, tinea nigra**). It comes from the Latin word for a "worm, grub, larva." Like lupus, it began to be used for skin diseases in the 14th century. The ring-shaped appearance of these fungal infections bears a slight resemblance to a worm (Fig. 6.18); hence, tinea is also called a "ringworm."

One would guess that the practice of coining skin pathological in such theomorphic terms has fallen out of favor thanks to the advancements of modern medicine. However, modern medicine has somewhat continued this tradition of animal metaphors for skin lesions. **Ichthyosis** (Gr. *ichthys*, fish + -*osis*, condition), which was coined in 1815, is used for dry, scaly skin that resembles fish scales. **Keratosis** (Gr. *keras*, horn + -*osis*, condition) is used for an abnormal growth of the horny layer of the skin (e.g. **keratoma, actinic keratosis, seborrheic keratosis**).

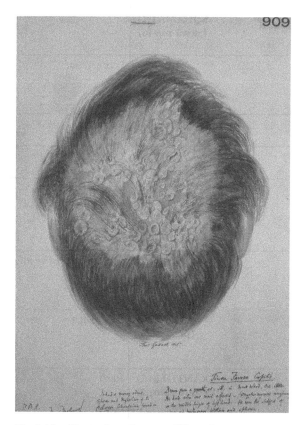

Fig. 6.18 Illustration of a case of Tinea favosa capitis (honeycomb ringworm of the head). *Source:* Wellcome Collection/CC BY 4.0.

Some Suggested Readings

Celsus. *On Medicine, Volume II: Books 5-6.* Translated by Walter G. Spencer. Loeb Classical Library 304. Cambridge: Harvard University Press, 1938.

Jouanna, Jacques. "*Disease as Aggression in the Hippocratic Corpus and Greek Tragedy: Wild and Devouring Disease.*" In *Greek Medicine from Hippocrates to Galen.* Edited by Philip van der Eijk, 81–96. Leiden: Brill, 2012.

Verbov, Julian. "Celsus and His Contributions to Dermatology." *International Journal of Dermatology* 17, no. 6 (1978): 521–523.

In addition to and including the aforementioned loan words for skin diseases, the following word elements are commonly used in medicine to describe skin lesions and other conditions:

Greek or Latin word element	Current usage	Etymology	Examples
CRYPT/O (krip-tō)	Hidden, covered, secret	Gr. *kryptos*, covered, hidden	**Crypt**olith, **crypt**ocephalous
ICHTHY/O (ĭk-thē-ō)	Fish, fish-like (e.g. scaly)	Gr. *ichthys*, fish	**Ichthy**osis, **ichy**otoxin
LEPID/O (lĕ-pĭd-ō)	Scaly	Gr. *lepis, lepidos*, scale, scaly	**Lepid**ic, **lepid**otrichia
SQUAM/O (skwā-mō) **SQUAMAT/O** (skwā-mă-tō)	Scale, scaly	L. *squama, -ae*, f. a scale (i.e. of a fish/reptile)	**Squam**ocellular, **squamat**ization Loan word: **Squama** (skwā'mă) pl. **Squamae** (skwā'mē")
LEPR/O (lĕp-rō)	Leprosy, scaly	Gr. *lepra*, scaly, scaly disease	**Lepr**ology, **lepr**oma Loan word: **Lepra** (lĕp'ră)
XER/O (zer-ō)	Dry	Gr. *xeros*, dry	**Xer**oderma, **xer**ostomia
SICC/O (sĭk-ō)	Dry	L. *siccus, sicca, siccum*, dry	**Sicc**ant, de**sicc**ate
PSOR/O (sō'rō) **PSORIAS/O** (sŏ-rī'ă-sō)	Itch, psoriasis	Gr. *psoros*, itch Gr. *psoriasis*, itch, mange	**Psoria**siform, **psor**elcosis Loan word: **Psoriasis** (sŏ-rī'ă-sĭs)
SCABI/O (skā-bē-ō)	Scabies (caused by mites)	L. *scabies, -ei*, f. scabies/itch	**Scabi**ophobia, **scab**icite Loan word: **Scabies** (skā'bēz)
PRURIT/O (proo-rĭ-tō)	Severe itch	L. *pruritus, -i*, m. itch	**Prurit**ogenic, **prurit**ic Loan word: **Pruritus** (proo-rīt'ŭs)
EXANTHEM/O (eg-zan-thĕm-ō)	Rash	Gr. *exanthema*, eruption, pustule fr. Gr. *anthos*, flower fr. Gr. *anthein*, to blossom, erupt	**Exanthem**atous Loan word: **Exanthema** (eg"zan"thē'mă) / **Exanthem** (eg-zan'thĕm)
ANTH/O (an-thĕm-ō)	Flower	Gr. *anthos*, flower	**Anth**ology, **anth**ophobia

Greek or Latin word element	Current usage	Etymology	Examples
HERPET/O (hĕr-pet-ō)	Reptile, herpes (spreading blisters)	Gr. *herpes, herpetos*, a creeping thing	**Herpet**ic, **herpet**ology Loan word: **Herpes** (hĕrp′ēz″)
LUP/O (loo-pō)	Wolf, lupus	L. *lupus, -i*, m. wolf	**Lup**iform, **lup**oid Loan word: **Lupus** (loo′pŭs)
PEDICUL/O (pi-dik-yŭ-lō)	Louse, lice	L. *pediculus, -i*, m. a louse	**Pedicul**osis, **pedicul**ar Loan word: **Pediculus** (pi-dik′yŭ-lŭs)
NECR/O (nĕ-krō)	Dead, dead tissue	Gr. *nekros*, dead body, dead	**Necr**osis, **necr**obiosis
MYC/O (mī-kō) **MYCET/O** (mī-sĕ-tō)	Fungus, mold	Gr. *mykes, myketos*, mushroom	**Myc**obacterium, **mycet**oma
FUNG/O (fŭng-gō)	Fungus	L. *fungus, -i*, m. mushroom, fungus	**Fung**iform, **fung**iferous Loan word: **Fungus** (fŭng′gŭs) pl. **Fungi** (fŭn′jī, fŭng′gī″)
CARCIN/O (kar-sĭn-ō)	Cancer, crab, crab-like	Gr. *karkinos*, crab, type of skin lesion	**Carcin**oma, **carcin**oid
CANCR/O (kăng-krō)	Ulcer (rapidly spreading)	L. *cancrum, -i*, n. sore, lesion fr. L. *cancer, cancri*, m. crab, type of skin lesion	**Cancr**oid Loan word: **Cancrum** (kăng′krŭm) pl. **Cancra** (kăng′kră)
ONC/O (ong-kō) **-ONCUS** (ong-kus)	Swelling, tumor, abnormal mass	Gr. *onkos*, a mass, tumor	**Onc**ology, cheil**oncus** Loan word: **Oncus** (ong′kŭs)
TUM/O (tū-mō)	Tumor, swelling	L. *tumor, tumoris*, m. tumor, swelling	**Tum**escence, **tum**ifacient Loan word: **Tumor** (too′mŏr)
PY/O (pī-ō)	Pus	Gr. *pyon*, pus	Anti**py**ogenic, **py**orrhea
PUR/O (pū-rō) **PURUL/O** (pūr-ū-lō)	Pus, consisting of pus	L. *pus, puris*, n. pus L. *purulentus*, full of pus	**Pur**omucous, **purul**ence
RHYTID/O (rit-ĭ-dō)	Wrinkle	Gr. *rhytis, rhytidos*, wrinkle	**Rhytid**ectomy, **rhytid**oplasty Loan word: **Rhytide** (rĭ′tĭd)
RUG/O (roo-gō)	Crease, fold	L. *ruga, -ae*, f. crease, wrinkle	**Rug**ose, cor**rug**ator Loan word: **Ruga** (roo′gă) pl. **Rugae** (roo′gē″)

Review	Answers
Suppuration is the production of pus. The combining forms for "pus" are _____, _____, and _____.	**PY/O, PURUL/O, PUR/O**
The root in rhytidectomy means _____. The Latin loan word _____ means "a fold, wrinkle, and crease."	**wrinkle** **ruga**
The term xeroderma literally means "_____ skin."	**dry**
Pediculosis capitis is a condition of lice of the _____. Based on the Latin loan word, a louse is called a _____.	**head** **pediculus**
Psoriasis is a chronic, episodic skin disease characterized by silvery plaques that result in a thickening of the skin cells, particularly at the elbows, knees, arms, and legs. The root PSOR- in this word can mean _____ and _____.	**itch, psoriasis**
Pruritus is a Latin loan word for the symptom of a severe _____.	**itch**
A contagious infestation of the skin with mites that causes a severe itch is called _____.	**scabies**
A condition where there is a hypersecretion of sebum is known as seborrhea. The technical term for dandruff is seborrhea sicca, which literally means _____ seborrhea.	**dry**
Ringworm is a term for a fungal disease affecting the skin that is known by its Latin loan word, _____. The combining forms for 'fungus' are _____, _____, and _____.	**Tinea** **MYC/O, MYCET/O, FUNG/O**
The chronic autoimmune disease characterized by inflammation and ulceration of the body, whose name is derived from the Latin word for "wolf," is called _____.	**Lupus**
Necrotic tissue is _____ tissue. The name of "gnawing" disease in which there is a growth of necrotic tissue associated with a loss of blood supply to an area is _____.	**dead** **gangrene**
Ichthyosis is a pathological condition that makes the skin appear to look like _____ scales.	**fish**
The combining form _____ is used for leprosy. It originally meant "scaly." Consequently, the loan word _____ is used today for the scaly, nodular lesions that occur with leprosy.	**LEPR/O** **lepra**
In medicine, the loan word _____ is used for a scale from the epidermis or a thin plate of bone. The combining forms associated with this term are _____ and _____.	**squama** **SQUAM/O, SQUAMAT/O**
Lepidic lesions are a wide variety of _____ lesions.	**scaly**
An oncus is a loan word used for "a _____."	**tumor**
According to Taber's Cyclopedic Medical Dictionary, a carcinoma is "a malignant tumor that occurs in epithelial tissue and may infiltrate local tissues or produce metastases." The shared root in carcinoma and carcinoid term means _____, _____, and _____.	**cancer, crab, crab-like**
Herpetic lesions are vesicular eruptions that are associated with the virus called Herpes. These terms both come from a Greek word that meant a _____ thing.	**creeping**
The root that is used for "a rash" is _____. The root ANTH- in this root means _____.	**EXANTH-** **flower**
_____ is the name of the contagious bacterial infection of the skin around the mouth and nostrils that produces pustules causing weeping and crusted yellowish lesions. This is an ancient medical term that comes from the Latin verb "to attack."	**Impetigo**

Lessons from History: Cosmetics and Plastic Surgery in Ancient Greek Medicine

Food for Thought as You Read:

What are Galen's views on cosmetic medicine? What do Celsus' surgical descriptions reveal about plastic surgery in antiquity?

Cosmetics were used in the Greek and Roman world, particularly by women, to preserve, restore, or enhance beauty. Ancient Greek medicine's involvement in cosmetics was primarily in the form of the restoration of beauty. One of the earliest examples of medicine's involvement in cosmetics comes from the Hippocratic treatise *Diseases of Women II* (*Mul.* 2.185-191), which are remedies for the loss of hair and changes in complexion affecting women.

By the 2nd century AD, a long list of medical and nonmedical authors had contributed to the list of cosmetic recipes. Renowned for her beauty, Cleopatra's expertise in the domain of cosmetics was legendary. Although the ancient work entitled *Cleopatra's Cosmetics* was probably not written by her, the drug recipes in this book appear in numerous medical works of antiquity, which also contributed to her fame as an expert in cosmetics. In Galen's lists of medical recipes for **alopecia** (Gr. baldness, fox mange), Galen quotes *Cleopatra's Cosmetics*:

> Another remedy against alopecia. The power of this remedy is better than that of all the others, as it works also against falling hair and, mixed with oil or perfume, again incipient baldness and baldness of the crown; and it works wonders. One part of the burnt domestic mice, one part burnt remnants of vine, one part of burnt horse teeth, one part of bear fat, one part of deer marrow, one part of reed bark. Pound them dry, then add a sufficient amount of honey until the thickness of honey is convenient, and then dissolve the fat and the marrow, kneed and mix them. Place the remedy in a copper box. Rub the alopecia until new hair grows back.
>
> *Composition of Medicines According to Places* K. 12.404.
> Translation by Laurence Totelin in "Cold, Dry and Bald."
> *The Recipes Project.* Accessed 11/2020 https://recipes.hypotheses.org/2945.

That cold and/or dryness of the head could cause alopecia are two of the common theoretical explanations found in ancient authors. One would suspect on a theoretical level that this recipe was believed to counteract such qualities. Therefore, the burnt ingredients could be interpreted as having warming and drying qualities, while the fat and marrow would have been something that moistens the scalp. However, as Totelin points out, the rational for this recipe may be less rational than a humoral explanation. She argues that the *materia medica* in this recipe could have been seen as fertilizing ingredients that would counteract the effects of the Autumn of life when a man loses his hair. Although modern medicine has come to a better understanding of the causes of the different types of alopecia, the numerous forms of treatments for hair loss reveal that this disease continues to attract both medical and nonmedical "experts" in cosmetics.

In his discussion of cosmetic recipes, Galen suggested that medicine and cosmetics had a rather tangential relationship:

> In what way the cosmetic (*kosmetikos*) part of the medicine differs from the art of adornment (*kommotikos*): For the art of adornment (*kommotikos*), the goal is to produce an acquired beauty, but for the cosmetic part of medicine, the goal is to preserve everything naturally in the body that corresponds to its beauty by nature. The head that has alopecia looks unfitting, just when the eyelashes and the hairs of the eyebrows fall from the eyes, but what is even more important is what these hairs contribute to the health of the parts ... however to make of the appearance of the face whiter by drugs, or redder, or the hairs of the head curly, or yellowish, or black, or just as women, lengthening them as far as possible, these are the sort things of depravity of cosmetics, not the works of medicine.
>
> *Composition of Medicines According to Places* K. 12.434

In the above passage, Galen uses two Greek words, *kommotikos* (the art of embellishment) and *kosmetikos* (the art of arranging/adorning), that have similar meanings to create a terminological distinction that matches his belief that medicine's role in cosmetics is limited to the restoration of the natural state of beauty, particularly with disfiguring diseases such as alopecia. In this respect, it differs from cosmetics, whose goal, according to Galen, was to produce beauty that is not natural to the body. Interestingly, today, we use the root from the latter Greek word (*kosmetikos*) for surgeries that aim to improve the natural appearance of the body, i.e. **cosmetic surgery**. The other subset of **plastic surgeries** is called **reconstructive surgery** whose aim is to restore the appearance and function of damaged parts. The goal of this surgery is more in line with the goals Galen ascribes to the cosmetic (*kosmetikos*) part of medicine.

In addition to medications, ancient Greek physicians also used surgery to treat skin diseases and disfigurements. Typically, this involved cauterizing or excising a lesion. In some cases, surgery was the preferred option. For instance, Celsus (VII.9.10) states that polyps of the nostrils are best removed with a knife. Ancient Greek physicians also began to perform surgeries to correct mutilations of the body. Celsus (VII.9.1) describes how nostrils, earlobes, lips, and wounds that are not healing could be treated to help correct what is deformed and unsightly. In respect to such wounds, he notes that

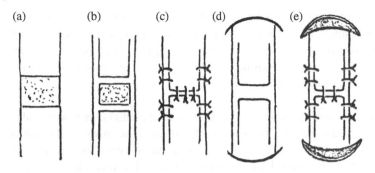

(a) (b) (c) (d) (e)

Fig. 6.19 Image and description of operation for the correction of mutilation in Celsus. (a) Quadrilateral incisions for the excision of the mutilation. Parallel incision carried from the four angles in opposite directions, (b) skin and underlying tissue raised as flaps on opposite sides of the excited area, (c) flaps drawn together and sutured to cover over the area, (d) semilunar incisions to relieve tension, (e) relaxed flaps drawn together, leaving two lunate raw areas to heal by ulceration. *Source:* Spencer 1979/Harvard University Press.

when new skin is not produced in the place of the wound, it can be drawn from neighboring parts, and when the change is small this does not rob the other parts and is hardly noticed. One method is to enclose the mutilated part with a square of skin drawn from the two neighboring sides of the wound site. This involves cutting the neighboring skin into two square flaps, making two semilunar cuts at the anchoring points of these skin flaps, and then drawing the skin flaps over the wound site and suturing their edges (Fig. 6.19).

Celsus' description of creating skin flaps to correct mutilation reveals that ancient Greek medicine performed minor plastic surgeries. In modern healthcare, **plastic surgery** is a branch of medicine dealing with operative procedures to correct deformities and defects as well as repair injuries. Some of these surgeries require the use of a **graft**. In modern medicine, tissue that is transplanted to another part of the body to repair a defect is called a graft. Skin grafts are commonly used to treat areas of skin loss due to burns, infections, trauma, and surgery. The term "graft" comes from the Greek verb, *graphein*, which means "to write" or "to scrape." Writing and scraping shared some common ground in antiquity in that writing on wax tablets involved using a stylus to scrape the letters into the wax tablet.

Some Suggested Readings

Manjo, Guido. *The Healing Hand: Man and Wound in the Ancient World.* Cambridge, MA: Harvard University Press, 1975.

Totelin, Laurence. "*The Third Way. Galen, Pseudo-Galen, Metrodora, Cleopatra and the Gynaecological Pharmacology of Byzantium.*" In *Collecting Recipes. Byzantine and Jewish Pharmacology in Dialogue.* Edited by Lennart Lehmhaus, and Matteo Martelli, 114–119. Berlin: *De Gruyter*, 2017.

Totelin, Laurence. "*From technē to kakotechnia: Use and Abuse of Ancient Cosmetic Texts.*" In *Knowledge, Text, and Practice in Ancient Technical Writing*, Edited by Marco Formisano, and Philip J. van der Eijk, 138–162. Cambridge: Cambridge University Press, 2017.

Etymological Explanations: Grafts

There are a variety of word elements used to denote from where a graft is derived. The relationship between the literal and the medical meanings is not always clear. That said, the roots used to form these words appear frequently in medical terminology.

Skin grafts
Homograft and **Allograft** – A homograft (Gr. *homos*, same), also called an allograft (Gr. *allos*, other [of a group], different than normal) is a graft of material taken from another individual of the same species.
Heterograft and **Xenograft** – A heterograft (Gr. *heteros*, other [of two], different from) also called a xenograft (Gr. *xenos*, foreign) is a graft of material from an individual of another species.
Isograft – An isograft (Gr. *isos*, equal) is graft material derived from an individual who is the same genotype as the patient.
Autograft – An autograft (Gr. *autos*, self) is a graft of material from another part of the patient's body.

Vocabulary

Greek or Latin word element	Current usage	Etymology	Examples
ALL/O (al-ō)	Other, different, abnormal	Gr. *allos*, other (of a group), different, foreign	**All**ograft, **all**oplast
HETER/O (hĕt-ĕr-ō)	Different, other	Gr. *heteros*, other (of two), different	**Heter**ograft, **heter**ogeneous
AUT/O (ot-ō)	Self, same	Gr. *autos*, self, by itself	**Aut**ograft, **aut**omobile
HOM/O (hō-mō) **HOME/O** (hō-mē-ō)	Same, like	Gr. *homos*, like, same Gr. *homoios*, like similar	**Hom**ograft, **home**oplasia
IS/O (ī-sō)	Equal	Gr. *isos*, equal	**Is**ograft, **is**omerous
XEN/O (zen-ō)	Foreign	Gr. *xenos*, foreign, strange, guest/host	**Xen**ograft, **xen**ogamy
COSM/O (kŏz-mō) **COSMET/O** (kŏz-mĕ-tō)	Universe, world, beautification, cosmetic	Gr. *kosmos*, world, order, adornment Gr. *kosmetikos*, the art of dress and ornament	**Cosm**esis, **cosmet**ic
-PLASTY (plas-tē)	Surgical reconstruction	Gr. *plastos*, formed, molded	Rhino**plasty**, cheilo**plasty**
-GRAFT	Tissue transplant	Gr. *graphis*, a style for writing, a needle for embroidering	Allo**graft**, xeno**graft**

Review	Answers
A graft is a surgical transplantation or implantation of tissue. In terms of grafts, the terms allograft and _____ are both used for a tissue transplantation from one species of an animal to another animal of the same species (i.e. human to human graft). The combining form HOM/O means _____ or _____. The combining form ALL/O means _____, _____, and _____.	**homograft** **same, like** **other, different, abnormal**
In terms of grafts, the terms heterograft and _____ are both used for a tissue transplantation from one species of animal to a different species of animal. The combining form HETER/O means _____ and _____. The combining form _____ means "foreign."	**xenograft** **different, other** **XEN/O**
The combining form in. autograft means _____ or _____. An autograft is a transplantation of tissue from one area of the patient's body to another area of the same patient's body.	**self, same**
The combining form in isograft means _____. An isograft is a transplantation of tissue between two individuals who are genetically the same.	**equal**
Cosmesis is consideration of the effect a procedure will have on the appearance of the patient. The root in cosmesis has multiple meanings: _____, _____, and _____.	**world, universe, beautification**
The branch of surgery that deals with correcting deformities and defects is called _____ surgery. The repair of a part that has been damaged is called reconstructive surgery. The other form of plastic surgery is cosmetic surgery, which is a surgical technique directed toward improving the appearance of a person. A surgical reconstruction of a nose is called a rhino_____.	**plastic** **plasty**

7

Musculoskeletal System

CHAPTER LEARNING OBJECTIVES
1) You will gain a better understanding of the Greek and Latin word elements that are fundamental to the musculoskeletal system.
2) You will learn about ancient Greek medicine's understanding of the musculoskeletal system, as well as orthopedic concepts and practices.

Etymological Explanations: Common Terms and Word Elements for the General Parts of the Musculoskeletal System

The musculoskeletal system is made up of bones, joints, muscles, tendons, ligaments, bursae, and soft tissue. The function of the musculoskeletal system is to provide support, structure, protection, and movement to the human body. In the following discussion, the nominative and genitive singular forms of the anatomical Latin terms are provided in the parenthesis. The Greek and Latin roots are in all caps and emboldened.

General parts of the musculoskeletal system

Bone (L. *os, ossis*) – Bones not only protect and give form to the body but they also store minerals and produce blood cells within the bone marrow. The roots **OSTE-** and **OSS-** are derived respectively from the Greek *osteon* and the Latin *os, ossis*. Today, **osteon** is used as a loan word for a "microscopic unit of compact bone." In ancient Greek medicine, bones were considered the hardest and driest parts of the body due to the belief that their elemental composition was mostly of earth. The notion that they were composed of earth is probably also derived from the manner in which bones decompose into "dust." The dust resulting from the breakdown of the minerals and fibers of bones may also explain why in some creation stories "earth" is a material from which human beings are said to have been made. In Greek mythology, the Greek god Prometheus is sometimes said to have created humans out of water and earth (Apollodorus 1.7.1–1.7.3), and in Hesiod's *Theogony*, the first woman (Pandora) is said to have been made from clay by the Greek god of the forge, Hephaestus.

Joint (L. *junctura, juncturae* or *articulatio, articulationis*) – The bones are joined together by a variety of different types of joints (Fig. 7.1). In medical terminology, the roots **JUNCTUR-**, **ARTICUL-**, and **ARTHR-** which are, respectively, derived from the Latin *junctura* and *articulare* and the Greek *arthron*, means "a joint." Because **ARTICUL-** comes from the Latin verb *articulare*, it also means "to segment" and "to speak distinctly." With respect to speech, "to articulate" is to speak with a clear enunciation of words, but in a physical sense, "to articulate" is to join something together. This connection between speech and joints is also evident in the use of **ARTHR-**. The term dysarthria is defined in medicine as an impairment in speaking due to a muscular impairment of the mouth, tongue, or pharynx. One of our earliest examples of an individual attempting to rectify a speech impediment of this nature comes from Plutarch's *Parallel Lives*. Plutarch relates how the famous Greek orator Demosthenes (384–322 BC) had a "weakness of voice and indistinctness of speech and shortness of breath which disturbed the sense of what he said by disjoining his sentences." One of the methods Demosthenes used to overcome this was to place pebbles in his mouth and then repeat verses. To this day, the story of the "Pebbles of Demosthenes" is commonly cited as an early example of speech therapy.

In *Bones for Beginners*, Galen places joints into two major categories: diarthrosis and synarthrosis. These ancient Greek medical terms for different types of joints in the body are still used today in medicine. A **diarthrosis** is a joint with visible motion, and a **synarthrosis** is a joint that lacks visible motion.

Greek and Latin Roots of Medical and Scientific Terminologies, First Edition. Todd A. Curtis.
© 2025 John Wiley & Sons, Inc. Published 2025 by John Wiley & Sons, Inc.
Companion website: www.wiley.com/go/Curtis

Fig. 7.1 Anatomical Latin terms for the *Junctura synovialis* (synovial joint) and the parts of the musculoskeletal system: *os* (bone), *caput articulare ossis* (articular head of the bone), *musculus* (muscle), *tendo* (tendon), *bursa* (bursa), *capsula articularis* (articular capsule), and *cartilage articularis* (articular cartilage). *Source:* Drawing by Chloe Kim.

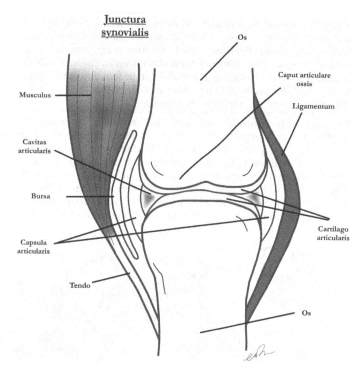

A **suture** (L. *sutura, suturae*) is one example of synarthrosis. The bones of the cranium and face are joined by bony sutures. The Greek and Latin roots for "suture" or "seam" are **RAPH-** and **SUTUR-**, respectively. The Greek loan word **raphe** is used today in medicine for an anatomical seam or crease that joins two halves of a part. Sutura is the anatomical Latin term used for the immovable fibrous or cartilaginous joints.

A diarthrosis is also called a synovial joint. Formed from Latin and Greek word elements (Gr. *syn-* together + L. *ovum*, egg), synovial derives its name from the consistency and egg white-like appearance of the viscous fluid that lubricates the interior of joints. The term is believed to have been coined by the 16th century physician Paracelsus. Today, **synovia** (L. *synovia, synoviae*) is the anatomical term used for the fluid in the joint (i.e. synovial fluid), but **synovium** (L. *synovium, synovii*) is the term for the connective tissue that lines these joints (i.e. synovial membrane).

Ligament (L. *ligamentum, ligamenti*) – Ligaments are passive fibrous structures that connect bones and support joints. The roots used for "ligament" are **DESM-** and **LIGAMENT-**, which respectively are derived from the Gr. *desmos* and L. *ligamentum*. The Greek word *desmos* was used for anything that was binding (e.g. fetters, band, door-latch), which explains why, in addition to "ligament," the root **DESM-** is used for "bonding" or "band." In ancient Greek medicine, the word *syndesmos* was the specific term for an anatomical ligament. The compound root **SYNDESM-** continues to be used for "ligament" today in words such as syndesmectomy, syndesmography, and syndesmophyte. Ligamentum is derived from the Latin verb *ligare*, which means "to bind or tie." Consequently, in modern medicine, the root **LIG-** means "to bind or tie something," for example the ligation of a blood vessel.

Cartilage (L. *cartilago, cartilaginis*) – Cartilage is a specialized type of connective tissue that is a structural component of the rib cage, forms the intervertebral discs, and protects the ends of long bones at the joints. The roots **CARTILAG-** and **CHONDR-** are used in medicine for "cartilage." Ancient Greek medicine recognized that cartilage was distinct from bone, sinew/ligaments, and flesh. In his *Bones for Beginners*, Galen also notes that bones can be joined by what he calls a "growing together" symphysis. There are three types of symphyses according to Galen: (i) a *synchondrosis*, as its name implies, is a symphysis formed by cartilage (Gr. *chondros*); (ii) a *synsarkosis* is joined by flesh (Gr. *sarkos*); and (iii) a *synneurosis* is a symphysis joined by sinew (Gr. *neuron*, nerve, sinew). Their word elements, **CHONDR-**, **SARC-**, and **NEUR-** are commonly used today for "cartilage," "flesh/muscle," and "nerve," respectively. Thanks to publicized injuries of modern professional athletes, the meniscus is perhaps the most famous cartilage in the human body. There are two *menisci* at the top of the tibia: a medial meniscus and a lateral meniscus. Meniscus is a loan word that comes from the Greek word for "a crescent," which is the shape of this cartilage. Thus, the root **MENISC-** refers to this cartilage of the knee; it is also used for anything that is "crescent-shaped" (Fig. 7.2).

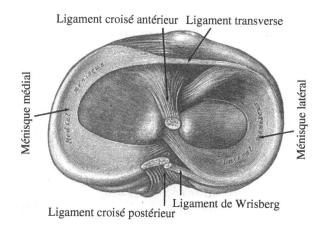

Fig. 7.2 The right tibia, as seen from above, showing the lateral and medial menisci. Image from Henry Gray, *Anatomy of the Human Body*, 1918. *Source:* Bartleby/Wikimedia Commons/Public domain.

Muscles (L. *musculus, musculi*) – Muscles are attached to the bones primarily via fibrous tissue called tendons, and together they provide movement to the body. The roots used for "muscles" in medicine are **MUSCUL-**, **MY-**, **MYS-**, and **MYOS-**, which are from the Latin *musculus* and the Greek *mys*. In addition to carrying the meaning "muscle," both the Latin *musculus* and the Greek *mys* also mean "mouse." The taxonomic term *Mus musculus* encompasses all the subspecies of the "house mouse." The etymological connection between "mouse" and "muscle" can be found in other languages as well (German *maus* mouse; "muscle"; Arabic *adalah* "muscle," *adal* "field mouse"). Some have speculated that the reason for the connection between a mouse and a muscle is that a biceps muscle resembles a mouse when flexed.

Tendon (L. *tendo, tendinis*) – A tendon attaches a muscle to a bone. The roots used for "tendon" are **TEN-**, **TENONT-**, and **TENDIN-**. The etymologies of the roots for tendons suggest that it comes from a stem for "something stretched." The most famous tendon in the body is perhaps the "Achilles' tendon," which is a combined tendon that joins the calf muscles (i.e. soleus, gastrocnemius, and plantaris) to the heel bone (i.e. calcaneus). The German surgeon Lorenz Heister (1683–1758) was the first to link this tendon to the Greek hero of the Trojan War, Achilles. In Greek myth, Achilles was killed by the arrow of Paris (guided by Apollo), piercing Achilles' ankle, leaving him mortally wounded (Fig. 7.3). The most popular account of the vulnerable spot of Achilles is found in Statius' *Achilleid* (c. 1st century AD). According to this account, Achilles' mother, Thetis, held him by the heel when she dipped him in the River Styx to render him invulnerable. The *Iliad* and the *Odyssey* make no mention of this story.

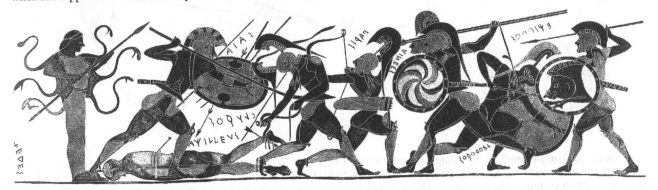

Fig. 7.3   The battle for the body of Achilles in a 6th century BC Chalcidian vase-painting. The corpse of Achilles lies in the middle with an arrow in his heel. The mother of Achilles, the goddess Thetis, stands at the far left. The Greek hero Ajax (to the immediate left of Achilles' body) thrusts his spear at the Trojan hero Glaucus (to the immediate right of Achilles' body) as Glaucus attempts to pull away Achilles' body by means of a rope tied around the ankle. Paris (right of Glaucus), the Trojan hero who killed Achilles, is shooting an arrow at Ajax. *Source:* The Inscription Painter, Chalkis/Wikimedia Commons/Public domain.

Fascia (L. *fascia, fasciae*) – Fascia is a broad band of connective tissue that envelops and separates muscles. The term fascia is a loan word from the Latin word meaning "band, bandage, or ribbon," which explains why this is the term for the decorative band that hangs at the side of a Roman Catholic priest's garments. The root of this Latin word is **FASCI-**.

Bursa (L. *bursa, bursae*) – A bursa is a fibrous fluid-filled sac that occurs near joints that reduces friction of tendons gliding over bones. The root for bursa is **BURS-**. The Latin word *bursa* originally meant "sack, bag for money," which is why this root appears in terms that have to do with "money," such as "bursary" and "reimburse."

Greek or Latin word element	Current usage	Etymology	Examples
OSTE/O (os-tē-ō)	Bone	Gr. *osteon*, bone	Periosteum, osteotome Loan word: **Osteon** (os′tē-on″)
OSS/O (ŏs-ō) **OSSE/O** (ŏs-ē-ō)	Bone	L. *os, ossis*, n. bone L. *osseus, -a, -um*, bony	Ossicle, interosseous Loan word: **Os** (os) pl. **Ossa** (os′ă)
JUG/O (jū-gō) **JUNCTUR/O** (jŭngk-too-rō)	Joint, a joining	L. *jungere (jugere), junctum*, to join L. *jugum, -i*, n. a yoke L. *junctura, -ae*, f. a joining	**Juncture, jug**al Loan word: **Junctura** (jŭngk-toor′ă) pl. **Juncturae** (jŭngk-toor′ē″)

Greek or Latin word element	Current usage	Etymology	Examples
ARTICUL/O (ar-tik-yŭ-lō)	Joint, to join, to speak clearly	L. *articulatio, articulationis,* f. joint, knuckle fr. *articulare,* to segment, to speak distinctly	Extra-**articul**ar, dis**articul**ate Loan word: **Articulatio** (ar-tik″yŭ-lā′shē-ō) pl. **Articulationes** (ar-tik″yŭ-lā′shē-nēz)
ARTHR/O (ar-thrō)	Joint	Gr. *arthron,* joint	**Arthr**algia, **arthr**oplasty
LIGAT/O (lī-gā-tō) **LIGAMENT/O** (lig-ă-men-tō)	To bind, tie Ligament	L. *ligare, ligatum,* to bind, tie L. *ligamentum, -i,* n. ligament	**Ligat**e, **ligament**opexy Loan word: **Ligamentum** (lig″ă-ment′ŭm) pl. **Ligamenta** (lig″ă-ment′ă)
DESM/O (dez-mō)	Ligament, band, bond	Gr. *desmos,* band, bond, ligament fr. Gr. *deein,* to tie	Syn**desm**osis, **desm**orrhexis
CARTILAG/O (kăr-tĭ-lă-gō)	Cartilage	L. *cartilago, cartilaginis,* f. gristle, cartilage	**Cartilag**inification, **cartilag**inous Loan word: **Cartilago** (kăr″tĭ-lă′gō) pl. **Cartilagines** (kăr″tĭ-lă′je-nēz)
CHONDR/O (kŏn-drō)	Cartilage	Gr. *chondros,* granule	**Chondr**omalacia, costo**chondr**itis
MENISC/O (mĕn-ĭs-kō)	Meniscus, crescent	L. *meniscus, -i,* m. meniscus fr. Gr. *meniskos,* crescent	**Menisc**ocyte, **menisc**ectomy Loan word: **Meniscus** (mĕ-nis′kŭs) pl. **Menisci** (mĕ-nis′kī″)
SYNOVI/O (sĭ-nō-vē-ŏ) **SYNOV/O** (sĭn-ō-vŏ)	Synovial fluid	L. *synovia, -ae,* f. synovial fluid (new L. *synovia,* albuminous joint fluid)	**Synov**ectomy, **synovi**al Loan word: **Synovia** (sĭn-ō′vē-ă) pl. **Synoviae** (sĭn-ō′vē-ē″)
CAPSUL/O (kăp-sŭ-lō) **CAPS/O** (kă-′sŏ)	Capsule	L. *capsula, -ae,* f. little chest or box L. *capsa, -ae,* f. box	Intra**capsul**ar, **caps**itis Loan word: **Capsula** (kăp′sŭ-lă) pl. **Capsulae** (kăp′sŭ-lē″)
BURS/O (bŭr-sō)	Bursa (anatomical), bag, pouch	L. *bursa, -ae,* f. a sack, purse, anatomical pad-like sac associated with joints	**Burs**itis, intra**burs**al Loan word: **Bursa** (bŭr′să) pl. **Bursae** (bŭr′sē″)
FASCI/O (făsh-ē-ō)	Fascia, band	L. *fascia, -ae,* f. a broad band, bandage, a broad band of connective tissue enveloping muscle	Myo**fasci**tis, **faci**otomy Loan word: **Fascia** (fash′ē-ă) pl. **Fasciae** (fash′ē-ē)
MUSCUL/O (mŭs-kyŏ-lō)	Muscle, mouse	L. *musculus, -i,* m. muscle, mouse	**Muscul**ocutaneous, **muscul**ar Loan word: **Musculus** (mŭs′kyŭ-lŭs) pl. **Musculi** (mŭs′kyŭ-lī″)

Greek or Latin word element	Current usage	Etymology	Examples
MY/O (mī-ō) **MYOS/O** (mī-ō-sō) **MYS/O** (mī-sō)	Muscle, mouse	Gr. *mys*, *myos*, muscle, mouse	**My**oatrophy, epi**mys**ium, **myos**itis
TENDIN/O (ten-dĭ-nō)	Tendon	L. *tendo*, *tendinis*, m. tendon fr. L. *tenere* to stretch	**Tendin**itis, **tendin**opathy Loan word: **Tendo** (ten′dō) pl. **Tendines** (ten′dĭ-nēz)
TEN/O (ten-ō) **TENONT/O** (tĕn-ŏn-tō)	Tendon	Gr. *tenon*, *tenontos*, tendon, sinew	**Ten**odesis, **tenont**odynia

Review	Answers
Osteoarthritis is the chronic deterioration of cartilage in synovial joints and vertebrae. The combining form OSTE/O means _____ and the root means _____ in this term.	**bone, joint**
A tenodesis is a surgical fixation of a _____.	**tendon**
Myositis ossificans is an inflammation of a _____ that is associated with the pathological formation of _____.	**muscle, bone**
The broad fibrous connective tissue that envelops and separates muscle is called _____ because it resembles a broadband.	**fascia**
According to its word elements, the musculocutaneous nerve innervates _____ and _____.	**muscle, skin**
According to its word elements, myofascitis is an inflammation of the _____ and the _____.	**muscle, fascia**
An inflammation of the fibrous fluid-filled sac near a joint is called _____itis.	**burs**
The term for the albuminous fluid occurring in joints is _____, and likewise, the term for the membrane in synovial joints is _____.	**synovia, synovium**
A meniscoid structure resembles a _____ moon. The surgical excision of a torn meniscus is called a _____.	**crescent meniscectomy**
Chondromalacia is the pathological softening of articular _____.	**cartilage**
A desmorrhexis is a rupture of a _____.	**ligament**
Also known as a "frozen shoulder," adhesive capsulitis is an inflammation of the glenohumeral joint _____ that produces fibrous adhesions.	**capsule**
The anatomical Latin plurals for muscles, bones, tendons, ligaments, cartilage, and joints are _____, _____, _____, _____, _____, and _____.	**musculi, ossa, tendines, ligamenta, cartilagines, juncturae (or articulationes)**
Based on its root, a ligature is a surgical filament that can _____ or _____ blood vessels or other structures.	**bind, tie**

Etymological Explanations: Greek and Latin Roots for the Parts of Bones

In the following discussion of the anatomical terms associated with the parts of bones, the nominative and genitive singular forms of the anatomical Latin term are provided in parenthesis. The Greek and Latin roots are formatted in all caps and emboldened.

In modern osteology, human bones are categorized according to their shape and length, most notably: **long bones (L. *ossa longa*)**, **short bones (L. *ossa brevia*)**, **flat bones (L. *ossa plana*)**, and **irregular bones (L. *ossa irregularia*)**. The following terms are used for the parts of bones (Fig. 7.4).

Fig. 7.4 Anatomical Latin terms for the parts of the *os logum* (long bone), which are the *epiphysis, metaphysis, diaphysis, facies articularis* (articular surface/face), *caput ossis* (head of the bone), *collum ossis* (neck of the bone), *corpus ossis* (body of the bone), *medulla ossis flava* (yellow marrow of the bone), *medulla ossis rubra* (red marrow of the bone), *line epiphysialis* (epiphysial line), *lamina epiphysialis* (epiphysial plate), periosteum, and endosteum. *Source:* Drawing by Chloe Kim.

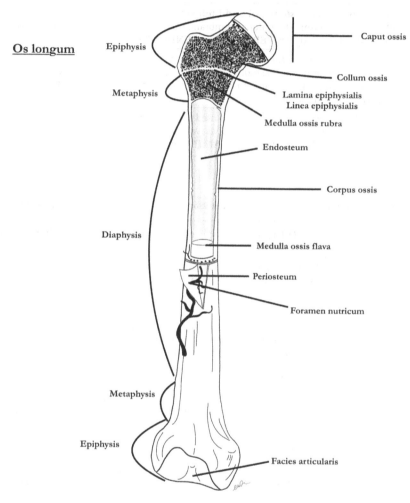

Os longum

Epiphysis
Metaphysis
Diaphysis
Metaphysis
Epiphysis

Caput ossis
Collum ossis
Lamina epiphysialis
Linea epiphysialis
Medulla ossis rubra
Endosteum
Corpus ossis
Medulla ossis flava
Periosteum
Foramen nutricum
Facies articularis

Parts of bones

Head of the Bone (L. *caput ossis*), Neck of the Bone (L. *collum ossis*), and Body of the Bone (L. *corpus ossis*) – Long bones are often said to have a head, which is where the articulates with another body, neck, which the part that connects the head to the body of the bone, and body, which is the shaft of the bone. The roots for the head, neck, and body of a bone are correspondingly: **CAPIT-**, **COLL-**, and **CORPOR-**.

Growth Plate (L. *physis, -is*) – For long bones, the suffix **-PHYSIS** refers to the growth plate. The prefixes (**APO-, DIA-, META-, EPI-**) found in apophysis, diaphysis, metaphysis, and epiphysis refer to the part of the bone in relation to the growth plate. The term **epiphysis (EPIPHYS-)** is used for the ends of bones and the ossification centers derived from the growth plate. Modern osteological terminology defines an **apophysis (APOPHYS-)** as being a bony prominence apart from the growth plate. Modern terminology for the parts of a long bone includes the **diaphysis (DIAPHYS-)**, which is the shaft of a long bone between the growth plates, and the **metaphysis (METAPHYS-)**, which is the area of bone development between the diaphysis and the epiphysis. In ancient Greek, *physis* was a term that spoke to the "nature" or "natural qualities" of something. It is derived from the Greek verb *phyein*, which means "to grow or arise." From this verb is derived a collection of important roots used in medicine and science. **PHYT-**, from *phyton*, is used for "a growth, plant," **PYSI-** is used for "nature" and "physical," and the suffix **-PHYMA** is used for "a growth, plant, or tumor."

Marrow of the Bone (L. *medulla ossis*) – Based on the Latin *medulla* and the Greek *myelos*, the roots **MEDULL-** and **MYEL-** are used for "bone marrow." However, **MYEL-** is also used for the "spinal cord," which is the column of nervous tissue proceeding from the brain down the spine. This dual meaning goes back to ancient Greek medicine. Galen makes a distinction between the *myelos* of bones and the *myelos* of the spinal cord by saying that unlike the *myelos* of the spinal cord, the *myelos* of bones lack sensation. The reason for this dual usage comes from *myelos* core meaning being the soft inmost part of something. Thus, bone marrow and the spinal cord are the soft inner parts "within" a bone, the latter being present in the large hole in the vertebrae known as the vertebral foramen (L. *foramen vertebrale*). As to the purpose of marrow, Galen put forward that Nature created the hollow in the bone for marrow because marrow is the proper nutriment for the bones. Today, we recognize that **red marrow** (L. *medulla ossium rubra*) produces red blood cells, and that **yellow marrow** (L. *medulla ossium flava*) consists primarily of fat cells and does not participate in hematopoiesis.

Periosteum (L. *periosteum, -i*) and Endosteum (L. *endosteum, -i*) – The membrane lining the marrow cavity of the bone is called the endosteum. The fibrous membrane that covers the exterior of bones is called the periosteum. The compound roots for these parts of the body are **PERIOSTE-** and **ENDOSTE-**.

Foramen (L. *foramen, foraminis*) – A hole or passageway into a bone, which typically carries blood vessels and/or nerves, is usually called a foramen. The root **FORAMIN-** comes from the Latin word for "hole" or "aperture." Foramen is derived from the Latin verb *forare*, which means "to bore or pierce." The roots **FOR-** and **FORAT-** mean "a hole" or "to bore/drill," and they appear in words such as perforation and biforate.

Lamina (L. *lamina, -ae*) – Lamina is used for a flat layer of a structure. It is also used for the flat part on both sides of the arch of a vertebra. In classical Latin, a *lamina*, as well as a *lamella*, was "a plate or a thin piece of metal or marble." Thus, the loan words, **lamina** and **lamella**, and the roots, **LAMIN-** and **LAMELL-**, are used for a "thin plate, layer."

Greek or Latin word element	Current usage	Etymology	Examples
MYEL/O (mī-ĕ-lō)	Bone marrow, spinal cord	Gr. *myelos*, marrow	**Myel**ogram, osteo**myel**itis
MEDULL/O (mĕd-ū-lō)	Bone marrow, the innermost part of an organ	L. *medulla, -ae*, f. marrow	**Medull**itis, **medull**ary Loan word: **Medulla** (mĕ-dŭl′ă) pl. **Medullae** (mĕ-dŭl′ē″)
PHYSI/O (fĭz-ē-ō) **-PHYSIS** (fĭ-sĭs)	Nature, natural function growth, growth plate	L. *physis, -is*, f. growth plate fr. Gr. *physis*, nature, growth	**Physi**ology, epi**physis**
PHYT/O (fī-tō) **-PHYTE** (fīt)	A growth, plant	Gr. *phyton*, growth, plant	Osteo**phyte**, **phyt**ochemistry
-PHYMA (fī′mă)	A growth, tumor	Gr. *phyma*, tumor, growth	Tarso**phyma**, rhino**phyma**
CAPIT/O (ka-pĭ-tō)	Head, head of a long bone	L. *caput, capitis*, n. head	**Capit**ate, **capit**al Loan word: **Caput** (kap′ut″) pl. **Capita** (kap′ĭ-ta″)
COLL/O (kŏl-lō)	Neck, neck of a long bone	L. *collum, -i*, n. neck	Torti**coll**is, **coll**ar Loan word: **Collum** (kŏl′lŭm) pl. **Colla** (kŏl′lă)
CORPOR/O (kor-pŏ-rō)	Body	L. *corpus, corporis*, n. body	**Corpor**eal, **corpor**ality Loan word: **Corpus** (kor′pŭs) pl. **Corpora** (kor′pŏ-ră)

Greek or Latin word element	Current usage	Etymology	Examples
FORAMIN/O (fŏ-ram-ĭ-nō)	A hole or passageway in a bone (foramen)	L. *foramen, foraminis,* n. hole	**Foramin**al, **foramin**otomy Loan word: **Foramen** (fŏ-rā′mĕn) pl. **Foramina** (fŏ-ram′ĭ-nă)
LAMIN/O (lă-mĭn-ō)	Plate (lamina)	L. *lamina, -ae,* f. plate	**Lamin**ated, **lamin**opathy Loan word: **Lamina** (lam′ĭ-nă) pl. **Laminae** (lam′ĭ-nē″)

Review	Answers
A subcapital fracture is under the _____ of a bone.	**head**
Corpus vertebrae is best translated the _____ of the vertebra.	**body**
An osteophyte is an abnormal bone _____.	**growth**
The surgical excision of the flat parts of the vertebral arch is called a _____.	**laminectomy**
The intervertebral foramen is a _____ or _____ between the vertebrae.	**hole, passageway**
In respect to bones, a myelogram is a count of _____ _____ cells. In respect to the nervous system, a myelogram is an image of the _____ _____.	**Bone marrow** **Spinal cord**
Medullitis is an inflammation of bone _____.	**marrow**
In respect to long bones, the suffix -PHYSIS is associated with the _____ _____. An inflammation of the end of a bone is a _____itis. Inflammation of the shaft of a long bone is a _____itis. Inflammation of the portion of the bone that includes the growth plate and slightly beyond is a _____itis.	**growth plate** **epiphys** **diaphys** **metaphys**

Lessons from History: Galen's Bones for Beginners and the Teaching of Anatomy

Food for Thought as You Read:

Why were the bones of the skeleton important to ancient medical education? How are they important to modern medicine?

Written in the 2nd century AD, Galen's *Bones for Beginners* reveals that many of our technical terms for bones and joints are ultimately derived from Greek anatomical writings. Unlike his more advanced works on anatomical dissection, *Bones for Beginners* is written for novices who want to learn anatomy. In the introductory remarks to *Bones for Beginners*, Galen points out that the knowledge of bones is fundamental to the treatment of fractures and joint dislocations. For Galen, bones are the first structures to be studied in anatomical dissections. In *On Anatomical Procedures*, a work for more advanced students, Galen advises that a physician should first study the bones of the body before moving to the muscles. Having studied the bones and muscles, the physician should then proceed to the arteries, veins, and nerves, and lastly, one should study the viscera and glands.

There are 206 bones that make up the human skeleton. Galen calls the aggregate of bones in the human body the *skeletos* (dried-up, withered), from which we get the anatomical Latin term **skeleton**. *Bones for Beginners* reveals that Galen was not always using a human skeleton when writing about the human body. In his introduction to *On Anatomical Procedures*, Galen notes that outside of Alexandria, where the study of bones was via demonstrations using human skeletons, it was quite difficult to have access to a human skeleton. He advised his readers that if they cannot visit Alexandria, they may be able to gain access to human bones via the serendipity of an abandoned corpse or by prying into a grave (Fig. 7.5).

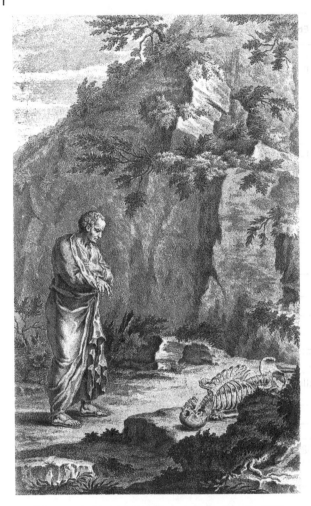

Fig. 7.5 Image of Galen finding a skeleton found in William Cheselden, *The Anatomy of the Human Body*. VIIth Edition. London, 1756. *Source:* Wellcome Collection/Public domain.

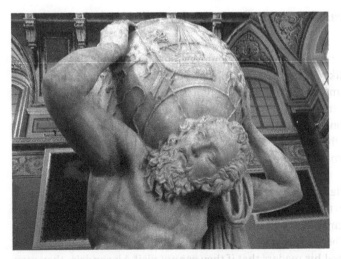

Fig. 7.6 2nd century AD Roman sculpture of Atlas holding a celestial dome with the constellations of the heavens depicted on it. *Source:* Dr.Conati/Wikimedia Commons/Public domain.

That said, he recommends using ape (Gr. *pithekos*) skeletons since they are closest to humans, and it appears that Galen used the Barbary macaque (L. *Macaca sylvanus*) in some of his descriptions of bones in *Bones for Beginners*.

After discussing the nature of bones and joints, Galen's *Bones for Beginners* makes *a capite ad calcem* (literally "head to heel") survey of the bones of the skeleton. Galen gives far more lines of text to describing the skull than to any other part of the body, perhaps because of its intimate association with the brain. He begins with a discussion of the dome-like structure of the skull known as the *kranion* (L. *cranium, cranii*). The gloss he provides to these bones explains the origins of the terms used for bones today. When discussing the sutures of the cranium, he describes how the *lamboeide* (L. *sutura lambdoidea*) located at the back of the cranium looks like the Greek *lambda* (Λ), and the *stephanaia* (L *sutura coronalis*) gets its name from its location since this is part of the head where the *stephanos* (crown, wreath) is placed. Having described the cranium in some detail, he then moves to the other major and minor bones of the skull (e.g. L. *maxilla* [upper jawbone], L. *mandibula* [lower jawbone], *zygoma* [cheek bone, nasal bones]).

Galen moves next to the *spondyloi* (= L. *vertebrae*), the word from which we get the root for "vertebra, a backbone," **SPONDYL-**. He notes that the typical human spine has 24 vertebrae (7 cervical, 12 thoracic, and 5 lumbar). Galen accurately describes the differences between the types of vertebrae of the lumbar, thoracic, and cervical spine, as well as the bones *kokkyx* (L. *os coccygis* or simply *coccyx*) and the *hieron osteon* (L. *os sacrum* or simply *sacrum*). From this, we recognize that the sacrum's Greek name, *hieron osteon* (holy bone) explains why the Latin adjective for "sacred" is used for the name of this bone. As to the rationale for the coccyx's name, it comes from the Greek word for "cuckoo" due to it resembling the shape of the beak of this bird. The whole spine is called the ***rhachis*** by Galen, which today is the loan word for the vertebral column. Today, each vertebra has a specific letter (i.e. cervical = C, thoracic = T, and Lumbar = L) and number attached to it (i.e. C1-7, T1-12, L1-5) to identify which vertebra a physician is referencing. This is done from superior to inferior. For example, the most superior cervical vertebra is referred to as C1, and the most inferior cervical vertebra is termed C7. Today, C1 is also termed the "**Atlas**" after the Titan in Greek mythology who was punished by Zeus for his involvement in the war between the Olympians and the Titans. Ancient Greek physicians did not call the C1 vertebra the Atlas; the term was coined centuries later. The reason for this vertebra being called the "Atlas" comes from the false belief that Atlas held up the Earth on his shoulders, much like C1 holds up the skull. In Greek myth, Atlas held up the column that separates the heavens from the earth, so he actually held up the heavens on his shoulders (Fig. 7.6). The reason for the mistaken belief that Atlas held up the earth is that 16th century map makers included an image of Atlas holding up a celestial sphere (a device for tracking the constellations in the heavens) on his back. The constellations were used for sea and land navigation, so it made sense to include a map of the figure of Atlas holding up the heavens. Over time, the celestial sphere was conflated with the image of the globe of the earth, which also explains why a collection of maps is also called an "Atlas" today.

The rib cage is the next set of bones that *Bones for Beginners* discusses. In Greek, the ribs are called *pleura* (L. *costa, costae*). The root **PLEUR-** is used today for "rib," "side," and the serous membrane known as the "pleura." There are twelve ribs, and they are numbered 1–12, superior to inferior. Galen identifies the breastbone to which the ribs are attached as the *sternon* (L. *sternum, sterni*), which was the Greek word for "chest." According to Galen, the sternum was also called the *xiphoeides* because the sternum looks like a *xiphos* (sword). Today, the tip of the sternum bears the name xiphoid process.

The Greek name for the shoulder blade was *omoplata* (L. *scapula, scapulae*) which is a compound term formed from *omos* (shoulder) + *plata* (flat surface). The root **OM-** is used today for "shoulder." It appears in the name for the triangular part of the spine of the scapula, the *acromion* = Gr. *acros* (top) + *omion* (little shoulder). Galen calls the beak-shaped process of the scapula the *korakoeide* (L. *processus coracoideus*) because it is crooked like the beak of a *korax* (raven). In Greek, the phrase "*es korakas*" (to the ravens) was a curse word meaning roughly "go hang yourself" or "go to hell" since ravens pick the carcasses of dead bodies. The only bony attachment of the shoulder girdle, the collarbone, was called the **kleida** (L. *clavicula, claviculae*) by Galen, assumedly because it looked like a "key" or "latch," which bears the same name. Consequently, **CLEID-** is used today for the "collarbone."

Galen uses the term *brachion* (L. *humerus, humeri*) for the bone of the arm. Today, the brachium is a term for the arm, rather than for the bone. He names the bones of the forearm the *pechys* (L. *ulna*) and the *kerchis* (L. *radius, -i*). *Pechys* was the Greek term for the "forearm," as well as a unit of length since it was the distance between the point of the elbow to the tip of the finger. The bones of the wrist were collected called the *karpoi* (L. *carpus, carpi*), and the five ray-like bones making up the palm were termed the *metakarpoi* (L. *metacarpus, metacarpi*). In modern anatomy, they are numbered lateral to medial or thumb to pinky, 1–5. Like today, Galen identifies the bones of the fingers as *phalanges* (L. *phalanx, phalangis*). A *phalanx* was also a Greek word for a rectangular type of battle formation brought to perfection by Philip of Macedon (382–336 BC), the famous Macedonian king who was the father of Alexander the Great. The fingers themselves were referred to as *daktyloi*, which is why we use the root **DACTYL-** for "finger" today.

Turning to the bones of the lower extremity, Galen divides the pelvis into three parts: the **lagon** (L. *os ilium*), which means "loin," the *ischion* (L. *os ischium*), which means "hip-joint," and the *hebe* (L. *os pubis*). *Hebe* is the Greek word for youth or the time before manhood (it is also the name of the Greek goddess of youthful beauty). Assumedly, this is because this is the area where adolescence is evident by the growth of pubic hair. Today, **HEB-** is still used for pubic bone in terms of hebotomy.

Galen calls the bone of the thigh the *meros* (L. *femur*). The large medial bone of the leg he calls the **kneme** (L. *tibia, tibiae*) and the lateral bone is termed the *perone* (L. *fibula*). The roots **KNEM-** and **PERONE-** are respectively used today for the "leg" and "fibula." Like the Latin word *fibula*, the Greek word *perone* was the term for a "brooch," or the "tongue of a buckle," and it was used for the lateral bone of the leg because the fibula resembles this type of fastener with respect to the tibia (Fig. 7.7).

Fig. 7.7 Bronze Roman fibula (broach).
Source: Wellcome Collection/CC BY 4.0.

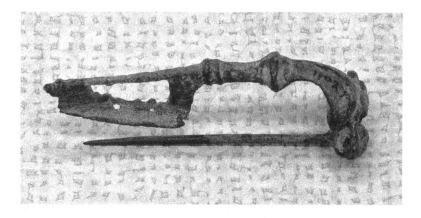

The kneecap was termed the **myle (L. patella)** because it supposedly looked like a "millstone" (*myle*). **MYL-** is used for the "molar"(grinder) rather than for the "patella" today. The kneecap was also called the **epigonatis** because it is located "upon" (*epi-*) the knee (*gony*). Today, **GONY-** is used for "knee," but not for the "kneecap."

Galen calls the top bone of the ankle the *astragolas* (L. *talus*), perhaps because it looked like a die (*astragalos*). The large bone of the heel is called the *pterna* (L. *calcaneus, calcanei*), which means "heel." **PTERN-** is used today for the "heel." While Galen names the cube-shaped bone called the **kuboeides** (L. *os cuboideum*) and the boat-shaped bone called the **skaphoeides** (L. *os naviculare*) of the tarsus, he does not specifically call the five bones of the sole of the foot as the **metatarsi.** Similar to today, Galen calls the bones of the toes and the fingers **phalanges**.

Some Suggested Readings

Agrawal, Anuj. "Musculoskeletal Etymology: What's in a Name? *Journal of Clinical Orthopaedics and Trauma* 10, no. 2 (2019): 387–394.

Goss, Charles M., and Chodkowski, Elizabeth G. "On Bones for Beginners by Galen of Pergamon." *American Journal of Anatomy* 169 (1984): 61–74.

Panourias, Ioannis G., et al. "The Hellenic and Hippocratic origins of the Spinal Terminology." *Journal of the History of Neuroscience* 20, no. 3 (2011): 177–187.

Singer, Charles. "Galen's Elementary Course on Bones." *Proceedings of the Royal Society of Medicine* 45 (1952): 767–776.

Etymological Explanations: Greek and Latin Roots for the Skeletal Bones

In the following discussion of the anatomical terms associated with the skeletal bones (Fig. 7.8), the nominative and genitive singular forms of the anatomical Latin term are provided in parenthesis. The Greek and Latin roots are formatted in all caps and emboldened.

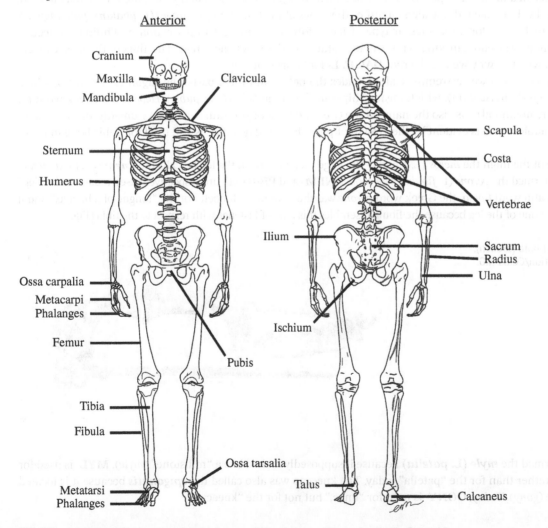

Fig. 7.8 Anatomical Latin terms for the bones of the skeleton. *Source:* Image by Chloe Kim.

Skeleton (L. *skeleton, -i*) – There are 206 bones that make up the human skeleton. The common root for the skeleton is **SKELET-**. The skeleton is divided into the axial skeleton and the appendicular skeleton. The axial skeleton is comprised of the skull, spine, and rib cage. The appendicular skeleton is comprised of the bones of the upper and lower limbs.

Cranium (L. *cranium, -i*) – The dome-like structure of the skull is known as the cranium. The modern root for the cranium is **CRANI-**.

Maxilla (L. *maxilla, -ae*) and Mandibula (L. *mandibula, -ae*) – The jawbones are the maxilla, which is the upper jawbone, and the mandibula, which is the lower jawbone. The corresponding roots for the jawbones are **MAXILL-** and **MANDIBUL-**.

Spine (L. *spina, -ae*) – The individual bones of the backbone are collectively called the spine. The spine derives its name from the thorn-like processes at the posterior aspect of the vertebrae, which are called the spinous processes. The root **SPIN-** is derived from the Latin noun for "thorn," *spina*. The root **SPIN-** is used for the "whole spine" (i.e. backbone, vertebral column, spinal column), "thorn," or "thorn-like structure." Thus, in botany, a cactus could be called a spinose plant because it is full of thorns, and the numerous spinous processes of the vertebral column make it look "thorny" as well. The spinal column is called the rhachis, which is a loan word from Greek. The root **RHACH-** generally uses the combining vowel -I when being joined to other word elements.

Vertebra (L. *vertebra, -ae*) – The individual bones of the spine/backbone are called vertebrae (Figs. 7.9 and 7.10). The roots **SPONDYL- and VERTEBR-** are used for these bones. The typical human spine has 24 vertebrae (7 cervical, 12 thoracic, and 5 lumbar). Today, each vertebra has a specific letter (i.e. cervical = C, thoracic = T, and Lumbar = L) and number attached to it (i.e. C1-7 [CI-VII], T1-12 [TI-XII], L1-5 [LI-V]) to identify which vertebra a physician is referencing. This is done from superior to inferior. For example, the most superior cervical vertebra is referred to as C1, and the most inferior vertebra is termed C7.

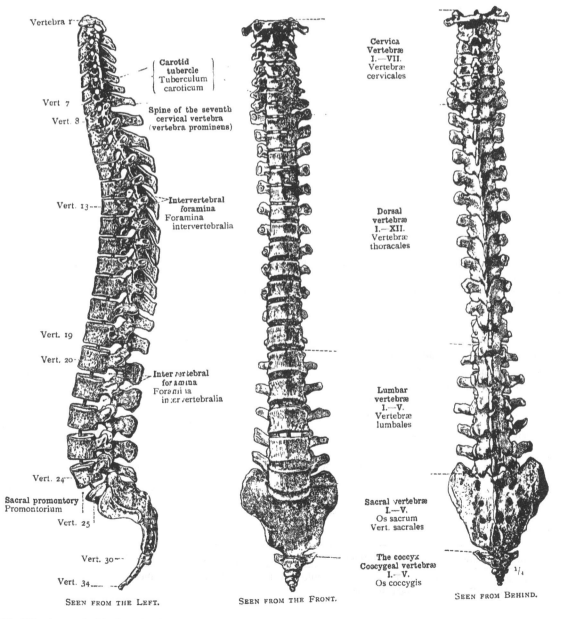

Fig. 7.9 Anatomical Latin terms for the vertebral column, image from Fig. 37 on p. 24. *Source:* Carl Toldt, *An Atlas of Human Anatomy.* 1919.

Vertebra

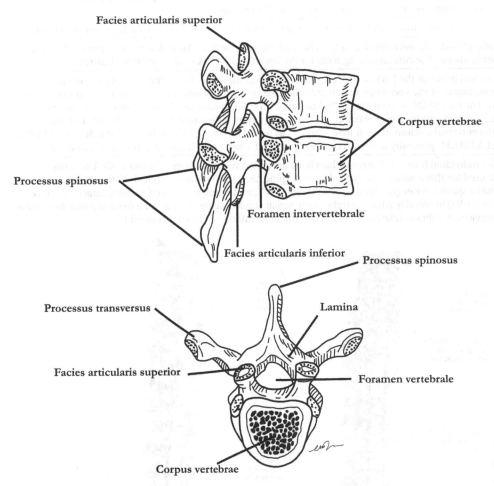

Fig. 7.10 Anatomical Latin terms for the parts of a vertebra: *Corpus vertebrae* (body of the vertebra), *Lamina* (lamina), *Processus transversus* (transverse process), *Processus spinosus* (spinous process), *Facies articularis superior* (superior articular facet), *Facies articularis inferior* (inferior articular facet), *Foramen vertebrae* (Foramen of the vertebra), and *Foramen intervertebrale* (intervertebral foramen). *Source:* Drawing by Chloe Kim.

Sacrum (L. *os sacrum* or simply *sacrum*) – The triangular bone under L5 is called the sacrum. It is composed of five fused vertebrae (S1–S5). The root for this bone is **SACR-**. **SACR-** can also mean "sacred."

Coccyx (L. *os coccygis* or simply *coccyx*) – The vestigial bones at the end of the sacrum are collectively called the coccyx. As noted, the coccyx's name, it comes from the Greek word for "cuckoo" due to it resembling the shape of the beak of this bird. The roots for coccyx in modern medical terminology are **COCCYG-** and **COCCY-**. **COCCYG- and COCCY-** are used for cuckoos and similar birds. Hence, the bird known as the "roadrunner" is classified as a Geococcyx.

Rib (L. *costa*, *-ae*) – There are twelve ribs, and they are numbered 1–12, superior to inferior (Fig. 7.11). The root commonly used for "rib" is **COST-**.

Sternum (L. *sternum*, *-i*) – The ribs are attached to the breastbone, which is called the sternum. The commonly used root for sternum today is **STERN-**.

Appendicular skeleton – upper extremity

Scapula (L. *scapula*, *-ae*) – The bone known as the shoulder blade is called the scapula, and its root is **SCAPUL-** (Fig. 7.12).

Clavicle (L. *clavicula*, *-ae*) – The only bony attachment of the shoulder girdle, the collarbone, was called the clavicle or clavicula. **CLEID-**, **CLAVICUL-**, and **CLAVIC-** are used today for the clavicle.

Fig. 7.11 Anatomical Latin terms for the ribcage. *Source:* Carl Toldt et al. (1919)/Rebman Company/Public domain.

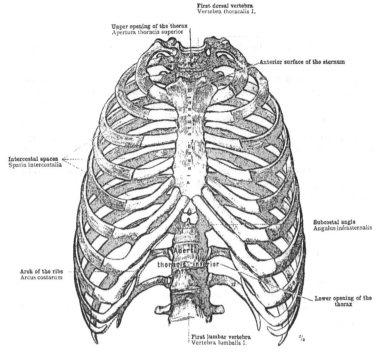

First dorsal vertebra.
Vertebra thoracalis I.

Upper opening of the thorax
Apertura thoracis superior

Anterior surface of the sternum

Intercostal spaces
Spatia intercostalia

Subcostal angle
Angulus infrasternalis

Arch of the ribs
Arcus costarum

Apertura thoracis inferior

Lower opening of the thorax

First lumbar vertebra
Vertebra lumbalis I.

(1—7, Costæ veræ, sternal or true ribs ; 8—12, Costæ spuriæ, asternal or false ribs ; 11 and 12, Costæ fluctuantes, floating ribs.)

Fig. 7.12 Anatomical Latin terms for the bones of the upper extremity, image from Fig. 231 on p. 106. *Source:* Carl Toldt et al. (1919)/Rebman Company/Public domain.

THE APPENDICULAR SKELETON

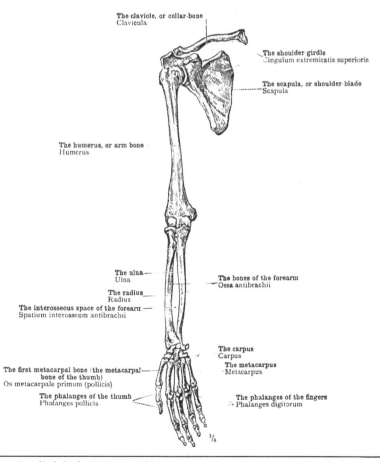

The clavicle, or collar-bone
Clavicula

The shoulder-girdle
Cingulum extremitatis superioris

The scapula, or shoulder-blade
Scapula

The humerus, or arm bone
Humerus

The ulna
Ulna

The bones of the forearm
Ossa antibrachii

The radius
Radius

The interosseous space of the forearm
Spatium interosseum antibrachii

The carpus
Carpus

The metacarpus
Metacarpus

The first metacarpal bone (the metacarpal bone of the thumb)
Os metacarpale primum (pollicis)

The phalanges of the thumb
Phalanges pollicis

The phalanges of the fingers
Phalanges digitorum

Humerus (L. *humerus*, -i) – The bone of the upper arm is called the **humerus**, and its corresponding root is **HUMER-**. The etymological origin of humerus is a Latin word for "shoulder" (*umerus*).

Radius (L. *radius*, -i) – The term radius and its root **RADI-** are used for the lateral bone of the forearm (according to the human anatomical position of the hand/forearm, which is palm forward). **RADI-** comes from the Latin word for "staff, rod, and ray," and therefore, it also carries the meaning of "radiation" and "ray."

Ulna (L. *ulna, -ae*) – The ulna, which is a Latin word that originally meant "elbow," is used today for the medial bone of the forearm, and its root is **ULN-**.

Carpal bone (L. *os carpale*) – Each bone of the wrist is called a carpal bone. The carpus, or wrist, is made up of eight carpal bones, which are aligned in two rows. As described in Taber's, "the proximal row contains (from the thumb to the little finger) the scaphoid, lunate, triquetral, and pisiform bones. The distal row contains (from thumb to little finger) the trapezium, trapezoid, capitate, and hamate bones." The root **CARP-** is a homomorph that can mean both "wrist" or "fruit."

Metacarpal bone (L. *os metacarpale*) – The five ray-like bones making up the palm are called the metacarpi. In modern anatomy, they are numbered lateral to medial or thumb to pinky, 1–5. The root for these bones is **METACARP-**.

Phalanx (L. *phalanx, phalangis*) – The bones of the fingers are called the phalanges. A single bone of the finger is a phalanx. The root for a finger bone or a toe bone is **PHALANG-**. There are 56 phalanges in the human body, 14 for each hand and foot. Like the metacarpals, they are numbered lateral to medial 1–5, according to human anatomical position.

Appendicular skeleton – lower extremity

Pelvis (L. *pelvis, -is*) – The term pelvis and its root **PELV-** comes from the Latin word for "basin." Similar to today, the pelvis is divided into three parts: the **ilium (L. *ilium, -i*)**, the **ischium (L. *ischium, -i*)**, and the **pubic bone (L. *os pubis*)**. The corresponding roots for these parts of the pelvis are **ILI-**, **ISCHI-**, and **PUB-**. Based on its etymology, PUB- can be used for the "pubic bone," as well as "young adult" and "puberty. (Fig. 7.13)"

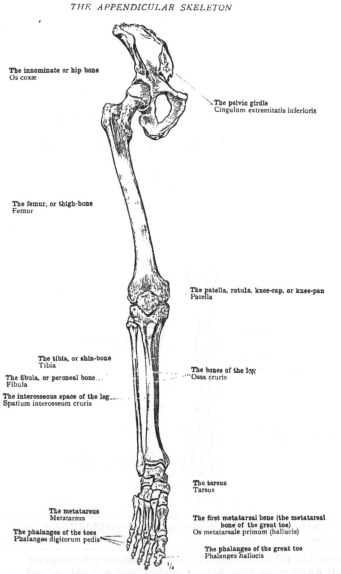

THE APPENDICULAR SKELETON

Fig. 7.13 Anatomical Latin terms for the bones of the lower extremity, image from Fig. 232 on p. 107. *Source:* Carl Toldt et al. (1919)/Rebman Company/Public domain.

The innominate or hip bone
Os coxæ

The pelvic girdle
Cingulum extremitatis inferioris

The femur, or thigh-bone
Femur

The patella, rotula, knee-cap, or knee-pan
Patella

The tibia, or shin-bone
Tibia

The fibula, or peroneal bone
Fibula

The bones of the leg
Ossa cruris

The interosseous space of the leg
Spatium interosseum cruris

The tarsus
Tarsus

The metatarsus
Metatarsus

The first metatarsal bone (the metatarsal bone of the great toe)
Os metatarsale primum (hallucis)

The phalanges of the toes
Phalanges digitorum pedis

The phalanges of the great toe
Phalanges hallucis

Femur (L. *femur, femoris*) – The anatomical Latin word for the thigh and the large bone of the thigh is the same, femur. Thus, the root **FEMOR-** has both of these meanings.

Tibia (L. *tibia, -ae*) – The large medial bone of the leg is called the tibia. The root for the tibia is **TIBI-**.

Fibula (L. *fibula, -ae*) – The lateral bone of the leg is termed fibula, and its root is **FIBUL-**. The Greek roots **KNEM-** and **PERONE-** are used today respectively for the "leg" and "fibula."

Patella (L. *patella, -ae*) – The anatomical Latin name for the "kneecap" is the patella, and its root is **PATELL-**. The term comes from the Latin word for a "dish" or "platter."

Tarsal bone (L. *os tarsale*) – Tarsus and its root **TARS-** are used for the "ankle." The tarsal bones are seven bones of the ankle, hindfoot, and midfoot, consisting of the talus, calcaneus, navicular, cuboid, and three cuneiform bones. The top bone of the ankle is called the talus, and it sits on the bone known as the calcaneus. The roots **TAL-** and **ASTRAGAL-** are used for the talus. **PTERN-** is used today for the "heel." **CALCANE-** is used for the calcaneus.

Metatarsal bone (L. *os metatarsale*) – We use the root **METATARS-** for the ray-like bones of the plantar foot in a similar fashion to how we use **METACARP-** for the palmar bones of the hand. As noted, the root for a finger bone or a toe bone is **PHALANG-**. Both the phalanges and the metatarsal bones of the foot are numbered in similar manner to the metacarpals and phalanges of the hand, except it is done medial to lateral, 1–5.

Greek or Latin word element	Current usage	Etymology	Examples
SKELET/O (skĕl-ĕ-tŏ)	Skeleton	L. *skeleton, -i*, skeleton fr. Gr. *skeletos*, dried-up	Muculo**skelet**al, **skelet**ization
CRANI/O (krā-nē-ō)	Cranium (portion of the skull that encloses the brain)	L. *cranium, -i*, n. skull fr. Gr. *kranion*, skull	**Crani**otomy, **crani**oclast Loan word: **Cranium** (krā′nē-ŭm) pl. **Crania** (krā′nē-ă)
MAXILL/O (mak-sil-ō)	Maxilla	L. *maxilla, -ae*, f. upper jaw	**Maxill**ofacial, naso**maxill**ary Loan word: **Maxilla** (mak-sil′ă) pl. **Maxillae** (mak-sil′ē″)
MANDIBUL/O (man-dib-yŭ-lō)	Mandible	L. *mandibula, -ae*, f. lower jaw	Sub**mandibul**ar, **mandibul**opharyngeal Loan word: **Mandibula** (man-dib′yŭ-lă) pl. **Mandibulae** (man-dib′yŭ-lē″)
VERTEBR/O (vĕr-tĕ-brō)	Vertebra, backbone	L. *vertebra, -ae*, f. a joint	Intra**vertebr**al, in**vertebr**ate Loan word: **Vertebra** (vĕrt′ĕ-bră) pl. **Vertebrae** (vĕrt′ĕ-brē″)
SPIN/O (spī-nō)	Spine, thorn, vertebral column	L. *spina, -ae*, f. thorn	**Spin**algia, **spin**ose Loan word: **Spina** (spī′nă) pl. **Spinae** (spī′nē″)
RACH/O (rāk-ō) **RACHI/O** (rā-kē-ō)	Vertebral column, spinal cord	Gr. *rachis*, backbone	**Rach**icele, **rachi**algia Loan word: **Rachis** (rā′kĭs)

Greek or Latin word element	Current usage	Etymology	Examples
SPONDYL/O (spŏn-dĭ-lō)	Vertebra	Gr. *spondylos*, vertebra	**Spondyl**odynia, **spondyl**osis
CERVIC/O (sĕr-vĭ-kō)	Neck, cervical	L. *cervix, cervicis*, f. neck	**Cervic**al, **cervic**algia Loan word: **Cervix** (sĕr'viks) pl. **Cervices** (sĕr'vĭ-sēz")
THORAC/O (thŏ-ră-kō)	Thorax	L. *thorax, thoracis*, m. thorax fr. Gr. *thorax*, breastplate	**Thorac**oabdominal, **thorac**ocentesis Loan word: **Thorax** (thŏr'aks") pl. **Thoraces** (thŏr'ă-sēz")
LUMB/O (lŭm-bō)	Loin, lumbar	L. *lumbus, -i*, m. loin, lumbar	**Lumb**osacral, **lumb**ago Loan word: **Lumbus** (lŭm'bŭs) pl. **Lumbi** (lŭm'bī")
SACR/O (să-krō)	Sacrum bone, sacred	L. *sacrum, -i*, n. posterior triangular bone of the pelvis fr. L. *os sacrum*, holy bone	Lumbo**sacr**al, **sacr**ad Loan word: **Sacrum** (sā'krŭm) pl. **Sacra** (sā'kră)
COCCYG/O (kŏk-sĭ-gō) **COCCY/O** (kŏk-sē-ō)	Coccyx, tailbone	L. *coccyx, coccygis*, m. coccyx, cuckoo, tailbone fr. Gr. *kokkyx*, a cuckoo, particularly its beak, which is what the coccyx bone looks like	**Coccy**algia, **coccyg**eal Loan word: **Coccyx** (kok'siks) pl. **Coccyges** (kŏk'sĭj-ēz)
COST/O (kŏs-tō)	Rib	L. *costa, -ae*, f. rib	**Cost**ochondral, sterno**cost**al Loan word: **Costa** (kŏs'tă) pl. **Costae** (kŏs'tē)
STERN/O (stĕr-nō)	Sternum, breastbone	L. *sternum, -i*, n. sternum, breastbone fr. Gr. *sternon*, chest	**Stern**ocleidal, **stern**odynia Loan word: **Sternum** (stĕr'nŭm) pl. **Sterna** (stĕr'nă)
XIPH/O (zif-ō)	Xiphoid process, sword-like	Gr. *xiphos*, sword	**Xiph**opagotomy, **xiph**oid Loan word: **Xiphoid** (zī'foyd")
SCAPUL/O (skăp-ū-lō)	Scapula, shoulder blade	L. *scapula, -ae*, f. scapula, shoulder blade	**Scapul**ohumeral, **scapul**ar Loan word: **Scapula** (skap'yŭ-lă") pl. **Scapulae** (skap'yŭ-lē")
OM/O (ō-mō)	Shoulder	Gr. *omos*, shoulder	**Om**ohyoid, acr**om**ion
CLAVICUL/O (klă-vĭk'ū-lō) **CLAVIC/O** (klăv-ĭ-kō)	Clavicle, collarbone	L. *clavicula, -ae*, f. little key, collarbone	Sterno**clavicul**ar, **clavic**otomy Loan word: **Clavicula** (klă-vĭk'ū-lă) pl. **Claviculae** (klă-vĭk'ū-lē)

Greek or Latin word element	Current usage	Etymology	Examples
CLEID/O (klī-dō)	Clavicle, collarbone	Gr. *kleis, kleidos,* key, collarbone	**Cleid**orrhexis
HUMER/O (hūmĕ-rō)	Humerus	L. *humerus, -i,* m. bone of the upper arm	**Humer**oulnar, sub**humer**al Loan word: **Humerus** (hū′mĕ-rŭs) pl. **Humeri** (hū′mĕ-rī″)
RADI/O (rād-ē-ō)	Radius, ray, radioactive	L. *radius, -i,* m. staff, rod, ray, outer bone of the forearm	**Radi**oulnar, **radi**ology Loan word: **Radius** (rād′ē-ŭs) pl. **Radii** (rād′ē-ī)
ULN/O (ŭl-nō)	Ulna	L. *ulna, -ae,* f. elbow, inner bone of the forearm	**Uln**ocarpal, radi**ouln**ar Loan word: **Ulna** (ŭl′nă) pl. **Ulnae** (ŭl′nē)
CARP/O (kăr-pō)	Wrist, carpal bone(s)	L. *carpus, -i,* m. wrist, bone of the wrist fr. Gr. *karpos,* wrist	**Carp**optosis, **carp**al Loan word: **Carpus** (kăr′pŭs) pl. **Carpi** (kăr′pī)
METACARP/O (met-ă-kar-pō)	Metacarpal bone(s)	L. *metacarpus, -i,* m. metacarpus, bone of the palm fr. Gr. *meta-* beyond + *karpos,* wrist	**Metacarp**ectomy, **metacarp**al Loan word: **Metacarpus** (met″ă-kar′pŭs) pl. **Metacarpi** (met″ă-kar′pī)
PHALANG/O (fal-ăn-gō)	Phalanx	L. *phalanx, phalangis,* f. phalanx, a finger or toe bone fr. Gr. *phalanx,* a finger and a finger-like battle formation	Brachy**phalang**ia, **phalang**ectomy Loan word: **Phalanx** (fă′langks″) pl. **Phalanges** (fă-lan′jēz″)
DACTYL/O (dak-tĭ-lō)	Finger, toe	Gr. *daktylos,* finger	**Dactyl**edema, syn**dactyl**ia
ILI/O (il-ē-ō)	Ilium bone	L. *ilium, -i,* n. groin, flank, upper bone of the pelvis	**Ili**ocostal, **illi**ocaudal Loan word: **Ilium** (il′ē-ŭm) pl. **Ilia** (il′ē-ă)
ISCHI/O (is-kē-ō)	Ischium bone	L. *ischium, -i,* n. lower, posterior bone of the pelvis fr. Gr. *ischion,* hip joint	**Ischi**oanal, **ischi**ococcygeal Loan word: **Ischium** (is′kē-ŭm) pl. **Ischia** (ĭs′kē-ă)
PUB/O (pū-bō)	Pubic bone, adult, puberty	L. *pubis, -is,* m. pubic bone, anterior inferior bone of the pelvis fr. L. *pubes,* arrived at the age of puberty, adult, *(os) pubis,* pubic bone	**Pub**ofemoral, **pub**ic Loan word: **Pubis** (pū′bĭs) pl. **Pubes** (pū′bēz″)
FEMOR/O (fem-ŏ-rō)	Femur bone, thigh	L. *femur, femoris,* n. thigh, bone of the thigh	Inter**femor**al, **femor**otibial Loan word: **Femur** (fē′mŭr) pl. **Femora** (fem′ŏ-ră)

Greek or Latin word element	Current usage	Etymology	Examples
PATELL/O (pă-tĕl-ō)	Patella bone	L. *patella, -ae*, f. dish, platter, kneecap bone	Infra**patell**ar, **patell**ofemoral Loan word: **Patella** (pă-tel′ă) pl. **Patellae** (pă-tel′ē)
GONY/O (gŏn-ĭ-ō)	Knee	Gr. *gony*, knee	**Gony**campsis, **gony**oncus
TIBI/O (tib-ē-ō)	Tibia bone	L. *tibia, -ae*, f. pipe, flute, medial bone of the lower leg	**Tibi**otarsal, pre**tibi**al Loan word: **Tibia** (tib′ē-ă) pl. **Tibiae** (tib′ē-ē)
CNEM/O (nē-mŏ)	Leg	Gr. *kneme*, leg, tibia	**Knem**ometry, gastro**cnem**ial
FIBUL/O (fĭb-yŭ-lō)	Fibula bone	L. *fibula, -ae*, f. a brooch, pin, lateral bone of the lower leg	Tibio**fibul**ar, calcaneo**fibul**ar Loan word: **Fibula** (fĭb′yŭ-lă) pl. **Fibulae** (fĭb′yŭ-lē)
PERONE/O (pĕr-ō-nē-ō)	Fibula bone	Gr. *perone*, a pin or brooch	**Perone**otibial, **perone**al Loan word: **Perone** (pĕ-rō′nē)
ASTRAGAL/O (ă-stra-gă-lō)	Talus bone	Gr. *astragalos*, talus, die	**Astragal**ectomy, sub**astragal**ar Loan word: **Astragalus** (ă-strag′ă-lŭs)
TAL/O (tā-lō)	Talus bone, ankle	L. *talus, -i*, m. talus, the ankle bone	**Tal**ocrural, **tal**ofibular Loan word: **Talus** (tā′lŭs) pl. **Tali** (tā′lī″)
CALCANE/O (kal-kā-nē-ō)	Calcaneus bone	L. *calcaneus, -i*, m. heel, heel bone fr. L. *calx, calcis*, heel, *os calcis*, bone of the heel	**Calcane**ofibular, **calcane**al Loan word: **Calcaneus** (kăl-kā′nē-ŭs) pl. **Calcanei** (kăl-kā′nē- ī″)
PTERN/O (tĕr-nŏ)	Heel	Gr. *pterna*, heel	**Ptern**algia
SCAPH/O (skaf-ō)	Scaphoid, shaped like the hull of a boat	Gr. *skaphe*, boat	**Scaph**ocephalism, **scaph**oid
METATARS/O (met-ă-tar-sō)	Metatarsus bone	L. *metatarsus, -i*, m. metatarsus fr Gr. *meta-* beyond + Gr. *tarsos*, flat of foot, ankle bones	**Metatars**ophalangeal, **metatars**al Loan word: **Metatarsus** (met″ă-tar′sŭs) pl. **Metatarsi** (met″ă-tar′-sī″)

Review	Answers
Pternalgia is a pain in the _____.	heel
The anatomical Latin name for the collarbone is _____. The combining forms for the collarbone are_____, _____, and _____.	clavicula CLEID/O, CLAVIC/O, CLAVICUL/O
The peroneal artery is near the perone, which in anatomical Latin is the bone known as the _____.	fibula
The breastbone is also called the _____ in anatomical Latin.	sternum
The letter and number for the topmost vertebra of the neck is _____. It is also named after the Greek Titan who held up the heavens, _____.	C 1 (C I) Atlas
The anatomical Latin name for the bone known as the kneecap is the _____.	patella
A fracture of the bone of the thigh is known as a _____ fracture.	femoral (Femur)
The intercostal muscles are located between the _____.	Ribs
Omalgia affects the _____.	shoulder
The anatomical Latin name for the bone located at the brachium is_____.	humerus
The anatomical position of a body is the palms anterior (supinated hand). In the anatomical position the lateral bone of the antebrachium is the _____ and the medial is the _____.	radius, ulna
A hebotomy is the incision at the _____ bone, which is the anterior inferior bone of the pelvis.	pubic (pubis)
Spondylitis is an inflammation of a _____.	vertebra
L 5 (L V) is the most inferior _____ vertebra.	lumbar
A fractured shoulder blade is known as a _____ fracture.	scapular (scapula)
A xiphophyllous plant has _____-shaped leaves.	sword
Knemometry measures the _____.	leg
In the anatomical position, the lateral bone of the leg is called the _____, and the medial bone is called the _____.	fibula, tibia
A bone of the finger or toe is called a _____. The combining forms for finger are _____ and _____.	phalanx dactyl/o, digit/o
An astragalectomy is a removal of the bone known in anatomical Latin as the _____, which is the top bone of the ankle.	talus
A gonyoncus is a tumor of the _____.	knee
In anatomical Latin, the upper bone of the pelvis is called the _____, and the lower posterior bone (the "sit bone") of the pelvis is called the _____.	Ilium, ischium
The small rows of bones of the wrist are collectively called the _____ bones.	carpal (carpi)
In anatomical Latin, the upper bone of the jaw is called the _____, and the lower part is called the _____.	maxilla, mandibula
The seven vertebrae of the neck are called the _____ vertebrae. The 12 vertebrae of the mid-back are called the _____ vertebrae. The five vertebrae of the lower back are called the _____ vertebrae.	cervical thoracic lumbar
The genus of the bird known as a "roadrunner" is Geococcyx, which literally means "Land _____." The combining forms for tailbone are _____ and _____.	cuckoo COCCYG/O, COCCY/O
The "*Hieron Osteon*" (Holy Bone) is called the _____ in anatomical Latin.	Os sacrum (Sacrum)
The five bones that make up the palm of the hand are called the _____. Similarly, the five bones that make up the sole of the foot are called the _____.	metacarpi (metacarpal bones) metatarsi (metatarsal bones)
The dome-shaped part of the skull is called the _____ in anatomical Latin.	cranium
The combining form for a boat-shaped or hollowed-out structure is _____.	SCAPH/O

Etymological Explanations: Greek and Latin Roots for the Parts and Movements of Muscles

In the following discussion of the anatomical terms associated with muscles, the nominative and genitive singular forms of the anatomical Latin term are provided in parenthesis. The Greek and Latin roots are formatted in all caps and emboldened.

Types and parts of muscles

Types of Muscles – The Greek and Latin roots commonly used for "muscle" are **MY-**, **MYS-**, **MYOS-**, and **MUSCUL-** (Fig. 7.14). Muscles are categorized into three groups in modern medicine: cardiac muscle, smooth muscle, and skeletal muscle. Smooth muscle is the contractile tissue of the viscera, such as the stomach, intestines, and arteries. The compound root used for "smooth muscle" is **LEIOMY-**. Cardiac and skeletal muscles are called striated muscles. The compound combining form used for "striated muscle" is **RHABDOMY-**. While skeletal muscle and cardiac muscle are both striated muscles, they differ in a number of ways. Unlike skeletal muscles, the contractions of cardiac muscle are involuntary, and its cellular composition is quite different from skeletal muscle. The root **LEI-** is also for anything that is "smooth," and **RHABD-** is used for anything that is "striated" or "rod-like."

Nomina generalia musculorum

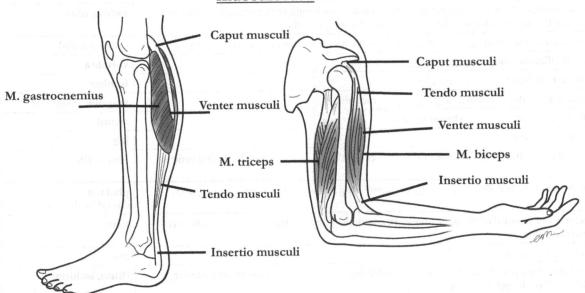

Fig. 7.14 Anatomical Latin terms for the muscles: *Caput musculi* (heat/origin of the muscle), *Insertio musculi* (insertion of the muscle), *Venter musculi* (belly of the muscle), and *Tendo musculi* (tendon the muscle). *Source:* Drawing by Chloe Kim.

Belly (L. *venter, ventris*) of a Muscle – At the macroscopic level, the thick fleshy part is called its "belly" or venter of a muscle, and its root is **VENTR-**.

Tendon (L. *tendo, tendinis*) – As noted, a skeletal muscle is often attached to a bone via a tendon, and the roots for "tendon" are **TEN-**, **TENONT-**, **TENDIN-**. The tendon that is attached to the bone that moves when a muscle contracts is called the **insertion** (L. *insertio, insertionis*). The tendon that does not move when a muscle contracts is called the **origin** or **head** (L. *caput, capitis*) of the muscle. The Latin suffix **-CEPS** is used for "head" and it appears sometimes in the names of muscles to indicate the number of origins a muscle has (e.g. biceps, triceps, uniceps).

Sarcomere and Sarcolemma – At the microscopic level (Fig. 7.15), skeletal muscles are made up of organelles called myofibrils that are arranged in cylindrical bundles in a muscle cell. The myofibrils are parceled at equal length by longitudinal endpoints called sarcomeres, which give this muscle its striated appearance under a microscope. The sarcolemma is the membrane that covers the myofibrils. The roots **MER-** and **LEMM-** are widely used in medicine and scientific vocabulary. **MER-**, which is from the Greek word for a part, *meros*. As noted earlier, **MER-** is used today for "part" or "partial." **LEMM-** is derived from the Greek word (*lemma*) for "something that could be peeled off or separated" (e.g. rind, husk). In modern anatomy, **LEMM-** is used for a "membrane" or "sheath-like structure." The root **SARC-** is used for "flesh" and "muscle."

Fig. 7.15 Internal parts of muscle.

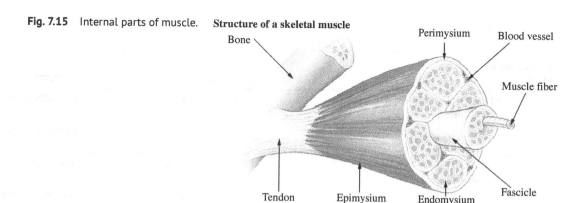

Structure of a skeletal muscle

Myofibers and Myofibrils – The cellular building block of a skeletal muscle is the myofiber. A myofiber (muscle cell) is a tubular cell composed of numerous myofibrils. The root **FIBR-** is used for "filament, fiber," which is not the Classical Latin meaning of *fibra*, from which this root is derived. In Classical Latin, *fibra* meant a section or termination of something (e.g. a lobe of the liver, viscera, a subdivision of a root). The "thread-like" meaning of this word appears to have occurred in the 16th century. Today, **fibra** (L. *fibra, fibrae*) is used as a loan word for "fiber" and **fibrilla** (L. *fibrilla, fibrillae*) for "little fiber, fibril."

Fascicle (L. *fasciculus, -i*) – A bundle of myofibers is called a fasciculus/fascicle. Fasciculus is the diminutive of the Latin term *fasces*, which meant "a bundle," particularly a bundle of sticks. In ancient Rome, the *fasces* were bundles of sticks that were carried by lictors before the chief Roman magistrates (Fig. 7.16). This bundle of sticks symbolized the "unity" of the Roman Republic, which is why this symbol also appeared on the back of dimes in the United States. The loan word **fasciculus** and its root **FASCICUL-** are used today for a small bundle of longitudinal rod- or fiber-like structures (e.g. bundle of axons, muscle fibers).

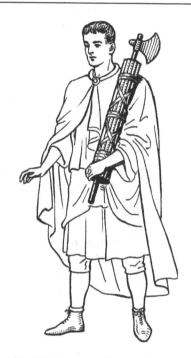

Fig. 7.16 Image of Roman fasces.

Endomysium (L. *endomysium, -i*), Epimysium (L. *epimysium, -i*), Perimysium (L. *perimysium, -i*) – Myofibers are bound together by a thin connective tissue called endomysium. Perimysium is the connective tissue that surrounds the fasciculi of a muscle. Muscles are made of numerous fasciculi. Epimysium is the outermost sheath of connective tissue that envelops a skeletal muscle.

Greek or Latin word element	Current usage	Etymology	Examples
MUSCUL/O (mŭs-kyŏ-lō)	Muscle, mouse	L. *musculus, -i*, m. muscle, mouse	**Muscul**ocutaneous, **muscul**ar Loan word: **Musculus** (mŭs′kyŭ-lŭs) pl. **Musculi** (mŭs′kyŭ-lī″)
MY/O (mī-ō) **MYOS/O** (mī-ō-sō) **MYS/O** (mī-sō)	Muscle, mouse	Gr. *mys, myos*, muscle, mouse	**My**oatrophy, epi**mys**ium, **myos**itis

Greek or Latin word element	Current usage	Etymology	Examples
RHABD/O (răb-dō)	Striated, rod, rod-like	Gr. *rhabdos*, rod, wand	**Rhabd**omyoma, **rhabd**olith
LEI/O (lī-ō)	Smooth	Gr. *leios*, smooth	**Lei**omyosarcoma, **lei**odermia
SARC/O (săr-kō)	Flesh, muscle	Gr. *sarx, sarkos*, flesh, fleshy pulp of fruit	**Sarc**openia, **sarc**omere
MER/O (měr-ō) **-MER** (měr) **-MERE** (měr)	Part, partial	Gr. *meros*, a part	**Mer**otomy, poly**mer**, sarco**mere**
LEMM/O (lěm-ō) **-LEMMA** (lem-ă)	Membrane, husk, sheath-like structure	Gr. *lemma*, a peel, husk; a membrane	**Lemm**ocyte, sarco**lemma**
FIBR/O (fī-brō) **FIBRILL/O** (fī-bril-ō)	Fiber, fibril (muscle fiber)	L. *fibra, -ae*, f. fiber, filament

L. *fibrilla, -ae*, f. small fiber, fibril | **Fibr**oadenia, **fibrill**arin

Loan word: **Fibrilla** (fī-bril′ă) pl. **Fibrillae** (fī-bril′ē) |
| **FASCICUL/O** (fă-sik-yŭ-lō) | A small bundle of rod-like structures, fascicle | L. *fasciculus, -i*, m. little bundle of sticks fr. L. *fasces*, bundle of sticks | **Fascicul**ation, **fascicul**ar

Loan word: **Fasciculus** (fă-sik′yŭ-lŭs) pl. **Fasciculi** (fă-sik′yŭ-lī″) |
| **TENDIN/O** (ten-dĭ-nō) | Tendon | L. *tendo, tendinis*, m. tendon fr. L. *tenere*, to stretch | **Tendin**itis, **tendin**opathy

Loan word: **Tendo** (ten′dō) pl. **Tendines** (ten′dĭ-nēz) |
| **TEN/O** (ten-ō) **TENONT/O** (těn-ŏn-tō) | Tendon | Gr. *tenon, tenontos*, tendon, sinew fr. Gr. *teinein*, to stretch | **Ten**odesis, **tenont**odynia |
| **TON/O** (tō-nō) | Tension, tone | Gr. *tonos*, a stretching, tightening | Hyper**ton**ic, myodys**ton**ia |
| **CAPIT/O** (kap-ĭ-tō) **CIPIT/O** (sip-ĭ-tō) **-CIPUT** (sĭp-ŭt) **-CEPS** (seps) | Head, origin of a muscle | L. *caput, capitis*, n. head, origin of a muscle | **Capit**ate, bi**cipit**al, sin**ciput**, bi**ceps**

Loan word: **Caput** (kap′ut″) pl. **Capita** (kap′ĭ-ta″) |
| **VENTR/O** (ven-trō) | Belly (of a muscle), cavity, abdomen | L. *venter, ventris*, m. belly, cavity | **Ventr**icle, **ventr**al

Loan word: **Venter** (vent′ĕr) pl. **Ventres** (ven′trēz″) |

Review	Answers
A sarcoma is a type of cancer that arises from mesenchymal tissue, e.g. muscles and bones. A sarcoma of striated muscles is called a _____myosarcoma. A sarcoma of smooth muscles is called a _____myosarcoma.	**rhabdo-, leio-**
The shared root in epimysium and perimysium means _____.	**muscle**
The venter of a muscle is also called the muscle _____.	**belly**
The combining form SARC/O means _____ and _____.	**muscle, flesh**
A tenodesis is a surgical fixation of a _____.	**tendon**
The movable attachment of a muscle to a bone is called its _____. The stable attachment of a muscle to a bone is called the _____.	**insertion (insertio) origin (caput, head)**
A fasciculus looks like a _____ of rod-like structures.	**bundle**
The membrane that covers myofibrils is the sarco_____. The unit/part of myofibrils that gives striated muscles their appearance is called the sarco_____.	**-lemma -mere**
A condition of increased resting tension in a muscle is called hyper_____icity.	**ton-**
Tendinitis is an _____ of a _____.	**inflammation, tendon**
A myofibroma is a tumor that contains _____ and _____ tissue.	**muscular (muscle), fibrous (fiber)**
A tenontoplasty is a surgical reconstruction of a _____.	**tendon**

Lessons from History: Muscles in Ancient Greek Medicine

Food for Thought as You Read:

> *What types of explanations were used by Galen to explain the movement of muscles?*
> *How did we arrive at our current nomenclature for the names of muscles?*

In ancient Greek medicine, the distinction between cardiac and skeletal muscles is evident in the writings of Galen. In his *On the Movement of Muscles*, Galen notes that heart muscle is not the same as skeletal muscle. Galen recognizes that the heart's movements are involuntary. He also claims that the heart is different than skeletal muscle with respect to thickness, form, texture, and hardness. For Galen, muscles are organs of voluntary motion, and therefore, the heart is not a muscle, which is quite different from the modern understanding of the heart having its own distinct type of striated muscle. Galen recognized that certain movements occur unconsciously. For example, a person does not think about which direction to move the tongue when speaking, the diaphragm when breathing, or the sphincter with excretion. However, for Galen, these are still movements that are voluntary since the soul (*psyche*) causes these to happen via nerves. To justify this position, Galen argues that movements during the night (e.g. sleepwalking, movements of the hands, breathing), when a person is obviously unconscious, occur because the *psyche* is actively causing muscles to contract. The notion that the *psyche* continues to be active during sleep is also found in explanations of the nature of dreams in Classical and Hellenistic philosophy (Aristotle's *On Dreams*) and medicine (Hippocrates, *Regimen IV*). Galen's definition of voluntary movement is part of his anatomical approach to physiology. Galen argues that the psychic source of these muscle contractions is located in the ventricles of the brain, and it is through the nerves that a muscle becomes an "instrument of the soul" (*psychikon organon*).

In *On the Movement of Muscles*, Galen recognizes that the muscles have tone, even during sleep. He notes that the nerves' connection to the encephalon (brain) is ultimately the reason for muscle tone, as well as the movement of muscles. While Galen suggests that tendons and nerves share some similarities in the physical constitution, he notes that a tendon injury will affect a muscle quite differently than a nerve injury. Damage to a tendon will affect the muscle's ability to move, but cutting a peripheral nerve or the spinal cord causes a loss of motion, tone, and sensation. Galen does not explain in this work exactly how the nerves are making muscles move. In other Galenic works, Galen explains that the ventricles of the brain are filled with *psychikon pneuma*, which appears to be a fine airy substance that Galen claims is the first instrument of the soul and that it communicates with muscles via nerves. Galen does not specifically address what, if any, physical effects the *psychikon pneuma* has on muscles. Suffice it to say that the movement of a muscle is ultimately a psychic phenomenon that affects the innate nature (*physis*) of a muscle. It should be said that, in some of Galen's anatomical discussions, the actions of nerves and tendons on muscles are explained in mechanical terms. In Galen's *On the Use of the Parts*, he attempts to show how the nature and purpose of the parts of the human body reveal that Nature is an intelligent and skillful Craftsman. For example, Galen notes that the looping of the recurrent laryngeal nerve under the arteries (Aorta and the Right Subclavian Artery) creates a reverse motion similar to a *glossocomion*, which is an instrument used for setting bones (Fig. 7.17). He states, "Just as in the instrument for the leg [the *glossocomion*] the source of the movement, which lies in our hands on the roller, draws on the legs of the noose as far as the pulleys, and from the pulleys the motion travels from above downward again to the part of the leg to be stretched, so the nerves of the larynx behave in the same way (trans. May, *Galen On the Usefulness of the Parts of the Body*, vol. 1, p. 368)." Here, Galen is suggesting that the nerves function as the cords of a device, which is part of his overall argument that Nature has created a device for movement similar to those made by "engineers" (*mechanikoi*) and those made by physicians called "tool makers" (*organikoi*).

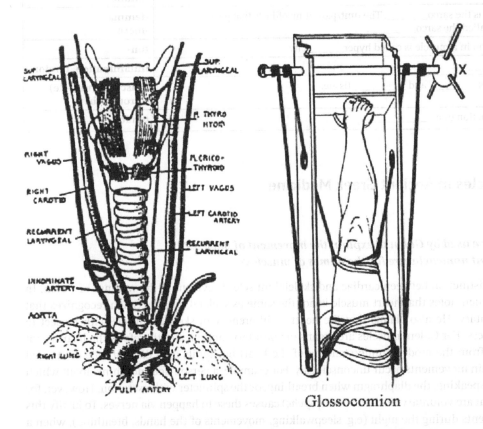

Fig. 7.17 Image of the glossocomion and the recurrent laryngeal nerve. The glossocomion was a tool used for reducing fractures via traction. Galen believed that the recurrent laryngeal nerve loops around the aorta and right subclavian artery are much like the pully system created by the cords of the glossocomion. *Source:* Oeuvres d'Oribase, (1862)/Imprimerie nationale/Public Domain.

Glossocomion

In *On the Movement of Muscles*, Galen correctly recognizes that complex movements are due to the shape of the joint and the presence of multiple muscles. He also recognizes that an individual muscle has specific motions. He notes that a muscle will be active both in its lengthening and in its shortening (i.e. eccentric and concentric movements). Galen sees this as evidence that a muscle is capable of both lengthening and shortening. Galen's physiological solution to this phenomenon is rational but wrong. He claims that a muscle has two parts. The internal part of a muscle contracts or flexes, and the external part of the muscle extends or lengthens. Thus, if there is a wound to the internal part of the muscle (biceps?), the muscle and part will remain in an extended position, but if there is a wound to the external part of the muscle, the muscle will assume a flexed position. Likewise, he hypothesizes that if a nerve is cut to the internal part of the muscle, the muscle will lengthen, and if the nerve is severed to the external part of the muscle, the muscle will shorten. However, Galen again makes a distinction between injuries to tendons and nerves. He notes that if a tendon of a muscle is cut, then the muscle will typically move to a shortened position. This is an observable phenomenon with tendon injuries, such as the bulging appearance of the biceps when its long head is torn, which is sometimes referred to as the "Popeye sign."

There are around 650 skeletal muscles in the human body. The identification of each muscle by a specific name was not a primary concern among ancient Greek physicians and anatomists. When identifying muscles, most of their attention was given to denoting the number of muscles at a given structure and their actions rather than providing a specific name for each muscle. This lack of attention to providing the specific names of muscles is evident in Galen's *Anatomy of Muscles*, which is a descriptive anatomical work similar to Galen's *Bones for Beginners*. In this work, Galen gives the number of muscles at a given body part and describes their actions.

Ancient Greek physicians occasionally named a muscle by its location. The author of the Hippocratic work *On Joints* calls the other muscles of mastication the *krotaphitai*, which is derived from the Greek word for the side of the forehead (i.e. the temple). Modern anatomical terminology will use Latin nouns and adjectives to denote the location of a muscle. The anatomical Latin name for this muscle is *musculus temporalis*. Temporalis is a Latin adjective that is formed from the Latin word *tempus, temporis,* which can mean "a division, section." In respect to location, it means "the temple of the head," but in respect to time, it signifies a "portion or period of time." Based on the aforementioned meanings, some have suggested that this area of the head is called the *tempus* because it is generally the first place that the hair turns gray as we get older. However, much like the connection between the meanings of "mouse" and "muscle" with respect to *musculus*, there is no definitive answer as to why this area of the head was called the *tempus*.

The origin of naming muscles according to their actions is also evident in some ancient Greek medical terms. The earliest reference to a muscle being named according to its action is found in the Hippocratic work *On Joints* (c. 5th century BC). This author calls the muscles of the lower jaw responsible for chewing the *masseteres* (singular *masseter*), which is a noun formed from the Greek verb meaning *massaomai* (to chew). The *sphincter* is another example of a muscle being named according to its action in ancient Greek medicine. Both Rufus of Ephesus and Galen make mention of this type of muscle, usually in reference to the *sphincter ani*. As a type of muscle, Galen recognizes that the function of sphincter muscles is to retain, not excrete something. The Greek *sphinkter* is derived from the Greek verb *sphingein*, which means "to squeeze, bind tight." It is believed that the Sphinx, the Greek mythical winged creature that plagued Thebes, is also derived from the verb *sphingein*, and therefore, its name literally means "Strangler." The Sphinx was a female monster with the body of a lion, the torso of a woman, and an eagle's wings who was defeated by the Greek mythological hero, Oedipus.

Written in Latin during the 16th century, Vesalius' *On the Fabric of the Human Body* is one of the seminal works for diagramming, labeling, and naming the muscles of the human body. Vesalius' work contains a series of images in which the layers of muscles are reflected layer by layer (Fig. 7.18), which today is termed "Vesalius Muscle Man." Vesalius' names are quite descriptive but differ significantly from the names used today for the same muscles. For example, the modern anatomical Latin name for the triceps muscle, *Musculus triceps brachii* (triceps muscle of the arm), identifies this muscle by its location and the three origins of the muscle. Vesalius identifies this same muscle as the *Musculus cubitum extendens* (Elbow-extending muscle), which is quite accurate given that this is the primary action of the triceps muscle that modern anatomists recognize. The modern names of muscles became standardized with the *Ninth Congress* of the *Anatomische Gesellschaft* (1895).

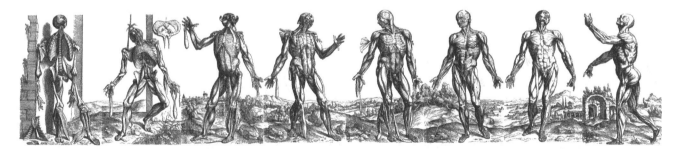

Fig. 7.18 Composite of the eight images that are collectively known as Vesalius' "Muscle Man." These plates created for Vesalius' *De fabrica* provide a layer-by-layer dissection of the muscles that hold the body up, and as they are removed, the body is artistically propped up. Images from Andreae Vesalii, *De humani corporis fabrica libri septem*, 1543. *Source:* Andreas Vesalius/Wikimedia Commons/Public domain.

The current names of skeletal muscles can be difficult to remember because many of these names are long and hard-to-remember Latin phrases. The principles for naming muscles found in *Nomina Anatomica* reveal that such anatomical terms reveal the action, shape, or location of a muscle. If you know the logic behind the name of muscles, it will help you to remember that muscle's name. When identifying a muscle in medical English, often the word *musculus* (muscle) is omitted from the terms in medical terminology because it is already understood that the term refers to a muscle.

Example:

> *Musculus vastus lateralis* = Vastus lateralis
> *Musculus flexor digit minimi* = Flexor digiti minimi

In modern Anatomical Latin, the Latin names for the actions of muscles have the *-or*, or sometimes the *-er* ending, such as *levator, sphincter,* and *flexor*. These suffixes are a common way for Latin to create a noun from a verb. In this way, the Latin **-OR** signifies that it is a doer of an action (he who does X, that which does X), which is evident in words in everyday English, such as "governor" and "accelerator." The following list has the roots for the names of muscles. These roots are derived from verbs, and therefore, they are quite common in medico-scientific terms. The image below contains the movements of the body for which muscles are named (Fig. 7.19).

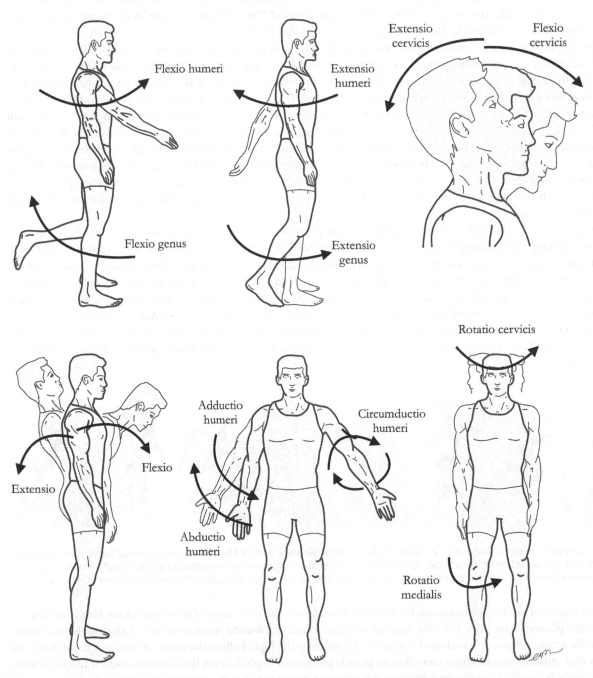

Fig. 7.19 Anatomical Latin terms for the movements of the body. *Source:* Image by Chloe Kim.

The location of a muscle is denoted in anatomical Latin by its general position and/or the bone that it is associated with.

> *musculus anterior tibialis* (or for short anterior tibialis) is located in the front (*anterior*) of the tibia (*tibialis*)
> *musculi intercostales interni* (or intercostales interni) is located at the inner part (*interni*) between the ribs (*intercostales*)

In some cases, the part of the body that it is being acted upon by the muscle appears in the name.

> *musculus flexor digitorum superficialis* (or flexor digitorum superficialis) reveals that this is a shallow (*superficialis*) bender (*flexor*) of the fingers (*digitorum*)
> *musculus flexor hallucis longus* (or flexor hallucis longus) reveals that this is a long (*longus*) bender (flexor) of the great toe (*hallucis*)

Another convention is to use a compound adjective that is formed from the names of bones associated with the muscle. The first word element in these adjectives denotes the origin of the muscle, and the second word element indicates the muscle's insertion.

> *musculus brachioradialis* (or brachioradialis) indicates that the origin of the muscle is the *brachium* (more specific the *humerus*), and its insertion is on the *radius* bone.

The first word in such compound adjectives is always the origin, but if the term has three-word elements, the second- and third-word elements could indicate the muscle has two origins and one insertion or that it has one origin and two insertions.

> *musculus sternocleidomastoideus* (or sternocleidomastoid) has two origins, the sternum and the clavicle. It inserts on the mastoid process.

Ligaments are also typically named according to the bones or structures that they bind together. The anterior talofibular ligament (L. *ligamentum talofibulare anterius*) is located at the front of the ankle, where it binds the talus to the fibula.

Muscles are often named with respect to their shape and size. The following list contains commonly used adjectives. The literal meanings of these terms appear in the parentheses. In general, the anatomical Latin term is left untranslated in medical English. For example, *musculus glutaeus minimus* is known simply as the "gluteus minimus," not the "smallest gluteus."

> *minor, minus*, minor (lesser, smaller, littler)
> *major, majus*, major (greater, larger)
> *minimus, -a, -um*, minimus (smallest, least, littlest)
> *maximus, -a, -um*, maximus (largest, greatest, biggest)
> *longus, -a, -um*, longus (long)
> *brevis, -e*, brevis (short)
> *planus, -a, -um*, planus (flat)
> *rectus, -a, -um*, rectus (straight)
> *vastus, -a, -um*, vastus (large, immense)

It is beyond the scope of this textbook to provide the adjectives used for all the muscles of the body. That said, it is a worthwhile endeavor to study the etymologies of the descriptive names for specific muscles because they often explain the shape of these muscles. The following are some of the interesting etymologies used to describe specific muscles of the human body.

> *deltoideus, -a, -um*, Gr. shaped like the Greek letter "delta" [Δ]
> *hyoideus, -a, -um*, Gr. shaped like the Greek letter "upsilon" [υ]
> *serratus, -a, -um*, L. having a jagged edge, saw-like
> *teres, teretis*, L. rounded, cylindrical
> *gracilis, -e*, L. slender, thin
> *splenius, -a, -um*, Gr. *splenion*, bandage
> *pectineus, -a, -um*, L. *pectin*, a comb, quill

Some Suggested Readings

Goss, Charles M. "On the Anatomy of Muscles for Beginners by Galen of Pergamon." *The Anatomical Record* 145 (1963): 477–501.

Goss, Charles M. "On Movement of Muscles by Galen of Pergamon." *American Journal of Anatomy* 123 (1968): 1–25.

Musil, Vladimir, et al. "The History of Latin Terminology of Human Skeletal Muscles (from Vesalius to the Present)." *Surgical and Radiologic Anatomy* 37, no. 1 (2015): 33–41.

Scarborough, John. ""Muscles" and "Bones"." In *Medical and Biological Terminologies Classical Origins*. Norman: University of Oklahoma Press, 1992.

Greek or Latin word element	Current usage	Etymology	Examples
DUC/O (doo-kō) DUCT/O (dŭkt-ō)	To lead, convey	L. *ducere, ductus*, to lead, draw or convey	**Duct**ile Ab**duc**ent
ABDUCT/O (ab-dŭk-tō)	To lead or convey away (midline)	*L. *abductor, -oris*, m. abductor fr. L. *abductio*, a leading away	**Abduct**ion Loan word: **Abductor** (ab-dŭk′tor) pl **Abductores** (ab-dŭk′to-rēz″)
ADDUCT/O (ă-dŭk-tō)	To lead or convey toward (midline)	*L. *adductor, -oris*, m. adductor fr. L. *adductio*, a leading toward	**Adduct**ion Loan word: **Adductor** (ad-dŭk′tor) pl. **Adductores** (ad-dŭk′to-rēz″)
ROT/O (rōt-ō) ROTAT/O (rō-tā-tō)	To turn around	L. *rotare, rotatum*, to cause to go around *L. *rotator, -oris*, m. rotator fr L. *rotatio*, f. a turning	**Rot**oblation Levo**rota**tion Loan word: **Rotator** (rō-tā′tor) pl. **Rotatores** (rō-tā′to-rēz″)
FLEX/O (fleks-ō) -FLEX (fleks)	To bend, flex	L. *flexor, -oris*, m. flexor fr. L. *flexio*, f. a bending	**Flex**ibility, circum**flex** Loan word: **Flexor** (fleks′or″) pl. **Flexores** (fleks′o-rēz″)
EXTENS/O (ek-sten-sō)	To stretch out, straighten, extend	L. *extensor, -oris*, m. extensor fr. L. *extensio*, f. a stretching out, straighten	**Extens**ion, **extens**or Loan word: **Extensor** (ek-sten′sŏr) pl. **Extensores** (ek-sten′so-rēz″)
PRON/O (prō-nō) PRONAT/O (prō-nā-tō)	Face down, lying prone	L. *pronator, -oris*, m. pronator fr. L. *pronatio*, f. a facing down	**Pron**ograde, **prona**tion Loan word: **Pronator** (prō-nā′tŏr) pl. **Pronatores** (prō-nā′tŏ-rēz″)
SUPIN/O (soo-pĭn-ō) SUPINAT/O (soo-pĭ-nāt-ō)	Face up, lying supine	L. *supinator, -oris*, m. supinator fr. L. *supernatio*, f. a facing up	**Supina**tion, **supina**tor Loan word: **Supinator** (soo″pĭ-nāt′ŏr) pl. **Supinatores** (soo″pĭ-nāt′ŏ-rēz″)

Greek or Latin word element	Current usage	Etymology	Examples
DILAT/O (dī-lăt-ō)	To spread out	L. *dilatator, -oris*, m. dilator fr. L. *dilatio*, f. a spreading out	**Dilat**ion, **Dilatat**or Loan word: **Dilatator** (dī-lăt′ŏr) pl. **Dilatatores** (dī-lăt′ŏ-rēz″)
SPHINCTER/O (sfĭngk-tĕr-ō)	To bind/constrict, ringlike muscle of an orifice (sphincter)	L. *sphincter, -eris*, m. sphincter fr. Gr. *sphinkter*, anything that binds tight, constricts	**Sphincter**algia, **sphinct**er Loan word: **Sphincter** (sfĭngk′tĕr) pl. **Sphincteres** (sfĭngk′tĕ-rēz″)
PON/O (pō-nō) **POS/O** (pō-sō) **POSIT/O** (pŏ-zi-tō)	To place, put	L. *ponere, positum*, to place, put	Com**pon**ent, decom**pos**er, **posit**ion
OPPON/O (ŏ-pō-nō) **OPPOS/O** (ŏ-pō-sō)	To place opposite (oppose)	L. *opponens, -entis*, opponens fr. L. *opponere*, to place opposite, oppose	**Oppon**ent, **oppos**ition Loan word: **Opponens** (ŏ-pō′nenz″) pl. **Opponentes** (op″ŏ-nen′tēz″)
PRESS/O (prĕs-ō)	To press	L. *premere, pressum*, to press	Com**press**ion, **press**ure
DEPRESS/O (dē-prĕs-ō)	To press down	L. *depressor, -oris*, m. depressor fr. L. *depressio*, f. a pressing down	**Depress**ion, **depress**or Loan word: **Depressor** (dē-prĕs′or) pl. **Depressores** (dē-prĕs′o-rēz″)
LEVAT/O (lĕ-vă-tō)	To lift, raise	L. *levator, -oris*, m. levator fr. L. *levatio*, f. a lifting up fr. *levare, levatum* to lift, raise	El**evat**ion, **levat**or Loan word: **Levator** (lĕ-vă′tor) pl. **Levatores** (lĕ-vă′to-rēz″)
RECT/O (rek-tō)	Straight, correct	L. *regere, rectum*, to make straight L. *rectus, recta, rectum*, straight	**Rect**ification, **rect**olabial
ERECT/O (ĕ-rek-tō) **ARRECT/O** (ă-rek-tō)	To lift up	L. *erector, -oris*, m. erector fr. L. *erectio*, a raising	**Erect**ion, **arrect**or Loan word: **Erector** (ĕ-rek′tŏr) pl. **Erectores** (ĕ-rek′tŏ-rēz″) **Arrector** (ă-rek′tŏr) pl. **Arrectores** (ă-rek′tŏ-rēz″)

Review	Answers
The *M. arrector pili* ____ up the hair to which it is attached. Based on its name, the *M. erector spinae* moves the _____. The common root in this anatomical word RECT- means _____ and _____.	**lifts (raises)** **spine** **straight, correct**
The *M. levator scapulae* is a muscle that _____ the _____.	**lifts (raises), scapula (shoulder blade)**
The *M.* _____ *pollicis* leads the thumb toward midline, the *M.* _____ *pollicis brevis* leads the thumb away from midline.	*adductor* *abductor*

Review	Answers
The muscle that turns the palm of the hand face up is called the M. _____. A muscle that turns something face down is called a _____.	*supinator* **pronator**
The *M. extensor carpi ulnaris* is a muscle that _____ the _____ toward the ulnar side of the forearm.	**extends (straightens, stretches out), wrist**
The *M. flexor digitorum profundus* is a deep muscle that _____ the _____ of the hand.	**flexes (bends), fingers**
The _____ *ani* is a ring-like muscle that constricts the orifice of the anus.	**sphincter**
The *M. opponens* is a muscle that places a part _____ to another. The combining form meaning "to place" is _____.	**opposite PON/O**
A triceps muscle has three _____.	**origins (heads, capita)**
The literal translation of *M. rectus* is the _____ muscle.	**straight**
The literal translation of *M. brevis* is the _____ muscle. The anatomical antonym of *M. brevis* is the *M.* _____.	**short** *longus*
The literal translation of *M. planus* is the _____ muscle.	**flat**
The anatomical antonym of *M. minor* would be the *M.* _____.	*major*
The anatomical antonym of *M. maximus* would be the *M.* _____.	*minimus*
A muscle that turns something around an axis is called a *M.* _____.	*rotator*
The combining forms meaning "to place" are _____, _____, and _____.	**PON/O, POS/O, POSIT/O**
M. depressor anguli oris is a muscle that presses the angle of the _____ in a _____ direction.	**mouth, downward**

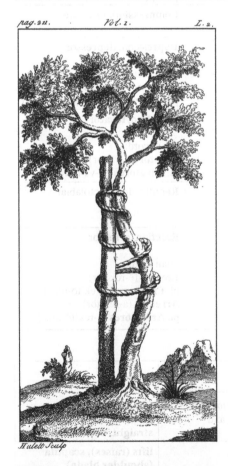

Hulett Sculp

Fig. 7.20 Frontispiece of Nicolas Andry de Bois-Regard, *Orthopédie*, 1741. *Source:* Nicolas Andry/Wikimedia Commons/Public domain.

Lessons from History: History of Orthopedics and Hippocratic Medicine

Food for Thought as You Read:

To what extent was the practice of orthopedics a part of Hippocratic medicine?

The primary field of modern medicine that deals with musculoskeletal injuries is called **Orthopedics**. Speaking of "Hippocratic orthopedics" is somewhat anachronistic because the term orthopedics did not exist in the 5th and 4th century BC. The term "orthopedics" was coined in 1741 by a French physician, Nicolas Andry, who entitled his book *Orthopédie*. Andry's book was translated into English in 1743 with the title *Orthopaedia* (Fig. 7.20). Written for parents and practitioners, the book addresses how to recognize and correct musculoskeletal deformities in children. In respect to the title of his work, Andry states, "of two Greek Words, viz. Orthos, which signifies straight, free from deformity, and Pais, a Child. Out of these two words I have compounded that of Orthopaedia, to express in one term the design I propose, which is to teach the different methods of preventing and correction of deformities of children (Andry, Nicolas. *Orthopaedia: or the art of correcting and preventing deformities in children: by such means, as may easily be put in practice by parents themselves, and all such as are employed in educating children. To which is added, a defense of the orthopaedia, by way of supplement / by the author. Translated from the French of M. Andry. 1743. London: Printed for A. Millar)."* Rather than meaning "child," the compound suffix **-PEDIA** (American spelling) or **-PAEDIA** (British spelling) is commonly used with the meaning "the education in X" (e.g. encyclopedia, pharmacopedia, gymnopedia, macropedia). This usage closely follows the Greek word *paideia* which means "the training of the mental and physical faculties of youths." **PED-** (**PAED-**) is the root used for "child" in modern medicine, and **ORTH-** appears in numerous words with the meanings "straight, correct, normal, and upright".

Hippocratic texts such as *On Joints* and *On Fractures* attest to 5th and 4th century BC medical texts writing specifically about the treatments for musculoskeletal injuries. However, there was not a formal field of Hippocratic medicine for the treatment of musculoskeletal problems. Such practices would have fallen under the broader category of *cheirourgikos* (**CHIR-**, **CHEIR-** hand + **ERG-** work), a term whose meaning is etymologically similar to the term chiropractic (**CHIR-**, **CHEIR-** hand + **PRACT-** fit for action). *On Joints* and *On Fractures* are two technical treatises that appear to have been written by the same author. Despite their apparently distinct titles, both texts address fractures and dislocated joints. Likewise, the author of the work *Head Wounds* shows that he is familiar with a wide variety of fractures of the skull. While the treatments in these 5th–4th century BC texts are not up to the standards of modern orthopedics, they do reveal a high level of practical experience in dealing with the treatment of joint dislocations and fractures. This is particularly true with respect to the manual techniques of moving fractures and joints back into their normal position, which are described in *On Joints* and *On Fractures*. The restoration of a bone or joint into its normal position is called a **reduction** (L. *reductio*, leading back) in modern medicine. The restoring of a bone into its normal position is also called "setting" a bone. Today, the terms "open reduction" and "closed reduction" speak to whether or not one needs to surgically cut to access the fracture. The term "internal fixation" is the use of screws and/or metal plates to hold a bone together internally.

On Fractures contains pragmatic information in regard to the treatment of a wide variety of fractures according to their type and location. The author begins with the basic principle that with fractures and dislocations, one must reduce the bone or joint back to its most natural position. The work is written from the perspective of a confident practitioner who recognizes the errors of some physicians in the reduction and immobilization of limbs. The work is ordered loosely according to the nature of the fracture and its location. As to the nature of fractures, he recognizes that different types of fractures must be treated differently. Although using different terminology, there is a recognition of the different therapeutic measures and problems in addressing a **closed** (or **simple**) **fracture** (i.e. the bone is not protruding out of the skin) versus a **compound fracture** (i.e. the bone protruding outside of the skin). Other types of fractures, such a **comminuted fracture** (i.e. a bone that is fractured into three or more pieces), are taken into consideration. In addition to indications and techniques for the reduction of a fracture, he provides advice on diet, wound care, and splinting. The number of days to change dressings or diet is discussed, and likewise, the time for different bones to heal is taken into consideration. To immobilize a fractured bone after reduction, in addition to bandages, the author describes a type of splint called a *narthekes*, which is an **orthosis** (i.e. any type of external orthopedic devices, braces, or splints applied to the body part to stabilize) made of wood rods. Some of the treatments of fractures described in *On Fractures* and *On Joints* are often praised by modern orthopedists for their correctness. That said, it is important to bear in mind that all of these reductions would have been enormously painful because ancient Greek surgery did not involve anesthesia, and patients who had compound fractures would have died at a high rate due to sepsis, as the ancient Greek physicians lacked an understanding of infections. The root for the Greek word for "fracture" *agmos* is rarely used in medical terminology (e.g. neuragmia). Instead, the Latin roots **FRANG-** and **FRACT-** are commonly used in medical and scientific terms for "break, broken."

On Joints discusses the indications and techniques for correcting **luxed** (i.e. dislocated) and **subluxed** (i.e. partial dislocation) joints. The author also addresses other orthopedic problems that require "surgery," such as correcting deviations in the spine and fractures of the nose. From the least to the most forceful technique, the author describes different methods of relocating a specific dislocated joint. Some of these techniques require assistants and specific devices to help create the force necessary to move the joint back into place. For instance, the author provides different methods of reducing a dislocated shoulder (with the physician's hand, with his heel, with the physician's shoulder in the armpit of the patient, with a pole, with a ladder, with a Thessalian chair), which appears to be somewhat common in a culture that values wrestling as a form of exercise (Fig. 7.21). The modern practitioner who is familiar with relocating joints will recognize similarities between these ancient techniques and modern methods, such as manipulation techniques for a dislocated jaw and the closed reduction of a deviated nasal fracture. The Latin root **LUX-** and the derivative **luxation** are used today for "dislocation." The author of *On Joints* uses the term *olisthanon* for "dislocation," which is a Greek word derived from the verb *olisthanein*, "to slip." Today, we use the suffix derived from this work, **-OLISTHESIS**, for "a slippage," typically of one vertebra on another.

In addition to braces and splints, some of the tools used in ancient Greek "orthopedics" have modern counterparts. The Hippocratic work entitled *Mochlion* (= *Instruments of Reduction*) is a surgical work that deals with the reduction of fractures and dislocations. Its title suggests that this work concerns itself with a lever-like tool used to reduce fractures and dislocations, the *mochlos*. The *mochlos*, or *mochliskos*, looks and functions similarly to a device called the "bone lever" in modern orthopedics (Fig. 7.22). The ancient Greek *ostagra* is another example of an ancient Greek surgical tool that is

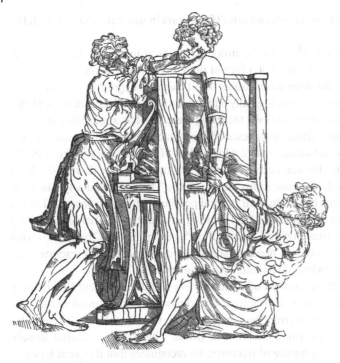

Fig. 7.21 16th century woodcut depicting one of the Hippocratic methods for relocating a dislocated/luxed shoulder.

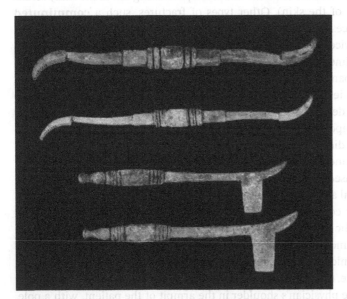

Fig. 7.22 *Mochliskos* (top two surgical instruments) and *Osteotome* (bottom two surgical instruments) from the collection of surgical instruments found at Pompeii after the eruption of Mount Vesuvius (79 AD). *Source:* Courtesy of Claude Moore Health Sciences Library, University of Virginia.

similar in appearance and use to its modern counterpart. The *ostraga* was a plier-like instrument used for picking out bone fragments at fracture sites (Fig. 7.23). Its modern counterpart is a tool called the bone forceps. *Agra* was a Greek word meaning "taking, catching." Today, the suffix **-AGRA** is commonly used for "a sudden, severe pain," particularly "gout" (e.g. cleidagra). Some ancient and modern tools share the same name but have different appearances. Ancient Greek medical texts discuss the use of an *osteotome* (bone-cutter). These tools had a small axe-like blade at one end to help cut fragmented edges of bones. Looking more like a file or chisel, the modern tool called an **osteotome** does not resemble its ancient Greek namesake. As noted previously, the compound suffix **-TOME** is commonly joined to an anatomical root to create a term that indicates what the surgical tool is used to cut. Some ancient Greek orthopedic devices were quite elaborate but worked on similar principles to those used in modern medicine. The famous *scamnon*, which is known as the "Hippocratic Bench," was a large, adjustable wood bench with ropes and wenches that was used for pulling a dislocated limb back into position or to correct abnormal spinal curvature. The modern devices used for pulling limbs or straightening the spine are distant cousins to this 5th century BC device, but all of them are based on the principle of using **traction** to help correct deformity. The root **TRACT-** is used quite commonly for things that "drag or draw something".

With respect to the spine, the author of *On Joints* recognizes that a practitioner should be aware of abnormal curvatures of the spine. He notes how the spine becomes bent (*skolioomai*) naturally or with old age. However, unnatural spinal curves should be corrected. The author provides a rather long discussion on how to correct a spinal deformity he calls *kyphosis* (hump-backed, hunchbacked) of the spine, which he states is due to a fall. The term **kyphosis** is used with a slight difference in modern orthopedics. Rather than being strictly used for a pathological curve, kyphosis also indicates that the spine has a natural anterior–posterior curve to it. In a normal spine, the thoracic and sacral areas of the spine are said to be **kyphotic** (**KYPH-** bent forward, a spine that is convex posteriorly) and the lumbar and cervical as **lordotic** (**LORD-** bend backward, a spine that is convex anteriorly). An abnormal anterior posterior curve would be one that is excessive (e.g. hyperkyphotic) or out of place (e.g. lumbar kyphosis). Based on the Greek word for "bent" (*skolioomai*), the term **scoliosis** is used for a side-bending curve of the spine. The direction of a scoliotic curve is determined by which side of the body the convexity of the curve is facing. **Levoscoliosis** is a left-bending curve (i.e. convex to the left), and **dextroscoliosis** is a right-bending curve (i.e. convex to the right). **LEV-** comes from the Latin word *laevus*, which means "left," and **DEXTR-** comes from the Latin adjective for "right," dexter. **SCOLI-** is the Greek root used for "crooked" or "bent." **ANKYL-** is a Greek root with a similar meaning to **SCOLI-**. **ANKYL-** means "crooked," but its more common medical meaning is "stiff" or "fused." **TORT-** is

Fig. 7.23 *Ostagra* from the collection of surgical instruments found at Pompeii after the eruption of Mount Vesuvius (79 AD). *Source:* Courtesy of Claude Moore Health Sciences Library, University of Virginia.

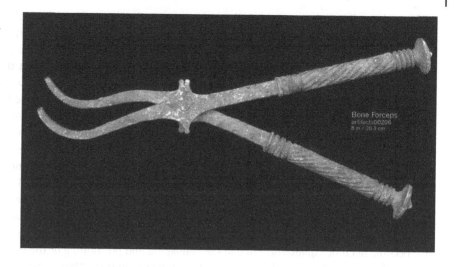

a Latin root with a similar meaning to **SCOLI-** in respect to the spine. **TORT-** means "twisted" or "turned," and it shows up in medial terms such as torticollis.

In addition to the curvature of the spine, the author of *On Joints* also addresses pathologies with an individual *spondylos* (vertebra). He notes how if one or more vertebrae are displaced forward, the patient may lose strength in the extremities, have urine retention, and/or die. However, if one or more vertebrae are displaced backward, the patient is less at risk. One can surmise that he is probably speaking of fractures of the spine. However, he may also be discussing what is termed today **spondylolisthesis**, which is a slippage forward or backward of one vertebra on another. As was noted above, the Greek root for "vertebra" is **SPONDYL-**. Thus, a breakdown of the vertebral structure is a **spondylolysis**, and degenerative changes at a vertebra are called **spondylosis.**

On Joints also has sections that address dislocations of lower extremity joints and their ramifications on gait and the development of the limbs. In the author's discussion of the different forms of dislocations of the hip, he provides a detailed description of the gait abnormalities of a person with a hip dislocation. He also points out the deleterious effects an unaddressed hip dislocation will have on the muscles and bone growth in children who are still growing, noting that the muscles will be less muscular, and the bones would not grow as long. To support this claim, he turns to Greek legends, stating that some storytellers say that the Amazons dislocate the joints of their male children at the hip so that the males would be maimed, and therefore, would not conspire against their female rulers. He notes that the ability to stand is worse if the hip is dislocated inward versus outward. This follows with the rest of the limb. Today, the terms **varus** (L. bent inward) and **valgus** (L. bent outward) are used to describe deformities of the lower extremities. These meanings for valgus and varus are straightforward for most joints, but it gets somewhat confusing with respect to knees because a "knock-kneed" leg position is said to be **genu valgum** and a "bowlegged" knee position is said to be **genu varum**. However, it is important to bear in mind that in modern medicine it is the most distal part of the bone involved in the joint that is the reference point (Fig. 7.24).

Fig. 7.24 Genu valgum and varum.

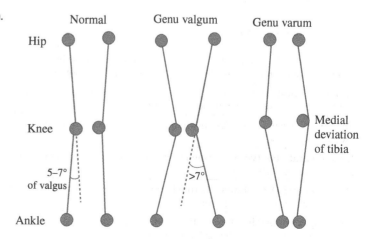

The author of *On Joints* recognizes that early intervention is necessary for children with congenital foot deformities. The author advises the reduction of the joint back into a midline position, followed by bandaging to hold it in place and different types of corrective shoes. Thus, like today, ancient Greek physicians created specialized splinting and foot orthoses to help with congenital foot deformities. By using the term *kullos*, the foot defect that the author of *On Joints* is speaking about appears to be what is called "club foot," a birth defect in which a foot is turned inward and downward. **Talipes** is a Latin word used today for foot deformities, particularly what is known as "club foot." It is formed from the word elements *talus*, ankle + *pes*, foot. A variety of Latin adjectives are used to indicate the type of foot deformity: **Pes cavus** (exaggerated arch of the foot), **Pes planus** (no arch of the foot, flat), **Pes valgus** (the foot is turned outward), and **Pes varus** (the foot is turned inward).

While ancient Greek physicians would have had some success with bone fractures, dislocated joints, and abnormal deformities, they were unaware of the bone and cartilage diseases that are commonly diagnosed today, thanks to radiographic studies. Without X-rays, bone scans, and MRI's, it would be impossible for an ancient Greek physician to diagnose diseases such as **osteopenia, osteoporosis, osteomalacia, chondromalacia, osteomyelitis, osteofibroma**, and **osteosarcoma**. That said, they recognized observable pathological changes in the bone. For instance, the author of *On Fractures* warns his readers about the dangers of fractures of the heel caused by jumping from a high place. He states that one of these dangers is that the heel bone may become necrotic (*sphakelisai*) due to the bandaging and positioning of the patient's leg. Thus, he seems to recognize that bone can become necrotic, similar to the skin becoming gangrenous. **Osteonecrosis** is the death of bone tissue due to a loss of blood supply. Sometimes, a fragment of dead bone will separate from the healthy bone, which is called a **sequestrum**.

Arthritis is the inflammation of one or more joints. There are over 100 different types of arthritides. Ancient Greek physicians' reliance on humoral pathologies to explain cause and to develop treatments would have made their therapeutic measures largely ineffective with respect to the different arthritides. The modern names of some of these types of arthritis bear witness to the humoral pathological model. **Gout** is derived from the Latin word *gutta* (drop), which reflects the ancient belief that an infiltration of a pathological humor was to blame for this type of arthritis. The root **RHEUMAT-** in **Rheumatoid arthritis** (RA) comes from a Greek word meaning "flow" or "discharge." The Greek words *rheumatikos* and *rheumatismos* were used by ancient Greek physicians such as Galen for effects of the pathological flow or discharge of the humor. Hence, today, the term for a catarrh, discharge, or flow is **rheum/rheuma**, and the study and treatment of joint and tissue inflammation is called **rheumatology**.

Some Suggested Readings

Craik, Elizabeth M. *"The Teaching of Surgery,"* In *Hippocrates and Medical Education. Selected Papers at the XIIth International Hippocrates Colloquium, Universiteit Leiden, 24–26 August 2005.* Edited by Manfred Horstmanshoff, 223–34. Leiden and Boston: Brill, 2010.

Hippocrates. *On Wounds in the Head. In the Surgery. On Fractures. On Joints. Mochlicon.* Translated by E. T. Withington. Loeb Classical Library 149. Cambridge, MA: Harvard University Press, 1928.

Livingston, M. C. "Hippocratic Principles in Orthopaedics." *Orthopedic Reviews* 17, no. 11 (1988).: 1122–1127.

Etymological Explanations: Greek and Latin Roots for Orthopedic Terms

General orthopedic terms
Atrophy and Hypertrophy – Atrophy is a marked decrease in the size of a muscle. Hypertrophy is a marked increase in the size of a muscle. Both use the root for "nourishment" and "growth," which is **TROPH-**.
Hypotonia and Hypertonia – Hypotonia is a marked reduction in the resting tension of a muscle. Hypertonia is a marked increase in the resting tension of a muscle. Both terms use the root for "tension" and "tone," **TON-**.
Spasm – A spasm is a sudden involuntary contraction of a muscle. The root for this is **SPASM-**, which comes from a Greek word for "wrenching, convulsion."
Myalgia and Myodynia – Formed from the compound suffixes for "painful condition," **-ALGIA** and **-ODYNIA**, myalgia/myodynia are terms for muscle pain.
Ostealgia and Osteodynia – Formed from the compound suffixes for "painful condition," **-ALGIA** and **-ODYNIA**, ostealgia/osteodynia are terms for bone pain.
Arthralgia and Arthrodynia – Formed from the compound suffixes for "painful condition," **-ALGIA** and **-ODYNIA**, arthralgia/arthrodynia are common terms for joint pain.
Ankylosis – Ankylosis is a stiff or immobile joint. The compound word is formed from the root for "stiff," "fused," and "crooked," **ANKYL-**.

Crepitus – Crepitus/crepitation is the grating/crackling sound that a dysfunctional joint can make. These terms are formed from the root for the sounds "creak" and "crackle," **CREPIT-**.

Strain – A strain is the result of trauma to a muscle, often causing pain and disability. While an English word, it is ultimately from the Latin verb *stringere*, to draw tight, bind tight.

Sprain – A sprain is the result of trauma to a ligament that causes pain and joint instability.

Dislocation – Derived from the Latin word for "place," *locus* (**LOC-**), a dislocation is a joint that is out of its normal anatomical place. Luxation is a completely dislocated joint. Subluxation is a partially dislocated joint. Both of these terms are derived from the Latin verb *luxare* (**LUX-**), to dislocate.

Reduction – Derived from the Latin verb *ducere* (**DUC-** and **DUCT-**), "to lead," reduction is the process of restoring the proper alignment of a joint or fractured bone.

Traction – Derived from the Latin verb *trahere* (**TRACT-**), "to drag, draw," traction is the pulling on a bone to help with alignment and proper healing.

Orthosis – Derived from the Greek word for "straight," *orthos* (**ORTH-**), orthosis is a term for a brace.

Prosthesis – Derived from the Greek word for "an addition," *prosthesis*, prosthesis is a term for an artificial limb.

Fractures

Fracture – Derived from the Latin verb *frangere* (**FRANG-**, **FRACT-**), "to break," a fracture is a break in a bone (Fig. 7.25).

Fig. 7.25 Types of fractures. *Source:* Adapted from Anatomy & Physiology, Connexions/http://cnx.org/content/coll1496/1.6/.

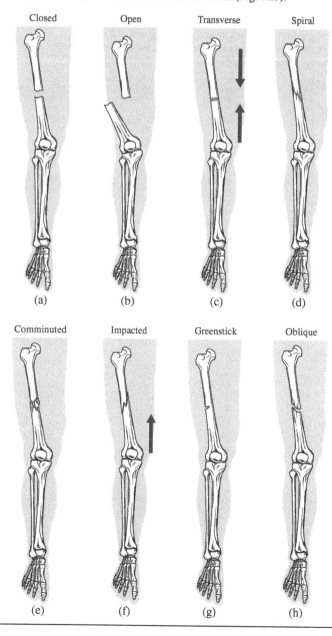

Closed   Open   Transverse   Spiral

(a)   (b)   (c)   (d)

Comminuted   Impacted   Greenstick   Oblique

(e)   (f)   (g)   (h)

Closed fracture is a broken bone with no open wound.

Fractures

Open fracture (or compound fracture) is a broken bone that has an open wound.

Transverse fracture is where the fracture line is at a right angle.

Spiral fracture follows a helical pattern along a long bone.

Comminuted fracture is where the bone is broken into little pieces.

Impacted fracture is where the broken end of a bone is wedged into the other end of the bone.

Greenstick fracture is a bending and incomplete fracture of the bone; and an oblique fracture is when the fracture line is at an angle.

Avulsion fracture is a pulling away of part of the bone, typically at the place of attachment of a ligament.

Spine pathologies

Kyphosis – Derived from the Greek word for "bent forward," *kyphos* (**KYPH-**), a kyphotic curve is convex posteriorly, and it is normal for the thoracic and sacral regions of the spine (Fig. 7.26). Kyphosis is sometimes used for an abnormal "hump" or excessive posterior convexity of the spine.

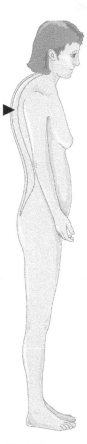

Fig. 7.26   Image of excessive kyphosis of the thoracic spine. *Source:* Adapted from Sevier Medical Art.

Lordosis – Derived from the Greek word for "bent backward," *lordos* (**LORD-**), a lordotic curve is convex anteriorly, and it is normal for the cervical and lumbar regions of the spine (Fig. 7.27). Lordosis is sometimes used for an abnormal "sway" or excessive anterior convexity of the spine.

Fig. 7.27 Image of excessive lordosis of the lumbar spine. *Source:* Adapted from Sevier Medical Art.

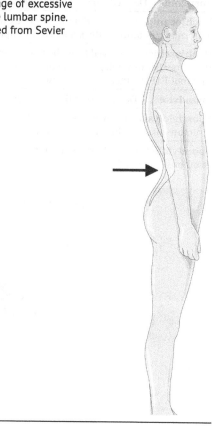

Scoliosis – Derived from the Greek word for "twisted, curved," *skolios* (**SCOLI-**), scoliosis is an abnormal lateral or side-bending curvature of the spine (Fig. 7.28).

Fig. 7.28 An anatomical illustration of scoliosis in the German edition of *Anatomie des Menschen: ein Lehrbuch für Studierende und Ärzte*, 1921. *Source:* Anatomie des Menschen, (1921)/Heidelberg University Library/ Public domain.

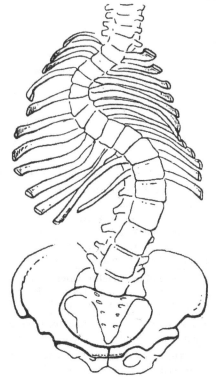

Torticollis – Derived from a Latin verb for "to twist, turn," *torquere* (**TORT-** and **TORS-**), torticollis is a stiff, side-flexed neck.

Rachiocampsis – Derived from the Greek word for "bent," *kamptos* (**CAMPT-, CAMPYL-, CAMPS-**), rhachiocampsis is an abnormal curvature of the spine. For example, scoliosis, torticollis, kyphosis, and lordosis.

Rachioschisis – Derived from the Greek verb for "to split," *schizein* (**SCHIZ-** and **-SCHISIS**), rachioschisis is a congenital split in the spine. For example, spina bifida is a split vertebra caused by the congenital failure of the vertebra to close around the spinal cord. The root **BIFID-** means "split in two."

Spondylosis – Derived from the Greek word for "vertebra," *spondylos* (**SPONDYL-**), spondylosis an ankylosing of vertebrae.

Spondylolysis – Derived from the suffix for "dissolution, breaking down," **-LYSIS**, spondylolysis is a breaking for the vertebral structure, usually the *pars interarticularis*.

Spondylolisthesis – Derived from the suffix for "a slipping," **-OLISTHESIS**, spondylolisthesis is the slippage of a vertebra on another vertebra (Fig. 7.29).

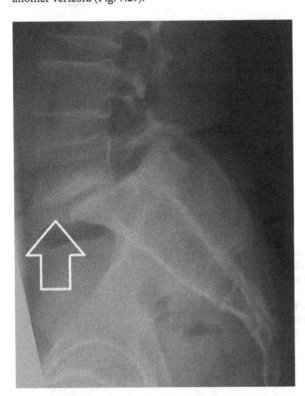

Fig. 7.29 X-ray of the lateral lumbar spine with a spondylolisthesis at L5-S1. *Source:* Lucien Monfils/Wikimedia Commons/CC BY-SA 3.0.

Joint, bone, and muscle pathologies

Varus and Valgus Deformities – The Latin adjectives varus (**VAR-**), "bent inward," and valgus (**VALG-**), "bent outward," are used to describe the bones' relationship to a joint. Coxa valga is a bent outward hip. Coxa vara is a bent inward hip. Genu valgum is commonly referred to as knock-kneed. Genu varum is commonly referred to as bowlegged. Hallux valgus is a lateral deviation of the great toe, also known as a bunion. Hallux varus is a medial deviation of the great toe.

Cavus and Planus Deformities – Cavus (**CAV-**), "hollow," and planus (**PLAN-**), "flat," are Latin adjectives used to describe abnormalities of position. Pes cavus is a high-arched foot. Pes planus is a flat foot. Talipes equinovarus is commonly referred to as a club foot. The root **TALIP-** is used for a deformity of the foot and ankle.

Osteoarthritis – Derived from the roots for "bone" and "joint," **OSTE-** and **ARTHR-** respectively, osteoarthritis is inflammation of weightbearing joints characterized by a progressive loss of cartilage.

RA – The root **RHEUMAT-** in RA comes from a Greek word meaning "flow" or "discharge." RA is a chronic, systemic inflammation of synovial joints causing deformation and loss of function (Fig. 7.30).

Fig. 7.30 Deformity of the hands, simulating rheumatoid arthritis. St Bartholomew's Hospital Archives & Museum. *Source:* Wellcome Collection/CC BY 4.0.

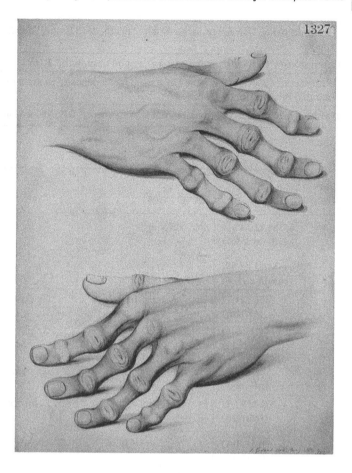

Gout – Derived from the Latin word for "a drop," *gutta*, gout is characterized by acute inflammation of a joint (typically the great toe) due to excessive uric acid in the blood. The suffix **-AGRA** is often used to denote the presence of gout in an area, e.g. cleidagra and podagra.

Myositis – Derived from one of the roots for "muscle," **MYOS**-, myositis is an inflammation of a muscle.

Tendinitis – Derived from one of the roots for "tendon," **TENDIN**-, tendinitis is an inflammation of a tendon.

Bursitis – Derived from the Latin term for a "purse or bag," *bursa*, bursitis is an inflammation of a bursa.

Epiphysitis – Derived from the compound root **EPIPHYS**-, which is used on the end part of a long bone, epiphysitis is an inflammation of the epiphysis of the bone.

Osteomyelitis – Derived from the roots for "bone" and "marrow," **OSTE**- and **MYEL**- respectively, osteomyelitis is an inflammation of bone and marrow.

Myeloma – Derived from the root for "marrow," **MYEL**-, a myeloma is a bone marrow tumor.

Osteoma – Derived from the root for "bone," **OSTE**-, an osteoma is a bone tumor.

Osteofibroma – Derived from the roots for "bone" and "fiber," **OSTE**- and **FIBR**- respectively, an osteofibroma is a tumor of bone and fibrous tissue.

Osteosarcoma – Derived from the compound suffix for a type of cancer, **-SARCOMA**, an osteosarcoma is a type of bone cancer.

Osteopenia – Derived from the suffix for "decrease, deficiency," **-PENIA**, osteopenia is a loss of bone mass/density.

Osteoporosis – Derived from the root for "a passage or pore," **POR**-, osteoporosis is a severe loss of bone mass/density characterized by the internal structure of the bone becoming more porous and making the bone prone to fractures.

Osteomalacia – Derived from the suffix for "an abnormal softening," **-MALACIA**, osteomalacia is a softening of the bone.

Chondromalacia – Derived from the root for "cartilage," **CHONDR**-, chondromalacia is a softening of the cartilage.

Osteonecrosis – Derived from the root for "death, dead tissue," **NECR-**, osteonecrosis is death of bone often due to lack of blood supply.

Osteophyte – Derived from the root for "a plant or growth," **PHYT-**, an osteophyte is a bony growth, also known as a bone spur.

Sequestrum – Derived from the Latin word for "a deposit," *sequestrum*, sequestrum is a bone fragment or other tissue that has separated from its original location.

Desmorrhexis – Derived from the root for "ligament," **DESM-**, a desmorrhexis is a ruptured ligament.

Greek or Latin word element	Current usage	Etymology	Examples
MALAC/O (mal-ă-kō) **-MALACIA** (mă-lā-shē-ă)	Soft, softening	Gr. *malakos*, soft	**Malac**osarcosis, chondro**malacia**
ORTH/O (or-thō)	Straight, correct, normal, upright	Gr. *orthos*, straight, correct, normal	**Orth**osis, **orth**otic
PED/O (pē-dō) **-PEDIA** (pē-dē-ă)	Child Education in X	Gr. *pais, paidos*, child Gr. *paideia*, education	**Ped**iatrics, pharmaco**pedia**
FRANG/O (frăn-gō) **FRACT/O** (frak-tō)	Break, broken	L. *frangere, fractum*, to break	**Frang**ible, **fract**ure
-RHEXIS (rek-sĭs)	A rupture	Gr. *rhexis*, burst, rupture	Karyo**rrhexis**, **desm**orrhexis Loan word: **Rhexis** (rĕk′sĭs) pl. **Rhexes** (rĕk′sēz″)
LUX/O (lŭks-ō)	Dislocated	L. *luxare*, to dislocate	Sub**lux**ation, **lux**ed
POR/O (pō-rō)	Passage, pore	Gr. *poros*, passage	Osteo**poros**is, neuro**pore**
-PENIA (pē-nē-ă)	Decrease, deficiency	Gr. *penia*, poverty; deficiency	Osteo**penia**, glyco**penia**
CREPIT/O (krep-ĭ-tō)	Creak, crackle	L. *crepare, crepitatum*, rattle, creak, crackle	**Crepit**ation, de**crepit**ate
-AGRA (ag-ră)	Gout, attack (of severe pain)	Gr. *agra*, a taking, catching	Pod**agra**, cleid**agra**
RHEUM/O (roo-mō) **RHEUMAT/O** (roo′mă-tō)	Flow, discharge, rheumatoid arthritis	Gr. *rheuma, rheumatos*, flow, current, stream	**Rheumat**oid Loan word: **Rheum** (room) **Rheuma** (room′ă)
ANKYL/O (ang-kĭ-lō)	Stiff, fused, crooked	Gr. *ankylos*, crooked, bent	**Ankyl**osis
SEQUESTR/O (sĕ-kwes-trō)	Fragment of bone/tissue	L. *sequestrum, -i*, n. a deposit	**Sequestr**ation, **sequestr**ant Loan word: **Sequestrum** (sĕ-kwes′trŭm) pl. **sequestra** (sĕ-kwes′tră)

Greek or Latin word element	Current usage	Etymology	Examples
TALIP/O (tal-ĭ-pō)	Deformity of foot and ankle	L. *talus, -i,* m. ankle + *pes,* foot	**Talip**omanus, **talip**edic Loan word: **Talipes** (tal′ĭ-pēz″)
PLAN/O (plā-nō)	Flat	L. *planus, -a, -um,* flat	**Plan**ula, **plan**ocellular
CAV/O (kā-vō)	Hollow	L. *cavus, -a, -um,* hollow	**Cav**otricuspid, con**cav**e
VALG/O (val-gō)	Bent outward	L. *valgus, -a, um,* bent	**Valg**oid, plano**valgus**
VAR/O (vă-rō)	Bent inward	L. *varus, -a, um,* bent	**Var**oid, equino**varus**
KYPH/O (kī-fō)	Bent forward (convex posteriorly)	Gr. *kyphos,* bent forward	**Kyph**oscoliosis, **kyph**osis
LORD/O (lor-dō)	Bent backward (convex anteriorly)	Gr. *lordos,* bent backward	**Lord**osis, **lord**otic
LEV/O (lē-vō)	Left	L. *laevus, -a, -um,* left	**Lev**ocardia, levo**scoli**otic
DEXTR/O (deks-trō)	Right	L. *dexter, -tra, -trum,* right	**Dextr**ad, **dextr**oscoliosis
SCOLI/O (skŏ-lē-ō)	Bent sideways, crooked	Gr. *skolios,* twisted, curved	Rachio**scoli**osis, **scoli**otic
TORS/O (tor-sō) **TORT/O** (tort-ō)	Twist, turn	L. *torquere, tortum, torsum,* to twist, turn	Sinistro**torsion**, **torti**collis
-OLISTHESIS (ŏ-lis-thē-sĭs)	Slipping	Gr. *olisthesis,* a slipping	Sacr**olisthesis**, spondyl**olisthesis**
BIFID/O (bī-fĭd-ō)	Split in two	L. *bifidus, -a, -um,* split in two	**Bifid**obacteria Loan word: **Bifid** (bī′fĭd)
SCHIZ/O (skĭ-zō) **-SCHISIS** (skĭ-sĭs)	A splitting, a cleft	Gr. *schizein,* to split, cleave	**Schiz**oblepharis, rhachi**schisis**
SPASM/O (spaz-mō)	Spasm	Gr. *spasmos,* a wrenching, convulsion	**Spasm**olytic, **spasm**odic
TRACT/O (trak-tō)	To draw, pull	L. *trahere, tractum,* to draw, drag	Con**tract**ure, ex**tract**
CAMPT/O (kămp-tō) **CAMPYL/O** (kăm-pĭ-lō) **-CAMPSIA** (kamp-sē-ă) **-CAMPSIS** (kămp-sĭs)	Bent, curved	Gr. *kamptos, kampylos,* bent	**Campt**odactylia, **campyl**obacter, gony**campsis**, a**campsia**

Review	Answers
Lordosis is a term for a spinal curve that is convex _____. Kyphosis is a term for a spinal curve that is convex _____.	**anteriorly** **posteriorly**
A stiff or immobile joint is termed ankylosis. The root in this term can mean _____, _____, and _____.	**stiff, fused, crooked**
The Latin word used for foot deformities is _____.	**talipes**
A hallux valgus is a deviation of the great toe _____. A hallux varus is a deviation of the great toe _____.	**outward (laterally)** **inward (medially)**
Pes cavus is a foot with a _____ arch. Pes planus is a foot with a _____ arch.	**hollow (cave-like, high)** **Flat**
A partially dislocated joint is called a _____.	**Subluxation (subluxed joint)**
Osteoarthritis (also known as degenerative joint disease, DJD) is a progressive disease that is associated with the cartilage in joints. It is often associated with the sign of a "creaking" sound with the movement of a joint; the root for this sign is _____. The softening of the cartilage that occurs with osteoarthritis is called chondro_____.	**CREPIT-** **-malacia**
Gout is a type of arthritis that is marked by painful attacks on a joint. It is linked to hyperuricemia. It typically affects one joint. The big toe joint is the most common joint affected by gout, which is called pod_____.	**-agra**
A slippage of a vertebra on another vertebra is called spondyl_____.	**-olisthesis**
A side-bending curve of the spine is called _____. If the curve is convex to the left, it is called _____, and if it is convex to the right, _____.	**scoliosis** **levoscoliosis** **dextroscoliosis**
The combining form in the term torticollis indicates that the neck is _____ or _____.	**twisted, turned**
Rheumatoid arthritis (RA) is an autoimmune disease that causes inflammation in multiple joints (typically hands and wrists) at the same time. The literal meaning of this term is that it "resembles rheum," which is a term for _____ or _____.	**flow, discharge**
Rachischisis is a _____ in the _____. Spina bifida is an example of rachischisis; spina bifida literally means a spine that is _____ in two. This can occur due to a congenital defect that leaves a vertebra without its laminae.	**split (cleft), vertebral column (spine)** **split**
A ruptured ligament is called a desmo_____. Trauma to a ligament due to excessive force is called a "sprain." Trauma to a muscle or tendon due to excessive force is called a "strain."	**-rrhexis**
Hypertonicity is excessive _____ or _____ in a muscle.	**tension, tone**
A "spasm" is a sudden, involuntary contraction of muscle due to trauma/irritation. The root for spasm is _____. A muscle cramp is a sudden, involuntary contraction of a muscle that is painful.	**SPASM-**
A fragment of necrotic bony tissue is termed a _____.	**sequestrum**
A decrease in the amount of bone mineral density is called osteopenia. If the bone mineral density loss exceeds 2.5 standard deviations, it is called osteoporosis. The root POR- in this term, indicates that the loss makes the bone look like it has _____ or _____.	**pores, passages**
The use of a "pulling" or "drawing" force to a dislocated joint or fractured bone is called _____. The moving or "leading back" of a joint or limb into its natural position is called _____.	**traction** **reduction**
A brace or splint used to support or maintain the position of a bone or joint is called an _____. The field of medicine that specializes in the treatment of musculoskeletal injuries is called _____. Both terms use the root ORTH-, which is a root that can mean _____, _____, _____, and _____.	**orthosis** **orthopedics** **straight, correct, normal, upright**
The roots CAMPYL- and CAMPT- mean _____ or _____.	**bent, curved**

8

Cardiovascular System, Blood, and Lymph

CHAPTER LEARNING OBJECTIVES

1) In this chapter, you will learn the Greek and Latin word elements for the anatomy, physiology, pathologies, and surgical interventions that pertain to the cardiovascular, blood, and lymphatic systems.
2) You will also become familiar with the ancient Greek concepts of the cardiovascular system and its function. You will gain a better understanding of the social and medical approaches to blood in the ancient Greek and Roman worlds.

Lessons from History: Galen's Theory of Blood Flow and the Circulation of Blood

Food for Thought as You Read:

To what extent is Galen's concept of blood flow based on theoretical speculations? To what extent is Galen's concept of blood flow based on experience (i.e. empirical)?
How is Harvey's discovery of the circulation a radical departure from Galenic physiology?

While most of the anatomical structures of the heart and blood vessels were recognized by anatomists such as Galen, the physiology of the cardiovascular system was far less understood.

Galen's physiology of the heart and blood vessels is an amalgamation of previous anatomical and physiological theories, primarily those of Aristotle. In Galen's physiological model, blood vessels carry nutriment and *pneuma* to the body. Like the theorists before him, Galen understood blood flow as unidirectional. Thus, Galen understood that blood flowed to the parts of the body where it is used by the body; it did not return to the heart. Like Erasistratus and Herophilus, Galen did make a distinction between arteries and veins. Galen recognized that venous blood was darker than arterial blood, and therefore, he rationalized that arterial blood had a different purpose than venous blood. For Galen, the concepts of *pneuma* (Gr. breath, air, spirit) and nutritive blood were fundamental to understanding the differences in venous and arterial blood, as well as the structure and function of the heart and blood vessels. Galen argued that venous blood served as the nutritive function of the body. The parts of the body attracted and used this nutritious blood in the appropriate quantities. Because arterial blood was invigorated with *pneuma*, it was lighter and warmer than venous blood, and he thought it served a vital function for the parts of the body that it supplied. In some respects, Galen's cardiovascular theories hinge on venous blood being understood as "food" for the body and arterial blood being the carrier of the "breath" and "warmth" that is vital to life.

Galen's theory links the origins of blood, veins, and arteries to the organs of the body (Fig. 8.1). Galen argues that the veins are formed from the liver. According to Galen, when food becomes liquified in the stomach, it is released into the intestines where the veins attract this liquified food into them. The food begins to take on the nature of blood via the intestinal veins, as this raw foodstuff blood continues to travel via the larger veins (today known as the mesenteric veins) and is further purified of waste material in it. The lighter waste materials go to the gall bladder, where they are turned into yellow

Greek and Latin Roots of Medical and Scientific Terminologies, First Edition. Todd A. Curtis.
© 2025 John Wiley & Sons, Inc. Published 2025 by John Wiley & Sons, Inc.
Companion website: www.wiley.com/go/Curtis

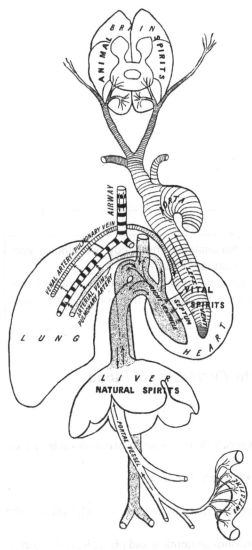

Fig. 8.1 Image of Galen's cardiovascular system form. *Source:* Singer, 1922/Springer Nature/ Public Domain.

bile, and the heavier ones are attracted by the spleen, where they become black bile. The refined blood is attracted to the liver via a large vein (known today as the **portal vein)** where it is ultimately purified into nutritive venous blood (Fig. 8.2). This nutritive venous blood is then carried away from the liver via a larger vein (today known as the **vena cava)** to the body via the veins so that each part of the body is supplied with its proper quantities of nutritive blood. Each part, in turn, attracts and assimilates what it needs from the blood. While Galen's theory is completely wrong with respect to the physiology of the body, as can be seen in this modern image of the splenic, mesenteric, and portal vessel, his theory is derived from the anatomy of the blood vessels supplying the intestines, spleen, gall bladder, and liver.

As to the origins of arteries and arterial blood, Galen links this to the heart. Galen describes how some of the venous blood travels to the heart via the major blood vessel that we now call the superior vena cava. It enters the right atrium and then passes to the right ventricle. In Galenic physiology, the nature of the right and left ventricles are quite distinct. The left ventricle contains an innate heat that rarifies and invigorates venous blood, thereby changing it into arterial blood. Rather than relying on the pulmonary arteries and veins to explain how venous blood gets to the left ventricle, Galen hypothesized that the venous blood in the right ventricle must travel through pores in the interventricular septum into the left ventricle. Once the venous blood is invigorated in the left ventricle, it leaves the heart via the aorta and the rest of the arteries. Thus, for Galen, the heart is the origin of the arteries, and its role is to supply the parts of the body with the life-giving force carried in the arterial blood. Some of this arterial blood makes its way to the head, where it is rarified in a psychic *pneuma* that is contained in the ventricles of the brain and it becomes the primary instrument of the soul's function with respect to sensation, movement, and the mental faculties of perception, reasoning, and memory. Although physiologically incorrect, Galen's cardiovascular model provided an explanation for the recognizable differences in the structure and distribution of veins and arteries, the differences in the appearance of venous and arterial blood, and blood's intimate relationship to both mental and bodily faculties.

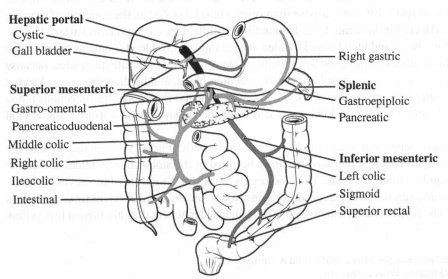

Hepatic portal
Cystic
Gall bladder
Superior mesenteric
Gastro-omental
Pancreaticoduodenal
Middle colic
Right colic
Ileocolic
Intestinal

Right gastric
Splenic
Gastroepiploic
Pancreatic
Inferior mesenteric
Left colic
Sigmoid
Superior rectal

Fig. 8.2 Image of the hepatic portal vein system. *Source:* Adapted from Anatomy & Physiology, Connexions./ http://cnx.org/content/col11496/1.6/.

Galen's theoretical conceptions of the physiology of the heart and blood were extremely influential on how generations of physicians and philosophers conceived of the anatomy and function of the body. Leonardo da Vinci's anatomical drawings have garnered much praise for their realistic depictions of the dissected body, and it is well known that Leonardo was involved in human dissection. That said, in numerous drawings, Leonardo incorporates anatomical features that he did not actually see in a human dissection. These unanatomical features are often overlooked by the casual observer of his artwork, but what they reveal is that Leonardo also saw the dissected human body through his "mind's eye." If you look closely at Leonardo's drawing of a heart, the septum between the ventricles has what appears to be holes or pores (Fig. 8.3). While this may be passed off as artistic shading, in some of Leonardo's other drawings of the human heart, these pores are even more evident. Although derived from anatomical dissections, Leonardo's drawings of the human heart reveal the influence of Galen's conception of the heart and the cardiovascular system.

Published in 1628, William Harvey's *Exercitatio Anatomica De motu cordis et sanguinis in animalibus* (*Anatomical Exercise Concerning the Movement of the Heart and Blood in Animals*) was pivotal in breaking the grip of Galen's physiological model. By vivisecting animals and dissecting human cadavers, Harvey performed a series of experiments that demonstrated that arterial and venous blood do not move in the unidirectional pattern that Galen put forth. Instead, blood runs in a continuous circuit throughout the body, which is why the cardiovascular system today is known as the circulatory system. In one experiment, Harvey measured the amount of blood in the left ventricle that a human heart could hold. He observed that with each contraction of the left ventricle, 2 ounces of blood left the heart. Based on the heart beating on

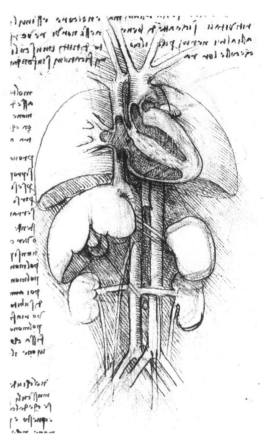

Fig. 8.3 Leonardo da Vinci's depiction of the ventricles and the septum of the heart. *Source:* Leonardo da Vinci/Wikimedia Commons/ Public domain.

average 72 times per minute, he calculated that 540 pounds of blood would be pumped per hour. Thus, it would be impossible for Galen's theory of food becoming venous blood to be correct since a human would have to eat 540 pounds of food every hour. Galen's invigorated arterial blood was dispelled by Harvey using the vivisection of animals. Harvey noted that the blood coming from the pulmonary vein into the right atrium was already a brighter red color before it reached the left ventricle, and therefore, Harvey's observation indicated that the left ventricle did not invigorate blood, as Galen had argued. In another experiment, Harvey observed that the blood in the veins does not move distally to the parts of the body, as Galen hypothesized, but instead, the venous blood moves toward the heart. To prove this, Harvey placed a tourniquet around an arm. He observed that when he attempted to move the blood distally, the valves in the veins prevented this, but if he moved it toward the heart, the blood moved more freely (Fig. 8.4). Thus, Harvey concluded that the valves of the veins were designed to allow blood to move toward the heart, which is the opposite direction of Galen's venous blood flow. Harvey's observations and experiments led him to argue that blood moves in a continuous circle via the blood vessels. Harvey, in turn, hypothesized that there must be a connection between the arteries and the veins for this to occur. The visible confirmation of the hairlike connections we now call **capillaries** was later made via a microscope by Marcello Malpighi in 1661. The use of the derivative of the Latin *capillus* (hair) for tiny blood vessels predates the discovery of the microscopic vessels we call capillaries today. Probably speaking to arterioles and venules, Andrea Cesalpinus (1523–1603) calls these hairlike structures *capillamenta*. The notion that arteries and veins are connected also predates Harvey and Malpighi. While Galen did not recognize that the blood circulated throughout the body, like his predecessor Erasistratus, Galen hypothesized that some venous and arterial vessels were connected by unseen *anastomoses* (outlets, openings). Today, a natural, surgical, or pathological connection between two blood vessels is referred to as an **anastomosis**, which is derived from the Greek verb meaning "to furnish a mouth". That said, Harvey's conception of a continuous physical movement of the

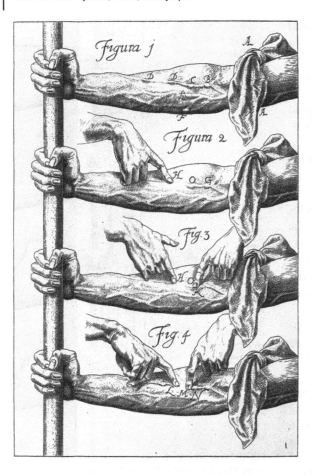

Fig. 8.4 Diagram illustrating William Harvey's experiments on the valves of the veins; drawing by S. Gooden for the Nonesuch edition of *De Motu Cordis*, London: 1928. *Source:* William Harvey/Wellcome Collection/CC BY 4.0.

blood throughout the body was a radical departure from Galenic physiology, providing a foundation for new physiological and pathological models to enter into medicine.

Some Suggested Readings

Singer, Charles. *The Discovery of Circulation of the Blood*. London: Wm. Dawson & Sons, 1956.
Wilkie, James S., and David Furley. *Galen on Respiration and the Arteries*. Princeton: Princeton University Press, 1984.

Etymological Explanations: Common Terms and Word Elements for the Anatomy of the Cardiovascular System

The cardiovascular system is made up of the heart and the network of vessels that move the blood throughout the body. Via the blood, it functions as a transport system for oxygen, nutrients, hormones, and metabolic wastes that are essential to life. It also plays an important role in regulating body temperature, protecting against microbes and foreign bodies, and preventing excessive blood loss. In the following discussion of the anatomical terms associated with the cardiovascular system, the nominative and genitive singular forms of the anatomical Latin term will be provided in the parenthesis. The Greek and Latin roots are formatted in all caps and emboldened.

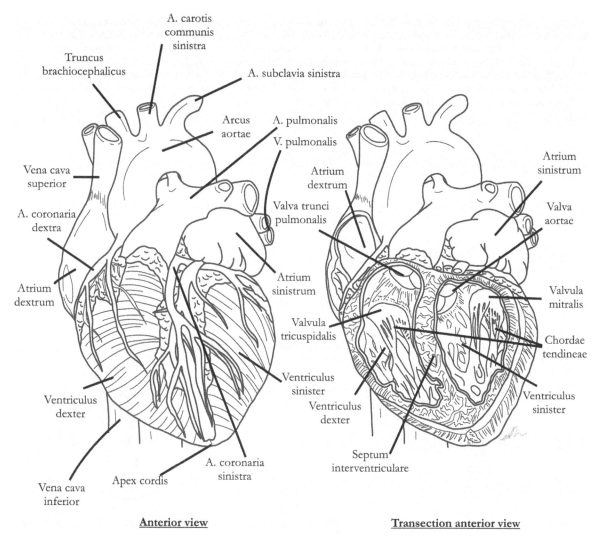

A. carotis communis sinistra

Truncus brachiocephalicus

A. subclavia sinistra

Arcus aortae

A. pulmonalis

V. pulmonalis

Atrium dextrum

Vena cava superior

Valva trunci pulmonalis

A. coronaria dextra

Atrium sinistrum

Atrium dextrum

Valvula tricuspidalis

Ventriculus sinister

Ventriculus dexter

Vena cava inferior

Apex cordis

A. coronaria sinistra

Atrium sinistrum

Valva aortae

Valvula mitralis

Chordae tendineae

Ventriculus sinister

Ventriculus dexter

Septum interventriculare

Anterior view

Transection anterior view

Fig. 8.5 Anatomical Latin for the heart. *Source:* Drawing by Chloe Kim.

The heart and its vessels (Fig. 8.5)

Heart (L. *cor, cordis*) – The heart is a muscular organ that acts like a pump, moving the blood throughout the body. The Latin root for the heart is **CORD-**. The root **CORD-** is sometimes confused with the root **CHORD-**, which is also sometimes spelled **CORD-**. In addition to their similar spelling, the potential confusion may be due to the *chordae tendinae*'s relationship to the heart. The *chordae tendinae* are a group of string-like tendinous structures that are attached to the cusps of the bicuspid and tricuspid valves. The Greek word *chord*, from which ultimately, we get the root **CHORD-**, meant "a string of a musical instrument." Consequently, the *chordae tendinae* are sometimes referred to as the heartstrings. The root CHORD- is used today for "string" or "cord" and is commonly used in medicine. *Kardia* is the Greek word for the heart, whose root is transliterated **CARDI-** or **KARDI-**. The differing transliterations of this root explain why the electrocardiograph's abbreviation can be ECG or EKG in medical terminology.

Myocardium (L. *myocardium, -i*), Epicardium (L. *epicardium, -i*), Pericardium (L. *pericardium, -i*) – The compound term used for the muscles of the heart is myocardium (Gr. *mys*, muscle + Gr. *kardia*, heart + -ium, tissue or structure). The heart's membranes are called the epicardium, endocardium, and pericardium, whose roots are **EPICARDI-**, **ENDOCARDI-**, and **PERICARDI-**. The epicardium is the membrane forming the outer layer of the heart, and the endocardium is the inner layer that lines the cavities of the heart. The pericardium is a protective sac that encloses the heart. The pericardial sac is composed of two layers: parietal pericardium and visceral pericardium. The outer layer is called the parietal pericardium because it is closest to the wall of the thorax. The inner layer is called the visceral pericardium because it is closest to the organ (i.e. the heart). The adjective "parietal" comes from the Latin word for the wall (L. *paries, parietis*), whose root **PARIET-** is typically used in anatomy for the "outer walls of a cavity." "Visceral" is derived from the Latin word for "organ" (L. *viscus, visceris*), and its root **VISCER-** is commonly used for "organ" in modern terminology.

Atrium (L. *atrium, -i*) – The upper two chambers of the heart are called the atria. The right atrium is the *atrium dextrum,* and the left atrium is the *atrium sinistrum*. The corresponding root for this part is **ATRI-**. The atrium of the heart takes its name from the lavishly furnished room found in ancient Roman homes. The term "atrium" was first used formally in medicine for the upper chambers of the heart around 1870. Prior to this usage, one can observe the conceptualization of the heart's atria as an arched architecture of a building in Leonardo da Vinci's (1452–1519) anatomical drawing (Fig. 8.6). The atria of the heart were commonly referred to as the auricles (little ears) because these upper chambers of the heart and their accompanying blood vessels resembled the handles of jars/storage vessels, which in turn looked like ears (Fig. 8.7).

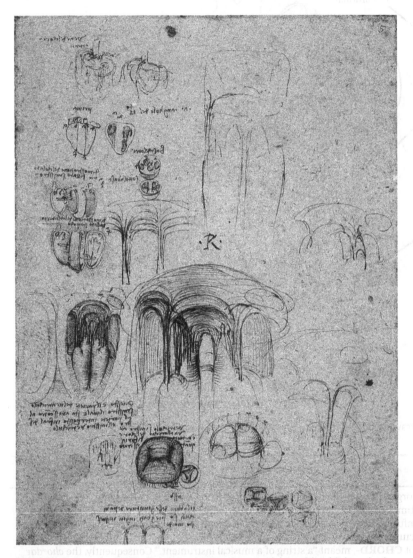

Fig. 8.6 Leonardo da Vinci's image depicts the ventricles with a high arched chamber, assumedly these columns are the *chordae tendinae,* sitting on top of the ventricles. *Source:* His Majesty King Charles III/The Royal Collection Trust/ Public domain.

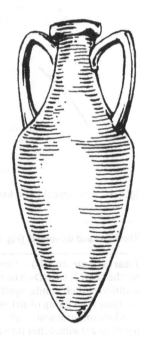

Fig. 8.7 Line drawing of an amphora with ear-like handles.

Ventricle (L. *ventriculus, -i*) – The lower two chambers of the heart are known as the ventricles. The right ventricle is the *ventriculus dexter,* and the left ventricle is the *ventriculus sinister*. In ancient Greek medicine, the ventricles were commonly referred to as the *koiliai,* which meant "belly." Today, roots derived from the Greek word *koilia,* **COELI-, CELI-, COEL-,** and **CEL-,** are used for "cavity" and "belly." The anatomical term "ventricle" comes from the Latin word for "little belly." The Latin root **VENTRICUL-** is used for "ventricle," a term that denotes a small anatomical cavity.

Septum (L. *septum, -i*) – The anatomical wall that separates the two atria from each other and the two ventricles from each other is called the septum. The root **SEPT-** is used in the natural sciences and medicine for "a wall-like structure that separates cavities."

Valve (L. *valva, -ae; valvulus, -i*) – The roots for **VALV-** and **VALVUL-**, which are used for "valve" and "valvule," ultimately come from a Latin word for "folding door." The heart has four major valves: the bicuspid and tricuspid valves are located between the atria and the ventricles, and the pulmonary valve and aortic valve are located between the ventricles and the major blood vessels leaving the heart. The right atrioventricular valve is called the tricuspid valve; the left atrioventricular valve is called the bicuspid valve. The root **CUSPID-** (L. *cuspis, cuspidis*) literally means "point," and therefore, it is used for structures that are pointed in appearance. The bicuspid valve is commonly referred to as the mitral valve. The term mitral is derived from the Greek word for a pointed hat worn by Persians, a *mitre*. The two-pointed Roman Catholic headdress worn by bishops, the miter, is derived from this Greek word (Fig. 8.8). Owing to this connection, the two-pointed bicuspid valve started to be referred to as the mitral valve around 1705. While cuspid valves are shaped like points, semilunar valves are shaped like half-moons, hence the root **LUN-** (L. *luna, -ae*, moon) in the term. The pulmonary valve and aortic valve are semilunar valves. The pulmonary valve (or pulmonic valve) lies between the right atrium and the pulmonary artery. The pulmonary valve opens up to allow the deoxygenated blood to travel via the pulmonary artery to the lungs. The aortic valve lies between the left ventricle and the aorta. The aortic valve ensures that oxygenated blood does not flow back into the left ventricle.

Fig. 8.8 Woodcut of Saint Nicholas receiving the mitre from angel. *Source:* Saint Nicholas/Wellcome Collection/CC BY 1.0.

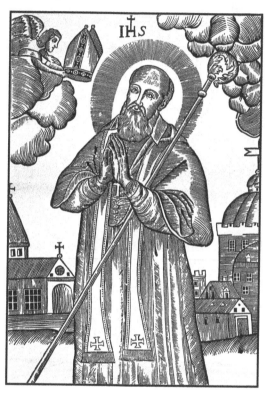

Pulmonary artery (L. *arteria pulmonalis*) and **Pulmonary vein** (L. *vena pulmonalis*) – The pulmonary artery carries deoxygenated blood from the right ventricle to the lungs. The pulmonary vein carries oxygenated blood from the lungs to the left atrium. The adjective used for the pulmonary artery and vein comes from the Latin word for a lung, *pulmo, pulmonis*. Both **PULM-** and **PULMON-** are used for "lung" in medicine.

Aorta (L. *aorta, -ae*) – The main trunk of arteries that arches over the top of the heart. The root for this vessel is **AORT-** The medieval Latin term *aorta* comes from the Greek *aorte* (fr. *aeirein*, to raise, lift). Aristotle was the first to use this term for this great artery of the heart, perhaps because the hook shape of the aorta made it appear to be suspended by the heart.

Brachiocephalic (*arteria brachiocephalica*), **left common carotid** (*areteria carotis communis sinistra*), **left subclavian arteries** (*arteria subclavia sinistra*) – Coming off of the aorta are the following major vessels, the brachiocephalic (Gr. *brachion*, arm + *kephalos*, head), the left common carotid, and the subclavian artery. Like other arteries and veins, the brachiocephalic and the subclavian are named according to the areas into which they travel. The left common carotid bifurcates (L. *bifurcus*, having two prongs) into the internal and external carotid arteries. The internal and external carotid arteries of the neck provide oxygenated blood to the brain. The Greek word *karotides* was used by Galen and other ancient physicians for these two arteries. In his *Doctrines of Hippocrates and Plato* (K. II. 6.4-17), Galen provides an etymology for *karotides*, claiming that the Greek word *karodes* ("voiceless" or "stupefied") became associated with these arteries because of the erroneous belief of physicians who held that the cutting or ligation of these vessels would lead to an animal becoming immediately voiceless. The other famous vessels of the neck are the jugular veins, which take the deoxygenated blood from the head back to the heart. There are two pairs of jugular veins, an external and internal. The jugular veins derive their name from the Latin word for "throat," *jugulum*. Jugulum is used as a loan word today for "neck" or "throat." In medicine, the roots **CAROTID-** and **JUGUL-** are commonly used for the carotid arteries and jugular veins, respectively.

Coronary artery (L. *arteria coronaria*) – The coronary arteries supply oxygenated blood to the muscles of the heart. Their name is derived from the Latin word for a "crown" or "garland," *corona* because these vessels form a crown around the top of the heart (Fig. 8.9). The root **CORON-** is used to today for "crown" or "crown-like" structures. *Corolla* is a Latin word that also means "crown," and its root **COROLL-** is used for crown-like structures. The term "coroner" is derived from the Latin *corona*. Originally, the coroner was a medieval county or municipal officer called the *custos placitorum coronae* ("the guard of the desires of the crown") who assessed taxes and protected the property of the king. The role of this position gradually changed over time; by the 17th century, the primary function of the coroner was to determine the cause of death in cases where it was not a natural death.

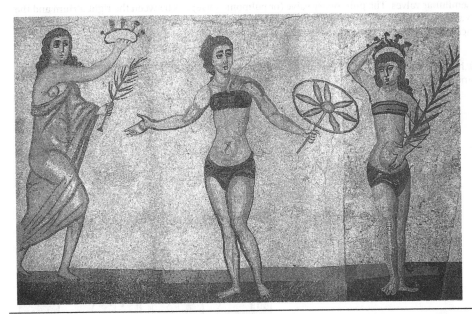

Fig. 8.9 The mosaic referred to as "ancient bikini girls," was excavated at the ancient Roman villa near Piazza Armerina in Sicily. The mosaics (other than this one) clearly show the athletic activities that women participated in. In this image it also shows a palm of victory and a corona. Such victory garlands/crowns were a common feature of Greek athletics that men participated in. *Source:* Gorup de Besanez/ Wikimedia Commons/CC BY-SA 4.0.

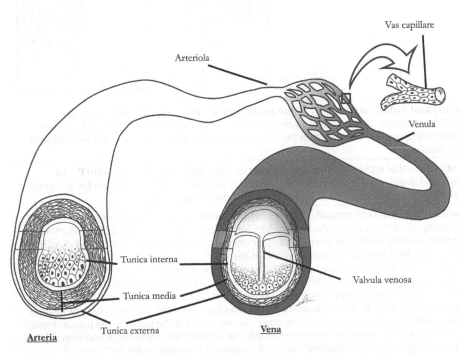

Fig. 8.10 Anatomical Latin terms for the blood vessels. *Source:* Drawing by Chloe Kim.

Blood vessels (Fig. 8.10)

Vessel (L. *vas, vasis*) – With respect to the types of vessels of the circulatory system, the Latin and Greek roots **VAS-**, **VASCUL-**, and **ANGI-** are commonly used for the "blood vessels," but it is important to bear in mind that these roots are also used for any tube, duct, or canal carrying a fluid. The Latin *vas* and the Greek *angeion* from which these roots are derived originally referred to any type of container that held liquids.

Artery (L. *arteria, -ae*) and Arteriole (L. *arteriola, -ae*) – The arteries are the vessels that carry the oxygenated blood from the heart to the body. The root used for "artery" is **ARTERI-**. The smaller and distal ends of arteries that feed into the capillaries are called "arterioles," for which **ARTERIOL-** is the root. The largest artery in the body is the **aorta**. The descending aorta (L. *aorta descendens*) begins at the end of the aortic arch and continues down into the abdomen.

Vein (L. *vena, -ae*) and Venule (L. *venula, -ae*) – The veins are blood vessels that carry blood back to the heart. The roots **PHLEB-** and **VEN-** are used for "vein" in medical terminology. The smaller distal end of the vein that is derived from the capillaries is called a "venule," and its root is **VENUL-**. The largest vein in the body is the inferior vena cava, which carries oxygen-depleted blood back to the heart from the lower part of the body. The second largest vein of the body is the superior vena cava, which carries oxygen-depleted blood to the heart from the upper part of the body.

Capillary (L. *vas capillare*) – As mentioned, the minute vessels that connect the arterioles to the venules are called capillaries. The root for capillary, **CAPILLAR-**, comes from the Latin adjective *capillaris, -e*, which means "hairlike." Hence, the anatomical term *capillus* means hair or filament, and the aforementioned root can be used for capillaries or for hairlike structures. Ancient Greek medicine did not conceive of capillaries; the term "capillary" began to be used for these minute hairlike blood vessels in the 1660s.

Parts of a blood vessel – The mouthlike opening of a blood vessel is referred to as the *ostium* (L. door, mouth) in anatomical Latin. Likewise, the three coats/layers of a blood vessel are referred to as *tunicae* (L. *tunica, -ae*, a Roman covering, tunic): *tunica externa* (also called *tunica adventitia*), *tunica media*, and *tunica interna* (also called *tunica intima*). The open space in the middle of a blood vessel is referred to as the lumen (L. *lumen, luminis*, light). The reason for this is that one can see light through this hole in the vessel. Consequently, the root **LUMIN-** can refer to the specific anatomical space in a vessel, or it can simply be used for "light."

Connections and divisions of blood vessels – Many of the connections and divisions of blood vessels come from Greek and Latin terms for everyday objects. An arch-like structure of a vessel is termed an arcus (L. *arcus, -us*, a bow, vault, arch). When a vessel splits into two or more vessels, it is said to have "forked," which is why the roots **FURC-** and **FURCAT-** (L. *furca, -ae*, a fork, prong) are used for these types of divisions in vessels. Where there is a major division in a vessel, such as a bifurcation, each of the vessels is called a ramus (L. *ramus, -i*, a branch). The root **RAM-** is commonly used in medico-scientific language for nerves, arteries, and veins. An interwoven network of blood vessels is commonly referred to as a plexus (L. *plexus, -us*, plexus, braided fr. L. *plectere*, to plait, interweave). A plexus of blood vessels is also sometimes referred to as a **rete** (L. *rete, retis*, net) because vessels look like "a net." Because these terms refer to everyday structures, the roots **FURC-/FURCAT-**, **ARC-**, **PLEX-**, **RAM-**, and **RET-** can also refer to anything that is "forked" (**FURC-/FUCAT-**), "arched" (**ARC-**), "interwoven" (**PLEX-**), "branched" (**RAM-**), and "net-like" (**RET-**).

Greek or Latin word element	Current usage	Etymology	Examples
CORD/O (kor-dō)	Heart	L. *cor, cordis*, n. heart	**Cord**ate, intra**cord**al Loan word: **Cor** (kor) pl. **Corda** (kor'dă)
CARDI/O (kard-ē-ō)	Heart	Gr. *kardia*, the heart	**Cardi**ology, endo**cardi**tis
VALV/O (val-vot-ō)	Valve	L. *valva, -ae*, f. a Roman folding door; valve	**Valv**otomy, **valv**iform Loan word: **Valva** (val'vlă) pl. **Valvae** (val've")
VALVUL/O (val-vyŭ-lō)	Valvule	L. *valvula, -ae*, f. a small *valva*, valvule	**Valvul**itis, **valvul**otome Loan word: **Valvula** (val'vyŭ-lă) pl. **Valvulae** (val'vyŭ-lē")

Greek or Latin word element	Current usage	Etymology	Examples
CUSPID/O (kŭs-pĭ-dō)	Cuspid, point	L. *cuspis*, *cuspidis*, f. a point	**Bicuspid**, **cuspid**ate Loan word: **Cuspis** (kŭs′pĭs) pl. **Cuspides** (kŭs′pĭ-dēz″)
MITR/O (mĭ′trō)	Mitral valve	L. *mitralis*, *-e*, mitral fr. Gr. *mitre*, a two-pointed hat	**Mitr**al
CHORD/O (kor-dō)	Cord, tendon	Gr. *chorde*, cord, rope, musical string	**Chord**itis, noto**chord**
LUN/O (loo-nō)	Moon	L. *luna*, *-ae*, f. moon	Semi**lun**ar, **lun**ate
CRESC/O (kres-ō) **CRET/O** (krē-tō)	Increasing, grow, crescent	L. *crescere*, to grow, increase	**Cresc**ent, con**cret**ion
ATRI/O (ā-trē-ō)	Atrium (a chamber of the heart), a central room	L. *atrium*, *-i*, n. a Roman foreroom; atrium (a chamber of the heart)	**Atri**oventricular, **atri**al Loan word: **Atrium** (ā′trē-ŭm) pl. **Atria** (ā′trē-ă)
VENTRICUL/O (ven-trik-yŭ-lō)	Ventricle, a small cavity	L. *ventriculus*, *-i*, m. a little belly; ventricle	Inter**ventricul**ar, **ventricul**oatriostomy Loan word: **Ventriculus** (ven-trik′yŭ-lŭs) pl. **Ventriculi** (ven-trik′yŭ-lī)
SEPT/O (sĕp-tō)	A wall dividing two cavities	L. *septum*, *-i*, n. a wall, barrier, an enclosure fr. L. *saepire*, to hedge, separate	**Sept**oplasty, **sept**ate Loan word: **Septum** (sep′tŭm) pl. **Septa** (sep′tă)
PARIET/O (pă-rī-ĕt-ō)	Wall	L. *paries*, *parietis*, m. wall	**Pariet**al, **pariet**otemporal Loan word: **Paries** (par′ē-ēz″) pl. **Parietes** (pă-rī′ĕ-tēz″)
VISCER/O (vis-ĕ-rō)	Organ	L. *viscus*, *visceris*, n. organ	**Viscer**al, e**viscer**ate Loan word: **Viscus** (vĭs′kŭs) pl. **Viscera** (vĭs′ĕr-ă)
CORON/O (kŏ-rō-nō)	Coronary vessels, a circular structure, crown	L. *corona*, *-ae*, f. a crown, garland also *corolla*, *-ae*, f. a crown	**Coron**ary, **coron**al Loan word: **Corona** (kŏ-rō′nă) pl. **Coronae** (kŏ-rō′nē″)
AORT/O (ā-or-tō)	Aorta	L. *aorta*, *-ae*, f. aorta fr. Gr. "what is lifts or hangs up"	**Aort**oclasia, **aort**algia Loan word: **Aorta** (ā-ort′ă) pl. **Aortae** (ā-ort′ē)
CAROTID/O (kă-rot-ĭd-ō)	Carotid	L. *carotis*, *carotidis*, f. carotid fr. Gr. *karodes*, causing stupor, soporific	**Carotid**ectomy, **carotid**al Loan word: **Carotid** (kă-rot′ĭd)

Greek or Latin word element	Current usage	Etymology	Examples
JUGUL/O (jŭg-yŭ-lō)	Jugular vein, throat	L. *jugulum, -i*, n. throat	**Jugul**ar, **jugul**ate Loan word: **Jugulum** (jŭg′ū-lŭm) pl. **Jugula** (jŭg′ū-lă)
PULM/O (pŭl-mō) **PULMON/O** (pul-mŏ-nō)	Lung	L. *pulmo, pulmonis*, m. lung	**Pulmon**ary, **pulm**oaortic
SAPHEN/O (săf-ĕ-nō)	Saphenous vein	L. *saphena, -ae*, f. saphenous vein, fr. Gr. *saphenes*, clear, manifest	**Saphen**ectomy, **saphen**ous Loan word: **Saphena** (să-fē′nă) pl. **Saphenae** (să-fē′nē)
PORT/O (port-ō)	Gate, entrance (Port of entry of a vessel or nerve into an organ)	L. *porta, -ae*, f. gate, entrance	**Port**ography, **port**al
OSTI/O (os-tē-ō)	Orifice, opening	L. *ostium, -i*, n. door, mouth	**Osti**al, **osti**ole Loan word: **Ostium** (os′tē-ŭm) pl. **Ostia** (os′tē-ă)
VAS/O (vā-zō)	Vessel	L. *vas, vasis*, n. a receptacle, vessel	**Vas**ospasm, **vas**odilation Loan word: **Vas** (vas) pl. **Vasa** (va′să)
VASCUL/O (vas-kyŭ-lō)	Vessel (a little vessel)	L. *vasculum, -i*, n. a small vessel	**Vascul**itis, **vascul**ar
ANGI/O (an-jē-ō)	Vessel	Gr. *angeion*, vessel	**Angi**oma, **angi**otomy
ARTERI/O (ar-tēr-ē-ō)	Artery	L. *arteria, -ae*, f. artery fr. Gr. *arteria*, "air carrier," windpipe, artery	**Arteri**orrhaphy, **arteri**ogram Loan word: **Arteria** (ar″tēr′ē-ă) pl. **Arteriae** (ar″tēr′ē-ē″)
ARTERIOL/O (ar-tēr-ē-ō-lō)	Arteriole	L. *arteriola, -ae*, f. arteriole, little artery	**Arteriol**onecrosis, **arteriol**osclerosis Loan word: **Arteriola** (ar-tēr″ē-ō′lă) pl. **Arteriolae** (ar-tēr″ē-ō′lē″)
PHLEB/O (flĕ-bō)	Vein	Gr. *phleps, phlebos*, vein	**Phleb**otomist, **phleb**angioma
VEN/O (vĕ-nō)	Vein	L. *vena, -ae*, f. vein	**Ven**osclerosis, **venoven**ostomy Loan word: **Vena** (vē′nă) pl. **Venae** (vē′nē″)
VENUL/O (ven-yŭ-lō)	Venule	L. *venula, -ae*, f. venule, little vein	**Venul**ose, **venul**itis Loan word: **Venula** (ven′yŭ-lă) pl. **Venulae** (ven′yŭ-lē″)

Greek or Latin word element	Current usage	Etymology	Examples
CAPILLAR/O (kap-ĭ-ler-ō)	Capillary	L. *capillaris, -e*, hairlike; capillary fr. L. *capillus, -i*, m. a hair	**Capillar**itis, **capillar**ectasia Loan word: **Capillary** (kap′ĭ-ler″ē)
ARC/O (ar-kō)	Arch, a curved structure, a bow	L. *arcus, -us*, m. a bow, vault, arch	**Arc**uate, **arc**iform Loan word: **Arcus** (ar′kŭs)
RAM/O (rā-mō)	Ramus (a branching of vessels), branch, branchlike	L. *ramus, -i*, m. a branch	**Ram**ose, **ram**ification Loan word: **Ramus** (rā′mŭs) pl. **Rami** (rā′mī″)
FURC/O (fŭr-kō) **FURCAT/O** (fŭr-kā-tō)	A forking, splitting	L. *furca, -ae*, f. a fork, prong	Bi**furc**ation, **furc**al Loan word: **Furca** (fŭr′kă) pl. **Furcae** (fŭr′kē″)
PLEX/O (plek-sō)	Plexus (an interwoven network of vessels or nerves), to plait, interweave	L. *plexus, -us*, m. plexus, braided fr. L. *plectere*, to plait, interweave	**Plex**opathy, **plex**itis Loan word: **Plexus** (pleks′ŭs)
RET/O (rē-tō)	Net, network	L. *rete, retis*, n. net	**Ret**operithelium, **ret**ial Loan word: **Rete** (rē′tē) pl. **Retia** (rē′tē-ă)
LUMIN/O (loo-mĭ-nō)	Light, lumen (the open space between walls of a vessel)	L. *lumen, luminis*, n. light	Trans**lumin**al, **lumin**iferous Loan word: **Lumen** (loo′měn) pl. **Lumina** (loo′mĭ-nă)

Review	Answers
The root in visceral and viscerad is _____ and it means _____.	**VISCER-** organs
The loan word for "a unit of light" and the open space between walls of a vessel is _____. The combining form derived from this word is _____.	**lumen LUMIN/O**
The roots in bifurcation and furcal mean _____. A bifurcation in a vessel means that the vessel splits into two different vessels. A ramus is the term used for one of the divisions of a forked structure. The literal meaning of the combining form RAM/O and the loan word "ramus" is _____.	**forked branch**
The arcuate artery is derived from the anatomical Latin term arcus, which means _____.	**arch**
The Greek root meaning "heart" is typically _____, but it can also be spelled _____, which explains why an echocardiogram can be abbreviated ECG or EKG.	**CARDI-, KARDI-**
Coronoid would be used for a _____ structure that resembles a _____. The loan word for this root is _____. With respect to the cardiovascular system, the CORON- is used in the word for the _____ arteries and veins. The Latin synonym of CORON- is _____.	**circular, crown corona coronary COROLL-**
The "hypertrophy or failure of the right ventricle resulting from disorders of the lungs, pulmonary vessels, chest wall, or respiratory control center" is termed *cor pulmonale*. The root PULMON- refers to the _____. The anatomical Latin term *cor* means _____. The root formed from Cor is _____. This root should not be confused with the Greek root for "cord/tendon," which is typically spelled _____.	**lungs heart CORD- CHORD-**
Based on its root, phlebitis is an inflammation of a _____.	**vein**

Review	Answers
The *rete cutaneum* is a _____ of blood vessels supplying the skin. The combining form from this anatomical Latin term is _____.	net/network RET/O
The *vena cava* is the anatomical Latin term that literally means the cavernous _____. Thus, a radiographic image of the veins is called a _____gram.	vein veno
A venous plexus is filled with anastomosing vascular channels and located in the dura that covers the clivus of the skull. The loan word _____ and the combining form _____ refer to a structure that looks like its parts are "interwoven."	plexus, PLEX/O
The anatomical Latin for a small vein is _____, and its combining form is _____. The anatomical Latin for a small artery is _____, and its combining form is _____.	venula, VENUL/O arteriola, ARTERIOL/O
The excision of part of an artery is an _____ ectomy.	arteri
The three combining forms for the vessel are _____, _____, and _____. The anatomical Latin term for the vessel is _____; thus, a capillary vessel is termed a _____ *capillare*.	ANGI/O, VAS/O, VASCUL/O vas, vas
The root PORT- in portal and portography in the cardiovascular system refers to the "portal vein," but its literal meaning is _____ and _____.	gate, entrance
Aortoclasia is a rupture of the _____.	aorta
"Carotid endarterectomy is a surgical procedure to remove a build-up of fatty deposits, which cause narrowing of a _____ artery." The adjective jugular, as in jugular vein, literally means _____.	carotid throat
The surgical formation of an opening in the wall between the atria would be termed an atrial _____ plasty. The wall between the chambers of the heart is referred to as the _____.	septo septum
The root for the upper two chambers of the heart is _____. The combining form for the lower two chambers of the heart is _____.	ATRI- VENTRICUL/O
The combining form for "valve" is _____, and for valvule, the combining form is _____. The valve between the left atrium and left ventricle is termed the bicuspid valve because it has two _____. It is also called the _____ valve. The valve between the right atrium and the right ventricle is called the _____ valve because of its three points. The aortic and pulmonary valves are called semilunar valves because they are shaped like a crescent _____.	VALV/O, VALVUL/O points mitral tricuspid moon

Lessons from History: The Pulse and the Diagnosis of Disease

Food for Thought as You Read:

What made diagnosing disease via the pulse attractive to physicians, patients, and society?

> In comparing the time (*chronos*) of the diastole (*diastole*) < of the pulse (*sphygmos*) > to the time of its systole (*systole*), as Herophilus required, it can be recognized that the sick person has an abnormal pulse-rate. For great deviations from the natural rhythm (*rhythmos*) into what is contrary to nature indicate great harm ...
>
> Galen, *Synopsis of my books on the Pulse* (K. 9.470)

The above quote is from Galen's *Synopsis of his own Books on the Pulse*, which, as the title implies, provides a summary of books that Galen wrote on the diagnostic value of the pulse. As can be seen in this quote, the origin of the use of the pulse as a diagnostic tool commonly ascribed to Herophilus of Chalcedon (335–280 BC), who is also famous for human dissection. Much of our modern cardiac terminology, such as **diastole** (Gr. *diastole*), **systole** (Gr. *systole*), **sphygmus** (Gr. *sphygmos*), and **rhythm** (Gr. *rhythmos*), is derived from ancient Greek words found in Herophilus' writings. That said, the ancient medical understanding of the pulse was quite different from our modern medical concepts. For example, when ancient physicians spoke of "systole" (contraction) and "diastole" (expansion), they were referencing the contraction and expansion of the blood vessels rather than the heart. Herophilus and other ancient Greek physicians referred to the expansion/contraction of the artery as the *sphymos*. The root **SPHYGM-** and the Latinized loan word **sphygmus** used in medicine today for "a pulse" are derived from the Greek word for "a throbbing or pulsation," *sphygmos*. The modern usage of **systole** and **diastole** refers to the contraction and expansion of the heart, and these two terms are closely linked to corresponding changes in blood pressure, which Greek physicians did not quantitatively measure. When speaking about blood pressure, modern medicine often uses the root **TENS-**, which means "stretch" since the vessels are being stretched by the volume of blood in them. Thus, hypertension and hypotension are used for high blood pressure and low blood pressure, respectively.

While Herophilus and other Greek physicians often pointed to the connection between the heart and the expansion/contraction of the arteries, their physiological theories and anatomical observations led to erroneous notions about the mechanism causing this expansion/contraction of the arteries. For example, since the arteries do not collapse in a cadaver, Herophilus and other anatomists may have mistaken this normal position of the artery to be its maximum, and therefore, they hypothesized that some faculty other than blood, usually *pneuma*, must be present to cause the artery to contract more. Erasistratus understood that only *pneuma* was present in the arteries, and therefore, pneuma was responsible for the movement of the arteries. It is possible that his error lies with what he observed with the dissection of dead bodies, since typically the blood is more readily observed in the veins in a cadaver, and there is a gravitational settling of the blood after death that is associated with *livor mortis*. It should be pointed out here that Erasistratus did recognize that blood would come out of a severed artery. His explanation for this was that the *pneuma* that escaped from the severed artery left a void artery. Because of the ancient physical principle that nature hates empty spaces (*horror vacui*), this void in the arteries was immediately filled by pouring in from the veins through the supposed natural anastomoses between the arteries and the veins. Broadly speaking, ancient theories of the expansion and contraction of the vessels incorporated mechanical explanations for the pulse as well as theories that spoke in terms of an "energy" or "faculty" that was responsible for this perceptible sign of human physiology.

The cardiac term **rhythm** is derived from the Greek word *rhythmos*, which means a "proportion, order, measured time or motion," or as the peripatetic philosopher Aristoxenus (f. 370 BC) defined it in his work *On Rhythm*: "rhythm arises whenever the distribution of time intervals takes on some definite arrangement." It seems likely that Herophilus was influenced by music and poetry when he chose *rhythmos* to be the term for the regular movement of blood vessels. Given that Herophilus would have interacted with numerous poets, musicians, and philosophers in the Hall of the Muses (*Mouseion*) in Alexandria, an institution that brought together the best scholars in the Hellenistic world and whose name is preserved in our word "museum," it seems likely that Herophilus had the Greek metric rhythm of poetry in mind when he considered how the pulse had a repetitive pattern. In Greek poetry, the repetitive patterns of long and short syllables within each verse of a poem were one of the ways in which different forms of Greek poetry were identifiable. Philosophical discussions of rhythm reveal that the concept was also used to speak to the function of the soul and nature. Given that rhythm was used to define different types of poetry and music in Greek philosophical circles, and given the connection between *pneuma* and cardiovascular physiology in medical literature, it seems quite plausible that Herophilus drew from this criterion in poetry and music when he began to speak of how the deviations from the measured pattern of pulses of a vessel could be used by a physician to determine what was abnormal and indicative of disease. While modern authors have made much of Marcellinus' (2nd century AD) *On Pulses* description of Herophilus using a clepsydra (water clock) to measure the pulse, Marcellinus' claim is unverifiable, and for this reason, scholars find it somewhat dubious despite water clocks being a part of Greek technology around 325 BC. However, Herophilus did indeed distinguish pulses that were divergent from the natural rhythm, broadly classifying them according to how deviant they were from a normal rhythm, size, speed, and strength, as well as labeling specific types of pulses.

The notion that pulses could change in rhythm due to age and the health of an individual led to a wide variety of terminology and diagnostic concepts. Galen systematized the wealth of knowledge about the pulse inherited from Herophilus and Galen's predecessors, creating introductory literature and theoretical tomes on the pulse: *On the Use of the Pulse, Causes of Pulses, Different Kinds of Pulses, Diagnosis by the Pulse, Prognosis by the Pulse, On the Pulse for Beginners,* as well as his *Synopsis of my Books on the Pulse.* In this literature, one will find very descriptive names for types of pulses. He uses the term *myrmekizon* for a rapid feeble pulse, likening it to an ant crawling, which is formed from the Greek word for an ant, *myrmex*. While we do not associate this with the pulse, the root **MYRMEC-** is still used for "ant" or "ant-like" in medical and scientific terminology. The term *dorkadizon* was used for a pulse that is irregular in its expansion, and therefore, it is said to be "capering" like a deer or gazelle (Gr. *dorkas*, deer, gazelle). It is possible that what was being referenced to here is what today is called a "bounding pulse," which according to Taber's Cyclopedic Medical Dictionary, is "a pulse that reaches a higher intensity than normal, then disappears quickly." While some of the pulse terms found in ancient Greek pulse literature seem to be derived from the physician's mind's eye, a plethora of these pulses were derived from the experience of an ancient Greek physician palpating a patient's pulse.

It should be said that the pulse is quite important in modern medicine, and there are similarities with respect to the terms used and the ways in which the pulse is described. In modern medicine, we sometimes use vivid terms, such as the "pistol-shot pulse" and "running pulse," to describe a type of pulse. We often tend to speak to the location of a pulse, for example the dorsal-pedal (*dorsalis pedis*) pulse. We also speak to the strength and the phase of a pulse (for example the term presphygmic speaks to the period before a pulse wave.) We also measure the force, pressure, and volume of pulse with devices such as the sphygmobolometer [Gr. *sphygmos*, pulse + Gr. *bolos*, mass + meter], sphygmomanometer [Gr. *sphygmos*, pulse + L. *manu*, hand + meter], and sphygmoplethysmograph [Gr. *sphygmos*, pulse + Gr. *plethysmos*, to increase + graph]. When we talk about the pulse being "regular," we are referring to its force and frequency being the same. However, the heart is of central importance to the modern conception of the pulse; for example this can be observed when a rapid pulse rate is called **tachycardia,** and a slow pulse rate is called **bradycardia**. The roots **TACHY-** and **TACH-** are used for "quick" and "rapid," and **BRADY-** is used for "slow." The SA node and AV node, and their associated structures, such as the branches and Purkinje fibers, can be the source of these arrhythmias. Today, heart arrhythmias are treated with medications and surgery. In some cases, **cardiac ablation** is used to remove pathological tissue. The root **LAT-** means to "bear" or "convey." Cardiac ablation is a surgical procedure that uses a catheter in the heart to make scars in the tissue of your heart to block the irregular electrical signals it is sending. Named after the fibers that cause this (the root **FIBRILL-** means "fiber" or "fibril"), the quivering of the heart muscle commonly associated with arrhythmias is called **fibrillation**. A-fib (atrial fibrillation) is one of the conditions that a cardiac ablation is used for.

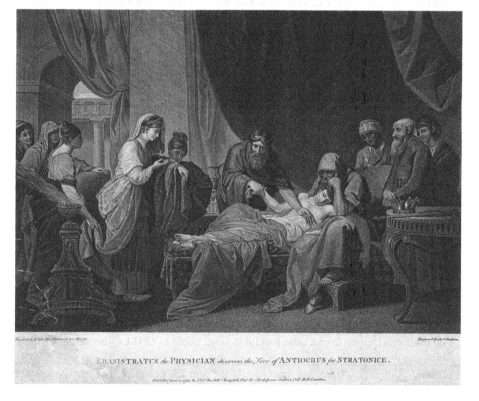

Fig. 8.11 Erasistratus recognizing Antiochus' lovesickness for Stratonice. Stipple engraving by G. Graham, 1793, after Benjamin West. *Source:* Erasistratus / Wellcome Collection / Public domain.

Thanks to Galen and his predecessors, the use of the pulse became a mainstay in the diagnostic repertoire of physicians for centuries, and therefore, in popular culture it often shows up in images and stories of the diagnostic ability of a physician. This is particularly true with respect to the diagnosis of "lovesickness." Valerius Maximus' *Memorable Deeds and Sayings* (5.7.3. ext. 1), Plutarch's in his *Life of Demetrius* (38), Appian's *Roman History* (11.10), Lucian's *The Syrian Goddess* (17-18), Galen's *On Prognosis* (1.4), and Julian's *Misopogon* (347), all mention Erasistratus successfully making the diagnoses of lovesickness (Fig. 8.11). Legends require big names, and therefore, in this legend, Seleuces I, one of Alexander the Great's generals and a namesake of the Seleucid Empire, had a wife named Stratonice, who was the stepmother to Seleuces' son, Antiochus. In the legend, Antiochus fell in love with Stratonice, but because he could not act upon this love, he became very ill to the point that Seleuces called Erasistratus to diagnose and treat Antiochus' illness. At first, it was thought due to the signs and symptoms that Antiochus was suffering from a disease caused by black bile (i.e. melancholic disease). In addition to observing the color of the face, most of these accounts have Erasistratus using the pulse to determine the real pathos of this prince. Erasistratus noticed that whenever Stratonice walked into the room, Antiochus' face became flush and his pulse changed, and therefore, Erasistratus recognized that this was not a *nosos* (disease) of the body, but indeed a *pathos* (affection) of the *psyche* (soul). The legend of Erasistratus diagnosing a prince with lovesickness via the pulse became the genesis for Galen claiming to have done the same thing with a woman who had fallen in love with a dancer. That said, Galen pointed out that there is no pulse that is specific to lovesickness. The inclusion of the pulse also points to how the use of the pulse had become a "sexy science" in that the method of "seeing" inside the body via the pulse had captured the imagination of society. In many respects, this still occurs today when society becomes fascinated and somewhat overly trusting of a new method or technology for diagnosing disease.

Some Suggested Readings

Amundsen, Darrel W. "Romanticizing the Ancient Medical Profession: The Characterization of the Physician in the Graeco-Roman Novel" *Bulletin of the History of Medicine* 48, no. 3 (1974): 320–337.

Berrey, Marquis. "*Herophilus' Pulse and Archimedes' Mechanized Mathematics*." In *Hellenistic Science at Court*. 191–126. Berlin: De Gruyter, 2017.

Johnston, Ian, and Niki Papavramidou. *Galen on the Pulses: Four Short Treatises and Four Long Treatises*. Berlin: De Gruyter, 2023.

Etymological Explanations: Common Terms and Word Elements for the Physiology of Cardiovascular System

Pulse and blood pressure
Diastole and Systole – Derived from Greek words for "relaxation" and "contraction," diastole is the period of cardiac muscle relaxation, and systole is the period of contraction of the chambers of the heart.
Hypertension and Hypotension – Derived from the Latin root for "stretched," **TENS-**, hypertension is high blood pressure, and hypotension is low blood pressure.
Arrythmia/Dysrhythmia – Derived from the Greek root for "regular" and "rhythm," **RHYTHM-**, cardiac arrhythmia/dysrhythmia is an irregularity or loss of rhythm of the heart.
Bradycardia and Tachycardia – Derived from the root for "slow," **BRADY-**, bradycardia is a slower than normal resting heart rate (i.e. less than 60 beats per minute). Derived from the root for "rapid" and "fast," **TACHY-**, tachycardia is a faster than normal resting heart rate (i.e. greater than 100 beats per minute).
Paroxysm – Derived from a Greek word for "irritation" and "exasperation," *paroxusmos*, a paroxysm is a sudden, periodic attack or recurrence of disease or symptom. It is also used for sudden spasms or convulsions of any kind.
Fibrillation – Derived from a Latin root for "a small fiber," **FIBRILL-**, fibrillation is twitching, quivering, or random contractions of the myocardium.
Flutter – A flutter is a tremulous movement of the ventricle or atrium. The term is derived from an Old English term meaning "to be tossed into confusion."
Premature ventricular contraction (PVC's) – A PVC is a common disturbance of the rhythm that can be indicative of myocardial damage.
Sphygmus – A single pulse is called a sphygmus. Thus, the root for "pulse" is **SPHYGM-**, and a pathological pulse will have the suffix **-SPHYGMIA**.

Pathologies of the cardiovascular system

Aneurysm – The term aneurysm comes from the Greek word Gr. *aneurysma*, a widening. It is used for a localized abnormal widening of a vessel due to weaknesses in the walls of the vessel (Fig. 8.12). Such a pathological feature can rupture and cause massive blood loss and death. The root of an aneurysm is **ANEURYSM-**. Consequently, the root of aneurysm is **EURY-** meaning "wide" and is commonly used in medicine and the natural sciences in terms such as eurytherm and eurycephalic. This root should not be confused with **EUR-**, which is used for Europe. The etymology of *eurys* "wide" and *ops* "face" is often given as an explanation for the word Europe. Traditionally, the connection between the two roots may hark back to the Greek myth of Europa. In Greek mythology, Europa was a Phoenician princess who was whisked away by Zeus, who disguised himself as a beautiful bull, to Crete where she bore his children who became the great heroes of Crete, particularly Minos (Fig. 8.13). Her father, Agenor or Phoenix, depending on the account, sent his sons to look for her. They were charged to never come back if they did not find Europa. These sons settled in the lands around the Mediterranean Sea.

Fig. 8.12 Image of abdominal and thoracic aneurysms provided by the National Institute for Health. *Source:* National Institute for Health/ U.S. Department of Health and Human Services/Public Domain.

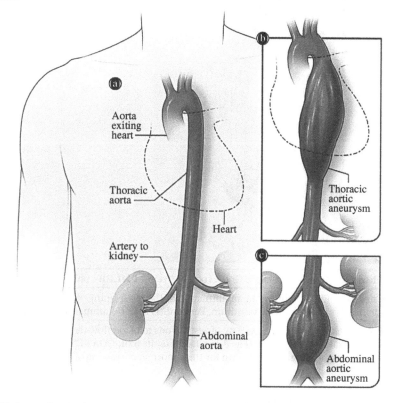

Fig. 8.13 Since 2002, Greece has had an image of Europa riding a bull (Zeus) on its Euro coins. *Source:* efilippou/Getty Images.

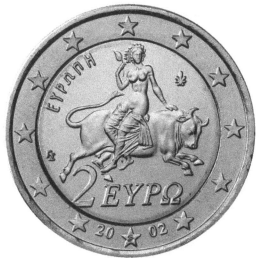

Ectasis and Varicosis – An abnormally dilated vein is called venectasia or phlebectasis. The root **DILAT-** means "expand." The different suffix forms in venectasia and phlebectasis mean "dilated" and "expanded." Generally, these terms refer to varicosis. The root for this pathological condition is **VARIC-**, which derives its Latin word for "a swollen, twisted vein," varix. The etiology of varices is far ranging. The image to the right is a marble relief depicting a man offering a votive to the Greek god of medicine, Asclepius (Fig. 8.14). Typically, votives dedicated to Asclepius were terracotta images of body parts indicating the area of the affliction Asclepius healed. They do not actually depict the disease. However, this votive is different because it contains an image of a swollen, tortuous vein that reveals that this individual had a varix.

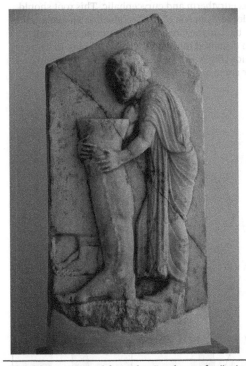

Fig. 8.14 Marble votive relieve dedicated to Asclepius in Athens, c. 4th century BC. *Source:* Gary Todd/Wikimedia Commons/CC0 1.0.

Phlebitis – Formed from the Greek root for "vein," **PHLEB-**, phlebitis is an inflammation of a vein.

Carditis – Endocarditis is an inflammation of the inner lining of the heart or the endocardium. Myocarditis is an inflammation of the heart muscle or the myocardium. Pericarditis is an inflammation of the sac around the heart or the pericardium.

Coarctation – There are a variety of restrictions to blood flow that can cause cardiopathies. The compression of the walls of a vessel is referred to as coarctation (Fig. 8.15). Based on its root, **COARCTAT-**, a coarctated structure is described as "confined." *Coarctatio aortae* is a pathological Latin term for the abnormal narrowing of the aorta often caused by a birth defect.

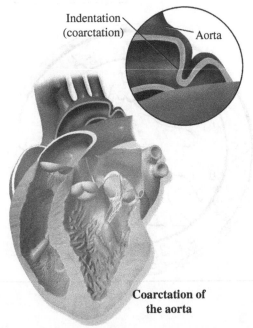

Indentation (coarctation)

Aorta

Coarctation of the aorta

Fig. 8.15 Image of aortic coarctation. *Source*: Adapted from Blausen.com staff, 2014.

Tamponade – Elevated pressure in the pericardium that impairs the filling of the heart is called cardiac tamponade (Fig. 8.16). The term is derived from a French word for a "rag" or "plug." The term tampon is used for cotton plugs used to absorb and stop the outflow of vaginal blood during menses, and it is the origin of the name for the company Tampax. The pathological or intentional compression of a part is referred to as tamponade or tamponage. The three signs used to recognize cardiac tamponade are low blood pressure (hypotension), bulging jugular veins, and muffled heart sounds.

Fig. 8.16 Image of cardiac tamponade. *Source:* Adapted from Blausen.com staff, 2014.

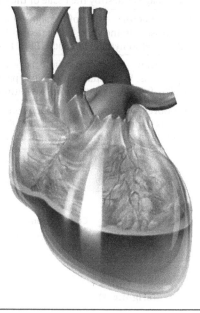

Stenosis – Likewise, the narrowing of an artery or valve can also lead to a cardiomyopathy. The root **STEN-**, which means "narrow" is used in terms such as stenotic and stenosis. A stenotic valve can be treated via percutaneous valvuloplasty, which involves inserting and inflating a balloon in the stenotic valve to reduce the constriction. Inflammation of the inner lining of the heart, called endocarditis, can restrict blood flow. **STRING-** and **STRICT-** are two roots that mean "to narrow, bind, and compress."

Ischemia – The holding back of blood causing diminished oxygenation of tissue is called ischemia. The root **ISCH-** in this word means "to hold back" and the suffix **-EMIA** is used for "a pathological condition of blood."

Claudication – Derived from Latin adjective *claudus*, which means "limping," claudication is a limp or spasm (typically in the calf) that occurs with walking due to inadequate blood supply.

Occlusion – The blocking of a blood vessel is called an occlusion. The root **CLUS-** means to "shut" or "close off," and is used in terms such as malocclusion. The other form derived from the same Latin word and having the same meaning is **CLUD-**. There are a wide variety of conditions that can lead to a heart attack. The blockage of coronary arteries due to a buildup of fat, cholesterol, and other substances in these vessels is often a predisposing condition for a heart attack.

Infarction – An occlusion of a coronary artery causing tissue death is called an infarction (Fig. 8.17), as in the term for a heart attack, myocardial infarction (MI). The term infarction comes from the Latin verb *infarcire*, which means "to stuff in."

Fig. 8.17 Image of myocardial infarct. *Source:* Adapted from Blausen.com staff, 2014.

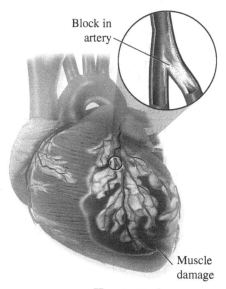

Block in artery

Muscle damage

Heart attack

Arteriosclerosis and Atherosclerosis – The process of plaque buildup is called atherosclerosis. Based on its root **SCLER-**, arteriosclerosis is a hardening of the arteries. Atherosclerosis is a form of arteriosclerosis. The root **ATHER-** indicates that fatty plaques are responsible for the hardening of the artery. If a plaque ruptures and completely blocks blood flow, the lack of blood flow can damage or destroy the tissue of the heart muscle.

Angina pectoris – One of the signs of a heart attack is called angina pectoris. The term angina pectoris refers to the oppressive pain and pressure in the chest associated with a heart attack. This chest pain can be confused with other conditions that affect the chest, such as stethomyitis. The roots **STETH-** and **PECTOR-** both mean "chest."

Palpitation – Another symptom associated with heart attacks is the feeling of one's "heart racing," this symptom is referred to as palpitations. Panic attacks also cause palpitations, which lead people with anxiety to believe that they are having a heart attack. The term "palpitation" comes from the Latin verb *palpitare*, which means "to move quickly, tremble."

Diaphoresis/Sudoresis – Another sign of a heart attack is profuse sweating. Excessive sweating, which is one of the signs of cardiac arrest, is termed diaphoresis. The root of this word **PHOR-** means to "bear" or "convey." Its suffix form, **-PHORESIS**, is commonly used for the "transmission" of something. Likewise, the suffix forms, **-PHORE** and **-PHOR**, mean the "bearer" of something.

Greek or Latin word element	Current usage	Etymology	Examples
SPHYGM/O (sfĭg-mō)	Pulse	Gr. *sphygmos*, pulse	**Sphygm**omanometer, micro**sphygmia**
-SPHYGMIA (sfĭg-mē-ă)			Loan word: **Sphygmus** (sfĭg′mŭs) pl. **Sphygmi** (sfĭg′mī″)
RHYTHM/O (rith-mō)	Rhythm	Gr. *rhythmos*, regular, measure, rhythm	Ar**rhythm**ia, dys**rhythm**ia
			Loan word: **Rhythm** (rith′ĭm)
SYSTOL/O (sis-tŏ-lō)	Contraction	Gr. *systole*, contraction	**Systol**ic, peri**systole**
			Loan word: **Systole** (sis′tŏ-lē)
DIASTOL/O (dī-as-tŏ-lō)	Expansion	Gr. *diastole*, expansion	**Diastol**ic, brady**diastole**
			Loan word: **Diastole** (dī-as′tŏ-lē)
TACHY- (tak-ē)	Quick, rapid	Gr. *tachys*, swift, quick, rapid	**Tachy**cardia, cardio**tach**ometer
TACH/O (tak-ō)			
BRADY- (brăd-ē)	Slow	Gr. *bradys*, slow	**Brady**cardia, **brady**asystolic
STETH/O (steth-ō)	Chest	Gr. *stethos*, chest, breast	**Steth**oscope, **steth**omyitis
TENS/O (tĕn-sō)	Stretch	L. *tendere, tensum*, to stretch	Hyper**tens**ion, hypo**tens**ion
DILAT/O (dī-lăt-ō)	Expand	L. *dilatare*, to spread out	Vaso**dilat**or, **dilat**ion
-ECTASIA (ĕk-tā-sē-ă)	Dilated, expanded	Gr. *ektasis*, stretching, tension	Ven**ectasia**, cardi**ectasis**
-ECTASIS (ĕk-tā-sis)			
STRICT/O (strĭk-tō)	To narrow, bind, compress	L. *stringere, strictum*, to draw tight, press together	Con**strict**or, **string**ent
STRING/O (strĭn-gō)			

Greek or Latin word element	Current usage	Etymology	Examples
SPASM/O (spaz-mŏ) **SPASMOD/O** (spaz-mŏ-dŏ)	Convulsion, spasm	Gr. *spasmos*, a wrenching, convulsion	Vaso**spasm**, **spasmod**ic Loan word: **Spasmus** (spaz′mŭs)
FIBRILL/O (fĭ-bril-ō)	Fibril, fiber, *quivering of the heart	L. *fibrilla, -ae*, f. small fiber, fibril	**Fibrill**ation, de**fibrill**ator Loan word: **Fibrilla** (fĭ-bril′ă) pl. **Fibrillae** (fĭ-bril′ē)
PALPIT/O (păl-pĭ-tō)	Sensation of rapid beating of the heart	L. *palpitare*, to tremble, move quickly	**Palpit**ation, **palpit**ate
ANGIN/O (an-jĭ-nō)	Angina pectoris, choking	L. *angina*, a choking, strangling	**Angin**oid, **angin**ophobia Loan word: **Angina** (an-jī′nă)
ATHER/O (ath-ĕ-rō)	Fatty plaque	Gr. *athere*, porridge, cereal, gruel	**Ather**osclerosis, **ather**ectomy
SCLER/O (sklĕ-rō)	Hard	Gr. *skleros*, hard	Arterio**scler**osis, **scler**otic
ISCH/O (is-kō)	Hold back	Gr. *ischein*, to hold back	**Isch**emia, **isch**uria
COARCT/O (kŏ-ărk-tō) **COARCTAT/O** (kŏ-ărk-tāt-ō)	To confine	L. *coarctare*, to confine, draw together	**Coarct**ation, **coarct**otomy
VARIC/O (var-ĭ-kō)	A swollen, tortuous vein	L. *varix, varicis*, f. enlarged vein	**Varic**osis, **varic**ation Loan word: **Varix** (var′iks) pl. **Varices** (var′ĭ-sēz″)
ANEURYSM/O (an-yŭ-rizm-ō)	Abnormal widening of a vessel	Gr. *aneurysm*, dilation of a vessel	**Aneurysm**oplasty, **aneurysm**al Loan word: **Aneurysm** (an′yŭ-rizm)
EURY- (ū-rē)	Wide	Gr. *eurys*, wide	**Eury**cephalic, **eury**thermal
CLUS/O (kloo-sō) **CLAUD/O** (klod-ō)	Shut, closed off	L. *claudere, clausum*, to shut, close	Oc**clus**ion, **claud**ent
CLAUDIC/O (klod-ĭ-kō)	Limping	L. *claudicare*, to limp	**Claudic**ation
PHOR/O (fŏ-rō) **-PHOR** (phŏr) **-PHORE** (phŏr) **-PHORESIS** (fŏ-rē-sĭs)	To bear, convey; (-phor, -phore) bearer; (-phoresis) transmission	Gr. *phoros*, bearing, carrying, bringing	Eu**phor**ia, phromato**phore** dia**phoresis**
LAT/O (lā-tō)	To bear, convey	L. *ferre, latum*, to bear, carry	Ab**lat**ion, col**lat**e

Review	Answers
The term aneurysm comes from the Greek word Gr. *aneurysma*, a widening. It is used for a localized abnormal widening of a vessel due to the weaknesses in the walls of a vessel. Such a pathological feature can rupture and cause massive blood loss and death. The root for aneurysm is _____. Consequently, the root inaneurysm is EURY-, meaning _____, and it is commonly used in medicine and the natural sciences in terms such as eurytherm and eurycephalic.	**ANEURYSM-** **wide**
The root TENS- in hypertension and hypotension, which are terms used for high blood pressure and low blood pressure, means _____ since the vessels are being stretched by the volume of blood in them.	**stretch**
A rapid heart rate (>100 bpm in an adult) is called _____cardia, and a slow heart rate (<60 bpm in an adult) is called _____cardia.	**tachy** **brady**
The combining form for _____ is SPHYGM-, which appears in terms such as anisosphygmia and sphygmomanometer. The Latinized loan word associated with the root is _____.	**pulse** **sphygmus**
The contraction of the chambers of the heart is called _____ and the dilation of the chambers of the heart is called _____. Both terms are commonly used in the assessment of blood pressure today. The combining forms for these terms are _____ and _____.	**systole,** **diastole** **SYSTOL/O,** **DIASTOL/O**
Excessive sweating, which is one of the signs of cardiac arrest, is termed diaphoresis. The root in this word PHOR- means to _____ or _____. Its suffix form, _____, is commonly used for the "transmission" of something. Likewise, the suffix forms -PHORE and -PHOR mean the _____ of something.	**bear, convey** **-PHORESIS** **bearer**
A swollen, twisted vein is called a _____. The combining form for this pathological sign is _____.	**varix,** **VARIC/O**
The temporary diminished blood flow to an organ is called _____. The root ISCH- in this word means to _____, and it is used in terms such as ischuria.	**ischemia** **hold back**
An obstruction of a vessel can cause ischemia. An occlusion of a vessel causing tissue death is called an infarct, as in the term for a heart attack or myocardial infarct. The root CLUS- means _____ or _____, and it is used in terms such as malocclusion. The other root derived from the same Latin word and having the same meaning is _____.	**shut, close off** **CLUD-**
The root _____ is found in the word used to describe the predictable limping/cramping after a distance walked caused by a peripheral vascular disease.	**CLAUDIC-**
Based on its root SCLER-, arteriosclerosis is a _____ of the arteries. Atherosclerosis is a common form of arteriosclerosis. The root ATHER- indicates that _____ is responsible for the hardening of the artery.	**hardening** **fatty plaques**
The root STEN-, which means _____ is used in terms such as stenotic and stenosis. STRING- and STRICT- are two roots that mean to _____, _____, and _____.	**narrowing** **narrow, bind,** **compress**
The term _____ pectoris refers to the oppressive pain and pressure in the chest associated with a heart attack. This pain can be easily confused with other conditions that affect the chest, such as stethomyitis. The combining form STETH/O means _____.	**angina** **chest**
The compression of the walls of a vessel is referred to as coarctation. Based on its root, a coarctated structure is described as being _____. The pathological or intentional compression of a part is referred to as _____. Elevated pressure in the pericardium that impairs the filling of the heart is called cardiac tamponade.	**confined** **tamponade**
Another symptom associated with heart attacks is the feeling of one's "heart racing"; this symptom is referred to _____.	**palpitations**
The root DILAT- means _____. The different suffix forms in venectasia and cardiectasis mean _____ and _____.	**expand** **dilated,** **expanded**
The medicinal term defibrillation refers to the use of an electroshock to stop fibrillation of the heart. Fibrillation of the heart is associated with cardiac arrest and arrythmias. The root FIBRILL- means _____ or _____. The SA node and AV node, branches, and their associated structures, such as the Purkinje fibers, can be the source of arrythmias. In some cases, cardiac ablation is used to remove pathological tissue. The root LAT- means to _____ or _____.	**fibril, fiber** **bear, convey**

Lessons from History: Changing Concepts of Blood

Food for Thought as You Read:

Why is blood important to religions of the ancient world? To what extent do medical theories represent a secularization of blood?
Why is blood important to ancient medicine?
How did the discovery of blood cells change medicine's approach to blood?

The roots **HEM-**, **HEMAT-**, and **SANGUIN-** used in modern medicine are derived from the Greek and Latin words for "blood," *haima* and *sanguis, sanguinis*. While we share the same terms for blood, our understanding of blood differs from the ancient cultures in which the Greeks and Romans lived. The connection between blood and life made blood fundamental to both religious practices and medical treatments in these cultures. While the rationale undoubtedly varied among the diverse cultures of the Mediterranean, a basic connection between blood and life seems to underpin religious practices and prohibitions. While the pouring out of animal blood was a common type of sacrifice offered to the gods in Mediterranean cultures, it was not considered the same as any other fluid of an animal's body. Passages from the Bible reveal that blood was multivalent in Judeo-Christian religious practices. In the book of Leviticus (17:13-14 NIV translation) in the Bible, which contains Jewish religious rituals and laws, one finds the following religious prohibition: "you may not eat of the blood of any creature, because the life of every creature is its blood; anyone who eats it will be cut off." This passage articulates how the consumption of animal blood can be a source of defilement. That said, blood is also seen in the context of purification. This can be observed in the Jewish high priest's sacrifice and sprinkling of goat's blood in the Holy of Holies to purify his people of their sins during the annual high holy day known as Yom Kippur. The concept of purification also underpins the Christian drinking of wine in remembrance of Jesus Christ's blood being poured out as a sacrifice for the forgiveness of humanity's sins. Being misrepresented as the actual act of drinking blood, this symbolic drinking of blood became a point of criticism used by Romans and Jews against the followers of the Christian faith. Thus, what was considered acceptable and what was not varied based on one's religious perspective. The famous *taurobolium* of the Romans, which was practiced from the 2nd through the 4th century AD, is another rather striking religious use of blood, commonly referred to as a blood bath. Originating in Asia Minor, the *taurobolium* was closely connected with the cults of Attis, but more specifically with the Cybele/*Magna Mater* ("Great Mother of the Gods"). Though he does not refer to the *taurobolium* by name, the best-known description of this practice comes from Prudentius, a Christian apologist of the 4th century AD:

> The high priest, you know, goes down into a trench dug deep in the ground to be made holy ... Above him they lay planks to make a stage ... When the beast for sacrifice has been stationed here, they cut his breast open with a consecrated hunting-spear and the great wound disgorges a stream of hot blood, pouring on the plank-bridge below a steaming river which spreads billowing out. Then through the many ways afforded by the thousand chinks it passes in a shower, dripping a foul rain, and the priest in the pit below catches it, holding his filthy head to meet every drop and getting his robe and his whole body covered with corruption ...
>
> Prudentius, Crowns of Martyrdom, X.1005-1050, translation from Prudentius.
Against Symmachus 2. Crowns of Martyrdom. Scenes From History. Epilogue.
Translated by H. J. Thomson. Loeb Classical Library 398. Cambridge: Harvard University Press, 1953.

Writing from a Christian perspective, this sacrifice was indicative of the disdainful elements of pagan worship. It can be observed from ancient inscriptions that this ritual was a mystery cult prevalent among Romans, and its practice was believed to confer some blessing on the initiate, perhaps with respect to the afterlife, but exactly what was the nature of this blessing remains rather unclear. While the numerous inscriptions found in the Roman cities attest to the popularity of this mystery cult, the specific details about this bloody ritual and its purpose are lacking in ancient sources outside of Prudentius. Similar to the famous Eleusinian mysteries of Greece, the *Magna Mater* cult's infamous secrecy is partly responsible for this lack of information, which, unfortunately, has left the details of the rituals and their purposes lost to history.

While the connection between life and blood has not been lost over time, the religious notions of purification and defilement are somewhat foreign to the modern mind due in part to the secularization of this life-giving fluid of the body. The secular approach to blood can be recognized in the ancient Greek medical theories of blood's relationship to life. In ancient Greek medicine, *haima* was often described as one of the fluids, or humors, fundamental to health and disease. The humors of the body were considered natural, and broadly speaking, they were essential to the health and function of the body. Disease was regularly associated with these fluids, particularly when they became peccant for a variety of reasons, such as being out of place, unbalanced, poorly mixed, or becoming corrupted. The explanations as to how many and which humors were responsible for diseases varied among the humoral explanations found in the Hippocratic Corpus. As Craik points out, of the humors discussed in the Hippocratic Corpus, *phlegma* (where we get our modern term for the "phlegm" associated with the respiratory system) and *chole* (a term used today for "gall" and "bile") were the fluids most regularly described as an engendering disease. Craik goes on to point out that "different accounts are given of their nature and importance ... typically, it is supposed by Hippocratic writers that unwanted or excessive moisture gathers in the head, then disperses in flux to some bodily part – eyes, ears, chest etc. – which becomes affected by disease ... there is a particular danger if the matter should dry up and become stuck in the bodily ducts or if it cannot be arrested in its progress from the head to other parts of the body. This danger is evident in, for example, *Places in Man* and *Internal Affections*." While the famous theory of the four humors, which speaks to phlegm, bile, black bile, and blood being the fundamental fluids of the body, became the dominant pathophysiological model into the 16th century thanks primarily to the writings of Galen, it is a mistake to call this Hippocratic because it is only articulated in the "Hippocratic" work, *On the Nature of Man*, and therefore, it is neither pervasive nor fundamental to the humoralism found in the Hippocratic Corpus.

In *On the Nature of Man*, the four humors are recognizable with respect to their appearance, qualities, and association with different seasonal diseases. With respect to phlegm, the author claims, "phlegm increases in a man in winter; for phlegm, being the coldest constituent in the body, is closest akin to winter (*Nat. Hom.* VII, Loeb translation)." He goes on to explain that is why this humor is prevalent in the sputum and nasal discharges found in the diseases associated with winter. Blood, on the contrary, is associated with moisture and warmth. Blood is, therefore, more prevalent in the body in the spring because the spring is very moist and somewhat warm, and it is for this reason that men are commonly affected with dysentery and hemorrhages from the nose in the spring. He then links the qualities of the four seasons with the qualities of the four humors, and in so doing, he accounts for the presence of seasonal diseases. Bile is associated with disease of the summer because this humor is very hot and somewhat dry like the season; black bile, being very dry and somewhat cold, is most prevalent in autumn. Using the theory of opposites, which entails treating a disease using therapeutic measures that were believed to create opposite qualities (e.g. treat a hot and wet disease with a specific regimen to create a cold and dry effect in the body), the author creates a theoretical explanation to justify the validity of the therapeutic measures he is using to treat diseases in the body. This theory also serves as the basis for preventative medicine since one can prescribe a particular regimen or evacuate a humor to prevent the seasonal diseases associated with a specific humor. *On the Nature of Man* and other ancient medical works reveal that their pathophysiological model of blood was qualitative and empirical in that it was derived from the experience of touching and observing blood in nature. That said, the fundamental association of life and blood can be recognized by blood being commonly linked to health, disease, procreation, and the nature of human beings.

The popular perception that Greek medicine was irrational because it relied heavily on bloodletting, known as venesection or phlebotomy, to cure diseases is somewhat erroneous. Perhaps this misunderstanding is derived from ancient Greek and Roman iconography for medicine (Fig. 8.18). Much like the stethoscope today, the depiction of the brass cup used in venesection was often used to signify someone was an *iatros* or *medicus*. While the practice of venesection was iconic for medicine in the Greek and Roman world, it was just one of many therapeutic measures used to treat patients, and there was a greater tendency in ancient Greek medicine to use regimen over venesection in the treatment of patients. Furthermore, some physicians, particularly the followers of Erasistratus, did not practice venesection.

As to the rationality of this practice, Galen's *On Treatment by Venesection* provides a list of indications for bloodletting that reveals the criteria such as age, health, body type, and type of disease that must be taken into consideration prior to performing venesection. Broadly speaking, venesection was used as an evacuative remedy, which involved removing peccant blood, and the diversion of blood, which was employed when one was attempting to stop unnatural bleeding of a body part. There were different types of bad blood. Galen held that blood, which was intrinsically bad owing to a faulty mixture of humors, which he called **dyscrasia**, should be removed. If a humor becomes excessively hot or cold, such as in the case of **cacochymia**, this humor also must be removed due to its deleterious effect. Galen's understanding of cacochymia and dyscrasia is derived from the belief that other humors were potentially present in blood. Excess blood in an area known as *plethos* or *plethora*, was another indication for the evacuation of blood. Galen claimed that there were two different types of *plethos*, a dynamic *plethos* and a passive type of *plethos* that he termed *plethos* by filling. *Plethos* by filling is a mechanical type of overabundance of blood that occurs when blood rushes down into a part, causing overfilling. This type of *plethos* can lead to the rupture of vessels, and therefore, Galen advises that it be evacuated quickly. The dynamic *plethos* is linked to Galen's notion of the faculties of the parts. Galen believed that each organ had specific "powers" or "faculties" that he described in terms of attraction, assimilation, and evacuation. For

Fig. 8.18 Relief for a 2nd-century-AD physician. The child with the distended abdomen appears to be his patient, and the large vessel to the left is an oversized bronze cup, which was typically used with bloodletting. *Source:* Carole Raddato / Wikimedia Commons / CC BY-SA 2.0.

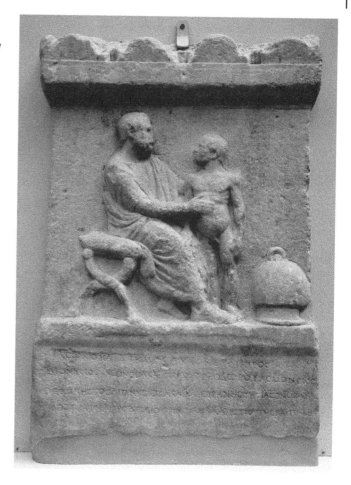

instance, if a part's faculty was weak with respect to evacuation, then the humor would begin to oppress the part. He links this type of *plethos* to inflammations. Like other physicians of the time, Galen's notion of inflammation was partially derived from the concept of putrefaction of blood. The putrefaction of blood was thought to produce heat; perhaps this belief is derived from the observation of how rotting fruit is warm to the touch, or perhaps it was simply observed in the connection between *tumor* and *calor* experienced with inflammations of the body. Localized inflammation was termed a *phlegmone*. Owing to their belief that this heat could in fact progress to the rest of the blood in the body, inflammation was believed to be the source of some bodily fevers. This explains the medical rationale for bleeding a patient suffering from fever, which was practiced well over a millennium in medicine. Thus, the identity of physicians was closely linked not only to their ability to remove blood from the body but also to their ability to provide a theoretical rationale for this practice.

That said, the diversion of blood was perhaps the most irrational indication for bleeding a patient in antiquity. Galen and other physicians believed that one could control the unnatural loss of blood from a part by simply diverting the blood from the part via cutting another approximate or supply vessel. In so doing, they believed that they were able to control the flow of blood, and hopefully, stop the diseased part from drawing blood to it. Perhaps the rationale for such a practice stemmed from the observation of how the flow of water could be diverted to lessen its flow to another area. Regardless of its rationality or not, this practice undoubtedly had deleterious effects on the vast majority of patients who received this treatment. The lack of effectiveness of this treatment is perhaps the reason for the Christian Gospels in 3 separate places mentioning Jesus healing a woman who suffered from bleeding for 12 years, claiming that she suffered and spent much of her money on physicians (Matthew 9:20–22, Mark 5:24–34, and Luke 8:42–48).

Our current cellular conception of the nature of blood had its origins with the invention of the microscope and the subsequent investigation into the nature of blood by Marcello Malpighi, Jan Swammerdam and Anthony van Leeuwenhoek. The roots used for "cell" today **CYT-** (Gr. *kytos*, a hollow receptacle, a vessel) and **CELLUL-** (L. *cellula*, little chamber) speak to the simplistic understanding of the cell as being a tiny "room" or "receptacle." The classical cell theory that all organisms were made of cells and they are the basic units of life was proposed by Theodor Schwann and Matthias Schleiden in 1839.

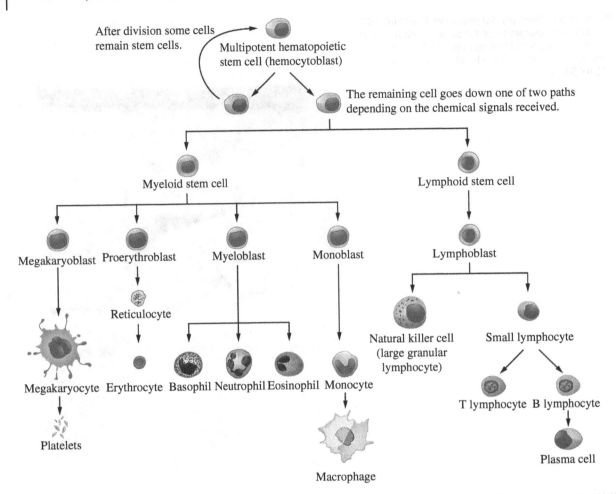

Fig. 8.19 Image of hematopoiesis. *Source:* Adapted from Anatomy & Physiology, Connexions/http://cnx.org/content/coll1496/1.6/.

The modern understanding that the various cellular components of blood come from embryonic blood cells embodies the scientific principle of *Omnis cellula e cellula* (all cells come from cells) that was articulated by Rudolph Virchow in his work *Cellular Pathologies* (1858). Virchow's cellular pathological theories seem to be the final nail in the coffin for the humoral pathological model of disease because the hidden causes of health, disease, and life could now be explained via a very different building block. Nevertheless, humoral concepts remain pervasive in modern medical terms (e.g. choleric, phlegm, melancholy, plethora, rheumatoid, etc.) due to the long life of this pathological theory in medical literature.

The above image illustrates how the "*omnis cellula e cellula*" is central to our understanding of hematopoiesis, blood making, and how it differs vastly from the Galenic nutriment-humoral model for the formation of blood (Fig. 8.19). The **hemocytoblast** is the stem cell for all other cellular components of blood. The root **BLAST-**, which is derived from the Greek word *blastos* (a bud, shoot), is used in science and medicine for "an embryonic/stem cell." Hemocytoblast can create either **lymphoid** or **myeloid** cells. The myeloid cells, broadly speaking, are **erythrocytes**, **leukocytes**, or **platelets**. As noted in the earlier chapters, **MYEL-** is a root used for the "spinal cord" and "bone marrow," and therefore, the myeloid cells derived their name from the bone marrow that creates red blood cells. Lymphoid cells ultimately become **lymphocytes**, which are cells that are fundamental to our immune system.

Some myeloid cells become megakaryocytes. A **megakaryocyte** is a large bone marrow cell with a lobated nucleus. The root **KARY-** in megakaryocyte refers to the "cell nucleus." Thus, both **NUCLE-** and **KARY-** are used for "cell nucleus" in medicine and science. The etymologies of **NUCLE-** and **KARY-** reveal that they are derived from Latin and Greek words for "a nut/kernel." Megakaryocytes develop into **platelets**, which are also called **thrombocytes**. Because these cells are necessary for blood clotting, the root **THROMB-** (Gr. *thrombos*, a clot) is used to describe these cells' primary action. **THROMB-** is also often used for pathological clots. The physiological process of stopping blood flow after a vascular injury, **hemostasis**, requires a complex interaction between endothelial cells, platelets, and coagulation factors. The term **coagulation** is from the Latin word for anything that causes milk to curdle, *coagulum*. The correlation between curdling of milk and blood coagulation is evident in the Hippocratic wound care that involved placing sap from a fig tree on a plug of wool that was used to supposedly stop hemorrhaging. The belief in the efficacy of this medication was derived from the observation that the sap from a fig tree would curdle milk, so it stood to reason that it would do the same thing to blood; it has been demonstrated that fig tree sap actually has the opposite effect on blood.

Myeloid cells can also become **erythrocytes** (red blood cells). Erythrocyte formation (**erythropoiesis**) in adults takes place in the bone marrow. The primary function of erythrocytes is to carry oxygen. Via **hemoglobin**, red blood cells carry oxygen to tissue and organs and contribute to the movement of carbon dioxide away from the tissue and organs. The **GLOB-** in hemoglobin means "ball" or "sphere," which is what hemoglobin looks like at a molecular level. A **reticulocyte** is the last cellular stage of the formation of an erythrocyte. The immature **erythrocytes** are called **reticulocytes** (**RETICUL-**, little net), owing to the netlike features of these cells. Reticulocyte counts in blood increase as a normal response to **anemia**, which is typically caused by a reduction of red blood cells. The old and fragile erythrocytes are later removed from circulation by macrophages in the liver, spleen, and bone marrow.

Turning to the other major division of hematopoiesis, as mentioned before, hemocytoblasts also can become **lymphoid cells**. Via **lymphoblasts**, these lymphoid cells ultimately become **lymphocytes**. The bone marrow, thymus, spleen, and lymph nodes also contribute to the body's lymphocytes. The lymphocytes are associated with the body's immune response to infection. Immunity is the protection from disease, particularly infectious disease. The term immunity is commonly said to have come from the Latin term for "exempt from duty, fees, taxation," *immunis*. The medical sense of this word, "protection from disease," seems to have started around 1879 among French and German authors. In the Roman world, *immunitas* could be granted to classes of individuals, taking the form of an exemption from a particular burden(s) imposed on others. Taken in this sense, immunity frees one from the burdensome effects of a particular disease.

In modern medicine, **phlebotomy** or **venesection** is rarely used therapeutically. Phlebotomy is now an incision or puncture of the vein to withdraw blood for testing. HCT or Hct stands for hematocrit, which is used to measure the percentage of red blood cells in a given volume of blood. The suffix in this term means "separate," it also can mean "to judge" as in the word "critical." The cellular counts in blood are a central feature of drawing blood to diagnose pathologies. Thus, one will find a plethora of acronyms for blood counts. For example, the acronym CBC is used for complete blood count; RBC is used for red blood count; WBC is the white blood count; HGB is used for the blood level of hemoglobin; and MCV is the mean corpuscular volume, which is the calculation of the volume of red blood cells using HCT and RBC results. Another important aspect of blood that is tested is the coagulation of blood. PT speaks to prothrombin time, which measures the activity of this clotting factor, and PTT refers to the partial thromboplastin time. Thromboplastin and prothrombin are clotting factors that are necessary for blood to coagulate. While the concept of blood cells has affected the practice of venesection, there are a number of similarities between ancient Greek medicine and modern medicine when it comes to hematological concepts and terminology, particularly with respect to the concepts of bad mixture, abnormal filling, or losing of blood. For example, coming from the Greek word for a faulty mixture of humors, **dyscrasia** is used today as a synonym for hematologic disease. The root **CRAS-** and its suffix form **-CRASIA** is used for "mixture."

Unlike ancient Greek medicine's technique of redirecting blood flow via venesection, modern medicine uses a device called a **hemostat** to stop excessive bleeding or a medication that stops the flow of blood; such medication is termed a **hemostatic**. The root **STAT-** in these terms, can mean "standing" or "stoppage." When used as a suffix, **-STAT**, is "a device for stopping, ceasing something." In addition, we are capable today to regulate blood flow via medications. A type of drug that causes the narrowing of a blood vessel, and therefore reducing blood flow, is termed a **vasoconstrictor**. A drug that causes the expansion of a blood vessel is called a **vasodilator**.

Some Suggested Readings

Brain, Peter. *Galen on Bloodletting: A Study of the Origins, Development and Validity of his Opinions, with a Translation of the Three Works*. Cambridge: Cambridge University Press, 1986.

Craik, Elizabeth. "Hippocratic Bodily "Channels" and Oriental Parallels." *Medical History* 53, no. 1 (2009): 105–116.

Duffin, Jacalyn. *"Why Is Blood Special? Changing Concepts of a Vital Humour."* In *History of Medicine: A Scandalously Short Introduction*, Third Edition. 204–230. Toronto: University of Toronto Press, 2021.

Scarborough, J. *"Vascular Matters: Heart and Blood, 'The Liquids of Life'."* In *Medical and Biological Terminologies*. 213–235. Norman: University of Oklahoma Press, 1992.

Etymological Explanations: Common Terms and Word Elements for Blood and Lymph

Blood and its parts

Blood (L. *sanguis, sanguinis*) – In modern medicine, blood is understood as being composed of both liquid and solid material. When separated from each other, 52–62% of the blood is a liquid material called blood plasma, and the remaining part is solid material called blood corpuscles. The blood corpuscles are the white blood cells (leukocytes), red blood cells (erythrocytes), and platelets (thrombocytes). Derived from the Latin word for "small body" *corpusculum*, the term corpuscle is typically used for any small, rounded body, particularly cells suspended in a medium. It began to be applied to blood in 1845. The roots for blood are **SANGUIN-**, **HEM-**, and **HEMAT-**.

Plasma (L. *plasma, -ae*) – Blood plasma is 91.5% water and 7% proteins, including albumin, globulin, and clotting factors. Coming from the Greek verb *plassein* "to form or mold," the loan word plasma and its root **PLASM-** literally mean "something formed or molded." Hence, we have terms such as cytoplasm for the formed part of the gelatinous fluid that fills the cell.

Serum (L. *serum, -i*) – The viscous flood left over after blood coagulation is appropriately called serum. In Latin, *serum* was the watery part of curdled milk, which we also refer to as "whey": "Little Miss Muffet, she sat on her tuffet, eating her curds and whey." In medicine, **SER-** refers to the serum, and it is associated with both the viscous liquid left over after blood coagulation and the pale, watery substance produced by serous membranes.

Thrombocytes/Platelets – Formed from the root for "a clot," **THROMB-**, thrombocytes' (platelets') primary function is to help with hemostasis.

Erythrocytes – Erythrocytes are called red blood cells. Erythrocytes' primary function is the transportation of oxygen to the tissue. In the context of blood, **ERYTHR-** (Gr. red) typically refers to "red blood cells." Derived from the root for "a small ball," **GOBUL-**, hemoglobin is a ball-shaped molecule in red blood cells that transports oxygen and carbon dioxide.

Leukocytes – Leukocytes are called white blood cells. Leukocytes' primary function is to provide protection against infection. In the context of blood, **LEUK-** (Gr. white) typically refers to "white blood cells." Distinguished by the presence or absence of granules in the cytoplasm, leukocytes are divided into granulocytes and agranulocytes. Granulocytes include basophils, eosinophils, neutrophils, and mast cells; agranulocytes are lymphocytes and monocytes. The term "granule" comes from the Latin diminutive *granulum*, "small grain." Thus, words such as "granite" and "granuloma" that use the roots **GRAN-** or **GRANUL-** are ultimately referring to something that has a "grain-like" appearance.

Basophils, Neutrophils, and Eosinophils – Basophils, neutrophils, and Eosinophils are granulocytes. The suffix **-PHIL** in these terms is used to indicate what type of dye these cells are attracted to. The root **BAS-** in basophil is used for "basic solutions" in this term, but the root can be used for a "base," "foundation," "step," and "a walking." Meaning "neither," **NEUTR-** in neutrophil is used for a solution that is neither basic nor acidic. **EOSIN-** in eosinophil refers to a red-florescent dye called eosin. It is derived from the Greek word for "dawn," eos. Likewise, the Greek goddess of the dawn, Eos, often has the epithet, "rosy fingered dawn," which speaks to the red-hued beauty of a sunrise (Fig. 8.20). Consequently, **EO-** and **EOS-** are used for "dawn" in compound terms. Eos and her siblings Helios (Sun) and Selene (Moon) were listed among the second-generation of Greek gods, known as the Titans. Like some of the Titans and the Protogenoi (first-born gods), her name indicates that she is a personification of important features in the physical world. Eosinophils, basophils, and neutrophils are identified as polymorphonuclear leucocytes, which are cells that are released in response to infections and asthma. The root **MORPH-** means "shape" and "form," which is used in polymorphonuclear to refer to the varied shapes of the nuclei in these cells.

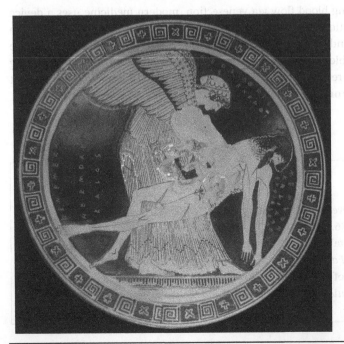

Fig. 8.20 The Greek goddess Eos is holding her son Memnon, who has been killed by Achilles. Attic red-figure, c. 490–480 BC. *Source:* Bibi Saint-Pol/Wikimedia Commons/Public domain.

Monocytes – Monocytes are a type of agranulocytic leukocyte. The root **MON**- means "one," and it appears as a combining form in the word monocyte. Monocytes are one of the phagocytic parts of the immune system's response to infection. Presence of an abnormally high number of mononuclear leukocytes in the blood in infectious mononucleosis is why the dreaded "kissing disease" is called "mono" for short.

Lymphocytes – Lymphocytes are a type of agranulocytic leukocyte. Lymphocytes are white blood cells that account for much of the body's immunity. Less than 1% are present in the circulating blood. The majority of lymphocytes are found in the spleen, lymph nodes, and other lymphoid organs.

Fig. 8.21 The anatomical Latin terms for the lymphatic system. *Source:* Drawing by Chloe Kim.

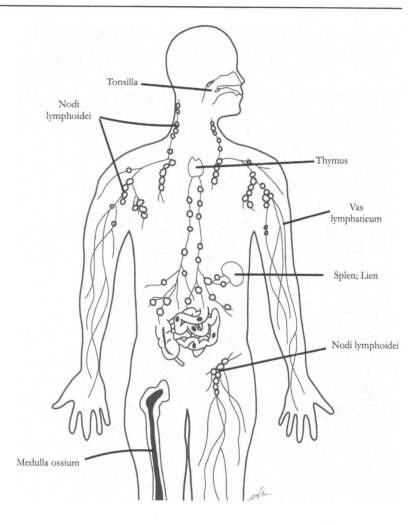

Tonsilla

Nodi lymphoidei

Thymus

Vas lymphaticum

Splen; Lien

Nodi lymphoidei

Medulla ossium

Lymph and the lymphatic system (Fig. 8.21)

Lymph (L. *lympha, -ae*) – Lymph is a thin clear fluid that is central to the body's immune response. John Hunter (1728–1793) is generally credited with discovering the lymphatic system since he recognized that vessels and nodes of the lymphatic system were distinct from the veins and arteries, and he believed that the purpose of these lymphatics was to absorb foreign material. The term lymph (**LYMPH**-) is derived from the medieval Latin word for "clear water" *lympha*. This medieval Latin word is said to derive from the Greek *nymphe*, which was a Greek word used to describe a goddess of a spring, a "nymph." The lymphatic system is a network of organs, lymph nodes, and lymph vessels that transport lymph from tissue into the bloodstream. Lymph originates from interstitial fluid of tissue that is drawn into lymph capillaries. In addition to fighting infections, the lymphatic system also regulates the interstitial fluids of the body. Therefore, an impairment of the lymphatic vessels can cause swelling in the body's appendages known as lymphedema.

Chyle (L. *chylos, -i*) – When lymph carries emulsified fats from the lacteals in the digestive tract, it becomes thick and milky; this milky lymph is called chyle. Chyle comes from the Greek word for a "fluid" or "humor" of the body, *chylos*. The root **CHYL**- is used for chyle in modern medicine.

Lymph vessels (L. *vasa lymphatica*) – Vessels that receive lymph from lymph capillaries and circulate it to lymph nodes. The lymph vessels terminate into lymph ducts which channel the lymph to the veins. An infection of a lymph vessel is termed lymphangitis. The compound root **LYMPHANGI**- is commonly used for lymph vessels.

Lymph nodes (L. *nodi lymphoidei*) – Lymph nodes are small ovoid structures that, along with the spleen, act as important filters in the lymphatic system. The lymph node's palpable knot-like consistency is why the Latin word *nodus* (knot) is used to describe this gland. They are typically found in the cervical, axillary, and groin areas. The description of the location and nature of an *aden* (**ADEN-**, gland) in the Hippocratic text *On Glands* reveals that the lymph node was often what an ancient Greek physician was referring to when he used the term *aden*. Today, the compound root **LYMPHADEN-** is used for "lymph node," and therefore, a disease that affects a lymph node is called lymphadenopathy. An infected, swollen lymph node is called a **bubo** (pl. buboes). *Yersinia pestis*, the bacterium that is often pointed to as being the cause of the deadliest pandemic in history, the Black Death, can cause a lymph gland/node to become swollen and pus-filled, which is why it is sometimes referred to as the Bubonic plague (Fig. 8.22). The late Latin term **bubo** used to describe such swellings appears to have been derived from the Greek word *boubon*, which was used for any swollen gland, particularly those in the groin. The root **BOUBON-** is used for the "a swollen lymph node".

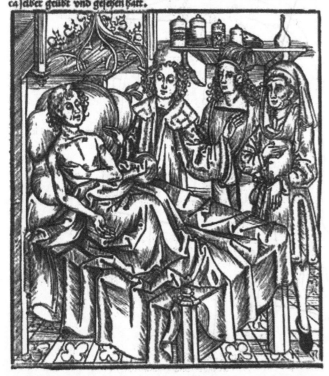

Fig. 8.22 Plague victim in bed pointing out to three physicians the swelling or bubo under his armpit, *Pestbuch*, by Hieronymus Brunschwig, 1500. *Source:* Hieronymus Brunschwig/Wikimedia Commons/Public domain.

Thymus (L. *thymus, -i*) – The thymus is responsible for the maturation of specialized lymphocytes called "thymocytes" or "T-cells." The root **THYM-** is used for the thymus gland, while it appears in anatomical Latin as *thymus*. The Latin anatomical term thymus originally came from the Greek word *thymos*, which was a word used in medicine for an excrescence looking like a bud of a thyme plant (Gr. *thymon*). The term was used for this gland in the neck by ancient Greek medical authors of the Roman period, such as Dioscorides, Galen, and Rufus of Ephesus.

Bone Marrow (L. *medulla ossium*) – About 60–70% of lymphocytes are formed in the marrow of the bones, particularly the red marrow of the bones. The "B-cell" lymphocytes are from the bone marrow, and they become plasma cells in an immune response to a virus. Other immature lymphocytes leave the red marrow to become fully formed in the spleen and lymph nodes, where they are stored to fight against infections. The roots for bone marrow are **MEDULL-** and **MYEL-**.

Spleen (L. *splen, splenis; lien, lienis*) – The spleen is a small organ locate in the left rib cage, just above the stomach. The spleen filters blood and makes white blood cells that protect the body from infection. The roots **SPLEN-** and **LIEN-** are used for the "spleen."

Tonsil (L. *tonsilla, -ae*) – Situated near the entrance to the digestive and respiratory tracts, the palatine tonsils, pharyngeal tonsils (adenoids), and lingual tonsils form a ring of lymphoid tissue that plays a key role in our immune response by stopping germs entering the body. The root **TONSILL-** and loan word tonsil are derived from the Latin word for an "almond," *tonsilla*, owing to this lymphatic tissue resembling an almond.

Greek or Latin word element	Current usage	Etymology	Examples
SANGUIN/O (sang-gwi-nō)	Blood	L. *sanguis, sanguinis*, m. blood	Con**sanguin**ity, **sanguin**eous Loan word: **Sanguis** (săng′gwĭs)
HEM/O (hē-mō) HEMAT/O (hēm-ă-tō) -EMIA (ē-mē-ă)	Blood	Gr. *haima, haimatos*, blood	**Hem**othorax, **hemat**ology, erythr**emia**
PLASM/O (plăz-mō) -PLASM (plă-zm)	Fluid portion of blood (plasma), something formed or shaped	Gr. *plasma*, anything formed or molded fr. *plassein*, to form, mold	Cyto**plasm**, **plasm**atherapy Loan word: **Plasma** (plaz′mă)
PLAST/O (pla-stō) -PLAST (plast) -PLASIA (plă-zē-ă)	formed, molded forming cell or organelle condition of formation, growth	Gr. *plastos*, formed, molded fr. *plassein*, to form, mold	**Plast**id, chloro**plast**, neo**plasia**
SER/O (sēr-ō)	Fluid left over after blood clotting (blood serum), a watery fluid	L. *serum, -i*, n. watery part of curdled milk (whey)	**Ser**osanguineous, **ser**ous Loan word: **Serum** (sēr′ŭm) pl. **Sera** (sēr′ă)
-POIESIS (poy-ē-sĭs)	To make, produce	Gr. *poieein*, to make, produce	Erythro**poiesis**, cyto**poiesis**
BLAST/O (blă-stō) -BLAST (blăst)	Embryonic cell, formative cell or layer, bud or shoot	Gr. *blastos*, a bud, shoot	Homo**blast**ic, hemato**blast**
CYT/O (sī-tō) -CYTE (sīt)	Cell	Gr. *kytos*, a hollow receptacle, a vessel	Hemo**cyt**oblast, erythro**cyte**
THROMB/O (thrŏm-bō)	A clot	L. *thrombus, -i*, m. a clot fr. Gr. *thrombos*, clot	**Thromb**ocyte, **thromb**osis Loan word: Thrombus (throm′bŭs) pl. Thrombi (throm′bī″)
ERYTHR/O (ĕ-rĭth-rō)	Red, red blood cell	Gr. *erythros*, red	**Erythr**openia, **erythr**ocyte
LEUK/O (loo-kō) LEUC/O (loo-kō)	White, white blood cell	Gr. *leukos*, white	**Leuk**emia, **leuc**ocyte
RETICUL/O (rĕ-tĭk-yŭ-lō)	Net, network	L. *reticulum, -i*, n. little net	**Reticul**ocyte, **reticul**ated

Greek or Latin word element	Current usage	Etymology	Examples
GRANUL/O (gran-yŭ-lō)	Granule, small grain	L. *granulum, -i,* n. small grain, granule fr. L. *granum,* grain, seed	**Granul**ocyte, **granul**ar
CORPUSCUL/O (kor-pŭs-kū-lō)	Corpuscle, small mass or body	L. *corpusculum, -i,* n. small body fr. L. *corpus, corporis,* n. body	**Corpuscul**ar
GLOB/O (glō-bō) **GLOBUL/O** (glob-ū-lō)	Ball, sphere	L. *globulum, -i,* n. little ball fr. *globus,* ball or sphere	Hemo**glob**in, **globul**in Loan word: **Globus** (glō′bŭs) pl. **Globi** (glō′bī″)
MORPH/O (mŏr-fō)	Shape, form	Gr. *morphe,* shape, form, figure	Poly**morph**onuclear, iso**morph**ism
NUCLE/O (nū-klē-ō)	Center of cell (nucleus), nut, kernel	L. *nucleus, -i,* m. kernel, nut	Mono**nucle**osis, **nucle**ar Loan word: **Nucleus** (noo′klē-ŭs) pl. **Nuclei** (noo′klē-ī″)
KARY/O (kar-ē-ō)	Center of cell (nucleus), nut, kernel	Gr. *karyon,* nut, kernel	**Kary**otype, **kary**olysis Loan word: **Karyon** (kar′ē-on″) pl. **Karya** (kar′ē-a″)
NEUTR/O (noo-trō)	Neutral, neither	L. *neuter, neutra, neutrum,* neither	**Neutr**ophil, **neutr**openia
BAS/O (bā-sō)	Base, foundation, step, a walking	L. *basis, -is,* f. fr. Gr. *basis,* foundation, base, step, a walking	**Bas**ophil, **bas**ad Loan word: **Basis** (bā′sĭs) pl. **Bases** (bā′sēz″)
EOSIN/O (ē-ō-sĭn-ō)	Red dyes used in histology (Eosine)	Gr. *eos,* dawn + chemical suffix *-in*	**Eosin**ophil, **eosin**oblast Loan word: **Eosine** (ē′ŏ-sēn″)
EOS/O (ē-ōs-ō) **EO-** (ē-ō)	Dawn, early, morning red	Gr. *eos,* dawn	**Eo**cene, **eos**ophobia
PHIL/O (fĭ-lō) **-PHIL** (fil) **-PHILE** (fil)	Attraction, love	Gr. *philein,* to love, affinity for	Eosino**phil**, iodino**phil**ous, meso**phile**
LYMPH/O (lim-fō) **LYMPHAT/O** (lim-fa-tō)	Lymph, water	L. *lympha, -ae,* f. clear water; lymph	**Lymph**edema, **lymphat**ic Loan word: **Lymph** (limf)
NOD/O (nō-dō)	Node (lymph), swollen, knot-like	L. *nodus, -i,* m. knot	**Nod**ose, **nod**ular Loan word: **Nodus** (nŏd′ŭs) pl. **Nodi** (nō′dī″)

Greek or Latin word element	Current usage	Etymology	Examples
ADEN/O (ad-ĕ-nō)	Gland	Gr. *aden*, gland	Lymph**aden**opathy, lymph**aden**itis
SPLEN/O (splē-nō)	Spleen	Gr. *splen*, spleen	Micro**splen**ia, **splen**ectomy
LIEN/O (lī-ĕ-nō)	Spleen	L. *lien, lienis*, m. spleen	**Lien**ocele, gastro**lien**al Loan word: **Lien** (lī′ĕn)
TONSILL/O (ton-sĭ-lō)	Tonsil	L. *tonsilla, -ae*, f. almond	**Tonsill**itis, supra**tonsill**ar Loan word: **Tonsilla** (tŏn-sĭl′ă) pl. **Tonsillae** (tŏn-sĭl-ē)
THYM/O (thī-mō)	Thymus gland	L. *thymus, -i*, m. thymus fr. Gr. *thymos*, warty excrescence; thymus gland	**Thym**ectomy, megalo**thymus**
COAGUL/O (kō-ag-yŭ-lō)	Thickening of liquid into a gel or solid, particularly blood	L. *coagulum, -i*, n. that which causes to curdle	**Coagul**opathy, **coagul**ate Loan word: **Coagulum** (kō-ăg′ū-lŭm) pl. **Coagula** (kō-ăg′ū-la)
FIBR/O (fī-brō)	Fiber	L. *fibra, -ae*, f. fiber, filament	**Fibr**emia, **fibr**osis
BUBON/O (boo-bŏn-ō)	Swollen lymph node(s)	Gr. *boubon*, a swollen gland	**Bubon**adenitis Loan word: **Bubo** (boo′bō) pl. **Buboes** (boo′bō-ēz″)

Review	Answers
The loan word for a swollen or infected lymph node is _____ and its root is _____.	**bubo, BUBON-**
The combining form in granulocytes indicates that the cytoplasm of these cells looks like it contains small _____.	**grains**
The roots used for the "spleen" are _____ and _____.	**SPLEN-, LIEN-**
The compound combining form in lymphadenopathy and lymphadenocele refers to the anatomical structure of the lymphatic system known as a _____.	**lymph node**
The compound root in lymphangial and lymphangitis refers to the _____.	**lymph vessels**
The loan word and anatomical Latin term for tonsil is _____. Thus, an inflammation of a tonsil is spelled _____itis.	**tonsilla** **tonsill**
The surgical removal of the thymus gland is a _____ ectomy. The surgical removal of a lymph node is a _____ ectomy.	**thym** **lymphaden**
The fluid left over after the coagulation of blood is called _____, and its combining form is _____.	**serum, SER/O**
The fluid part of blood is referred to as _____. It's root PLASM- is used for something that is _____ or _____.	**plasma** **shaped, formed**
Coming from the Greek verb *plassein*, the suffix _____ is used for a "forming cell or organelle."	**-PLAST**
An embryonic cell that forms blood would be referred to as a hemato_____. The cellular process of forming blood is termed hemato_____.	**blast** **poiesis**
Based on its combining form, a reticulocyte looks like it has a little _____.	**net**
The combining forms for "nucleus" are _____ and _____.	**NUCLE/O, KARY/O**
The -phil in neutrophil, eosinophil, and basophil literally means _____ or _____. It is used in these terms because each cell shows up in a particular dye. Hence, a _____ phil is attracted to a basic dye.	**attraction, love** **baso**

Review	Answers
The root EO- that is used in words such as Eocene and eosine means _____, _____, and _____.	**dawn, early, morning red**
The loan word and anatomical Latin term for something that is knot-like is _____.	**nodus**
The combining form in neutrophil and the root in neutron literally means _____ or _____.	**neither, neutral**
The combining form in polymorphonuclear and morphogen means _____ or _____.	**shape, form**
The roots in hemoglobin and globulin mean _____ or _____.	**ball, sphere**
Blood cells are called corpuscles because they literally look like small _____. The combining form used for corpuscle is _____.	**bodies CORPUSCUL/O**
Red blood cells are called _____cytes, and white blood cells are called _____cytes.	**erythro, leuko**
A sanguiferous vessel carries _____.	**blood**
The suffix commonly used for pathological conditions of the blood is _____.	**-EMIA**
The loan word for a "thickening of liquid into a gel or solid, particularly blood" is _____. The name of the coagulating factor "fibrogen" literally means that it creates _____.	**coagulum fiber**
Platelets are also called _____cytes because these cells contribute to blood "clotting."	**thrombo**
ADEN/O is the combining form used for _____.	**gland**

Etymological Explanations: Pathologies of Blood and Lymph

The following is a summary of some of the modern diagnostic and symptomatic terms for blood and lymph pathologies:

Etymologies

Epistaxis – Epistaxis is a nose bleed. While it has Greek origins, epistaxis was not used for a "nosebleed" until 1793. The suffix **-STAXIS** is commonly used for a "dripping" or "oozing" of blood. Ultimately this term comes from the Greek word *stalaktos* "dripping, oozing out in drops," which is from the verb *stalassein* "to trickle," which is also where we get the word for the hanging formation in a cave called a stalactite.

Hemorrhage – Hemorrhage is an excessive discharge or flow of blood from the rupture of a blood vessel. As one would expect, excessive or unnatural loss of blood is considered pathological in ancient Greek medicine. Coming from the Greek word *haimorragia*, an excessive discharge or flow of blood typically from the rupture of a vessel is called a hemorrhage. The suffixes **-RRHAGIA** and **-RRHAGY** are, therefore, used for "condition of profuse bleeding."

Effusion – The movement of blood or another fluid into a cavity is called an effusion. For example, a hemothorax is an effusion of blood into the pleural space of the thoracic cavity. The root **FUS-**, which comes from the Latin verb *fundere, fusum*, to pour), means a "pouring" or "melting." Its homomorph is **FUS-**, which comes from the Latin word (*fusus*, spindle), and therefore, a fusiform aneurysm is in the shape of a spindle.

Transfusion – Modern medicine is also able to provide blood where there is a deficiency, which is termed a transfusion. The sense of "transferring of blood from one individual to another" was first recorded in the 1640s. The root **FUS-** in transfusion means "a pouring." Using the root meaning "self," **AUTO-**, a transfusion that involves using one's own blood is termed an autologous transfusion. Using the term meaning "same," **HOMO-**, the use of another's blood who is compatible (i.e. same blood time) is termed a homologous transfusion.

Plethora – As in ancient Greek medicine, the term plethora is used today for an excess of blood in the vessels. Similarly, a plethysmograph measures the amount of blood passing through or contained in the part. The roots **PLETH-** and **PLETHYSM-** are still used today for "excess" and "overfullness." As in ancient medicine, the movement of blood into an area in the body that it should not be is considered pathological.

Embolus – A piece of a clot that breaks off and travels to another area of the body where its "plugs" up the blood flow of a vessel is called an embolus, and the sudden obstruction/occlusion caused by this moving clot is called an embolism. In ancient Greek, an *embolos* "was anything pointed that could be thrust into something." Much like the "beak" or rostrum of a Roman naval ship, the pointed part of the battle prow of a Greek warship was called an *embolos* because it was thrown or thrust into a ship to damage and to sink the enemy vessel. The medical usage in reference to an obstruction of a blood vessel began in 1866, and it is used with non-blood material such as an aeroembolism. Derived from the Greek root "to throw" BAL- or BALL-, the root EMBOL- can also literally mean "anything that is thrust or thrown into something." For instance, in Taber's Cyclopedia, an embolalia is the "insertion of stammered sounds or fillers such as *ah, hmm, uh* in connected speech."

Thrombus – A DVT is an acronym that stands for "deep vein thrombosis." A thrombosis is a condition associated with a blood "clot." The loan word for a stationary clot is thrombus. Derived from the Greek word for a "clot," the Latinized thrombus is used for a pathological blood clot in a blood vessel or organ. As was discussed earlier, the root **THROMB-** is used for both pathological and normal clotting. The natural meaning is evident with terms such as prothrombin, which is a plasma protein coagulation factor II, and thromboplastin, which is a lipoprotein coagulation factor III.

Hemophilia – Coined in 1828, the X chromosome-linked bleeding disorder occurring only in boys and marked by deficiencies of blood-clotting proteins is called hemophilia (Gr. *haima* blood + *philia*, love, attraction, affection). Hemophilia is a term used today for a group of hereditary diseases affecting the clotting factors of blood that adversely affect its ability to coagulate.

Mononucleosis – Mononucleosis is a condition in which there is an abnormally high number of mononuclear leukocytes in the blood, typically caused by the Epstein-Barr virus.

Poikilocytosis – The compound suffix **-CYTOSIS** is used in hematological terms both for the presence of abnormal cells or the overabundance of a particular cell (Fig. 8.23). With respect to blood, the compound suffix **-CYTOSIS** typically refers to pathology involving red blood cells. Derived from the root for "irregular" and "diverse," **POIKIL-**, a condition of "irregularly" shaped red blood cells is called poikilocytosis.

Fig. 8.23 Image of the different types of blood cells associated with poikilocytosis. *Source:* Ed Uthman/Wikimedia Commons/ CC BY 4.0.

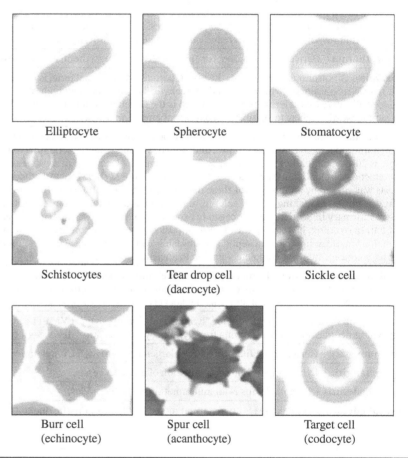

Elliptocyte   Spherocyte   Stomatocyte

Schistocytes   Tear drop cell (dacrocyte)   Sickle cell

Burr cell (echinocyte)   Spur cell (acanthocyte)   Target cell (codocyte)

Echinocytosis and Acanthocytosis – Echinocytosis and Acanthocytosis are both poikilocytic conditions in which the red blood cells have the appearance of having spines or thorns. Echinocytes tend to have smaller and more regular projections, while the projections of acanthocytes tend to be fewer, longer, and more irregular. The root **ECHIN-** means "spiny," and the root **ACANTH-** means "spiny," "thorn," and "spine."

Anisocytosis – Derived from the root for "unequal," **ANIS-**, a condition of "unequal"-sized red blood cells is called anisocytosis.

Macrocytosis – Derived from the root for "large," **MACR-**, a condition of "large"-sized red blood cells is called macrocytosis.

Microcytosis – Derived from the root for "small," **MICR-**, a condition of "small"-sized red blood cells is called microcytosis.

Reticulocytosis – Derived from the root for "little net," **RETICUL-**, an increased number of reticulocytes is called reticulocytosis.

Pleocytosis – Coming from the Greek root for "more" or "increased," PLE-, an excessive number of cells in a body fluid is called pleocytosis.

Erythrocytopenia – Derived from the Greek word for "poverty" and "need," *penia*, the suffix -**PENIA** is commonly used with hematological diseases where there is a diminished number of cells. Hence, a decrease in the amount of red blood cells in the body is called erythrocytopenia.

Lymphocytopenia – An abnormal reduction in the number of lymph cells is called lymphocytopenia.

Neutropenia – An abnormal reduction in the number of neutrophils is called neutropenia.

Thrombocytopenia – An abnormal reduction in the number of platelets is called thrombocytopenia.

Reticulocytopenia – Reticulocytopenia is a condition in which the number of reticulocytes is abnormally low.

Pancytopenia – Derived from the root for "all" and "every," **PAN-**, An abnormal reduction of all the cellular components in the blood is pancytopenia.

Anemia – Formed from the Greek word for blood *haima*, the compound suffix -EMIA is used for a pathologic condition of the blood. Literally meaning a "condition of no blood," the term anemia is a bit of a misnomer. Anemia is a general term used for a reduction in the mass of circulating red blood cells which leads to poor oxygenation of tissue. The hemoglobin levels of a patient are often tested to determine the presence of this disease. There are a wide variety of causes of anemia. For instance, aplastic anemia is a normocytic–normochromic type of anemia caused by the failure of blood marrow to produce enough red blood cells. This type of anemia can be linked to myelodysplasia. The term myelodysplasia is used for a hematological disease in which there is inadequate bone marrow production of normal blood cells. The compound suffix -**DYSPLASIA** means a "condition of faulty or painful formation or growth." Anemia can be caused by excessive blood cell destruction, which is associated with hemolysis. Anemia due to a genetic trait responsible for interference with hemoglobin synthesis is termed erythroblastic anemia.

Polycythemia – Derived from the root for "many," **POLY-**, Polycythemia is a condition in which there is an excess of red blood cells.

Toxemia – A poisonous substance in the blood, particularly from bacteria, is called toxemia. The root **TOX-** comes from the Late Latin *toxicus* "poisoned," which is from the Greek *toxikon pharmakon* which was a poison used on arrows. The *toxikon* is ultimately a Greek adjective that refers to the *toxon*, which is the Greek word for "bow and arrows." The bow and arrow sense **TOX-** is still present in words such as toxophilist, "a collector of bows and arrows."

Septicemia – Septicemia refers to sepsis of the blood. **Sepsis** is the body's extreme response to an infection, in which there is fever or hypothermia, tachycardia, tachypnea, and evidence of inadequate blood flow to internal organs. The risk of death from sepsis is as high as 30–50% depending on the severity. The ancient Greek concept of *sepsis* was associated with the theory of the rotting and putrefaction of blood that caused fevers. Louis Pasteur's (1822–1895) bacteria theory was essential to medicine recognizing that sepsis was caused by an infection of these microorganisms. Joseph Lister (1827–1912) is credited as the pioneer in antiseptic surgery that was pivotal to making surgery safer from infection, and therefore, more effective. While working as a surgeon at the Glasgow Royal Infirmary in Scotland, Lister began to experiment with the usage of carbolic acid to sterilize his surgical instruments and the patient. In so doing, he reduced the amount of postoperative infections and paved the way for other antiseptic techniques, which is why the American brand of antiseptic mouthwash is called Listerine. Today, the root **SEPTIC-** mostly refers to the bacterial notion of sepsis; a concept that was completely foreign to ancient Greek physicians.

Leukemia – Derived from the root used for "white" and "leukocytes," **LEUK-**, Virchow recognized and coined the term leukemia for this type of hematological cancer. Today, leukemia is used for a group of hematological cancers of the blood-forming organs characterized by the presence of abnormal leukocytes.

Lymphoma – Derived from the root for "lymph" and "lymphocyte," **LYMPH-**, Lymphoma is the term used for a collection of malignant neoplastic disorders coming from lymphocytes. Hodgkin's disease is a type of lymphoma.

Splenomegaly – Derived from the suffix for "enlargement," -**MEGALY**, splenomegaly is an enlargement of the spleen.

Lymphangitis – Lymphangitis is an inflammation of a lymph vessel.

Lymphadenitis – Lymphadenitis is an inflammation of lymph nodes.

Lymphedema – Lymphedema is an abnormal increase in fluids in tissue due to the disruption of the lymphatic system.

Greek or Latin word element	Current usage	Etymology	Examples
CRIT/O (krit-ō)	Separate, decide	Gr. *kritos*, fr. *krinein*, to separate, distinguish, judge	**Crit**ical, hemato**crit**
-**CRIT** (krĭt)			
CRAS/O (krā-sō)	Mixture, temperament	Gr. *krasis*, mixture, a mixing, temperament	Dys**crasia**, idiosyn**crasy**
-**CRASIA** (krā-zē-ă)			

Greek or Latin word element	Current usage	Etymology	Examples
MICR/O (mĭ-krō)	Small	Gr. *mikros*, small	**Micr**obe, **micr**ocytosis
MACR/O (mak-rō)	Long, large	Gr. *makros*, long, large	**Macr**ocytosis, **macr**opod
ANIS/O (an-ĭ-sō)	Unequal	Gr. *anisos*, unequal	**Aniso**cytosis, **aniso**sphygmia
POIKIL/O (poy-kĭ-lō)	Irregular, varied, spotted, mottled	Gr. *poikilos*, spotted, changeful, various	**Poikil**ocytosis, **poikil**oderma
ACANTH/O (ă-kan-thō)	Thorn, spine, spiny	Gr. *akantha*, thorn, spine	**Acanth**ocytosis, **acanth**olysis Loan word: **Acantha** (ă-kan'thă)
ECHIN/O (ĕ-kī-nō)	Spiny	Gr. *echinos*, sea urchin, hedgehog, spiny	**Echin**ocyte, **echin**oderm
PLE/O (plē-ō) PLEI/O (plī-ō) PLI/O (plī-ō)	More, increased	Gr. *pleion*, more, increase	**Ple**ocytosis, **plei**otropic, **pli**ocene
TOX/O (tok-sō)	Poison, bow, and arrow	Gr. *toxon*, a bow and arrows	**Tox**emia, **tox**ic
SEPTIC/O (sĕp-tĭ-kō)	Sepsis	Gr. *septikos*, putrid fr. *sepsis*, rotting, putrefaction	**Septic**emia, **septic** Loan word: **Sepsis** (sep'sĭs)
-RRHAGIA (rā-jē-ă) -RRHAGE (răj) -RRHAGY (rā-jē) RHAGAD/O (răg-ă-dō)	Rupture with profuse discharge of a fluid (typically blood) Tear, fissure, cleft	Gr. *rhegnynai*, to break, burst forth Gr. *rhagas*, *rhagados*, cleft, fissure	Gastro**rrhagia**, hemo**rrhage**, **rhagad**iform
-PENIA (pē-nē-ă)	Decrease, deficiency	Gr. *penia*, poverty, need	Cyto**penia**, thrombo**penia**
MEGA- (mĕg-ă) MEGAL/O (meg-ă-lō) -MEGALY (meg-ă-lē)	Enlargement, large	Gr. *megas, megalou*, large	**Mega**karyocyte, **megal**oblast, spleno**megaly**
-STAXIS (stăk-sĭs)	Dripping, oozing	Gr. *staxis*, a dripping, oozing	Epi**staxis**, broncho**staxis** Loan word: **Staxis** (stăk-sĭs)

Greek or Latin word element	Current usage	Etymology	Examples
STAS/O (stā-sō) STAT/O (stă-tō) -STASIS (stā-sĭs) -STAT (stăt)	A standing, stoppage, cause to stand -STAT =a device for stopping, ceasing something	Gr. *stasis*, standing, stoppage	**Stas**imorphia, **stat**olith, Meta**stasis**, hemo**stat** Loan word: **Stasis** (stā′sĭs) pl. **Stases** (stā′ēz″)
EMBOL/O (ĕm-bō-lō)	A moving clot in the blood (embolus), an interjection	L. *embolus*, *-i*, embolus Gr. *embolos*, that which is thrust into something, wedge, stopper	**Embol**ectomy, aero**embol**ism Loan word: **Embolus** (em′bŏ-lŭs) pl. **Emboli** (em′bŏ-lī″)
THROMB/O (thrŏm-bō)	A clot	Gr. *thrombus*, a clot	**Thromb**ophlebitis, **thromb**ocyte Loan word: **Thrombus** (throm′bŭs) pl. **Thrombi** (throm′bī″)
EDEMAT/O (ĕ-dē-mă-tō) -EDEMA (ĕ-dē-mă)	Swelling	Gr. *oidema*, *oidematos*, swelling	Myx**edemat**ous, lymph**edema** Loan word: **Edema** (ĕ-dē′mă)
FUS/O (fū-sō)	A pouring, melting	L. *fundere*, *fusum*, to pour	Ef**fus**ion, **fus**ion
PLETH/O (plĕth-ō) PLETHYSM/O (pleth-iz-mō)	Excess, overfullness	Gr. *plethora*, overabundance of a humor Gr. *plethysmos*, an increase	**Pleth**oric, **plethysm**ography Loan word: **Plethora** (plĕth′ō-ră)
IMMUN/O (ĭm-ū-nō)	Free from, safe	L. *immunis*, exempt from duty, fees, taxation	**Immun**otherapy, **immun**ity

Review	Answers
A hemothorax is an effusion of blood into the pleural space of the thoracic cavity. In the table above, the root FUS- means _____ or _____. Its homomorph FUS- comes from the Latin word (*fusus*, spindle), and therefore, a fusiform aneurysm is in the shape of a spindle.	**pouring, melting**
A DVT is an acronym that stands for "deep vein thrombosis." A thrombosis is a blood _____. The loan word for a stationary clot is _____.	**clot thrombus**
A piece of a clot that breaks off and then travels to another area of the body where in "plugs" up the blood flow of a vessel is called an _____ and the sudden obstruction/occlusion caused by this moving clot is called an embolism.	**embolus**
The X chromosome-linked bleeding disorders occurring only in boys and marked by deficiencies of blood-clotting proteins is called _____.	**hemophilia**
Meaning a "condition of no blood," _____ is a reduction in the mass of circulating red blood cells. The hemoglobin levels of a patient are often tested to determine the presence of this disease.	**anemia**
Leukemia is used for a group of hematological cancers of the blood-forming organs. It is characterized by the presence of abnormal _____cytes.	**leuko**
Lymphoma is a term used for a collection of malignant neoplastic disorders coming from _____cytes. Hodgkin's disease is a type of lymphoma.	**lympho**

Review	Answers
A nosebleed is called an _____. The suffix -STAXIS in this term means _____ or _____.	**epistaxis** **dripping, oozing**
Derived from the Greek word for "poverty" and "need," a decrease in the amount of red blood cells in the body is called erythrocyto_____. An abnormal reduction in the number of lymph cells would be _____ penia. An abnormal reduction in the number of neutrophils is _____ penia. An abnormal reduction in the number of platelets is _____ penia. An abnormal reduction of all the cellular components in the blood is_____ penia.	**penia** **lymphocyto** **neutro** **thrombocyto** **pancyto**
With respect to blood, the compound suffix -CYTOSIS is typically used for pathological changes to blood cells, particularly red blood cells. Thus, a condition of "irregular"-shaped red blood cells is called _____ cytosis; a condition of "unequal"-sized red blood cells is called _____ cytosis; a condition of "large"-sized red blood cells is called _____ cytosis; a condition of "small"-sized red blood cells is called _____ cytosis; and a condition of "spiny" is called _____ cytosis or _____ cytosis. An increased number of reticulocytes is _____ cytosis.	**poikilo, aniso,** **macro, micro,** **echino, acantho** **reticulo**
Coming from the Greek word for "more" or "increased," an excessive number of cells in a body fluid is called _____ cytosis. The other potential spelling for this could be _____ cytosis or _____ cytosis.	**pleo** **pleio, plio**
A device for stopping excessive bleeding would be called a hemo _____. Likewise, a medication that stops the flow of blood is termed a hemo_____ic.	**stat** **stat**
A poisonous substance in the blood, particularly from bacteria, is called _____emia.	**tox**
Inflammation of a lymph vessel is termed lymph_____. Swelling in an appendage caused by pathological changes to the flow of lymph is termed lymph_____.	**angitis (angiitis)** **edema**
Excessive discharge of blood typically from the rupture of a vessel is called a hemo_____. The suffixes _____ and _____ are used for "condition of profuse bleeding."	**rrhage** **-RRHAGIA,** **-RRHAGY**
Sepsis is the body's extreme response to an infection, in which there is fever or hypothermia, tachycardia, tachypnea, and evidence of inadequate blood flow to internal organs. Sepsis of the blood is termed _____emia.	**septic**
An enlargement of the spleen is termed spleno_____.	**megaly**
The term myelodysplasia is used for hematological diseases in which there is inadequate bone marrow production of normal blood cells. The compound suffix -dysplasia means a "condition of faulty or painful _____ or _____."	**formation,** **growth**
Erythroblastemia is an abnormal number of erythroblasts in the blood. The root in this word means _____ cell.	**embryonic**
Phlebotomy is an incision or puncture of a _____ to withdraw blood for testing.	**vein**
HCT or Hct stands for hematocrit. The suffix in this term means _____.	**separate**
A drug that prevents the clotting of blood is called an anti _____ant.	**coagul**
A drug that causes the narrowing of a blood vessel is termed a _____constrictor. A drug that causes the expansion of a blood vessel is called a _____dilator.	**vaso** **vaso**
A blood transfusion is a term used for "the giving of blood to a recipient who is deficient in blood." The root FUS- in transfusion means _____. Using the root meaning "self," the transfusion that involved using one's own blood is termed an _____logous transfusion. Using the term meaning "same," the use of another's blood who is compatible (i.e. same blood time) is termed a _____logous transfusion.	**pouring** **auto** **homo**
Coming from the Greek word for temperament/mixture, dys_____ is used today as a synonym for hematologic disease.	**crasia**
Coming from ancient Greek medicine, the term plethora is used today for an _____ or _____of blood in the vessels. Similarly, a plethysmograph measures the amount of blood passing through or contained in the part.	**overfullness,** **excess**
The Roman word for freedom from taxes is used in terms such as autoimmune and immunotherapy. In these terms, it literally means _____ and _____.	**free from, safe**

9

Respiratory System

CHAPTER LEARNING OBJECTIVES
1) You will learn the word elements and loan words associated with the respiratory system.
2) You will become familiar with ancient Greek concepts of respiration, air, and diagnosing respiratory pathologies.

Lessons from History: Aristotle's Theory of Respiration

Food for Thought as You Read:

What are some of the theories for the purpose of respiration in antiquity, particularly Aristotle's theory?
How do the lungs function in respiration, according to Aristotle?
How do the anatomical parts of respiration figure into Aristotle's classification of animals?

While ancient Greek and Roman conceptions of respiration differ vastly from our modern understanding of the physiology of the respiratory system, most of our modern medical vocabulary for the anatomical parts of the respiratory system can be found in the writings of Greco-Roman physicians and philosophers who worked on the question of respiration, particularly Aristotle, the Alexandrian anatomists Herophilus and Erasistratus, and Galen.

> What is the benefit provided for us by respiration (***anapnoes***)? Is it generation of the soul (***psyches***) itself, as Asclepiades says? Or, not generation, but a sort of strengthening of the soul, as Praxagoras...says? Or is it a sort of cooling of the innate heat (***emphytou thermotetos***), as Philistion and Diocles held?
>
> Galen, *On the Use of Respiration*, K. 4.471

Galen's statement reveals that there were a wide variety of theories on the purpose of respiration, which we also call **anapnea** (*ana-* again + *pnea*, breath). Asclepiades of Bithynia (c. 1st century BC), a famous physician who flourished in Rome, held that the soul itself was derived from our respiration. Praxagoras of Cos (c. 4th–3rd century BC), who is believed to have made the distinction between arteries and veins and whose theories on pulses and pneuma had an influence on subsequent anatomists such as Herophilus, appears to view respiration not as the genesis of the soul, but a means by which the soul is strengthened. The other famous physicians on Galen's list, Philistion of Locri (c. 4th century BC), also known as the Sicilian, and Diocles of Carystus (c. 375 BC–c. 295 BC), are both described as linking respiration to the cooling of the innate heat. What can be observed in this tour of medical theories of respiration is that the breath of humans is linked to life, particularly the soul and the heat of the body. Both observations are clearly derived from observing death. The last breath of a human being or animal signals the passing of life to death, which perhaps explains why the Greek word *pneuma* could mean both "breathed air" and "the spirit/soul of man." Likewise, the life and the heat of the body are intertwined. Today, this is termed *algor mortis* (coldness of death), which is the lowering of the body temperature after death.

The absence of Aristotle in Galen's list of theorists in the above passage from *On the Use of Respiration* is interesting given that Galen's own approach to respiration is quite reliant on the theories of respiration articulated by Aristotle in his treatise *On Respiration*, as well as in his "biological" works such as *On the Parts of Animals*. Aristotle's theory of respiration is

Greek and Latin Roots of Medical and Scientific Terminologies, First Edition. Todd A. Curtis.
© 2025 John Wiley & Sons, Inc. Published 2025 by John Wiley & Sons, Inc.
Companion website: www.wiley.com/go/Curtis

similar to the famous Diocles' and Philistion's in that Aristotle also believe that the purpose of respiration was to cool the innate heat of the body. In Aristotle's theory, the soul was responsible for the functions of living bodies (e.g. movement, sensation, growth, etc.), and these faculties of the soul were linked to a heat that was both innate and vital to life. Being cardiocentric, Aristotle locates the soul and its faculties in the heart. Using the analogy of the soul's heat being like a fire, he notes that if the soul's heat is not checked, it will become too hot and exhaust the fuel necessary for its maintenance, but if it becomes too weak, it is endangered of going out like a flame that has grown cold. He likens the lungs to bellows whose purpose is to maintain a proper heat of the heart. Like bellows used to stoke a fire, the lungs bring in air when they expand due to the heat of the heart. This action brings the cooler, outside air into the lungs, which in turn cools the heart. This chilling effect on the heart causes a decrease in the expansion of the heart and lungs, and like the action of a bellow, the contraction pushes the internal hot air outside of the body. For Aristotle, this continuous motion of respiration is fundamental to life (Fig. 9.1).

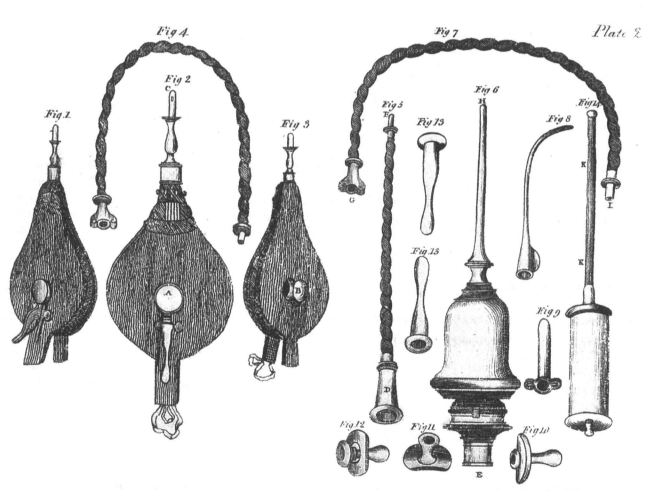

Fig. 9.1 Bellows have played a part in the history of medicine, as can be seen in this image of bellows (left) and clyster-pipes (right) for artificial respiration. *Source:* Bellows and clyster-pipes for artificial respiration / Wellcome Collection / Public domain.

Aristotle's approach to respiration was an integral part of his biological project of comparing the form and function of living things. For Aristotle, all living things need to cool off their innate, vital heat, but they do this in different ways. Fish, for example, use their gills to cool the heart with movement of water. For animals that have little heat, they require little to cool their innate heat, and this can be accomplished without lungs or gills. His criteria of respiring and non-respiring animals, lung and lungless animals, and bloody and bloodless lungs reveal Aristotle's anthropocentric approach to the differences in animal anatomy. Since, as Aristotle reasons, heat and the faculties of the soul were linked and since humans were the only living things possessing a rational faculty, their hearts were hotter than the other animals. Therefore, humans

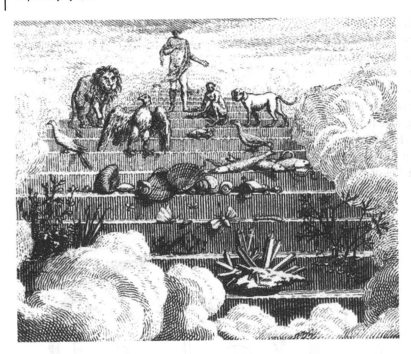

Fig. 9.2 Scala Naturae depicted in *Oeuvres d'histoire naturelle*, 1781. *Source:* Charles Bonnet / Wikimedia Commons / Public domain.

require a superior refrigeration system; humans use respiration via blood-filled lungs to effectively cool their hearts. As a consequence to this premise, Aristotle would classify animals who have lungs and respire as being more like humans in respect to the faculties of their soul. This "psychosomatic" approach to living things was the genesis for what later became known as the *Scala Naturae, The Ladder of Nature*, which was a classification system that arranged the entire natural world on a hierarchical continuum with human beings being at the apex (Fig. 9.2).

Suggested Readings

Bos, Abraham, and Rein Ferwerda. *Aristotle, On the Life-Bearing Spirit* (De Spiritu)*: A Discussion with Plato and his Predecessors on Pneuma as the Instrumental Body of the Soul.* Leiden: Brill, 2008.

Furley, David J., and James S. Wilkie. *Galen: On Respiration and the Arteries.* Princeton: Princeton University Press, 1984.

Hett, Walter S. Aristotle. *On the Soul; Parva Naturalia; on Breath.* Revised and reprinted Cambridge: Harvard University Press, 1957.

Lennox, James G. "Aristotle on Respiration: Framework Norms Meet Domain-Specific Norms." In *Aristotle on Inquiry: Erotetic Frameworks and Domain-Specific Norms*, 264–90. Cambridge: Cambridge University Press, 2021.

Etymological Explanations: Common Terms and Word Elements for the Anatomy of Respiratory System

The primary purpose of the respiratory system is twofold: (i) It brings air into the body through inhalation, which provides oxygen to the blood and tissues, and (ii) it removes carbon dioxide from the body via exhalation. In the following discussion of the anatomical terms associated with the respiratory system, the nominative and genitive singular forms of the anatomical Latin terms will be provided in parentheses. The Greek and Latin roots are formatted in all caps and emboldened. This discussion of the Greek and Latin word elements for the anatomical parts of the respiratory system will move from the **upper respiratory tract** (i.e. nose to larynx) to the **lower respiratory tract** (i.e. trachea to lungs), which will be followed by a discussion of the Greek and Latin word elements used for the organs, structures, and cavities associated with the respiratory system (Fig. 9.3).

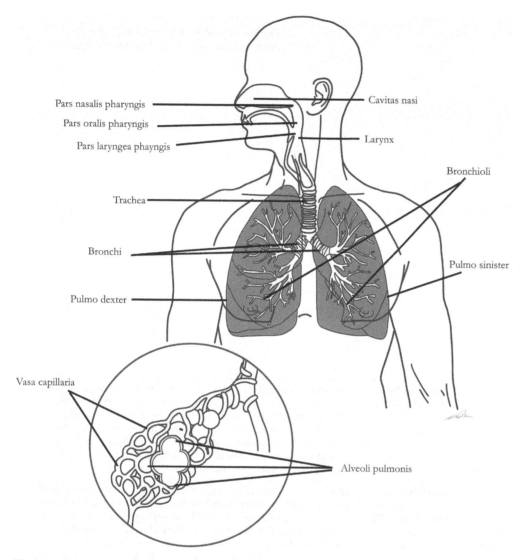

Pars nasalis pharyngis

Pars oralis pharyngis

Pars laryngea phayngis

Cavitas nasi

Larynx

Bronchioli

Trachea

Bronchi

Pulmo dexter

Pulmo sinister

Vasa capillaria

Alveoli pulmonis

Fig. 9.3 Anatomical Latin for the respiratory system. *Source:* Drawing by Chloe Kim.

Upper respiratory tract

Nose (L. *nasus, -i*) – In the respiratory system, the nose serves to moisten, warm, and filter air as it progresses to the respiratory tract. The Greek and Latin roots used for "nose" are **RHIN-** and **NAS-**. The anatomical Latin term for "nose" is *nasus*. Being such a prominent feature of the face, the nose is commonly used in symbolic language and idioms. For instance, the English idiom "to turn up one's nose at ..." refers "to refusing to take or accept something because it is considered inferior." This idiom appeared in English around 1749. The same idiomatic usage can also be found in ancient Greek and Latin. The Greek verb *muktrizein*, which is translated as "to turn up the nose, to sneer at," is derived from the Greek word for "nostril" *mukter*. In Latin, this idea is expressed by the idiom: *naso suspendere adunco*, which is translated "to sneer at." Perhaps these idioms reveal that raising one's nose was actually a common symbolic gesture used to demonstrate one's self-importance by showing utter disregard for another person or thing. The Greek word *mukter* and its derivatives are not used for "nostril" today. The Latin word *naris* (L. *naris, -is*), and its root **NAR-**, is the anatomical Latin term used for this passageway into the nose.

Sinus (L. *sinus, -us*) – The air-filled spaces in the skull that surround the nose are collectively called the paranasal sinuses. In ancient Latin, a sinus was a "curve," "fold," or "bending." Owing to its original meaning, any recess or cavity with a single opening could be called a "sinus." Thus, the roots **SIN-** and **SINUS-** have the meanings of "curve, cavity, socket, or sinus." The Latin term for a "cave," antrum, is used in a similar way to sinus when speaking about anatomical structures. An anatomical antrum refers to an almost closed cavity, especially in bone. Its root **ANTR-** can also be used for "cave, cavity, or sinus" in modern medico-scientific language. In respect to the respiratory system, the root **ANTR-** is specifically used for the maxillary sinus. For example, an antrotomy is a surgery that involves cutting into the maxillary sinus (Fig. 9.4).

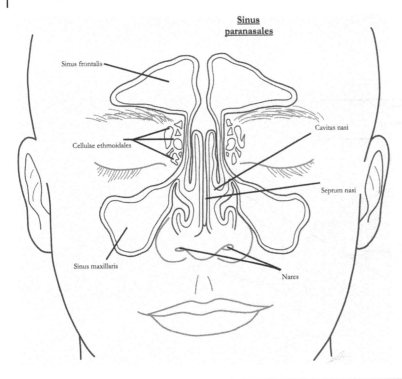

Sinus
paranasales

Sinus frontalis

Cellulae ethmoidales

Sinus maxillaris

Cavitas nasi

Septum nasi

Nares

Fig. 9.4 Anatomical Latin for the nose and paranasal sinuses. *Source:* Drawing by Chloe Kim.

Pharynx (L. *pharynx, pharyngis*) – The passageway by which food and air enter the body is called in everyday English the "throat." We have already seen that the Latin root **JUGUL-** can be used for "throat," and in fact, the Latin word jugulum appears as a loan word for "throat" in medical dictionaries. However, the more commonly used root and loan words for "throat" are, respectively, **PHARYNG-** and **pharynx**. Derived from the Greek word *pharynx*, pharynx is the anatomical Latin term for the throat. In addition to serving as a passageway for food and air, the pharynx contains lymphatic tissue known as the adenoids (Gr. *aden-*, gland + *-oid* resembling) and tonsils (L. *tonsilla*, almond) that are important to the immune system. The pharynx is divided into three areas that correspond to its association with the nose, mouth, and larynx: nasopharynx, oropharynx, and laryngopharynx.

Larynx (L. *larynx, laryngis*) – The last part of the upper respiratory tract is called the larynx, which is also called the "voice box" in everyday English. The combining form used for this anatomical part is **LARYNG-**, and similarly to how pharynx can be used as a suffix **-PHARYNX**, larynx is also used as a suffix **-LARYNX** in some terms. The similar spellings between larynx and pharynx may stem from both words being used in ancient Greek to refer to the "throat" rather than a specific anatomical structure. Today, the larynx refers to the anatomical passageway that allows air to travel to the trachea, and via the vocal cords, the larynx is also associated with production of the human voice. The epiglottis and glottis are two important structures of the larynx. The glottis is the opening between the vocal cords in the upper part of the larynx. The epiglottis is a valve-like structure that covers the glottis when one is swallowing, and thus, like the uvula's function for the nose, the epiglottis prevents food from entering the respiratory tract. In ancient Greek, *glottis, glotta,* and *glossa* all referred to the "tongue," and by extension, to "speech" and "language." The metaphorical meaning of speech as it applies to the tongue is still present in the roots **GLOSS-** and **GLOTT-**, which are used in words such as "glossary" (the "language" of a book) and "glottogonic" (pertaining to the creation of "language"). Although both roots can be used for "tongue" and "language," **GLOTT-** is the root that is used for the glottis and vocal cords of the larynx (Fig. 9.5).

Fig. 9.5 Anatomical Latin for the larynx. *Source:* Drawing by Chloe Kim.

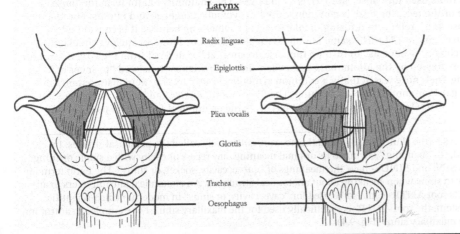

Larynx

Radix linguae

Epiglottis

Plica vocalis

Glottis

Trachea

Oesophagus

Lower respiratory tract

Trachea (L. *trachea, -ae*) – After leaving the larynx, we move into the lower respiratory tract, where the first anatomical structure that will be encountered is the large windpipe known as the trachea. This anatomical windpipe derives its name from its distinctively ribbed appearance. The cartilage in the trachea gives it a somewhat "rough" appearance, which is why the trachea was originally called the *tracheia arteria* "the rough artery" in ancient Greek. As noted previously in this textbook, the term *arteria* could be used somewhat indiscriminately for the blood vessel known today as the artery and for the airways of the respiratory tract since for some ancient Greek physicians, such as Erasistratus and Praxagoras of Cos (4th–3rd century BC), both structures were thought to carry air (or pneuma). Coming from the Greek adjective *trachys* for "rough," the adjective *tracheia* in *tracheia arteria* was used to distinguish the trachea from the other windpipes of the body. Medieval Latin shortened the Greek term to trachea, which is its current spelling and usage. In modern medical English, the root **TRACHE-** is used for the "trachea," but **TRACH-** and **TRACHY-** carry the meaning of "rough." All three of these roots have a similar spelling to the root for "neck," **TRACHEL-**, which adds to the potential for confusion considering the trachea's proximity to the neck (Fig. 9.6).

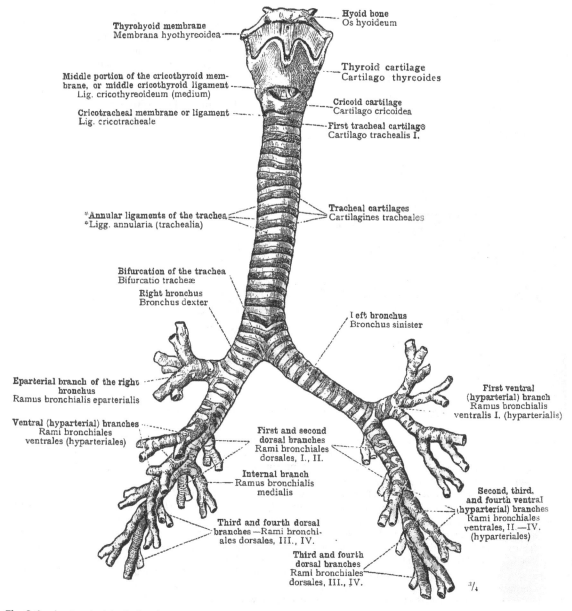

Fig. 9.6 Anatomical Latin for the trachea, bronchi, and bronchioles. *Source:* Carl Toldt et al. 1919/Rebman Company/Public Domain.

Bronchus (L. *bronchus*, *-i*) – Moving down the trachea, one encounters a ridged structure that creates a bifurcation in the respiratory tract. This ridged structure is called the carina of the trachea. It derives its name from the central ridge being likened to the keel of a ship (L. *carina*, keel of a ship). After the carina, the trachea becomes the right and left bronchi. Each bronchus enters a lung via the hilum (L. *hilum*, *-i*, little thing, trifle), which is a depression on the medial side of each lung where the major blood vessels also enter the lung. The anatomical term bronchus is a Late Latin word derived from the Greek word *bronchos*. The ancient Greek usage of the word *bronchos* differs from the way we use bronchus today. As Scarborough notes, "many Greek and Roman medical writers used bronchos as a synonym for the *tracheia arteria*, although occasionally medical Greek used bronchos to mean 'throat' as in the Hippocratic *Aphorisms*, VI, 37 (350 BC) and the *Acute Diseases*, I, 6, by Aretaeus of Cappadocia (about AD 100)." This ancient Greek usage of the term *bronchos* explains why Galen calls the cartilaginous rings of the trachea the *bronchia* and a tumor of the throat a *bronchocele*. The current meaning of **bronchus** and its root **BRONCH-** as one of the two terminal branches of the trachea began in the 1700s.

Bronchiole (L. *bronchiolus*, *-i*) – In modern medicine, the bronchi are the branched airways that come off the trachea and form tree-like structures via the smaller windpipes known as the brachioles. The bronchioles ultimately terminate into the microscopic air sacs known as the alveoli. This anatomical Latin term **bronchiolus** and its corresponding root **BRONCHIOL-**, which literally means "a small bronchial tube," began to be used in 1849.

Alveolus (L. *alveolus*, *-i*) – As noted, the respiratory tract terminates into small air sacs called alveoli. These thin-walled, microscopic air sacs of the lungs are fundamental to the exchange of oxygen from the lungs to the blood and vice versa in the case of carbon dioxide. Thanks to the invention of the microscope, Marcello Malpighi (1628–1694) was able to recognize the alveoli and their accompanying pulmonary capillaries. When recounting his observation that the lung contained alveoli, Malpighi stated the following: "By diligent investigation I have found the whole mass of the lungs, with the vessels going out of it attached, to be an aggregate of very light and very thin membranes, which, tense and sinuous, form an almost infinite number of orbicular vesicles and cavities, such as we see in the honey-comb alveoli of bees, formed of wax spread out into partitions." The anatomical Latin term alveolus is a diminutive of alveus, which meant "a hollow, cavity, and trough." Today, the loan word **alveolus** and its associated roots **ALVEOL-** and **ALVE-** refer to anatomical structures whose shapes are similar to this original Latin meaning. For instance, the bony socket that the tooth sits in is also called an "alveolus." (Fig. 9.7)

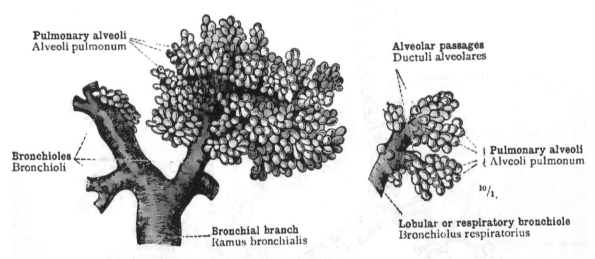

Fig. 9.7 Anatomical Latin for the bronchioles and alveoli. *Source:* Carl Toldt et al. 1919/Rebman Company/Public Domain.

Lung (L. *pulmo*, *pulmonis*) – The lungs are the organs of the lower respiratory tract. **PNEUM-** and **PNEUMON-** are the Greek roots commonly used for "lung" in modern medical English. The prevalence of this root is largely due to Aristotle's understanding of the purpose of respiration. At the time when Aristotle (384–322 BC) was teaching, the Greek word *pleumon* was the more commonly used term for "lung" and this word for "lung" can be traced back to Homer (c. 8th-7th century BC) in Greek literature. Instead of using *pleumon*, Aristotle chose to use the term *pneumon* when referring to the lung. He explains this choice in his work on *Respiration* (476.a.9 trans. G.R.T. Ross): "No animal yet has been seen to possess both lungs (*pneumona*) and gills (*branchia*), the reasons for this are that the lung is designed for the purpose of refrigeration by means of air (it seems to have derived its name (*pneumon*) from its function as a receptacle of the breath (*pneuma*)), while gills are relevant to refrigeration by water." For Aristotle the purpose of respiration was to cool the innate heat of the heart by the movement of *pneuma*, and the lungs were therefore termed "*pneuma*-things" owing to their connection with the Greek word for "breath," "breath of life," and "the soul," *pneuma*. Aristotle's influence on the naming of animal body parts is still evident today not only in our use of **PNEUM-** and **PNEUMON-** for "lung" but also in the modern technical usage of **BRANCHI-** for "gill." For instance, the adjective branchial refers to "gills or gill-like structures" in a body. Owing to its similar spelling, **BRANCHI-** can be is easily confused with **BRACHI-**, the latter of these two roots we have already seen carrying the meaning of "arm."

The anatomical Latin term for "lung," *pulmo*, is also the loan word used in medical English for "lung." Its etymology reveals that it was derived from the aforementioned Greek *pleumon* rather than Aristotle's *pneumon*. The connection between the Latin *pulmo* and Greek *pleumon* can be observed in these Greek and Latin words' shared meanings. In addition to the shared meaning of "lung," both *pulmo* and *pleumon* could also refer to lung-like creatures that we commonly refer to as jellyfish. The Latin adjective *pulmonarius*, *-a*, *-um*, from which we get our word for "pulmonary," originally meant "suffering from a disease of the lung." Today we use the roots **PULM-**, **PULMON-**, and **PULMONAR-** to refer to the "lungs." (Fig. 9.8)

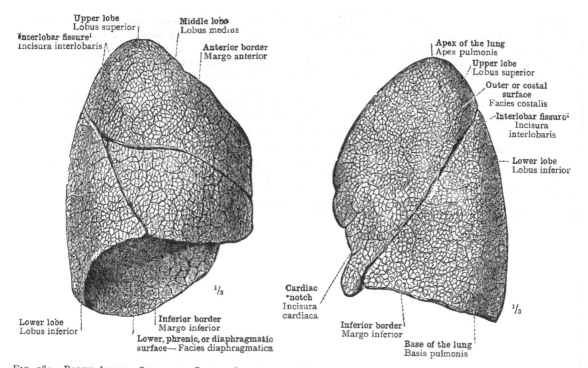

Upper lobe
Lobus superior

Middle lobe
Lobus medius

Interlobar fissure[1]
Incisura interlobaris

Anterior border
Margo anterior

Lower lobe
Lobus inferior

Inferior border
Margo inferior

Lower, phrenic, or diaphragmatic
surface— Facies diaphragmatica

FIG. 784.—RIGHT LUNG. OUTER OR COSTAL SURFACE.

Apex of the lung
Apex pulmonis

Upper lobe
Lobus superior

Outer or costal
surface
Facies costalis

Interlobar fissure[1]
Incisura
interlobaris

Lower lobe
Lobus inferior

Cardiac
notch
Incisura
cardiaca

Inferior border
Margo inferior

Base of the lung
Basis pulmonis

FIG. 785.—LEFT LUNG. OUTER OR COSTAL SURFACE.

* *Fissures of the Lung.*—The single fissure of the left lung, and the lower, more oblique, of the two fissures of the right lung, are sometimes distinguished as *great fissures* from the upper, nearly horizontal fissure of the right lung, which may he called the *supplementary fissure.*—TR.

Line of reflection of the pulmonary
pleura on to the root of the lung

Hilum of the lung
Hilus pulmonis

Anterior border
Margo anterior

Inner or mediastinal
surface
Facies mediastinalis

Ligamentum latum pulmonis, or broad ligament of
the lung—Lig. pulmonale

FIG. 786.—RIGHT LUNG. INNER OR MEDIASTINAL
SURFACE, WITH THE HILUM LAID BARE BY THE
REMOVAL OF THE STRUCTURES FORMING THE
ROOT OF THE LUNG.

Aortic groove
Sulcus aorticus

Bronchial arteries
Aa. bronchiales

Bronchial
lymphatic gland
Lymphoglandula
pulmonalis

Subclavian groove
Sulcus subclavius

Root of the lung
Radix pulmonis

Pulmonary artery
Arteria pulmonalis

Bronchus

Pulmonary veins
Vv. pulmonales

Ligamentum latum
pulmonis, or broad
ligament of the lung
Lig. pulmonale

Inferior border
Margo inferior

Lower, phrenic, or diaphragmatic
surface—Facies diaphragmatica

Boundary lines of the
pulmonary lobules

FIG. 787.—LEFT LUNG. INNER OR MEDIASTINAL
SURFACE, WITH THE ROOT OF THE LUNG CUT
ACROSS.

Pulmo—The lung.

Fig. 9.8 Anatomical Latin for the lungs. *Source:* Carl Toldt et al. 1919/Rebman Company/Public Domain.

Lobus (*lobus, -i*) – Perhaps the most recognizable features of the lungs are the "lobes," which in anatomical Latin are referred to as the **lobi**. The terms **lobe** and **lobus**, as well as the root **LOB-**, are ultimately derived from the Greek word *lobos*, which was used in medical literature in very similar ways as today. Much like today, the Greek word *lobos* and its diminutive *lobion* were used by ancient medical authors for anatomical features, such as the lobes of the liver and the lungs, as well as the earlobe. By using the word *lobos*, these ancient authors seem to be likening such anatomical structures to the capsule or pod of a leguminous plant. Today, a lobe is considered a well-defined part of an organ separated by deep grooves that are usually called fissures. The human lungs are one of the few places where asymmetry is prevalent, which can be observed in the different number of lobes. The left lung has two lobes (superior and inferior) and the right lung as three (superior, middle, and inferior). Furthermore, the right lung is shorter because of the liver, but the left lung is smaller because of the heart taking up some of its space.

Thoracic cavity (L. *cavitas thoracis*) – The lungs are situated in the thoracic cavity. The anatomical term **thorax** (L. *thorax, thoracis*) and its corresponding root **THORAC-** can be easily recognized as having come from the Greek word for the breastplate armor worn by soldiers, which is transliterated as the thorax. The Greek thorax was applied to the anatomical cavity partly due to Aristotle's classifications of animals. When discussing the morphology of viviparous animals in his *History of Animals* (493a5), Aristotle used the term *thorax* to describe the area between the neck and abdomen. His morphological usage of the term resembles how the word is used today in discussions of the parts of animals (Fig. 9.9).

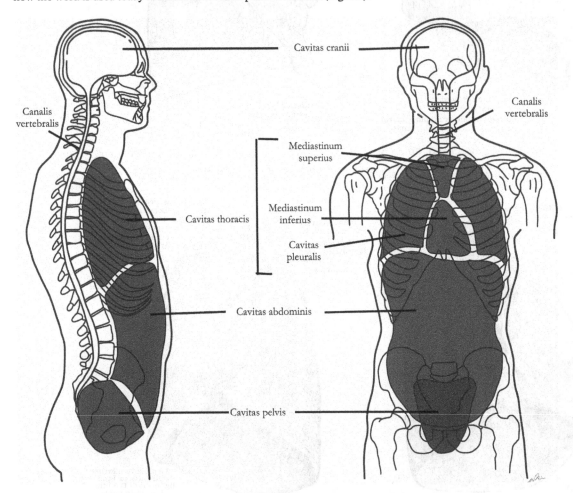

Fig. 9.9 Anatomical Latin for the cavities of the body. *Source:* Drawing by Chloe Kim.

Pleural Cavity (L. *cavitas pleuralis*) – In human anatomy, the thoracic cavity is further divided into the pleural cavities, the superior mediastinum, and the inferior mediastinum. The pleural cavities derive their name from **pleura** (L. *pleura, -ae*), whose root is **PLEUR-**, which is the serous membrane that encases each lung and enfolds on the wall of the thorax. The pleura has two parts, visceral and parietal. The **visceral pleura** encases the lung, and the **parietal pleura** lines the wall of the thorax. The serous secretions of the pleura allow it to lessen the friction of the lungs as the lung expands and contracts within the thoracic cavity. The term pleura first appeared in Latin in the 15th century. It was derived from the ancient Greek word *pleuron* (plural *pleura*) that carried the meaning "rib" or "side." When this word was adopted into Late Latin, they converted the singular into pleura, and therefore, the plural form became **plurae**, as it is today.

Mediastinum (L. *mediastinum, -i*) – The anatomical space between two cavities, particularly the space between the lungs, is referred to as the mediastinum. In respect to the thoracic cavity, the superior mediastinum cavity houses the aorta and its three accompanying major arteries, as well as the thymus, trachea, esophagus. The inferior mediastinum houses the heart. Originally, *mediastinus* was used for a "common servant" in Classical Latin. *Mediastinus* later came to mean "middling, middle" in Medieval Latin, and it is from this meaning that the neuter *mediastinum* began to be used in the 16ᵗʰ century for the aforementioned space between the lungs. The root for this space is **MEDIASTIN-**.

Diaphragm (L. *diaphragma, diaphragmatis*) – The thoracic cavity and the abdominal cavity are separated from each other by the diaphragm. Together with the muscles associated with the ribs, this muscular partition moves up and down to facilitate exhalation and inhalation of the lungs. Ancient Greek physicians, such as Galen, used the word *diaphragma* when writing about this structure. *Diaphragma* was also used in everyday Greek for any "partition wall" or "barrier." The latter meaning is recognizable from the diaphragm's constituent word elements: *dia-* across + *phragma*, a fence. Derived from the Greek *phragma*, the roots **PHRAGM-** and **PHRAGMAT-** refer to "a wall" or "obstruction" in modern medico-scientific language, and similarly, the suffix **-EMPHRAXIS** refers to a pathological "obstruction" of an anatomical part (e.g. pharyngemphraxis, nephremphraxis). The roots **DIAPHRAGM-** and **DIAPHRAGMAT-** are specifically used for the "diaphragm." In addition to **DIAPHRAGM-** and **DIAPHRAGMAT-**, the Greek root **PHREN-** is also used for "diaphragm." Oddly enough, **PHREN-** can also refer to the "mind" or the "mental faculties" (e.g. schizophrenia and the Latinized frenetic). The use of *phren* for the seat of the mind is evident in both Greek poetry and medicine. For example, the *Iliad* (9.185-7) depicts Achilles trying to divert his *phren* by playing music on a clear-sounding lyre, and ancient Greek medicine commonly used the term *phrenitis* to speak to a type of illness that affects the mental faculties. The reason for this odd pairing of mind and midriff may stem from the physical symptoms that are sometimes experienced at the midriff when one is consumed by intense emotions.

Greek or Latin word element	Current usage	Etymology	Examples
NAS/O (nā-zō)	Nose	L. *nasus, -i*, m. nose	Oro**nas**al, **nas**opharynx Loan word: **Nasus** (nā'sŭs) pl. **Nasi** (nā'sī″)
RHIN/O (rī-nō)	Nose	Gr. *rhis, rhinos*, nose	**Rhin**itis, **rhin**orrhea
NAR/I (nar-ē)	Nostril	L. *naris, -is*, f. nostril	Inter**nar**ial, **nar**icorn Loan word: **Naris** (nar'ĭs) pl. **Nares** (nar'ēz″)
SIN/O (sĭn-ō) **SINUS/O** (sī-nŭ-sō)	Curve; cavity, socket, or sinus	L. *sinus, sinus*, m. bending, curve, fold	Para**sin**oidal, **sinus**oid Loan word: **Sinus** (sī'nŭs) pl. **Sinus** (sī'nŭs) or English **Sinuses** (sī'nŭs-es)
ANTR/O (an-trō)	Cave; cavity or sinus	L. *antrum, -i*, n. cave	**Antr**ocele, **antr**ocele Loan word: **Antrum** (an'trŭm) pl. **Antra** (an'tră)
PHARYNG/O (fă-ring-gō) **-PHARYNX** (far-ingks)	Throat	L. *pharynx, pharyngis*, f. throat, fr. Gr. *pharynx*, throat	**Pharyng**eal, naso**pharynx** Loan word: **Pharynx** (far'ingks) pl. **Pharynges** (fă-rin'jēz″)
LARYNG/O (lăr-ĭn-gō) **-LARYNX** (lar-ingks)	Voice box, larynx	L. *larynx, laryngis*, m. larynx, organ of voices of the upper trachea fr. Gr. *larynx*	**Laryng**itis, electro**larynx** Loan word: **Larynx** (lar'ingks) pl. **Larynges** (lă-rin'jēz″)
EPIGLOTT/O (ĕp-ĭ-glŏ-tō) **EPIGLOTTID/O** (ĕp-ĭ-glŏt-ĭd-ō)	Epiglottis	L. *epiglottis, epiglottidis*, f. epiglottis, valve covering the larynx, fr. Gr. *epiglottis*	**Epiglott**itis, **epiglottid**ectomy Loan word: **Epiglottis** (ep″i-glot'ĭs) pl. **Epiglottides** (ep″i-glot'ĭ-dēz″)

Greek or Latin word element	Current usage	Etymology	Examples
GLOTT/O (glŏ-tō)	Vocal cords, tongue	L. *glottis, -is,* f. vocal cord, fr. Gr. *glotta,* tongue	**Glott**ic, **glott**ology Loan word: **Glottis** (glot′ĭs) pl. **Glottides** (glot′ĭ-dēz″)
TRACHE/O (trā-kē-ō)	Trachea	L. *trachea, -ae,* f. trachea, windpipe, fr. Gr. *traxeia arteria*	**Trache**otomy, **trache**al Loan word: **Trachea** (trā′kē-ă) pl. **Tracheae** (trā′kē-ē″)
TRACHEL/O (trak-ĕ-lō)	Neck	Gr. *trachelos,* neck	**Trachel**ocele, **trachel**ectomy
TRACH/O (trā-kō) **TRACHY-** (trā-kĭ)	Rough	Gr. *trachys,* rough	**Trach**oma, **trachy**phonia
BRONCH/O (brŏng-kō)	Bronchus	L. *bronchus, -i,* m. bronchus fr. Gr. *bronchos,* anatomical windpipe	**Bronch**odilating, **bronch**oblennorrhea Loan word: **Bronchus** (brong′kŭs) pl. **Bronchi** (brong′kī″)
BRONCHIOL/O (brong-kē-ō-lō)	Bronchiole	L. *bronchiolus, -i,* m. bronchiole, small bronchus fr. Gr. *bronchos,* anatomical windpipe	**Bronchiol**itis, **bronchiol**ectasis Loan word: **Bronchiolus** (brŏng-kē′ō-lŭs) pl. **Bronchioli** (brŏng-kē′ō-lī″)
HIL/O (hī-lō)	Hilum	L. *hilum, -i,* n. little thing, trifle	**Hil**itis, **hil**ar Loan word: **Hilum** (hī′lŭm) pl. **Hila** (hī′′lă)
PULM/O (pŭl-mō) **PULMON/O** (pŭl-mō-nō)	Lung	L. *pulmo, pulmonis,* m. lung	**Pulm**oaortic, **pulmon**ologist Loan word: **Pulmo** (pŭl′mō) pl. **Pulmones** (pŭl′mŏ-nēz″)
PNEUM/O (nū-mō) **PNEUMON/O** (noo-mŏ-nō)	Lung	Gr. *pneumon, pneumonos,* lung	**Pneum**ocentesis, **pneumon**ectasis
ALVEOL/O (al-vē-ŏ-lō) **ALVE/O** (al-vē-ō)	Alveolus, cavity, socket, sac	L. *alveolus, -i,* m. bucket, a little hollow	**Alveol**otomy, **alve**oalgia Loan word: **Alveolus** (al-vē′ŏ-lŭs) pl. **Alveoli** (al-vē′ŏ-lī″)
LOB/O (lō-bō)	Lobe, pod	L. *lobus, -i,* m. lobe, from Gr. *lobos,* lobe	**Lob**otomy, bi**lob**ate Loan word: **Lobus** (lō′bŭs) pl. **Lobi** (lō′bī″)
PLEUR/O (ploo-rō)	Pleura, rib, side	L. *pleura, -ae,* f. pleura, fr. Gr. *pleuron,* rib, side	**Pleur**ocentesis, **pleur**itis Loan word: **Pleura** (ploor′ă) pl. **Pleurae** (ploor′ē)
PHREN/O (fren-ō)	Diaphragm, mind	Gr. *phren,* midriff, seat of thought/emotion	**Phren**optosis, **phren**ic

Greek or Latin word element	Current usage	Etymology	Examples
DIAPHRAGM/O (dī-ă-frăg-mō) **DIAPHRAGMAT/O** (dī-ă-frăg-ma-tō)	Diaphragm	L. *diaphragma, diaphragmatis,* n. diaphragm fr. Gr. *diaphragma,* partition, barrier	**Diaphragm**itis, **diaphragmat**ic Loan word: **Diaphragm** (dī'ă-fram")
PHRAGM/O (frăg-maō) **PHRAGMAT/O** (frăg-ma-tō) **-EMPHRAXIS** (ĕm-frăks-ĭs)	Obstruction, wall	Gr. *phragma, phragmatos,* fence, partition; *emphrassein,* to block	**Phragmat**ic, meso**phragma**, nephr**emphraxis**
PECTOR/O (pĕk-tō-rō)	Chest	L. *pectus, pectoris,* n. chest	**Pector**iloquy, **pector**algia Loan word: **Pectus** (pek'tŭs) pl. **Pectora** (pek'tō-ră)
STETH/O (stĕth-ō)	Chest	Gr. *stethos,* chest	**Steth**omyitis, **steth**oscope
THORAC/O (thōr-ă-kō) **-THORAX** (thōr-aks)	Thorax	L. *thorax, thoracis,* m. thorax fr. Gr. *thorax,* breastplate	Pneumo**thorax**, **thorac**ostomy Loan word: **Thorax** (thōr'aks") pl. **Thoraces** (thōr'ă-sēz")
MEDIASTIN/O (mē-dē-ăs-tī-nō) **-MEDIASTINUM** (mē-dē-ăs-tī-nŭm)	Mediastinum	L. *mediastinum, -i,* n. mediastinum fr. L. *mediastinus,* a middling, a lowly servant	**Mediastin**itis, hemo**mediastinum** Loan word: **Mediastinum** (mē"dē-ăs-tī'nŭm) pl. **Mediastina** (mē"dē-ăs-tī'nă)

Review	Answers
In layman's terms, a nasopharyngoscopy is an examination of the _____ and the _____.	**nose, throat**
Rhinorrhea is a thin, watery discharge from the _____.	**nose**
The collection of fluid in the alveoli and interstitium that is associated with pulmonary edema can lead to serious problems with oxygen and carbon dioxide exchange. By its adjective, one recognizes that pulmonary edema affects the _____.	**lungs**
An inflammation of the major branches of the respiratory tract is termed _____itis. Dilation or expansion of the smaller branches of the respiratory tract is termed _____ ectasis.	**bronch** **bronchiol**
An inflammation of the anatomical "voice box" is termed _____itis. The loan word for this anatomical part of the respiratory tract is _____.	**laryng** **larynx**
Making a surgical opening in the thorax is termed a _____stomy.	**thoraco**
A cavity between two organs, particularly the lungs, is called a _____.	**mediastinum**
When speaking of an effusion into a cavity, the loan word for a cavity is used as a suffix. For instance, an effusion of blood in the mediastinal space is a _____mediastinum. The suffix -THORAX is used for an effusion into the pleural cavity. Thus, an accumulation of blood in the pleural cavity is called a hemo _____. An accumulation of pus in this cavity is a _____thorax, which is also termed empyema.	**hemo** **thorax, pyo**

Review	Answers
The phrenic nerve innervates the _____. The root PHREN- can mean _____, or _____.	**diaphragm** **diaphragm, mind**
A pneumonitis is an inflammation of a _____. The term pneumocentesis uses a variation of this root to create a term for a surgical puncture and aspiration of a _____.	**lung** **lung**
The device for listening to chest sounds is called a _____scope.	**stetho**
The surgical creation of an opening in the "windpipe" below the larynx is termed a _____ stomy. A trachelectomy is a surgical removal of an anatomical _____. The roots TRACHY- in trachyphonia and TRACH- in trachoma both mean _____.	**tracheo** **neck** **rough**
Expectoration is the coughing up of material out of the lungs. That said, the root in expectoration means _____, not lungs.	**chest**
The anatomical Latin term for "a nostril" is _____ and the plural form of this is _____.	**naris, nares**
An alveolar structure resembles a _____, _____, or _____. The root ALVEOL- is sometimes shortened to _____ as in alveoalgia, which is a pain in the socket of a tooth. The loan word for this thin-walled microscopic air sac of the respiratory tract is _____.	**cavity, socket, sac** **ALVE-** **alveolus**
The pod-like divisions of some organs such as the liver, lungs, and brain, are called a lobe. The anatomical Latin word for lobe is _____. The removal of a lobe of the lung would be a _____.	**lobus** **lobectomy**
The suffix _____ is used for a pathological obstruction. The roots for a wall or obstruction are _____ and _____.	**-EMPHRAXIS** **PHRAGM-, PHRAGMAT-**
The anatomical area of the pharynx associated with the nose is the _____pharynx. The area of the pharynx associated with the mouth is the _____pharynx. The area of the pharynx associated with the "voice box" is the _____pharynx.	**naso, oro, laryngo**
The serous membrane that encloses the lung and lines the wall of the thorax is called the _____. An inflammation of this structure is called _____itis.	**pleura** **pleur**
The space between the vocal cords is termed the _____. The fleshy valve-like structure that covers the larynx preventing food from getting into the lower respiratory tract is called the _____. The root GLOTT- can mean _____ or _____.	**glottis** **epiglottis** **vocal cords, tongue**
The anatomical Latin word for "a lung" is _____.	**pulmo**
Derived from the Latin word for a "bending," "fold," or "curve," the combining forms for the paranasal cavities are _____ and _____. That said, a sinusoidal wave is said to be _____.	**SIN/O, SINUS/O** **curved**
The combining form for a "cave" and the maxillary sinus is _____.	**ANTR/O**
Anatomical depression in the lungs by which the bronchus and blood vessels enter the lung is called the _____.	**hilum**

Lessons from History: Ancient and Modern Notions of Air

Food for Thought as You Read:

> *What is the relationship between aer/aither/pneuma in ancient Greek cosmological theories?*
> *What do they reveal about ancient concepts of the soul?*
> *How have these terms contributed to modern medical terminology?*

What material we breathe is fundamental to the understanding of human respiration. Three terms are quite important to ancient Greek approaches to this question: *aer*, *aither*, and *pneuma*. *Aer* was one of the elements that monists claimed to be the *arche* (first thing/element) of the universe. The Greek philosopher Anaximenes (c. 585–525 BC) appears to have put forward a monist theory of the universe in which *aer* is the element that is fundamental to all things, including breath (*pneuma*) and the soul (*psyche*): "Just as our *psyche*, being *aer*, constrains us, so *pneuma* and *aer* envelops the whole kosmos (DK 13 BC)." Thus, soul, breath, and air are intertwined in this cosmological theory. The connection between the soul and *aer* is also observed in Diogenes of Apollonia (5th century BC), and like Anaximenes, he held a monist theory in which *aer* was the primary element of the universe. Even among non-monists, *aer* played a prominent role as an element in the formation of the universe through its condensation and rarefaction. Empedocles (c. 495–c. 435 BC) was the first to specify "the four elements," identifying them as roots: air, fire, water, and earth. Empedocles' reasoning for there being four elements has been explained in the observation of fire. When a stick burns, it obviously has the element of fire in it; the black carbon left by the first must be earth; these ashes feel moist so water must be present; and the smoke produced by the fire indicates that *aer* is present.

Aristotle further developed Empedocles' and Plato' approaches to the four elements linking them to pairs of qualities: fire was dry and hot; earth was dry and cold; water was wet and cold; and air was wet and hot. Aristotle used a geocentric theory to explain the earth and its relationship to the cosmos. He saw the earth and the surrounding heavens as spherical or concentric circles. The four elements existed in what he called the sublunar sphere. They were arranged concentrically from the earth due to their qualities. He held that earth was the heaviest element, and therefore, it was most central in the cosmos/sublunar sphere and by extension, the universe. The water surrounding the earth was less heavy and therefore lies on the surface of the earth. Being lighter, the tendency for air and fire was to move upwards and away from the center. Air being wet and hot did not rise as high as fire, which was conceived of being lighter due to it being dry and hot. Beyond the layer of fire was the element *aither* which surrounded and formed the stars. The sublunar sphere was a place of change, and air was thought to be mutable depending on the forces at play in the sublunar realm. The sphere in which *aither* existed was considered unchanging and purer than air/fire. Aristotle's and other philosophers' theories about the divine properties and the fundamental nature of *aither* resulted in it being considered the "fifth element", which is where we get the term "quintessential."

That said, Aristotle did not invent the term *aither*. In Greek mythology, Aither was the personification of the bright upper sky. In Hesiod's *Theogony*, Aither was the child of Nyx (night) and Erebos (misty darkness). In the ancient cosmogonies, Aither was associated with the heavens and Erebos was associated with the dark mists of the underworld, and therefore, Aither serves as a contrast to his parents, just as light is the antithesis of darkness. Aither's name comes from the Greek verb *aithein*, which means "to burn, shine." Considering the stars were often thought to be burning and bright, one can surmise how the element *aither* became associated with the stars in Greek cosmologies.

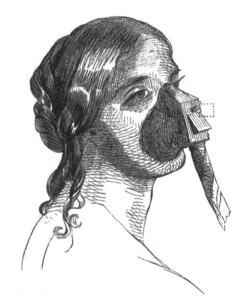

Today, the roots **ETHER-** and **AETHER-** are used for a modern gas called "ether." Ether is a chemical compound that has been recognized since the 14th century. It derived its name from its volatility and for its lightness. Its anesthetic properties were not fully recognized until 1842, when William T.G. Morton, a Boston dentist, began to use its anesthetic properties in his search to provide his patients with relief from the pain of dental procedures. It later came to be used for a wide variety of surgeries. The term for anesthetizing someone with the gas ether can be spelled **etherize** or **aetherize** depending on whether one is using an American or a British spellings (Fig. 9.10).

Suggested Readings

Bos, Abraham P. "'Pneuma' as Quintessence of Aristotle's Philosophy." *Hermes* 141, no. 4 (2013): 417–34.

Fenster, Julie M. *Ether Day: The Strange Tale of America's Greatest Medical Discovery and the Haunted Men Who Made It*. New York: HarperCollins, 2022.

Solmsen, Friedrich. "The Vital Heat, the Inborn Pneuma and the Aether." *The Journal of Hellenic Studies* 77 (1957): 119–23.

Fig. 9.10 Image of woman being etherized from John Snow's (1847) *On the Inhalation of the Vapour of Ether in Surgical Operations: Containing a Description of the Various Stages of Etherization, and a Statement of the Result of Nearly Eighty Operations in Which Ether has Been Employed in St. George's and University College Hospitals. Source:* Courtesy of the Wellcome Collection.

Etymological Explanations: Respiration and Air

The following is a summary of some of the modern diagnostic and symptomatic terms associated with air and respiration:

Respiration

Breathing/Respiration – The assessment of breathing is one of the diagnostic tools still used in medicine. Derived from the Greek verb *pneein* "to breath," the suffixes **-PNEA** and **-PNOEA** are used for "breathing" and "breath."

The Latin verb *spirare* "to breathe" is also commonly used in medicine in the form of the root **SPIR-**. The root **SPIR-**, as in inspiration (breathing in) and expiration (breathing out), means "breath" and "breathing"; the "s" is absorbed into the "x" in the latter term. The process of measuring breath is termed spirometry. Incentive spirometry is the therapeutic technique of improving the volume of breath. Incentive spirometry is commonly used in postoperative care to prevent atelectasis. A respirator literally is something that causes one to breathe again. The literal meaning of the terms aspirate and aspiration are somewhat misleading in respect to their medical usage. According to Taber's Medical Dictionary, aspiration in medicine has the following meanings: (i) the act of breathing; (ii) the inhalation of fluid or solid objects into the lower airways or lungs; (iii) withdrawal of fluid from a cavity by suctioning with an aspirator. Only number one fits the Latin meaning of *aspirare*, "to breath upon." It is important to bear in mind that the root SPIR- is a homomorph because the Greek root for "coil" or "coil-like" (Gr. *speira*, coil) shares the same spelling. Hence, a spirochaete is a genus of spiral-shaped, motile bacteria.

The Latin root **HAL-** in inhalation (breathing in) and exhalation (breathing out) means "breath" or "breathing." Halitus is a loan word from Latin that means "breath" or a "warm vapor" in medical English. Halitosis, the term for "bad breath," was coined in 1874, using the Latin *halitus*. Consequently, halitophobia is a fear of bad breath.

Anapnea – Formed from the prefix for "again," **ANA-**, anapnea is another term for respiration.

Eupnea – Formed from the prefix for "good," **EU-**, eupnea is normal breathing.

Dyspnea – Formed from the prefix for "faulty," **DYS-**, dyspnea is difficulty with breathing.

Apnea – Formed from the prefix for "not," **A-**, apnea is the inability to breathe for a period of time.

Tachypnea – Formed from the root for "fast," **TACHY-**, tachypnea is a rapid rate of respiration.

Bradypnea – Formed from the root for "slow," **BRADY-**, bradypnea is a slow rate of respiration.

Polypnea – Formed from the root for "many," **POLY-**, polypnea is the technical term for panting.

Hyperpnea – Formed from the prefix for "excessive," **HYPER-**, hyperpnea is breathing that is deeper than usual.

Hyponea – Formed from the prefix for "deficient," **HYPO-**, hypopnea is a decreased depth of breathing.

Orthopnea – Formed from the root for "upright," **ORTH-**, orthopnea is the condition in which one is able to breathe in an upright position but not in a flat position.

Platypnea – Formed from the root for "flat," **PLATY-**, platypnea is the condition in which one is able to breathe in a flat position but not in an upright position.

Air and other gases

Air – The root for air is **AER-**. The root **AER-** can be used for a variety of gases in the atmosphere. Thus, an aeroembolism literally is a moving clot that is composed of air, but the medical definition in Taber's is "a condition in which nitrogen bubbles form in body fluids and tissues due to an excessively rapid decrease in atmospheric pressure." Often, the root is used for the key gaseous element of life, oxygen. For instance, the root in "aerobic" and "aerobe" refers to oxygen; the **-BIC** and **-OBE** in the aforenoted words are derived from the Greek word for "life," *bios*. The root **BIO-** is often used in medicine for life/living organisms. For instance, an antibiotic is a medication used against "living" organisms called bacteria.

The roots based on the Greek word *pneuma, pneumatos* no longer carry the meaning of "breath" or "breath of life." The root **PNEUMAT-** is typically used for "wind," "gas," and "air," but on rare instances it can mean "respiration." Hence, pneumatology is the study of gases, and apneumatic refers to something without air. Owing to the use of the nominative of *pneumon* and *pneuma*, the root **PNEUM-** is a homomorph that can mean "lung" when it is derived from *pneumon*, but "wind," "gas," and "air" when it is derived from *pneuma*.

There are a variety of Greek and Latin word elements used for gases and atmospheric elements. The root **ATM-** is used for "vapor," "air," or "gas." It appears in words such as atmosphere, atmotherapy, and atmolysis. The root **PHYS-** means "air," "gas," or "air bubble." Thus, a physometra is air in the uterus. A physocele is a swelling caused by a gas. The root **ANEM-** is used for "wind," and therefore, an anemometer measures wind, and anemoclastic rocks are shaped by the fracturing forces of the wind. Derived from the Latin *nebula*, the root **NEBUL-** means cloud, cloud-like, and mist. The loan word **nebula** is used for the haziness on the cornea, cloudiness in the urine, and the substance used in an atomizer. A device for producing a fine spray or mist is called a nebulizer.

Oxygen – One of the fundamental gases of respiration is oxygen. This gaseous element of life was called "oxygen" in 1790 by Antoine-Laurent Lavoisier (1743–1794) because he erroneously believed that oxygen was essential in the formation of acids. Based on modern and ancient Greek meanings, the root **OXY-** can mean "oxygen," "acid," "sharp," "acute," or "rapid." While **OXY-** can mean oxygen, root **OX-** is more commonly used for oxygen. This can be seen in terms such as hypoxemia, which is a deficient amount of oxygen in the blood, and hypoxia, which is a deficient amount of oxygen in the tissue.

Carbon dioxide – The other fundamental gas of respiration is carbon dioxide. It received this name in 1869 because it consists of one carbon and two oxygen atoms. The roots **CAPN-** and **CARB-** are used for "carbon dioxide." Thus, hypercarbia and hypercapnia are synonyms in medical terminology because they both mean excessive carbon dioxide in the blood. The same can be said for hypocarbia and hypocapnia, which are terms for low amounts of carbon dioxide in the blood. That said, in addition to carbon dioxide, **CARB-** can also mean "carbon," and the root **CAPN-** can also mean "smoke."

Greek or Latin word element	Current usage	Etymology	Examples
PNE/O (nē-ō) -PNOEA (p-nē-ă) -PNEA (p-nē-ă)	Breath, breathing	Gr. *pnoia, pnoe,* breath, fr. *pneein,* to breath	**Pne**ocardiac, eu**pnea**
TACHY- (tak-ĭ) TACH/O (tak-ō)	Rapid, quick, speed	Gr. *tachys,* fast; *tachos,* speed	**Tachy**pnea, **tachi**stoscope
BRADY- (brăd-ĭ)	Slow	Gr. *bradys,* slow	**Brady**pnea, **brady**cardia
ORTH/O (or-thō)	Upright, straight, correct, normal	Gr. *orthos,* straight	**Ortho**pnea, **orth**orexia
PLATY- (plă-tĭ) PLAT/O (plă-tō)	Flat, broad	Gr. *platys,* wide, broad	**Platy**pnea, **platy**pod
POLY- (pŏl-ĭ)	Many, much	Gr. *polys,* many, much	**Poly**pnea, co**poly**mer
SPIR/O (spī-rō) SPIRAT/O (s-pĭ-răt-ō)	Breath, breathing	L. *spirare, spiratum,* to breathe, blow	**Spir**ometer, re**spirat**or
HAL/O (hăl-ō) HALIT/O (hăl-ĭ-tō)	Breath, breathing	L. *halare, halitum,* to breathe	In**hal**er, **halit**osis Loan word: **Halitus** (hal'ĭt-ŭs)
PNEUM/O (nū-mō) PNEUMAT/O (nū-măt-ō)	Wind, gas, air	Gr. *pneuma, pneumatos,* a breeze, breath, spirit	**Pneum**arthrosis, **pneumat**ocele
CARB/O (kăr-bō) CARBON/O (kar-bŏ-nō)	Carbon dioxide, carbon	L. *carbo, carbonis,* m. charcoal	**Carb**ohydrate, **carbon**ate
CAPN/O (kap-nō)	Carbon dioxide, smoke	Gr. *kapnos,* smoke	Hyper**capn**ia, **capn**ophobia
OXY- (ŏk-sē) OX/O (ŏk-sō)	Oxygen, acid, sharp, acute, rapid	Gr. *oxys,* acid, keen, sharp	**Oxy**phil, an**ox**ia

Greek or Latin word element	Current usage	Etymology	Examples
AER/O (ar-ō)	Air	Gr. *aer*, lower air, air	**Aer**obe, an**aer**obic
AETHER/O (ĕth-ĕr-ō) **ETHER/O** (ĕth-ĕr-ō)	Ether	Gr. *aither*, upper air, ether fr. *aithein*, to kindle, light, burn	**Ether**ize, **ether**eal
PHYS/O (fī-sō)	Air, gas, air bubble	Gr. *physa*, bellows, wind, air bubble; related to *physema*, that which is produced by blowing	**Phys**ometra, em**phys**ema
ATM/O (at-mō)	Vapor, air, gas	Gr. *atmos*, steam, vapor	**Atm**osphere, **atm**olyzer
NEBUL/O (neb-yŭ-lō)	Cloud, cloud-like, mist	L. *nebula*, -*ae*, f. cloud, mist	**Nebul**izer, **nebul**ous Loan word: **Nebula** (nĕb′ū-lă) pl. **Nebulae** (nĕb′ū-lī)
ANEM/O (a-nĕ-mō)	Wind	Gr. *anemos*, wind	**Anem**ometer, **anem**oclastic

Review	Answers
Derived from the Greek verb *pneein* "to breath," the suffixes _____ and _____ are used for "breathing" and "breath." Thus, respiration is _____pnea; normal breathing is _____pnea; painful or faulty breathing is _____pnea; the inability to breathe for short periods of time is _____pnea; rapid breath rate is _____pnea; slow breath rate is _____pnea; panting is _____pnea; being able to breathe in an upright position but not in a flat position is termed _____pnea; and the ability to breathe in a flat position but not in an upright position is _____pnea. Breathing that is deeper than that usually experienced during normal activity is termed _____pnea. A decreased rate and depth of breathing is termed _____pnea.	**-PNEA, -PNOEA** **ana, eu, dys, a, tachy, brady, poly, ortho, platy, hyper, hypo**
The root SPIR-, as in inspiration and expiration, means _____ and _____. The process of measuring breath is termed _____.	**breath, breathing spirometry**
The root PNEUMAT- means _____, _____, and _____. The root PNEUM- is a homomorph that can mean _____ when it is derived from *pneumon* but _____, _____, and _____ when it is derived from *pneuma*.	**gas, air, wind lung, gas, air, wind**
Hypercarbia and hypercapnia are used similarly in medical terminology in that they both mean excessive _____ in the blood. That said, in addition to carbon dioxide, the root in hypercarbia can also mean _____ and the root in hypercapnia can also mean_____.	**carbon dioxide carbon, smoke**
OXY- can mean _____, _____, _____, _____, or _____. The root OX- typically only refers to _____. This can be seen in terms such as hypoxemia, which is a deficient amount of _____ in the blood, and hypoxia, which is a deficient amount of_____ in the tissue. Similarly, pulse oximetry is the _____ of the percentage of oxygen at the site of an arterial pulse.	**oxygen, acid, sharp, acute, rapid oxygen, oxygen, oxygen measuring**
The combining form in atmosphere and atmolysis means _____, _____, or _____.	**vapor, gas, air**
Based on its combining form, an anemometer measures the _____.	**wind**
The combining form in physometra literally means that there is an _____, _____, or _____ in the uterus.	**air bubble, air, gas**
An _____embolism literally is a moving clot that is composed of air. The medical definition is "a condition in which nitrogen bubbles form in body fluids and tissues due to an excessively rapid decrease in atmospheric pressure."	**aero**
The term for anesthetizing someone with the gas ether can be spelled _____ize or _____ize depending on whether one is using an American or a British spelling.	**ether, aether**
The root in inhalation and exhalation means _____ or _____. Consequently, the term halitosis means bad _____, which is why halitophobia is a fear of bad _____.	**breath, breathing breath, breath**
A device for producing a fine spray or mist is called a nebulizer. Derived from the Latin *nebula*, the root NEBUL- means _____, _____, and _____. The loan word _____ is used for haziness on the cornea, cloudiness in the urine, and the substance used in an atomizer.	**Cloud, cloud-like, mist nebula**

Lessons from History: *Hippocratic Diagnosis and Treatment of Empyema*

Food for Thought as You Read:

> *What are some of the features of diagnosing and treating an empyema in Disease II?*
> *What role does auscultation fit into the diagnosis of empyema?*
> *In what important ways does Laënnec's approach to auscultation differ from the ancient Greek medical approach?*

An empyema is an effusion of pus into a body cavity. One of the more common varieties of empyema is empyema thoracis, which is also called a pyothorax and is an effusion of pus into the pleural space. Empyema thoracis is typically caused by bacterial suppuration of an organ, particularly the lungs (Fig. 9.11).

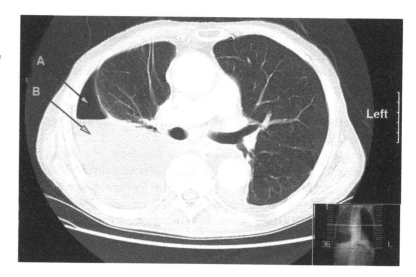

Fig. 9.11 CT transection of the thoracic space. Image and description from Drriad: "Arrow A- air, B- Fluid. Large hydro-pneumothorax, unilocular, some pleural thickening. Appearance suggestive of empyema. Associated collapse of right lung. Air in this patient is iatrogenic, from introduction of previous chest drain. Permission obtained from patient." *Source:* I, Drriad / Wikimedia Commons / CC BY-SA 3.0.

The below passage is taken from Hippocrates, *Disease II*, and it is part of a much longer account of how to diagnose and treat what the author calls *peripleumonia*. The original diagnosis seems to be based on the patient having a fever, violent coughing, and pyoptysis (expectorating pus). The author notes that the pus has become internal (*empyos*), which he sees as an important transition in this disease. The author relates the symptoms to specific days in order to suggest that the progression of the disease follows a recognizable pattern. The initial course of treatment is a regimen of food and infusions of medicaments, with the goal of moving and expectorating the pus from the lungs.

> ...When the fifteenth day after the pus has broken out into the cavity arrives, wash this patient in copious hot water, and seat him on a chair that does not move; have someone else hold his arms, and you shake him by the shoulders, listening on which of his sides there is a sound; prefer to incise on the left side, for it is less dangerous. If, because of the thickness and abundance of pus, there is no sound for you to hear – for sometimes this happens – on whichever side there is swelling and more pain, make an incision as low down as possible, behind the swelling rather than in front of it, in order that the exit you make for the pus will allow freedom of flow. First cut the skin between the ribs with a bellied scalpel; then wrap a lancet with a piece of cloth, leaving the point of the blade exposed a length equal to the nail of your thumb, and insert it. When you have removed as much pus as you think appropriate, plug the wound with a tent of raw linen, and tie it with a cord; draw off pus once a day; on the tenth day, draw all the pus, and plug the wound with linen. Then make an infusion of warm wine and oil with a tube, in order that the lung, accustomed to being soaked in pus, will not be suddenly dried out; discharge the morning infusion towards evening, and the evening one in the morning. When the pus is thin like water, sticky when touched with a finger, and small in amount, insert a hollow tin drainage tube. When the cavity is completely dried out, cut off the tube little by little, and let the ulcer unite before you remove the tube. A sign whether the patient is going to escape: if the pus is white and clean, and contains streaks of blood, he generally recovers; but if it flows out on the first day yolk-colored, or on the following day thick, slightly yellow-green, and stinking, when it has flowed out the patient dies.
>
> Hippocrates, *Diseases II* L. VII.171, trans. Potter pp. 242–245, Loeb V.

The above passage begins with a reassessment of the patient after 15 days. The passage reveals that **auscultation**, listening to internal sounds of the body, was one of the practices that ancient Greek physicians used to determine the nature of a disease in the thoracic cavity. The author discusses putting his ear up to the patient and listing to the thorax while the patient is being shook. In this passage, the physician's auscultation helps to determine which side to treat. This technique is in some respects similar to modern auscultation methods such as percussion since the goal is to determine the solidity of the effused material.

The root **AUSCULTAT-**, derived from the Latin verb *auscultare*, to listen, is used in the terms **auscultate** and **auscultation**. Modern **auscultation** is the "listening" to sounds of the body with a **stethoscope**. The term "stethoscope" is derived from its inventor, the famous French physician René Laënnec (1781–1826). Laënnec provides an account of how he came to invent the stethoscope in his book *De l'Auscultation Médiate*, which was published in August 1819:

> In 1816, I was consulted by a young woman laboring under general symptoms of diseased heart, and in whose case percussion and the application of the hand were of little avail on account of the great degree of fatness. The other method just mentioned [direct auscultation] being rendered inadmissible by the age and sex of the patient, I happened to recollect a simple and well-known fact in acoustics, ... the great distinctness with which we hear the scratch of a pin at one end of a piece of wood on applying our ear to the other. Immediately, on this suggestion, I rolled a quire of paper into a kind of cylinder and applied one end of it to the region of the heart and the other to my ear, and was not a little surprised and pleased to find that I could thereby perceive the action of the heart in a manner much clearer and more distinct than I had ever been able to do by the immediate application of my ear.

Based on this "discovery," Laënnec would go on to create a device that looked much like a telescope, which he later called the stethoscope. The device could be broken down, making it more portable. Using his new device, he investigated the sounds made by the heart and lungs inside the chests of patients, and later, he confirmed his findings by performing autopsies of the patients who passed away. Laënnec published *De L'auscultation Mediate* (On Mediate Auscultation) in 1819, and it quickly became a very influential text for the practice of medicine, making Laënnec's auscultation a fundamental tool for the physical examination of patients. Etymologically speaking, the term stethoscope is a bit of a misnomer since the word element -**SCOPE** implies one is using a device to "look" rather than "listen." (Fig. 9.12)

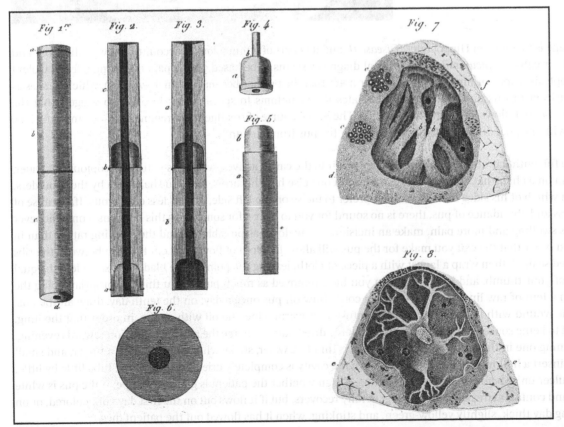

Fig. 9.12 Diagram of the stethoscope in Laennec's *De l'auscultation médiate, ou traité du diagnostic des maladies des poumons et du cœur, fondé principalement sur ce nouveau moyen d'exploration*, 1826. *Source:* Par R.T.H. Laennec/Wellcome Collection/Public domain.

Some breathing sounds have specific names. The snoring or snorting sound with laborious breathing heard during auscultation is called a **stertor**. The wheezing, snoring, or squeaking sound heard during auscultation is called **rhonchu**s, which consequently is also called a **wheeze** (Old Norse *hvoesa*, to hiss). A high-pitched, harsh sound occurring during inspiration heard during auscultation is called **stridor**. Popping sounds heard with inhalation are called **rales**. Derived from the suffixes meaning "voice" **-PHONY** and **-LOQUY**, the distinct transmission of vocal sounds during auscultation of the chest is called **pectoriloquy** or **pectorophony**. **PHON-** is a common root used for "voice" and "sound." For instance, a phonocardiogram is a record of heart sounds. **PHON-** commonly appears as the compound suffix **-PHONIA**. A rough-sounding voice or hoarseness is called **dysphonia** or **trachyphonia**.

The ability to see inside the respiratory tract is a great benefit to modern medicine, and today there are a wide variety of ways in which to visually examine the respiratory system. An **endoscope** is literally a device for viewing/looking inside the body. The process of looking inside the nose and throat with a flexible tube is called nasopharyngoscopy. A bronchoscope is a device used to look at the bronchi. Looking into the thorax using an endoscope is called a thoracoscopy. A pulmonary angiography is an X-ray imaging of the pulmonary vessels that is used to identify a pulmonary embolism. **CT** stands for **computed tomography**. The **TOM-** in tomography means "to cut." A CT is an X-ray scan that produces sectional anatomic images.

Turning back to the aforementioned Hippocratic discussion of empyema, the ancient surgical intervention used to treat this condition called for the cutting of an opening to gain access to the thoracic space. This procedure provides the physician with the ability to drain the pus and introduce medicaments into the cavity. The purpose of some of the medicaments was to mediate against a drastic change in the environment of the lungs so that the lungs do not dry out, immediately causing damage to these organs. In some respects, the pouring of wine and oil in the tube is similar to a lavage, a washing out of a cavity. Today, we use the suffix **-CLYSIS** for the lavage of a cavity. While rational by the standards of its day, the Hippocratic surgical procedure most likely did much more harm than good. Given ancient Greek physicians had no idea about bacterial infection, it is quite likely that they introduced more bacteria into the pleural space. What is worse, creating such a stoma would probably create a pneumothorax, leaving the patient worse off than before the heroic measure was taken.

Similar to Hippocratic treatment for empyema, one of the modern treatments for pleural effusion is to perform a surgical puncture and aspiration of the pleural space, which is called a **thoracocentesis**. Another is to create an opening, which is also called a **stoma**, and then insert a drainage tube. This surgery is called a **thoracostomy**. That said, the surgical techniques and aftercare used today are based on the understanding of how this type of surgery can create a pneumothorax.

Suggested Readings

Duffin, Jacalyn. *To See with a Better Eye: The life of R.T.H. Laennec.* Princeton: Princeton University Press, 1998.
Hippocrates. *Affections. Diseases 1. Diseases 2.* Translated by Paul Potter. Loeb Classical Library 472. Cambridge: Harvard University Press, 1988.
Laennec, R. T. H. *A Treatise on the Diseases of the Chest and on Mediate Auscultation.* Translated by John Forbes and W. J. Kelson Millard. Facsim. of the London, 1821 ed. New York: Hafner, 1962.
Stefanakis, Georgios et al. "Hippocratic concepts of acute and urgent respiratory diseases still relevant to contemporary medical thinking and practice: a scoping review." *BMC Pulmonary Medicine* 20, no. 1 (2020): 165.

Etymological Explanations: Pathologies of the Respiratory System

The following is a summary of some of the modern diagnostic and symptomatic terms for respiratory pathologies.

Signs and symptoms
Mucus – Fluids associated with the respiratory tract are mucus, phlegm, and sputum. The mucus is a viscid fluid secreted by mucous membranes and glands. The roots used for this fluid are **MUC-** and **BLENN-**.
Phlegm – Derived from one of the Greek terms for humor, phlegm is a thick mucus of the respiratory tract. The root of this word is **PHLEGMAT-**. Owing to its similarity, it is easily confused with the root **PHLEGMON-**. The latter combining form is used for "inflammation."
Sputum – Phlegm expelled from the lung by coughing is called sputum, which is a Latin loan word for "spit." The root for sputum is **SPUT-**.

Expectoration – Expectoration is the spitting of saliva or coughing up of material from the respiratory tract. The Greek root for "saliva" is **PTYAL-**. The suffix used for "spitting" is **-PTYSIS**. Thus, the expectoration of blood is hemoptysis, and the expectoration of pus is pyoptysis.

Dysphonia/Trachyphonia – Trachyphonia and dysphonia are both used for "a roughness or hoarseness of the voice."

Rhinorrhea – Derived from the suffix for "discharge," **-RRHEA**, rhinorrhea (or runny nose) is a thin, watery discharge from the nose.

Epistaxis – Formed from the suffix for "dripping" or "oosing," **-STAXIS**, epistaxis is a nosebleed. Likewise, bleeding inside of the walls of the bronchus is called a bronchostaxis.

Inflammations of the respiratory system

Sinusitis – Formed from the root for a "fold" or "sinus," **SINUS-**, sinusitis is an inflammation of the **sinuses**. Recall that the upper respiratory tract ends at the larynx and the lower respiratory tract begins at the trachea. Upper respiratory infections (URI or URTI) and lower respiratory infections (LRI or LRTI) are often denoted with the suffix for inflammation, **-ITIS**.

Rhinitis – Formed from the Greek root for "nose," **RHIN-**, rhinitis is an inflammation of the nasal passages, often associated with the common cold.

Pharyngitis – Formed from the Greek root for "throat," **PHARYNG-**, pharyngitis is an inflammation of the pharynx (or throat).

Laryngitis – Formed from the Greek root for "voice box," **LARYNG-** is an inflammation of the larynx (or voice box).

Tracheitis – Formed from the Latin root for the "trachea," **TRACHE-**, tracheitis is an inflammation of the trachea.

Bronchitis – Formed from the Greek root for "bronchus," **BRONCH-**, bronchitis is an inflammation of the airways known as the bronchi.

Pneumonitis – Formed from the Greek root for "lung," **PNEUMON-**, pneumonitis is an inflammation of the lungs, usually due to hypersensitivity to an allergen.

Pneumonia – Pneumonia is an inflammation of the lungs due to a bacterial, viral, or fungal infection.

Pleurisy or Pleuritis – Another term for pleurisy, which is an inflammation of the pleura, is pleuritis.

Types of respiratory pathologies

Effusion – An effusion is an accumulation of a gas or fluid into a cavity. The root **FUS-** in this word means "pour" or "melting." As noted earlier, pathological terms that denote an effusion are recognizable by a root or combining form for a fluid or gas being joined to a term for a cavity (e.g. **-THORAX**). For instance, an effusion of blood into the thorax, or more specifically the pleural space, is a hemothorax; an effusion of air into the pleural space is a pneumothorax; and an effusion of pus into this space is a pyothorax, which is also called empyema, based on the ancient Greek pathological term (Fig. 9.13).

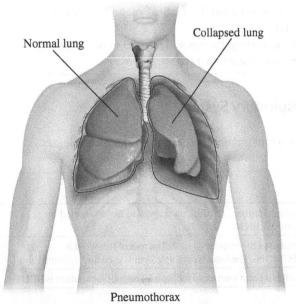

Fig. 9.13 Image of Pneumothorax. *Source:* From Blausen.com staff, 2014/Blausen Medical/CC BY-SA 4.0.

Pneumoconiosis – Pneumoconiosis is a restrictive disorder. A restrictive pulmonary disorder limits the intake of air into the lungs. The root **PNEUM-** in this term, means "lung" and the root **CONI-** means "dust." Any disease of the respiratory tract that is caused by the inhalation of dust particles could be called pneumoconiosis. The dust particles cause fibrotic tissue to form around the alveoli, restricting their ability to expand with inhalation.

Emphysema – Emphysema is a chronic obstructive pulmonary disorder (COPD). An obstructive pulmonary disorder blocks the flow of air moving into the lungs. The term comes from the Greek word *emphysema*, which means "inflation." Emphysema is a disease caused by an abnormal increase in the size of alveoli, which causes them to lose the elasticity necessary for proper exhalation. The root **PHYS-** in this term, means "air," "gas," and "air bubble." Other causes of COPD are chronic obstructive bronchitis, chronic bronchitis, and asthmatic bronchitis (Fig. 9.14).

Fig. 9.14 Image of Emphysema. Modified image, *source:* From Blausen.com staff, 2014/Blausen Medical/CC BY-SA 4.0.

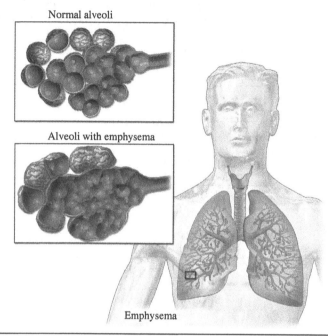

Normal alveoli

Alveoli with emphysema

Emphysema

Asthma – The disorder named after the Greek word for "panting, shortness of breath" is asthma, and its root is **ASTHMAT-**. As defined by Taber, asthma is an inflammatory disorder of the respiratory tract that causes periodic obstruction of airflow, usually in response to an allergen, a chemical irritant, an infection, or physical stimuli such as cold air or exercise. Obstruction of airflow is due to bronchospasms and excessive production of mucus. Patients will present with episodic wheezing, shortness of breath, and a cough. A prolonged state of an attack of asthma is called status asthmaticus.

Tuberculosis (TB) – TB is an infectious disease caused by the bacteria *Mycobacterium tuberculosis*. TB usually affects the lungs, but it can spread to other organs where it can cause caseous necrosis. Pulmonary TB produces chronic cough, sputum, fevers, sweating, and weight loss. TB gets its name from the characteristic tubercles that are present in the lungs. Consequently, the root **TUBERCUL-** is used for TB. The term tubercle is a diminutive of the Latin word *tuber*, which means "hump," "knob," and "swelling." Originally, TB could be used in reference to any disease characterized by tubercules. Thanks to the discovery of the *Mycobacterium tuberculosis* in 1882 by the German bacteriologist Robert Koch (1843–1910), TB is restricted to the disease caused by this type of bacterium. The ancient Greek term *phthisis* originally meant any "wasting" disease. It is still commonly used as a loan word and suffix for TB, **-PHTHISIS**. For example, nephrophthisis is TB of the kidneys and laryngophthisis is TB of the larynx (Fig. 9.15).

Fig. 9.15 "An anteroposterior X-ray of a patient diagnosed with advanced bilateral pulmonary tuberculosis. This AP X-ray of the chest reveals the presence of bilateral pulmonary infiltrate (white triangles) and "caving formation" (black arrows) present in the right apical region. The diagnosis is far-advanced tuberculosis." *Source:* Unknown author/Wikimedia Commons/Public domain.

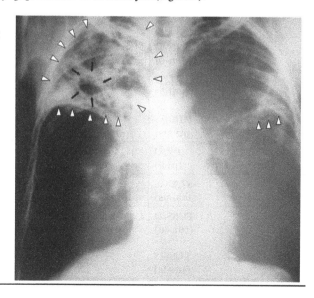

Atelectasis – A collapsed lung or an unexpanded lung of a fetus is called atelectasis. The suffixes **-ECTASIA** and **-ECTASIS** are used for "expansion" or "dilation." The **ATEL-** means "incomplete" or "imperfect." Thus, the abnormal expansion of the bronchus would be termed bronchiectasis.

Bronchospasm – **An** involuntary contraction of a bronchus is a bronchospasm, which is a constriction of the smooth muscles of the bronchi. An involuntary contraction of any muscle is often termed a spasm. **-SPASM** can be used as a suffix, as in bronchospasm. It can also be used as a root **SPASM-**. Thus, a spasmodic hiccup is called spasmolygmus (Gr. *lygmos*, hiccup, sob).

Pertussis – Whooping cough is also called pertussis. As noted in *Tabers' Cyclopedic Medical Dictionary*, pertussis is "an acute, contagious disease characterized by paroxysmal coughing, vomiting that follows the cough, and whooping inspiration." The root **TUSS-** in this term means "cough." Thus, an antitussive is a medication for "coughing."

Croup – Croup is an acute viral disease usually occurring from age 6 months to 5 years. It is recognized by a barking cough that is described as sounding "seal-like" and stridor, which is a high-pitched, harsh sound occurring during inspiration heard during auscultation. Croup is also called laryngotracheobronchitis, which indicates that it is an inflammation of the larynx, trachea, and bronchi.

Greek or Latin word element	Current usage	Etymology	Examples
AUSCULTAT/O (os-kŭl-tāt-ō)	To listen	L. *auscultare, auscultatum*, to listen to	**Auscultat**ion, **acuscultat**ory
PHON/O (fō-nō) **-PHONY** (fō-nē)	Voice, sound	Gr. *phone*, voice, sound	Tracheo**phony**, **phon**ograph
-LOQUY (lō-kwē)	Voice, speech	L. *loqui*, to speak	Pectori**loquy**, bronchi**loquy**
SPUT/O (spū-tō)	Sputum, spit	L. *sputum, -i*, n. spit	**Sput**ative, **sput**ation Loan word: **Sputum** (spūt′ŭm) pl. **Sputa** (spūt′ă)
PHLEGMAT/O (fleg-ma-tō)	Phlegm	Gr. *Phlegm*, a type of humor	**Phlegmat**ic, **phlegmat**ism Loan word: **Phlegm** (flem)
PHLEGMON/O (flĕg-mŏn-ō)	Inflammation	Gr. *phlegmasia; phlegmone*, inflammation	**Phlegmon**ous Loan word: **Phlegmon** (flĕg′mŏn)
MUC/O (mū-kō)	Mucus	L. *mucus, -i*, m. mucus	**Muc**ous, **muc**olytic Loan word: **Mucus** (mū′kŭs)
BLENN/O (blĕn-ō)	Mucus	Gr. *blennos*, mucus	**Blenn**ogenic, **blenn**adenitis
PTYAL/O (tī-ăl-ō) **-PTYSIS** (-ptĭ-sĭs)	Spit, spitting	Gr. *ptyein*, to spit	Hypo**ptyal**ism, hemo**ptysis** Loan word: Ptysis (tī′sĭs)
PY/O (pī-ō)	Pus	Gr. *pyon*, pus	**Py**othorax, em**py**ema
-STAXIS (stăk-sĭs)	A dripping/oozing of blood	Gr. *staxis*, a dripping of blood	Epi**staxis**, broncho**staxis**
TUSS/O (tŭs-sō) **-TUSSIS** (tŭs-ĭs)	Cough, coughing	L. *tussis, -is*, a cough	Anti**tuss**ive, per**tussis** Loan word: **Tussis** (tŭs′ĭs)

Greek or Latin word element	Current usage	Etymology	Examples
CONI/O (kŏ-nē-ō)	Dust	Gr. *konis, konios,* dust	Pneumono**coni**osis, **coni**ofibrosis
ASTHM/O (az-mō)	Asthma	Gr. *asthma, asthmatos,* panting, shortness of breath	Anti**asthmat**ic, **asthm**ogenic Loan word: **Asthma** (az′mă)
ASTHMAT/O (az-mă-tō)			
PHTHISI/O (thĭ-sĭ-ō)	Wasting, tuberculosis (TB)	Gr. *phthisis,* a wasting	**Phthisi**ogenesis, nephro**phthisis** Loan word: **Phthisis** (thĭ′sĭs)
-PHTHISIS (-f-thĭ-sĭs)			
TUBERCUL/O (tū-bĕr-kū-lō)	Tubercle, TB	L. *tuberculus, -i,* m. a little swelling, tubercle	**Tubercul**ocele, **tubercul**osis
ATEL/O (at-ĕl-ō)	Incomplete, imperfect	Gr. *ateles,* without end	**Atel**ectasis, **atel**ocardia
-ECTASIS (ek-tă-sĭs)	Dilation, expansion	Gr. *ektasis,* stretching out	Atel**ectasis**, telangi**ectasia** Loan word: **Ectasis** (ek-tă-sĭs)
-ECTASIA (ek-tă-zhē-ă)			
SPASM/O (spaz-mō)	Spasm	Gr. *spasmos,* a wrenching	Broncho**spasm**, phreno**spasm**, **spasm**odic
-SPASM (spazm)			Loan word: **Spasm**
FUS/O (fū-zō)	Pour, melt	L. *fundere, fusum,* to pour, melt L. *effusio, -onis,* a pouring forth	Ef**fus**ion, per**fus**ion,

Review	Answers
Pneumoconiosis is a restrictive lung disorder because it limits the intake of air into the lungs. The combining form in this term means _____ and the root means _____. Any disease of the respiratory tract that is caused by the inhalation of dust particles could be called pneumoconiosis. The dust particles cause fibrotic tissue to form around the alveoli, restricting their ability to expand with inhalation.	**lung, dust**
Emphysema is an obstructive lung disorder because it blocks the flow of air moving out of the lungs. The term comes from the Greek word *emphysema,* which means "inflation." The root PHYS- in this term means _____, _____, and _____. Emphysema is a disease caused by an abnormal increase in the size of alveoli, which causes them to lose the elasticity necessary for proper exhalation.	**Air, gas, air bubble**
The disorder named after the Greek word for "panting, shortness of breath" is _____ and its root is _____. As defined by Taber, asthma is an inflammatory disorder of the respiratory tract that causes periodic obstruction of airflow, usually in response to an allergen, a chemical irritant, an infection, or physical stimuli such as cold air or exercise. A prolonged state of an attack of asthma is called status asthmaticus.	**asthma, ASTHMAT-**
An effusion is an accumulation of a gas or fluid into a cavity. The root FUS- in this word means _____ or _____. As noted earlier, pathological terms that denote an effusion are recognizable by a root or combining form for fluid or gas being joined to a term for a cavity. For instance, an effusion of blood into the thorax, or more specifically the pleural space, is a _____ thorax; an effusion of air into the pleural space is a _____ thorax; and an effusion of pus into this space is a _____ thorax, which is also called empyema based on the ancient Greek pathological term.	**pour, melt** **hemo, pneumo, pyo**
One of the modern treatments for pleural effusion is to perform a surgical puncture and aspiration of the pleural space, which is called a thoraco_____. Another is to create an opening, which is also called a stoma, and then insert a drainage tube. This surgery is called thoraco_____. The looking into the thorax using an endoscope is called a _____scopy	**centesis** **stomy** **thoraco**
The surgical incision into the trachea for the purpose of removing a foreign body is called a _____ tomy. The creation of a surgical opening/mouth in the trachea is called a tracheo_____.	**tracheo** **stomy**

Review	Answers
The ancient Greek term *phthisis* originally meant _____ disease. It is still commonly used as a loan word and root for TB. For example, nephrophthisis is TB of the kidneys and _____phthsis is TB of the larynx.	**wasting** **laryngo**
TB gets its name from the characteristic granulomata (tubercles) that are present in the lungs due to the bacteria *Mycobacterium tuberculosis*. Consequently, the root _____ is used for TB. The term tubercle is a diminutive of the Latin word *tuber*, which means "hump," "knob," and "swelling."	**TUBERCUL-**
Recall that the upper respiratory tract ends at the larynx and the lower respiratory tract begins at the trachea. Upper respiratory infections (URI) and lower respiratory infections (LRI) are often denoted with the suffix for inflammation, -ITIS. Thus, an inflammation of the sinuses is _____itis; an inflammation of the tonsils is _____itis; an inflammation of the nose is _____itis; an inflammation of the bronchi is _____itis; an inflammation of the lungs is _____itis; an inflammation of the throat is _____ itis; an inflammation of the trachea is _____itis; and an inflammation of the voice box is _____itis. Pneumonia is also an inflammation of the lungs. Pneumonia differs from pneumonitis in that pneumonia is an inflammation due to bacterial, viral, or fungal infection, but pneumonitis is an inflammation due to hypersensitivity to chemicals or dust.	**sinus, tonsill,** **rhin, bronch,** **pneumon,** **pharyng, trache,** **laryng**
Another term for pleurisy, which is an inflammation of the pleura, is _____itis.	**Pleur**
Croup is also called laryngotracheobronchitis, which indicates that it is an inflammation of the _____, _____, and _____. It is recognized by a barking cough that is described as sounding "seal-like" and _____, which is a high-pitched, harsh sound occurring during inspiration heard during auscultation.	**larynx, trachea,** **and bronchi** **stridor**
The suffix forms _____ and _____ are used for "expansion" or "dilation." The abnormal expansion of the bronchus would be termed _____ ectasis. A collapsed lung or an unexpanded lung of a fetus is called atelectasis. The ATEL- means _____ or _____.	**-ECTASIA,** **-ECTASIS** **bronchi** **incomplete,** **imperfect**
An involuntary contraction of a muscle is termed a _____. -SPASM can be used as a suffix. Thus, an involuntary contraction of a bronchus is a broncho _____, which is a constriction of the smooth muscles of the bronchi. It can also be used as a root/combining form. Thus, a spasmodic hiccup is called a _____ lygmus (Gr. *lygmos*, hiccup, sob).	**spasm** **spasm** **spasmo**
Whooping cough is also called pertussis. As noted in Taber's, "pertussis is "an acute, contagious disease characterized by paroxysmal coughing, vomiting that follows the cough, and whooping inspiration." The root TUSS- in this term means _____. Thus, an antitussive is a medication for _____.	**cough** **coughing**
Formed from the suffix for "a dripping of blood," -STAXIS, the medical term for a nosebleed is _____. Likewise, a dripping of blood in a bronchus is termed broncho _____.	**epistaxis** **staxis**
Derived from one of the Greek terms for humor, _____ is a thick mucus of the respiratory tract. The combining form for this word is _____. Owing to its similarity, it is easily confused with the combining form PHLEGMON/O. The latter combining form is used for _____.	**phlegm** **PHLEGMAT/O** **inflammation**
The mucus is a viscid fluid secreted by mucous membranes and glands. The roots used for this fluid are _____ and _____. An _____ breaks up mucus and promotes coughing. Mucus expelled from the lung by coughing is called _____, which is a Latin loan word for "spit."	**MUC-, BLENN-** **expectorant** **sputum**
Expectoration is the spitting of saliva or coughing up of material from the respiratory tract. The Greek root for "saliva" is _____. The suffix used for "spitting" is _____. Thus, the expectoration of blood is _____ptysis, and the expectoration of pus is _____ptysis.	**PTYAL-** **-PTYSIS** **hemo, pyo**
Modern auscultation is the _____ to sounds of the body with a stethoscope, particularly with breathing. Some of the sounds have specific names. The snoring or snorting sound with laborious breathing heard during auscultation is called a _____. The wheezing, snoring, or squeaking sound heard during auscultation is called _____, which consequently is also called a wheeze (Old Norse *hvoesa*, to hiss). A high-pitched, harsh sound occurring during inspiration heard during auscultation is called _____. Popping sounds heard with inhalation are called rales. Derived from the suffixes meaning "voice," the distinct transmission of vocal sounds during auscultation of the chest is called pectori_____ or pectoro_____.	**listening** **stertor** **rhoncus** **stridor** **loquy, phony**
A rough sounding voice or hoarseness is called _____phonia or _____phonia.	**dys, trachy**
An endoscope literally is a device for _____ inside the body. The process of looking inside the nose and throat with a flexible tube is called _____scopy. A broncho_____ is a device used to look in the bronchi.	**viewing/looking** **nasopharyngo** **scope**
A pulmonary angiography is X-ray imaging of the pulmonary _____ that is used to identify a pulmonary embolism.	**vessels**
CT stands for computed tomography. The TOM- in tomography means _____. A CT is an X-ray scan that produces sectional anatomic images.	**cut/cutting**

10

Nervous System and Psychology

CHAPTER LEARNING OBJECTIVES

1) You will learn the word elements, loan words, and key terms associated with the nervous system and psychology.
2) You will become familiar with the historical concepts associated with ancient Greek ventricular theory and mental illnesses.

Lessons from History: Mental Faculties and the Ventricles Brain in Ancient Philosophy and Medicine

Food for Thought as You Read:

In what ways did ancient Greek concepts of "nature" and the "mental faculties" affect the way in which the anatomical structures of the brain were perceived?

In what ways do modern concepts of "nature" and "mental faculties" affect the way in which the anatomical structures of the brain are perceived?

Advancements in technology have contributed to a greater understanding of the anatomical locations of the mental faculties of the brain, which is commonly referred to as "brain mapping." Functional magnetic resonance imaging, also called an fMRI, creates images of brain functions by scanning the brain while a person is performing activities, such as listening to music. By showing which area is more active, the activity and the area of the brain are then "mapped." The electroencephalogram (EEG) has been used in neurofeedback studies, termed quantitative EEG analysis or EEG brain mapping, to monitor the electrical activities of parts of the cerebrum to determine what areas of the brain are playing a role in conditions such as ADHD, depression, and anxiety. However, such studies are not without issues with respect to methodology, measurement, and theory, and the tacit assumptions of cognitive researchers about the mind and its relationship to the body present numerous challenges not only to the locations of human cognitive and behavioral phenomena but also to its clinical applications.

Unlike modern brain mapping, which primarily focuses on the cerebrum as the locus of the higher brain functions, ancient Greek medicine focused on the ventricles of the brain as the location of the mental faculties in the brain. This ancient medical belief is rather striking given our modern conception of the ventricles as simply ependymal cavities that produce cerebral spinal fluid. The purpose of the following discussion of the ventricular theories in ancient medicine is to examine how assumptions about the mind–body relationship and nature led to influential but erroneous concepts as to the location of the mental faculties. Much of what I have to say here is derived from the writings of Phillip van der Eijk's work on Nemesius of Emesa.

> But since all the nerves throughout the body below the head arise from either the cerebellum (*parenkephalis*) or from the spinal cord (*notiaios myelos*), it was necessary for the ventricle (*koilia*) of the cerebellum to be of a respectable size and get a share of the psychic pneuma (*psychikon pneuma*) which had previously been prepared in the first ventricles (*prosthioai koiliai*).
>
> Galen, *De usu partium*, III.665

Greek and Latin Roots of Medical and Scientific Terminologies, First Edition. Todd A. Curtis.
© 2025 John Wiley & Sons, Inc. Published 2025 by John Wiley & Sons, Inc.
Companion website: www.wiley.com/go/Curtis

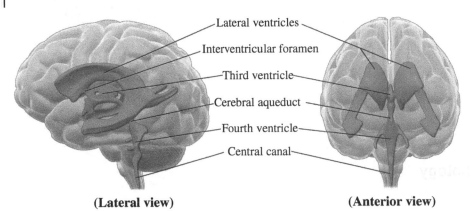

Fig. 10.1 Image of the four cerebral ventricles. *Source:* Adapted from Bruce Blausen, Medical Gallery of Blausen Medical 2014.

The above passage is taken from *On the Use of the Parts* (*De usu partium*), which is one of Galen's magna opera (great works) on human anatomy. Unlike some of his more technical anatomical writings that are geared towards actual dissection, such as *On Anatomical Administrations* (*De anatomicis administrationibus*), Galen's purpose for writing *On the Use of the Parts* is more philosophical. In this work, Galen uses his knowledge of anatomy to demonstrate how the form, location, and function of the parts of the human body reveal the providential character of Nature. It is important to bear in mind that when Galen claims that Nature does nothing in vain, his concept of Nature in many respects resembles Plato's Demiurge, which in Plato's *Timaeus* is a divine artisan-like figure who is responsible for fashioning the universe from pre-existing matter. Based in this conception of Nature, the main argument in the above passage is that the location of the ventricle (*koilia*) reveals that Nature has placed this ventricle close to the spinal cord (*notiaios myelos*) and cerebellum (*parenkephalis*) because it was the best place for the optimum function of the mental faculties. In modern medical and scientific terminology, the root **CELI-**, which is derived from the Greek word for a cavity, *koilia*, is typically used for "the abdominal cavity." The root **COEL-** (also spelled **CEL-**), which comes from the Greek word for "hollow," *koilos*, is used for any "cavity" or "hollow."

The ventricles of the brain were fundamental to Galen's anatomical explanation of the mental faculties in animals, particularly humans (Fig. 10.1). Why he did not focus on the cerebrum, or another prominent structure of the brain is perhaps due to the ventricles' central location in the brain and their hollowed-out appearance, which makes them appear to be of greater importance to the brain. Therefore, he theorized that the ventricles held the "psychic pneuma" (*psychikon pneuma*), which was important to the mental faculties of a human. As mentioned in Chapter 3, Galen understood *pneuma* as being an airy material that is the instrument of the soul. In Galenic physiology, the psychic pneuma is responsible for voluntary motion, sensation, as well as rational thought and memory. This psychic *pneuma* communicates sensation and voluntary motion to and from the ventricles through the spinal cord and the nerves. While Galen understood that there are four ventricles in the human brain, he referred to them differently than we do today. Galen spoke in terms of three ventricles in the brain: the anterior ventricle, the middle ventricle, and the posterior ventricle. What we term the first two ventricles, he generally lumped together and called them the anterior ventricle; our third ventricle appears to be his middle ventricle, and his so-called posterior ventricle is tantamount to the fourth ventricle in modern anatomy. Thus, in respect to the above passage in *On the Use of the Parts*, it makes sense for Nature to place the fourth ventricle close to the spinal cord and cerebellum since this ventricle would be able to better communicate with the body via the psychic pneuma in the nerves.

Galen's experiments on the ventricles of the brain reflect the same methodology and teleological approach to anatomy that he exhibits in many of his other anatomical works. In his descriptions of his experiments on living animals, he makes a distinction between the ventricles and their effect on the body. For example, in his *On the Opinions of Hippocrates and Plato* (*De placitis Hippocratis et Platonis*), he states the following:

> [Incising] the posterior ventricle harms the animal most, and next after that the middle ventricle. Incising each of the anterior ventricles causes less serious injury, but a greater degree in the older animals, a lesser degree in the young.
>
> Galen, *De placitis Hippocratis et Platonis*, V.605.

In regard to the Galen claim that the "harm" is caused by such an incision into the ventricle, Galen links this to a loss of sensation, motion, and consciousness, all of which the animal will potentially regain with the closure of the ventricle. A description of Galen's experiment on the ventricles can be found in *Anatomical Procedures* (IX.12). In *Anatomical Procedures*, he describes how he removed the dura mater from the brain and then made an incision into each of the ventricles. He notes that the incision would produce a degree of stupor in the animal. The stupor became more severe as he moved from the anterior to the posterior ventricle, noting that animals often did not recover from a cut to the posterior ventricle. Galen's experiment seems to suggest that the closer the ventricle is to the spinal cord, the more severe the loss of neurological function. While compression of the fourth ventricle has been shown to influence autonomic activity, it is unclear to what extent Galen's conclusions are derived from actual experimentation. It is conceivable that, via performing trepanation on humans or via the vivisection of animals, Galen may have arrived at some of these theories of the ventricles and the brain. However, Galen's experiment on the ventricles in *Anatomical Procedures* appears quite doubtful in my opinion. It appears to be a "thought experiment" that served to justify his preconceived understanding of the role of the ventricles in the body. Perhaps "experiment" is a misnomer since Galen does not appear to be using vivisection to find answers to questions about the body. While there is no doubt that Galen dissected dead and living animals and that he had a good understanding of anatomy, particularly for his time frame, here he seems to be using anatomy to justify his own anatomical and physiological theories.

One should bear in mind that Galen's focus on the ventricles of the brain is also part of the philosophical debate about the soul–body relationship. The location of the controlling part of the soul, which the Stoics referred to as the Hegimonikon, was of particular interest to philosophers. Aristotle and his followers argued that human thought and reason were located in the heart. This is somewhat surprising given Aristotle coined the Greek term word for the brain *enkephalos* (literally meaning "in the head") and he recognized that the mental faculties were disrupted by damage to the brain. Because Aristotle conceived of the brain's function as cooling the heart, he attributed the aforementioned phenomenon to the heart being affected by the brain in that the damaged brain was no longer able to cool the heart. Likewise, Stoic philosophers also put forward that the cognitive center of the soul was located in the chest rather than in the head. While it was common knowledge among anatomists that the brain was linked to mental faculties, such cardiocentric views persisted among these philosophical sects. Therefore, Galen used the ventricles as anatomical "proof" that the mental faculties are indeed located in the brain rather than the chest, and he goes on to claim that both Hippocrates and Plato held similar encephalocentric views in *On the Opinions of Hippocrates and Plato*.

Galen's ventricular theory was highly influential on subsequent theories about the location of the mental faculties. One reason for this may be that Galen's teleological approach to anatomy and his contextualization of Nature as a Demiurge was reconcilable to monotheistic views found among both religious and medical figures in Jewish, Christian, and Islamic societies. Galen's impact can be observed in our earliest example of brain mapping, which is found in the writings of Nemesius, who was a philosopher and Christian Bishop of Emesa. Writing in the 4th century AD, Nemesius wrote *On the Nature of Man* (*De natura hominis*), which was an influential work in both Christian theology and medicine. Pulling from theories found in ancient Greek philosophers and physicians, particularly Aristotle, Plato, Porphyry, and Galen, Nemesius argued that the human body and the faculties of the soul reveal humankind's place in the universe, particularly their relationship to God. Similar to Galen's teleological approach to anatomy in *On the Use of the Parts*, Nemesius argues that the parts of the human body reflect the work of a divine creator, and like Galen, Nemesius sees the ventricles and their relationship to psychic pneuma as evidence of the rationality of this creator. While his concept of psychic pneuma and the ventricles are Galenic, Nemesius' explanation goes further than Galen's by localizing specific mental faculties to each ventricle. He associates sensation and imagination with the anterior or "frontal cavities"; intellectual thought is in the middle cavity; and memory is located in the posterior cavity of the brain:

> If the frontal cavities are damaged in any way, the senses are impaired but thought remains unharmed. If the central cavity alone suffers, thought is overthrown but the sense-organs continue to preserve their natural power of sensation. If both the frontal and the central cavities suffer, reason is damaged together with the senses. But if the cerebellum suffers, memory alone is lost together with it, without sensation and thought being harmed in any way. But if the posterior cavity suffers together with the frontal and central ones, sense, reason and memory also are destroyed, in addition to the whole creature being in danger of perishing.
>
> Translation in *Nemesius, On the Nature of Man*, trans. and
> introduction R. W. Sharples and P. J. van der Eijk, p. 122.

Similar to Galen's ventricular experiments, in the above passage Nemesius supports his claims with "evidence" derived from observations. He also uses an account of a man suffering from phrenitis, which he ascribes to Galen, as evidence of the different functions of the ventricles. He relates how a certain wool worker standing on a building suddenly began throwing objects off the roof. When a crowd formed, he asked the people below if they wanted him to throw a fellow wool worker off the building, and thinking that the man was joking, the crowd said "yes." He then pushed his coworker off the building. This story is used to illustrate how the wool worker's behaviors reveal that his senses were sound in that he recognized what he was throwing from the building, but his intellectual capacity was diseased because he pushed another wool worker off a building for no reason. Nemesius suggests that a disease called phrenitis is the cause of the damage to the intellectual faculties of the woolworker. He then attributes hallucinations to damage to the frontal cavities, claiming that the central cavities remain unaffected when these phenomena occur.

Nemesius' localization of the mental faculties is quite similar to an account of the effects of phrenitis found in a fragment attributed to a 4th-century-AD medical author named Posidonius of Byzantium. Posidonius claimed that the location of the brain affected by phrenitis would manifest in the debilitation of specific mental faculties:

> Phrenitis is an inflammation of the membranes surrounding the brain during acute fever, causing insanity and loss of reason ... There are several different kinds of phrenitis, but the following three are most important. Either only imagination is affected and reasoning and memory are spared, or only reasoning is affected and imagination and memory are spared; or imagination and reasoning are affected and memory is spared. Furthermore, loss of memory due to febrile diseases usually destroys the faculties of reason and imagination as well. A disorder of the anterior part of the brain affects only the imagination; a disorder of the middle ventricle leads to aberration of reason; a disorder of the posterior part of the brain in the region of the occiput destroys the faculty of memory, usually together with the other two.
>
> Aëtius of Amida, *Medical Books* 6.2, translation by P. J. der Eijk
> in *Nemesius On the Nature of Man*, # 607, p. 121.

While the history of medicine reveals that physical trauma and disease have been used to speak to the localization of brain functions, it is impossible to know to what extent Posidonius' explanation is based on actual clinical observation and how much is purely speculation. This is especially difficult given what exactly constitutes as phrenitis varied widely among ancient medical writers. Furthermore, modern anatomical knowledge reveals that the ventricles are filled with cerebral spinal fluid and that they are not the anatomical location of cognition or sensation.

Other than medical accounts and empirical observations, there are other explanations for Nemesius' ventricular localization. The delineation between sensation, intelligence, and memory in Nemesius' account resembles the speculations of philosophers, particularly Aristotle, as to the phases of cognition and the soul. Aristotle's explanation of how sensations are processed into memories by the soul was taken up and expounded upon by both Peripatetic and Platonic philosophers, and therefore, it may have influenced Nemesius' brain mapping.

Another potential conceptional source for his localization of the brain, although not explicitly stated, could be the legal phases of a courtroom. The analogy would be that the anterior ventricles' faculties of sensation and imagination are likened to the first phase of a court proceeding in which the evidence is presented; the middle ventricle's faculty of intellectual thought is similar to the deliberation of a judge; and the posterior ventricle's faculty of memory is representative of the recording of the final judgment in the case. The use of metaphors and analogies were commonly used by philosophers and physicians in antiquity to conceptualize phenomena. The use of analogies, such as the modern convention of likening the brain to a computer, can be quite problematic and misleading since they often fall short of illustrating the complexities of the mind.

The localization of the mental faculties to the anterior, middle, and posterior ventricles became the dominant conceptional model for mental functions among medical and nonmedical writers up into the 16th century AD. In the 11th century, the famous Arabic philosopher–physician Ibn Sina (Avicenna) expounded upon the ventricular model by localizing specific Aristotelian concepts of sensation and cognition to specific ventricles. The influence of these ventricular theories led to Renaissance anatomists, such as Leonardo da Vinci (1452–1519), devoting a great amount of attention to these cavities of the brain. da Vinci describes how he poured wax into the ventricles of cadavers so that he could accurately map the size and shape of the ventricles (Fig. 10.2). However, da Vinci's pseudo-anatomical illustrations of the mind being a series of three cavities reflect how influential the ventricular theory was upon conceptions of the mind and its relationship to the body (Fig. 10.3).

In the 16th century, Vesalius' anatomical investigations and subsequent criticisms of Galen marked the beginning of the slow demise of ventricular theory (Fig. 10.4). Vesalius' recognition that the human brain does not have the so-called *rete mirabile* ("miraculous net" of blood vessels found at the base of the ox brains that was central to Galen's anatomical and physiological explanations for the mental faculties) did much to dispel the ventricular theory because it called into question Galen's anatomical explanation as to the source of psychic pneuma in the ventricles. Likewise, Vesalius observed that all the ventricles were full of aqueous humor rather than being only filled with psychic pneuma. Criticizing theologians who put forth the claim that the human ventricles differ from animals provides evidence that humans alone have a rational

Fig. 10.2 Leonardo da Vinci's images of the ventricles based on his wax-injections studies reveal a more anatomically correct depictions of the ventricles, modification of the original image. *Source:* Jan Voogd et al. 2020/Springer Nature/CC BY 4.0.

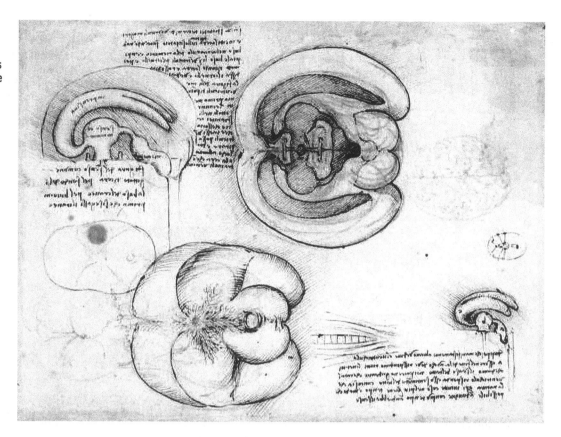

Fig. 10.3 Leonardo da Vinci's depiction of the ventricles as a series of cavities reflects the ventricular conception of the mind, modification of the original image. *Source:* Leonardo da Vinci / Wikimedia Commons / Public domain.

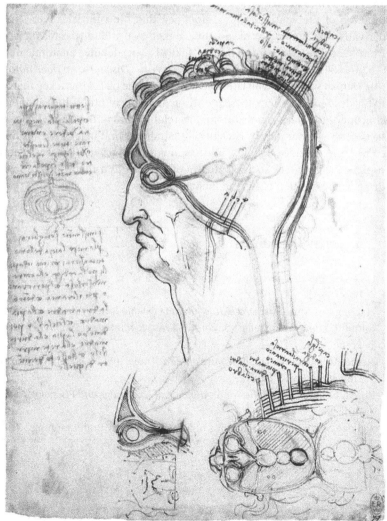

QVINTA SEPTIMI LIBRI FIGVRA

Fig. 10.4 Vesalius' *De humani corporis fabrica*, figure on plate 609, modification of the original image. *Source:* Unknown author/ Wikimedia Commons/Public domain.

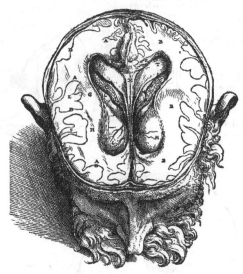

P RÆSENS figura quòd ad reliclam in caluaria cerebri portionē attinet, nulla ex parte uariat: atq̃ id folũ habet proprium, quod callofum corpus hic anteriori fua fe de à cerebro primùm liberauimus, ac dein eleuatum in pofteriora refleximus, feptum dextri ac finiftri uentriculorum di uellentes, & corporis inftar teftudinis extructi fuperiorem fuperficiem ob oculos pónetes.

Ab A ad Q *A, A, A itaq̃ & B, B, B, ac dein D, D, D, & E & F, & G & H eadem hic indicant, quæ in quarta figura. Sic quoque & L, L, & M, M, & O & P & Q eadem infinuant.*

R, R, R *Notatur inferior callofi corporis fuperficies. eft enim id à fua fede motum, atque in pofteriora reflexum.*

S,T,V Supe

soul, Vesalius noted that the human ventricles were not more numerous or significantly different from the ventricles of animals. While Vesalius was reticent to make any claims about the specific function of each ventricle when discussing the function of the ventricles, he maintained that the ventricles were the location of *spiritus animalis* (i.e. the theoretical derivative of Galenic psychic pneuma in medieval and renaissance science), and he claimed that rational thought was a gift from "God, the Creator of all things." Likewise, the detailed anatomical descriptions of the brain found in Nicolaus Stensen's (1638–1686) *Discours sur l'anatomie du cerveau* (*Discourse on the Anatomy of the Brain*) is why medical historians point to this Danish scientist, who later became a Catholic bishop, as a key figure in the demise of the ventricular theory. Adhering to his desire to base hypotheses "only on anatomical propositions that are obvious and certain," Stensen cast doubt on the concept of the *spiritus animalis* and its relationship to the brain. Instead of relying on such speculations, the brain should be described accurately by considering "all things that may cause any change to the actions of the brain, whether they may come from outside, as fluids, injuries, medicines; or be it internal causes, as diseases of which medicine counts a large number." Ultimately, such skepticism of the *spiritus animalis* led to scientists and physicians looking to other parts of the brain as the location of human mental faculties.

Suggested Readings

Galen. *Galen Psychological Writings*. Edited and translated by Peter. N. Singer. Cambridge: Cambridge University Press, 2013.

Harrington, Anne. *Medicine, Mind, and the Double Brain*. Princeton: Princeton University Press, 1987.

Cantani, Marco, and Stefano Sandrone. *Brain Renaissance: From Vesalius to Modern Neuroscience*. Oxford: Oxford University Press, 2015.

Nemesius of Emesa. *On the Nature of Man*, Translated by Robert W. Sharples and Philip J. van der Eijk. Liverpool: Liverpool University Press, 2008.

Rocca, Julius. *Galen on the Brain: Anatomical Knowledge and Physiological Speculation in the Second Century AD*. Leiden: Brill, 2003.

van der Eijk, Philip. J. "Nemesius of Emesa and Early Brainmapping." *The Lancet* 372, no. 9637 (2008): 440–441.

Etymological Explanations: Common Terms and Word Elements for the Anatomy of the Nervous System

The nervous system has three divisions: the central nervous system (CNS) (brain and spinal cord), the peripheral nervous system (PNS) (nerves that have left the CNS to innervate the parts of the body), and the autonomic nervous system (ANS) (responsible for the involuntary impulses that regulate, glands, smooth muscles, and cardiac muscles). In the following discussion of the anatomical terms associated with the nervous system, the nominative and genitive singular forms of the anatomical Latin term will be provided in the parenthesis. The Greek and Latin roots are formatted in all caps and emboldened.

Central nervous system (CNS)

Central Nervous System (*systema nervosum centrale*) – The **CNS** comprises the brain and spinal cord.

Cranium (L. *cranium, -i*) – The cranium is the dome-like structure of the skull that houses the brain.

Encephalon (L. *encephalon, -i*) – The encephalon is a loan word from the Greek word, *enkephalos*, that is commonly used for the "brain" (Fig. 10.5). Its root, **ENCEPHAL-**, is used for the "whole brain." As a suffix, encephalon is also used for the parts of the embryonic brain. There are three basic units of the brain: (i) The "forebrain" is called the **prosencephalon** [*pros-*, forward +], which is associated with the cerebrum, corpus callosum, and limbic system. (ii) The "midbrain" or **mesencephalon** [*mesos*, middle +] is the smallest of the three units, and its primary parts are the tectum and the paired cerebral peduncles. (iii) And at last, the "hindbrain," which comprises the brain stem and the cerebellum, is also called the **rhombencephalon** (rhomboid-shaped).

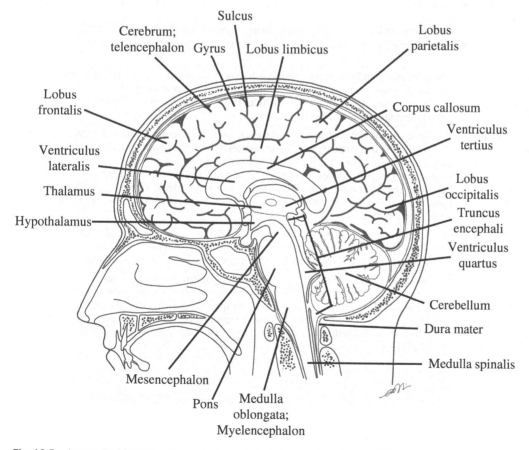

Fig. 10.5 Anatomical Latin for the brain (*encephalon*). *Source:* Drawing by Chloe Kim.

Meninges (L. *meninx, meningis*) – **Dura mater, arachnoid mater,** and **pia mater** are three membranes that envelop the brain and spinal cord. These membranes are collectively called the **meninges** (L. *meninx, meningis*). The singular form of meninges is **meninx,** and the root is **MENING-.** The thick outer membrane, known as the dura mater, is also called the **pachymeninx.** The root **DUR-,** which means "hard," is also used for the dura mater in medical terminology (e.g. subdural hematoma). The two thinner membranes are referred to as the **leptomeninges.** The arachnoid membrane is one of these thinner membranes. It derives its name from the root **ARACHN-,** which means "spider," because of its weblike formation. The membrane closest to the brain is called the pia mater. The Latin word for mother, *mater,* is used for the names of each of these membranes due to medieval Islamic medicine's influence on the Latin-speaking West. The term dura mater was derived from Latin translations of the Arabic phrase *umm al-dimagh as-safiqa,* which literally means "thick mother of the brain." The use of this phrase in medieval Islamic medicine denoted the membrane's relationship to the brain because words for "father" and "mother" were commonly used in Arabic to denote the relationship between things. Using the root for "thick," **PACHY-,** the dura mater is also referred to as the **pachymeninx.** In contrast, the root for "thin," **LEPT-,** is used for the pia mater and arachnoid mater in the term **leptomeninges.**

Cerebrum (L. *cerebrum, -i*) – The cerebrum, also known as the **telencephalon** (endbrain), is the largest portion of the brain. Because it is understood as the seat of consciousness and the center of the higher mental faculties, such as memory, learning, reasoning, judgment, intelligence, and emotions, the cerebrum takes precedence over the other parts of the brain in modern conceptions of the mind. Cerebrum was the Latin word for the anatomical brain. The word *cerebrum* also appears in Roman literature to express mental and emotional concepts, such as "understanding" and "anger," and therefore, these usages imply that there was a common understanding of the brain's connection to rational thought and emotion in the Roman intellectual world. Today, the cerebrum is associated with the interpretation of sensory impulses and all voluntary muscular activities, and its root **CEREBR-** can have the meaning of "understanding" in words such as cerebral.

Cerebral Cortex (L. *cortex cerebri*) – The outer layer of the cerebrum is called the cortex (L. *cortex, corticis*). The term cortex is often used to distinguish the outer layer of an organ from its soft inner part, which is commonly called the **medulla** (L. *medulla, -ae*). The root for the cerebral cortex is **CORTIC-,** which also means "outer layer" and "bark."

Cerebellum (L. *cerebellum, -i*) – Turning back to the externally recognizable parts of the brain, the portion of the brain located below the occipital lobe of the cerebrum is called the cerebellum. It is responsible for coordination and voluntary movements. Naturally, the root **CEREBELL-** is used for this part of the brain. Etymologically, the cerebellum is linked to the cerebrum; as noted, the cerebrum was originally used by the Romans for the "brain," and therefore, *cerebellum* originally meant "little cerebrum," which makes sense given that its hemispheric divisions and convolutions give it a somewhat similar appearance to the cerebrum.

Brainstem (L. *truncus encephali*) – Like the cerebellum and cerebrum, the brainstem is an externally visible structure that gives the brain its recognizable appearance. The brainstem connects the brain to the spinal cord, and it is responsible for basic bodily functions such as breathing, heart rate, and body temperature. The brainstem includes the midbrain, pons, and medulla oblongata. The most superior part of the brainstem is called the midbrain or **mesencephalon.**

Pons (L. *pons, pontis*) – The root **PONT-** is used for the rostral part of the brainstem known as the pons. That said, **PONT-** is used for any "bridge-like" structure of the body. This Latin root also appears in religious contexts, such as "pontificate." This religious connotation goes back to the ancient Roman religious figure known as the Pontifex Maximus (quite literally, greatest bridge-maker). Etymological speculations among ancient authors such as Plutarch seem to associate the origins of this Roman religious figure with the bridges of Rome, but others associate it with bridges in a more metaphorical sense, such as a bridge between the mortal and immortal world. The Pontifex Maximus became the most important position in the ancient Roman religion, which is probably why the Roman Catholic church uses the term Pontiff for a bishop.

Medulla (L. *medulla, -ae*) – The medulla or medulla oblongata is the caudal segment of the brainstem. The root used for this part, **MEDULL-,** is also used for "bone marrow" and "the inner part of an organ." The medulla oblongata is also called the **myelencephalon.** The medulla oblongata helps control the vital processes of heart rate, breathing, and blood pressure.

Lobes (L. *lobus, -i*) – The cerebrum is further divided into four lobes by the central sulcus, parieto-occipital sulcus, and lateral fissure (Fig. 10.6). The four lobes whose names correspond to the skull bones that they lie under are as follows: **frontal** (L. *lobus frontalis*), **parietal** (L. *lobus parietalis*), **temporal** (L. *lobus temporalis*), and **occipital** (L. *lobus occipitalis*). Each lobe is associated with different mental functions: the frontal lobe is linked to voluntary movement and personality; the parietal lobe is associated with sensations of pain, touch, and temperature; the temporal lobe is responsible for hearing, taste, and smell; and the occipital lobe's primary responsibility is vision (Fig. 10.6).

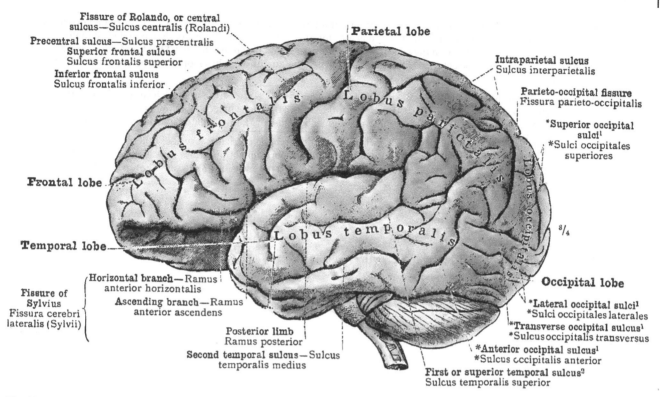

Fissure of Rolando, or central
sulcus—Sulcus centralis (Rolandi)
Precentral sulcus—Sulcus præcentralis
Superior frontal sulcus
Sulcus frontalis superior
Inferior frontal sulcus
Sulcus frontalis inferior

Parietal lobe

Intraparietal sulcus
Sulcus interparietalis

Parieto-occipital fissure
Fissura parieto-occipitalis

*Superior occipital
sulci[1]
*Sulci occipitales
superiores

Frontal lobe

Temporal lobe

Fissure of
Sylvius
Fissura cerebri
lateralis (Sylvii)

Horizontal branch—Ramus
anterior horizontalis
Ascending branch—Ramus
anterior ascendens

Posterior limb
Ramus posterior

Second temporal sulcus—Sulcus
temporalis medius

Occipital lobe

*Lateral occipital sulci[1]
*Sulci occipitales laterales
*Transverse occipital sulcus[1]
*Sulcus occipitalis transversus
*Anterior occipital sulcus[1]
*Sulcus occipitalis anterior
First or superior temporal sulcus[2]
Sulcus temporalis superior

Lobus frontalis — Lobus parietalis — Lobus temporalis — Lobus occipitalis

8/4

Fig. 10.6 Lobes and gyri of the cerebrum. *Source:* Carl Toldt et al. 1919 /Rebman Company/Public Domain.

Gyrus (L. *gyrus, -i*) – Each of the lobes contain convolutions known as gyri. The root **GYR-** comes from the Greek word for a "circle" or a "ring," which is also part of its modern meanings. Each gyrus of the cerebrum has an individual name (e.g. postcentral gyrus), and it is associated with specific functions within the lobe.

Fissure (L. *fissura, -ae*) – The root used for a "deep groove" or "fissure" is **FISSUR-**. The term fissure is derived from the Latin verb *findere*, which means "to split, cleave." The roots derived from this verb, **FIND-**, **FISS-**, and **FID-** all carry similar meanings and are frequently used in terms for the splitting of an object such as "fission" or "bifid."

Sulcus (L. *sulcus, -i*) – A sulcus is the Latin word for "a furrow," it is used for anatomical grooves, particularly those associated with gyri of the cerebrum. The root **SULC-** can be used for any groove-like structure. As to the different names for the grooves of the brain, fissures tend to be deeper than sulci.

Corpus Callosum (L. *corpus collusum*) – The hemispheres of the cerebrum are primarily interconnected by the corpus callosum, which literally means "tough/hard body." Composed of millions of nerve fibers, the corpus callosum is the largest of the three commissures of the brain.

Limbic System (L. *systema limbicum*) – The limbic system is associated with emotions and behavior. It is also involved with long-term memory and olfaction. The name "limbic" comes from the Latin word for "border," *limbus*, thus the root **LIMB-** and the loan word **limbus** are used for any "border-like" structure. The primary structures of the limbic system are the amygdala and the hippocampus.

Hippocampus (L. *hippocampus, -i*) – Internally, the cerebral hemispheres are united by three commissures: the aforementioned corpus callosum and the anterior and posterior hippocampal commissures. The hippocampus is part of the limbic system, and it is responsible for memory consolidation. The term hippocampus and its root **HIPPOCAMP-** are also used for the zoological genus of the seahorse: Gr. *hippokampos: hippos* "horse" + *kampos* "a sea monster." The use of the term for this area of the brain began in the 1700s. The reason for this usage is because, assumedly, the hippocampus of the brain looks like a seahorse. In Greek and Roman iconography, Poseidon's chariot is often depicted as being pulled by creatures that have horse torsos with fish tails, which is the original meaning of *hippokampos*. Poseidon's relationship with horses extends to the land as well, where he is known as the Greek god of horses. The root **HIPP-** is used today for "horse," for example hippotherapy and hippopotamus (river horse).

Amygdala (L. *amygdala, -ae*) – Like the hippocampus, the amygdalae are associated with memory; they are also important to social and emotional processes. Derived from the Greek word for an "almond," the root for these almond-shaped nuclei of the limbic system is **AMYGDAL-**. In addition to these neural structures, **AMYGDAL-** is used for anything associated with an almond, such as amygdalin.

Thalamus (L. *thalamus, -i*) – The thalamus is another important internal structure of the brain. The thalamus is an ovoid-shaped collection of nuclei found deep inside the brain that is responsible for processing almost all sensory signals and most motor programs to and from the cerebral cortex. Coming from the Greek word for an inner room, *thalamos*, the root **THALAM-** also can be used for an "inner room" or a "chamber-like" structure. Hence, in Botany, a pleiothalamous plant has more than the usual number of chambers or receptacles.

Nucleus (L. *nucleus, -i*) – As to the thalamus being identified as nuclei of the CNS, it is important to bear in mind that the original meaning of the nucleus is "kernel." The root **NUCLE-** is used for the central organelle of a cell, but in the CNS, a nucleus is a group of neuronal cell bodies that are clustered together, forming a recognizable mass or "kernel" that is associated with specific functions.

Ventricles (L. *ventriculus, -i*) – The root **VENTRICUL-** is used for the cerebral ventricles, as well as other small cavities of the body. There are four ventricles in the brain. The ventricles are where the cerebrospinal fluid (CSF) is generated continuously. The ventricles are interconnected with each other and the spinal cord, providing a pathway for CSF to move around the brain and spinal cord (Fig. 10.7).

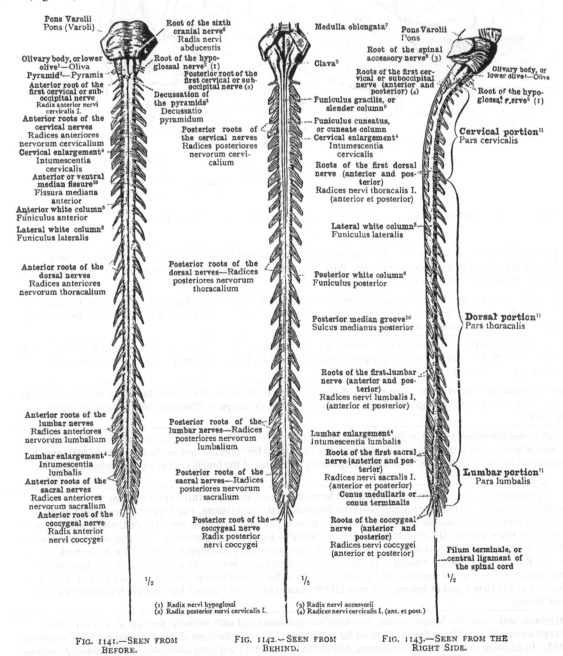

Fig. 10.7 Anatomical Latin for the spinal cord (*medulla spinalis*). *Source:* Carl Toldt et al. 1919/Rebman Company/Public Domain.

Cerebral Spinal Fluid (L. *liquor cerebrospinalis*) – The CSF supplies nutrients and removes waste products from the CNS. CSF also provides a watery cushion to the CNS. The watery nature of CSF is perhaps why the root for water, **HYDR-**, is often used for the cerebral spinal fluid, such as in the term **hydrocephalus**, which is an accumulation of excessive amounts of CSF in the ventricles.

Gray Matter (L. *substantia grisea*) and White Matter (L. *substantia alba*) – The cerebral cortex and the central part of the spinal cord consist of gray matter. The white matter forms the inner part of the cerebrum. The gray matter gets its appearance from the numerous neuronal cell bodies and the very limited amount of myelinated tissue. White matter is composed primarily of myelinated tissue, which gives it its characteristic color. The root **POLI-** is used for the color "gray," and by extension, the "gray matter of the brain." The root **ALB-** is used for "white," and it is infrequently used for the white matter of the brain.

Spinal Cord (L. *medulla spinalis*) – After the myelencephalon, the brain transitions into the spinal cord (Fig. 10.7). Coming from the Greek word for "marrow," the root for spinal cord and bone marrow is **MYEL-**. The spinal cord is a column of nerve tissue that connects the brain to the body. If one were to transect this cord, the division between gray and white matter would become quite evident. The gray matter is shaped like a butterfly, and its wings are called "horns." The anterior (ventral) horns are associated with motor function, and the posterior (dorsal) horns are interneurons, generally associated with conveying somato-sensory information. The white matter consists of myelinated axons that transmit impulses to and from the brain, as well as between the different levels of gray matter in the spinal cord.

Funiculus (L. *funiculus, -i*) – The white matter consists of myelinated axons that transmit impulses to and from the brain, as well as between the different levels of gray matter in the spinal cord. In respect to the spinal cord, the white matter is divided into three major divisions according to location (anterior, lateral, and posterior). Each division is called a funiculus. The root **FUNICUL-** is used for this division of white matter in the spinal cord. Derived from the Latin word for "rope" or "cord," **FUNICUL-** can also refer to any "rope-like" structure, such as the umbilical cord.

Fascicle (L. *fasculus, -i*) – Within each funiculus are tracts of nerve fibers called fascicles or fasciculi. As we have seen in the Chapter 7 on the musculoskeletal system, owing to its relationship to the Roman *fasces*, the root **FASICUL-** is used for a small bundle of longitudinal-running fibers.

Vertebral Column (L. *columna vertebralis*) – The spinal cord is protected by the collection of bones called the vertebral column. The spinal cord terminates into a pointed structure called the *conus medullaris* between the L1 and L2 vertebrae. Similar to how the term encephalon is used with respect to the embryonic brain, the notochord is a rod of embryonic cells that becomes the axial skeleton in chordate animals. In vertebrates, the notochord is replaced by the bodies of vertebrae. The root **NOT-** means the "back." The root **CHORD-** is used for "cord" or "tendon." As was discussed in the chapter on the musculoskeletal system, the roots **RHACHI-** and **SPIN-** share with **NOT-** the meaning of "back" or "vertebral column." The roots for a single bony segment of the vertebral column, a vertebra, are **SPONDYL-** and **VERTEBR-**.

Peripheral nervous system (PNS)

Peripheral Nervous System (L. *systema nervorum periphericum*) – The PNS is composed of nerves outside the CNS. A nerve (L. *nervus, -i*), the roots for "nerve" are **NERV-** and **NEUR-**, is a bundle of fibers (called axons) that convey sensory and motor impulses to and from the brain and spinal cord. This includes the cranial nerves (L. *nervi craniales*) and the spinal nerves (L. *nervi spinales*). The 12 pairs of peripheral nerves from the brain are called the cranial nerves. The peripheral nerves coming from the spinal cord are the spinal nerves (Fig. 10.8). There are 31 pairs of spinal nerves. Each pair of spinal nerves is identified by the level of the vertebrae they exit from the spine. More specifically, there are 8 cervical nerve pairs (C1–C8), 12 thoracic nerve pairs (T1–T12), 5 lumbar nerve pairs (L1–L5), 5 sacral (S1–S5), and 1 coccygeal nerve pair.

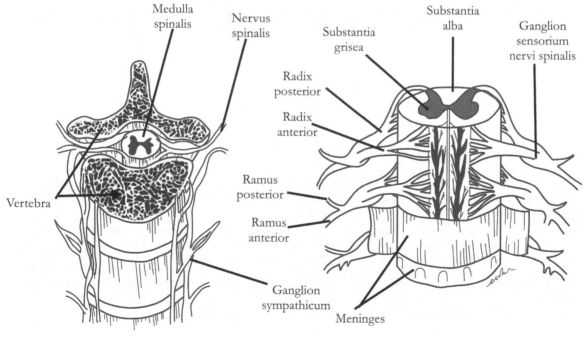

Fig. 10.8 Anatomical Latin for the spinal cord (*medulla spinalis*) and nerves (*nervi*). *Source:* Drawing by Chloe Kim.

Neuron (L. *neuron, -i*) – The loan word **neuron** is used in medicine for a "nerve cell." A neuron has three main parts. The body of the neuron is called the soma. As we have observed in the previous chapters , the word elements **SOMAT-, SOM-,** and **-SOME** are commonly used for "body," The tree-like/branched structure of a neuron is called a dendrite. The Greek root used for dendrite is **DENDR-** and it carries the potential meanings of dendrite, tree, or branched structure. The other projection off of the neuron is the axon. The root **AX-** can be used for "axon," "axle," and "axis."

Glial Cells – The other important cellular components of the nervous system are called glial cells. Gliocytes, or neuroglia, are the interstitial and supporting tissue of the nervous system. The root **GLI-** also means "glue," which is why gliocytes are sometimes called "glue cells." Oligodendrocytes are a type of gliocyte responsible for the myelination of the axon tracts in the CNS and the myelinated axons of the PNS.

Epineurium (L. *epineurium, -i*), Perineurium (L. *perineurium, -i*), and Endoneurium (L. *endoneurium, -i*) – Axons of peripheral nerves are joined together by delicate connective tissue called endoneurium. A collection of axons and their endoneurium that is ensheathed by perineurium is called a fasciculus. Nerve fasciculi and their blood vessels are in turn bound together by connective tissue known as epineurium. All of these layers collectively form the structure we term a peripheral nerve (Fig. 10.9).

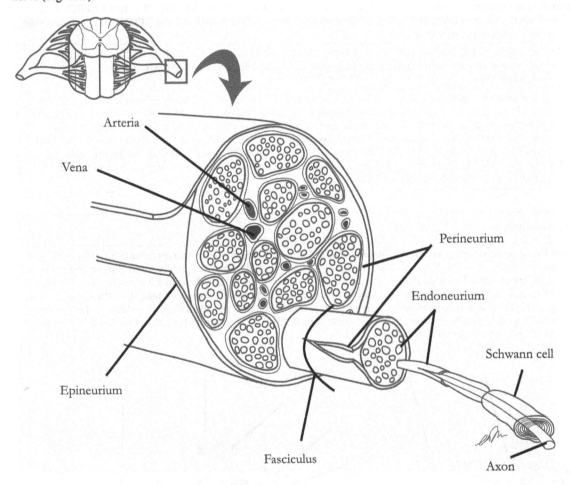

Fig. 10.9 Anatomical Latin for the parts of nerve (*nervus*). *Source:* Drawing by Chloe Kim.

Nerve Root (L. *radix, radicis*) – A nerve root is the first segment of a peripheral nerve leaving the spinal cord. The anterior root carries efferent (motor) stimuli and the posterior root carries afferent (sensory) stimuli. The roots for a nerve root are **RADIC-, RADICUL-,** and **RHIZ-.** The loan word for a nerve root is **radix.** In addition, all of these word elements could be used for any "root" or "root-like" structure in nature.

Nerve Branches (L. *ramus, -i*) – Where the nerve roots combine, they form a **ramus.** Being the primary branch of a spinal nerve that carries both motor and sensory information, it makes sense that this segment of the peripheral nerve is named after the Latin word for a "branch" on a "tree," and it also makes sense that the root **RAM-** is used for any branch-like structure. The anterior and posterior rami branch off, forming new nerves that carry the information for multiple levels of the nerve roots. These nerves will be identified by the object or area that they innervate. For example, the phrenic nerve innervates the diaphragm, and it comprises the C3–C5 nerve roots.

Plexus (L. *plexus, -us*) – The network of nerves (as well as blood, lymphatic vessels) is called a plexus.

Autonomic nervous system – Derived from the Greek word for independence, *autonomia* (Gr. *autos*, self + *nomos*, custom, rule), the root **AUTONOM-** means "self-controlling," "functioning independently," and the ANS. The ANS is part of the PNS that regulates involuntary physiological functions such as heart rate, blood pressure, respiration, and digestion. The ANS is composed of the sympathetic nervous system and the parasympathetic nervous system (Fig. 10.10).

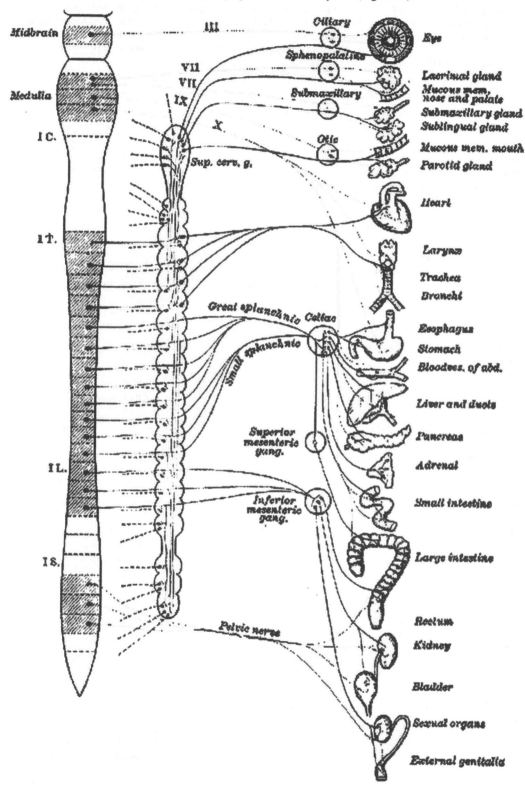

Fig. 10.10 Image of the innervation and function of the parasympathetic and sympathetic systems. *Source:* Adapted from Gray's Anatomy 20th edition. 1918.

Sympathetic nervous system – The sympathetic nervous system's primary function is to prepare a human for a stressful situation or an emergency, which is why it is linked with the phrase "fight-or-flight response." Thus, it creates a cascade of activities to maximize the performance of a human under stress: dilates pupils, increases heart rate, widens airways, increases circulation to skeletal muscles, decreases circulation to the gastrointestinal tract, and increases the availability of glucose. The use of the term sympathetic in respect to the body can be traced back to Aristotle who used the word *sympatheia* (suffering/affected together) to explain how when one part of the body suffers, another part will likewise be affected. This was used by Aristotle and his followers to justify their cardiocentric understanding of the controlling part of the mind. When faced with the evidence that damage to the brain causes deleterious changes to the mental faculties, the peripatetic response was to say that the heart suffered with the brain due to the heart's dependence on the brain to cool the innate heat of the heart.

Parasympathetic nervous system – The parasympathetic nervous system works alongside the sympathetic nervous system, being most active in ordinary, everyday conditions. It counterbalances the effects of the sympathetic nervous system.

Hypothalamus (L. *hypothalamus, -i*) – Located beneath the thalamus, the hypothalamus is the central controller of the preganglionic sympathetic and parasympathetic nervous systems; the hypothalamus also works with the pituitary gland to regulate the secretion of hormones.

Ganglion (L. *ganglion, -i*) – With respect to the ANS, a ganglion is a bundle of nerve cells that look like a tumor or cyst. They appear in both sympathetic and parasympathetic systems of the ANS. The root **GANGL-** comes from the Greek word *ganglion*, which literally means tumor or cyst. Thus, a ganglion can also be a swelling on the aponeurotic aspect of a tendon.

Greek or Latin word element	Current usage	Etymology	Examples of compound terms and loan words
NERV/O (nĕr-vō)	Nerve	L. *nervus, -i*, nerve, sinew	**Nerv**ous, **E**nerv**ate** Loan word: **Nervus** (nĕr'vŭs) pl. **Nervi** (nĕr'vī″)
NEUR/O (nū-rō)	Nerve, sinew	Gr. *neuron*, nerve, sinew, tendon	**Neur**algia, Peri**neur**ium Loan word: **Neuron** (noor'on″) pl. **Neura** (noor'ă″)
CRANI/O (krā-nē-ō)	Cranium (portion of the skull that encloses the brain)	L. *cranium, -i*, n. skull fr. Gr. *kranion*, skull	**Crani**otomy, Intra**crani**al Loan word: **Cranium** (krā'nē-ŭm) pl. **Crania** (krā'nē-ă)
CEPHAL/O (sĕf-ă-lō)	Head	Gr. *kephale*, head	**Cephal**ic, **Cephal**opod
ENCEPHAL/O (ĕn-sef-ă-lō) **-ENCEPHALON** (en-sef-ă-lŏn)	Brain	L. *encephalon, -i*, n. encephalon, brain fr. Gr. *enkephalos*, brain	**Encephal**omeningitis, Tel**encephal**on, Amyel**encephal**y Loan word: **Encephalon** (en-sef'ă-lŏn) pl. **Encephala** (en-sef'ă-lă)
CEREBR/O (sĕr-ĕ-brō)	Cerebrum (largest part of the brain), brain	L. *cerebrum, -i*, n. cerebrum, brain	**Cerebr**ifugal, Intra**cerebr**al Loan word: **Cerebrum** (sĕr'ĕ-brŭm) pl. **Cerebra** (sĕr'ĕ-bră)
CEREBELL/O (sĕr-ĕ-bĕl-ō)	Cerebellum	L. *cerebellum, -i*, n. cerebellum, little brain	**Cerebell**itis, **Cerebell**ipetal Loan word: **Cerebellum** (sĕr-ĕ-bĕl'ŭm) pl. **Cerebella** (sĕr-ĕ-bĕl'ă)

Greek or Latin word element	Current usage	Etymology	Examples of compound terms and loan words
PONT/O (pŏn-tō)	Pons (of the brain), bridge-like structure	L. *pons*, *pontis*, m. pons, bridge	**Pont**ine, **Pont**ibrachium Loan word: **Pons** (ponz) pl. **Pontes** (pon′tēz″)
LIMB/O (lim-bō)	Limbic system, border	L. *limbus*, *-i*, m. border	**Limb**ic, **Limb**o Loan word: **Limbus** (lim′bŭs) pl. **Limbi** (lim′bī″)
HIPPOCAMP/O (hip-ŏ-kam-pō)	Hippocampus, seahorse	L. *hippocampus*, *-i*, m. hippocampus, seahorse fr. Gr. *hippokampos*, *hippos* "horse" + *kampos* "a sea monster"	**Hippocamp**al Loan word: **Hippocampus** (hip″ŏ-kam′pŭs) pl. **Hippocampi** (hip″ŏ-kam′pī″)
THALAM/O (thăl-ăm-ō)	Thalamus (mass of gray matter located in the diencephalon), chamber, inner room	L. *thalamus*, *-i*, m. thalamus fr. Gr. *thalamos*, inner room, chamber	Hypo**thalam**us, **Thalam**olenticular Loan word: **Thalamus** (thăl′ă-mŭs) pl. **Thalami** (thăl′ă-mī″)
AMYGDAL/O (ă-mig-dă-lō)	Amygdala (almond-shaped nuclei in the temporal lobe), almond, tonsil	L. *amygdala*, *-ae*, f. amygdala fr. Gr. *amygdale*, almond	**Amygdal**in, **amygdal**itis, **amygdal**opathy Loan word: **Amygdala** (ă-mig′dă-lă) pl. **Amygdalae** (ă-mig′dă-lē″)
NUCLE/O (nū-klē-ō)	Nucleus (group of neuronal cell bodies), core, little nut or kernel	L. *nucleus*, *-i*, m. little nut, kernel, core, nucleus	**Nucle**ofugal, e**nucle**ation, **nucle**ar Loan word: **Nucleus** (noo′klē-ŭs) pl. **Nuclei** (noo′klē-ī″)
MENING/O (mĕn-ĭn-gō) -MENINX (mē-ningks)	Meninx (one of the three membranes enveloping the brain and spinal cord), membrane	L. *meninx*, *meningis*, f. meninx fr. Gr. *meninx*, *meningos*, membrane	**Mening**itis, **mening**ocele, **mening**eal Loan word: **Meninx** (men′ingks) pl. **Meninges** (mē-nin′jēz″)
LEPT/O (lĕp-tō)	Thin	Gr. *leptos*, thin, delicate	**Lept**omeninges, **lept**oderma, **lept**ophonia
PACHY- (pak-ē) PACH/O (pak-ō)	Thick	Gr. *pachys*, thick	**Pachy**meninx, **Pach**ometer, **pachy**dermia, acro**pachy**
ARACHN/O (ă-rak-nō)	Arachnoid membrane, spider, spider-like	Gr. *arachne*, spider	Sub**arachn**oid, **arachn**ophobia, **arachn**ids, **arachn**itis
DUR/O (dū-rō)	Dura mater membrane, hard	L. *durus*, *-a*, *-um*, hard	Sub**dur**al, **dur**able, in**dur**ation

Greek or Latin word element	Current usage	Etymology	Examples of compound terms and loan words
LOB/O (lŏ-bō)	Lobe	L. *lobus, -i*, m. lobe fr. Gr. *lobos*, a pod, lobe	**Lob**otomy, intra**lob**ular, multi**lob**ate Loan word: **Lobus** (lŏ'bŭs) pl. **Lobi** (lŏ'bī″)
GYR/O (jĭ-rō)	Gyrus (a convolution of the cerebrum), circle, ring	L. *gyrus, -i*, m. gyrus fr. Gr. *gyros*, circle, ring	A**gyr**ia, **gyr**oscope, **gyr**ation Loan word: **Gyrus** (jĭ'rŭs) pl. **Gyri** (jĭ'rī″)
SULC/O (sŭl-kō)	Sulcus (groove of brain), furrow, groove	L. *sulcus, -i*, m. furrow, groove	**Sulc**iform, **sulc**ate, Loan word: **Sulcus** (sŭl'kŭs) pl. **Sulci** (sŭl'kī″)
FISSUR/O (fi-shoor-ō)	Fissure, deep groove	L. *fissura, -ae*, f. cleft, fissure fr. L. *findere, fissum*, to split, cleave	**Fissur**al, super**fissur**e Loan word: **Fissura** (fi-soor'ă) pl. **Fissurae** (fi-soor'ē″)
FID/O (fĭ-dō) **FISS/O** (fĭ-sō)	Split, cleave	L. *findere, fissum*, to split, cleave	**Fiss**iparous, bi**fid**, **fiss**ipedia
VENTRICUL/O (ven-trik-yŭ-lō)	Ventricle, small cavity	L. *ventriculus, -i*, m. ventricle, little belly fr. L. *venter, ventris*, m. belly, cavity	**Ventricul**ography, **ventricul**itis, supra**ventricul**ar Loan word: **Ventriculus** (ven-trik'yŭ-lŭs) pl. **Ventriculi** (ven-trik'yŭ-lī″)
COEL/O (sē-lō) **CEL/O** (sē-lō)	Cavity, hollow	Gr. *koilos*, hollow	**Coel**osperm, hemo**cel**om
CORTIC/O (kor-tĭ-kō)	Cortex (cerebrum), outer layer, bark	L. *cortex, cortices*, m. bark, outer layer	Infra**cortic**al, **cortic**otropic, **cortic**ipetal Loan word: **Cortex** (kor'teks″) pl. **Cortices** (kort'ĭ-sēz″)
MYEL/O (mī-ĕ-lō)	Spinal cord, marrow	Gr. *myelos*, marrow, particularly bone marrow	**Myel**ogram, macro**myel**on, a**myel**encephalia
MEDULL/O (mĕ-dŭl-ō)	Medulla, marrow	L. *medulla, -ae*, f. marrow, pith	**Medull**ectomy, **medull**ispinal Loan word: **Medulla** (mĕ-dŭl'ă) pl. **Medullae** (mĕ-dŭl'ē″)
POLI/O (pōl-ē-ō)	Gray, gray matter of CNS	Gr. *polios*, gray (or grey)	**Poli**oencephalitis, **poli**osis, **poli**othrix
FASCICUL/O (fă-sik-yŭ-lō)	Fascicle, bundle of longitudinal fibers	L. *fasciculus, -i*, m. small bundle of rods, fascicle	**Fascicul**ar, **fascicul**ate Loan word: **Fasciculus** (fă-sik'yŭ-lŭs) pl. **Fasciculi** (fă-sik'yŭ-lī″)

Greek or Latin word element	Current usage	Etymology	Examples of compound terms and loan words
FUNICUL/O (fū-nĭk-yŭ-lō)	Funicle, rope-like	L. *funiculus, -i,* m. small rope, funiculus fr. L. *funis,* m. rope, cord	**Funicul**ar, **funicul**opexy Loan word: **Funiculus** (fū-nĭk′yŭ-lŭs) pl. **Funiculi** (fū-nĭk′yŭ-lī″)
FUN/O (fū-nō)	Rope, cord	L. *funis, -is,* m. rope, cord	**Fun**ic, **fun**iform Loan word: **Funis** (fū′nĭs)
RADICUL/O (ră-dĭk-ū-lō) **RADIC/O** (răd-ĭ-kō)	Nerve root, root	L. *radicula, radiculae,* f. little root fr. L. *radix, radicis,* f. root	**Radicul**itis, **radic**iform, e**radic**ate Loan word: **Radix** (ră′dĭks) pl. **Radices** (ră′dĭ-sēz″)
RHIZ/O (rī-zŏt-ō)	Nerve root, root	Gr. *rhiza,* root	**Rhiz**otomy, not**orhiz**al, **rhiz**ocarp
RAM/O (rā-mō)	Nerve branch, branch	L. *ramus, -i,* m. branch	**Ram**ose, **ram**iform, **ram**icorn Loan word: **Ramus** (rā′mŭs) pl. **Rami** (rā′mī″)
PLEX/O (pleks-ō)	Plexus (interwoven network of nerves, blood, lymphatic vessels)	L. *plexus, -us,* m. a braid, plexus fr. L. *plectere, plexum,* to plait, interweave	**Plex**opathy, **plex**iform Loan word: **Plexus** (pleks′ŭs)
GANGLI/O (gang-glē-ō)	Ganglion (groups of nerve cells)	L. *ganglion, -i,* n. ganglion fr. Gr. *ganglion,* tumor, cyst	**Gangli**oma, **gangli**ectomy Loan word: **Ganglion** (gang′glē-ŏn) pl. **Ganglia** (gang′glē-ă)
GLI/O (glī-ō)	Glia (supporting tissue of the nervous system), glue	Gr. *glia,* glue	**Gli**ocyte, **gli**osarcoma Loan word: **Glia** (glī′ă)
SOMAT/O (sō-măt-ō) **SOM/O** (sō-mō) **-SOME** (sōm)	Body (body of neuron)	Gr. *soma, somatos,* body	**Somat**ogenic, Di**som**us, Chromo**some** Loan word: **Soma** (sō′mă) pl. **Somata** (sō′măt-ă)
DENDR/O (dĕn-drō)	Dendrite (part of neuron), tree, branched structure	Gr. *dendron,* tree	**Dendr**oid, **dendr**ite, peri**dendr**itic Loan word: **Dendron** (den′drŏn)
AX/O (ak-sō)	Axon (long process of a neuron), axle, axis	Gr. *axon,* axle, axis	**Ax**olysis, peri**ax**onal Loan word: **Axon** (ak′son″)
NOT/O (nŏt-ō)	The back	Gr. *noton,* the back, a ridge	**Not**ochord, **not**omelus, **not**algia

Greek or Latin word element	Current usage	Etymology	Examples of compound terms and loan words
SPIN/O (spī-nō)	Spine, thorn, vertebral column	L. *spina, -ae,* f. thorn	**Spin**ose, juxta**spin**al, **spin**iferous Loan word: **Spina** (spī'nă) pl. **Spinae** (spī'nē″)
VERTEBR/O (věr-tě-brō)	Vertebra, back bone	L. *vertebra, -ae,* f. vertebra, joint	Inter**vertebr**al, in**vertebr**ate Loan word: **Vertebra** (věrt'ě-bră) pl. **Vertebrae** (věrt'ě-brē″)
SPONDYL/O (spŏn-dĭ-lō)	Vertebra	Gr. *Spondylos,* vertebra	**Spondyl**odynia, **spondyl**osis

Review	Answers
The roots for "nerve" are _____ and _____. That said, the loan word Neuron is used in medicine for a "nerve cell." A neuron has specific parts. The tree-like/branched structures are called dendrites. The root used for dendrite is _____ and it carries the potential meanings of _____, _____, or _____. The other projection off of the neuron is the axon. The root AX- can be used for _____, _____, and _____. The body of the neuron is called the _____.	**NERV-, NEUR-** **DENDR-** **dendrite, tree, branched structure,** **axon, axle, axis** **soma**
The cranium is the dome-like structure of the skull that houses the brain. The root for the cranium is _____	**CRANI-**
The technical term for a headache is a cephalalgia. The root CEPHAL- means _____.	**head**
Dura mater, pia mater, and arachnoid mater are three membranes that envelop the brain and spinal cord. These membranes are collectively called the meninges. The singular of meninges is _____, and the root used for the meninges is _____. The thick outer membrane, known as the dura mater, is also called the _____meninx. The root DUR- means _____ and _____. The two thinner membranes are referred to as the _____meninx. The arachnoid membrane is a one these thinner membranes. It derives is name from the root ARACHN-, which means _____, because of its weblike formation.	**meninx, MENING-** **pachy** **dura mater, hard** **lepto** **spider**
The brain is the portion of the central nervous system contained within the cranium. The root for the "brain" is _____. Derived from Greek, the loan word _____ is used for the "brain," and it is used as a suffix for the parts of the embryonic brain.	**ENCEPHAL-** **Encephalon**
The _____ is the largest part of the brain, and it is divided into right and left hemispheres.	**Cerebrum**
The outer layer of an organ is called the _____ to distinguish it from the inner part, which is called the _____. The root for the cerebral cortex is _____, which means _____, _____, or _____.	**cortex, medulla** **CORTIC-** **cortex, outer layer, bark**
The portion of the brain located below the occipital lobe of the cerebrum is called the _____, or "little cerebrum" in Latin. It is responsible for coordination and voluntary movements. The root _____ is used for this part of the brain.	**cerebellum** **CEREBELL-**
The brainstem connects the brain with the spinal cord. It includes the midbrain, pons, and medulla. The most superior part of the brainstem is called the midbrain, or _____. The root PONT- is used for the rostral part of the brainstem known as the pons. That said, PONT- is used for any _____ structure of the body. The medulla, or medulla oblongata, is the caudal segment of the brainstem. The root used for this part, MEDULL-, is also used for bone _____.	**mesencephalon** **bridge-like** **marrow**
The root _____ is used for the color gray, and by extension, the gray matter of the brain. The gray matter forms the outer part of the brain, and the white matter is the inner part. Gray matter is composed of numerous neuronal cell bodies with very little myelinated tissue. White matter is composed primarily of myelinated tissue, which gives it its characteristic color. The loan word _____ is used for the white matter of the brain.	**POLI-** **alba**

Review	Answers
Derived from the Latin word for a "kernel," the root _____ is used for the central organelle of a cell. In the central nervous system, a _____ is a group of neuronal cell bodies that are clustered together, forming a recognizable mass that is associated with specific functions.	**NUCLE-** **nucleus**
The thalamus is an ovoid-shaped collection of nuclei found deep inside the brain that is responsible for processing almost all sensory signal and most motor programs to and from the cerebral cortex. In addition to referring to the thalamus, the root THALAM- can be used for _____ or _____-like structures. The hypothalamus works with the pituitary gland to regulate the secretion of hormones.	**chamber, inner room**
The root LOB- means _____. Each cerebral hemisphere is divided into lobes, which are recognized by anatomical divisions and their functions.	**lobe**
The surface of the cerebral hemispheres is covered with numerous convolutions called gyri, which are separated by grooves called fissures or sulci. The root for GYR- can mean _____, _____, and _____. Like the lobes, the cerebral gyri have names and are associated with specific brain functions.	**gyrus, circle, ring**
Derived from the Latin verb for "cleaving," a fissure is a very deep groove in an anatomical structure. The root of a "deep groove" or "fissure" is _____. A sulcus is derived from the Latin word for a furrow, and, of the two grooves, is generally less deep. The root for sulcus is _____.	**FISSUR-** **SULC-**
The root _____ is used for the cerebral ventricles and other small cavities of the body. There are four ventricles in the brain.	**VENTRICUL-**
The limbic system is associated with emotions and behavior. It is also involved with long term memory and olfaction. The name "limbic" comes from the Latin word for border, *limbus*, thus the root _____ and the loan word _____ are used for a "border-like" structure.	**LIMB-, limbus**
The cerebral hemispheres are united by three commissures: the corpus callosum and the anterior and posterior hippocampal commissures. The root for the hippocampus is _____. Hippocampus is also used for the zoological genus of _____. The hippocampus is part of the limbic system and is responsible for memory consolidation.	**HIPPOCAMP-** **seahorse**
The root for the almond-shaped nuclei of the limbic system is _____. Like the hippocampus, the amygdalae are associated with memory; they are also important to social and emotional processes.	**AMYGDAL-**
Root for spinal cord and bone marrow is _____.	**MYEL-**
Gliocytes or neuroglia are the interstitial and supporting tissue of the nervous system. The combining form GLI/O also means _____.	**glue**
The notochord is a rod of embryonic cells in vertebrates that becomes the axial skeleton in chordates. In vertebrates, the notochord is replaced by the bodies of vertebrae. The combining form NOT/O means the _____. The root CHORD- means a _____ or _____. As was discussed in the Chapter 7 on the musculoskeletal system, the roots RHACHI- and _____ share the meaning of the back or vertebral column; the latter root also means spine and thorn.	**back** **cord, tendons** **SPIN-**
The roots for a vertebra are _____ and _____.	**VERTEBR-, SPONDYL-**
A nerve root is the first part of the peripheral nerve as it comes off the spinal cord. The anterior root carries efferent stimuli, and the posterior root carries afferent stimuli. The combining forms for nerve root are _____, _____, and _____. The loan word for a nerve root is _____. All of these word elements could be used for any "root" or "root-like" structure.	**RHIZ/O, RADICUL/O,** **RADIC/O** **radix**
The primary branch of a spinal nerve is called the _____, which is the Latin word for a branch on a tree.	**ramus**
The network of nerves (or blood, lymphatic vessels) is called a _____.	**plexus**
A _____ is a bundle of nerve cells that looks like a tumor or cyst. They appear in both sympathetic and parasympathetic systems of the autonomic nervous system.	**ganglion**
With respect to the spinal cord, a _____ is one of the three main divisions of the white matter (anterior, lateral, and posterior). The root FUNICUL- is used for this structure, as well as any _____-like structure. Within each funiculus are tracts of nerve fibers called _____, which is also the term used for a small bundle of longitudinal-running nerve (muscle) fibers.	**funiculus** **rope** **fasciculi**

Etymological Explanations: Common Terms and Word Elements for the Physiology and Pathophysiology of the Nervous System

Changes in memory, sensation, knowledge (perception), movement, speech, consciousness, and muscle health are all signs used for diagnosing pathologies of the nervous system. The following tables include the word elements used for these faculties of the nervous system, as well as other terms used for specific pathologies affecting the nervous system.

Memory, sensation, gnosia (perception)

Memory – According to Taber's, memory is the "mental registration, retention, and recollection of past experiences, sensations, or thoughts." The term "memory" comes from the Latin verb *memorare*, "to remind, recall to mind." The corresponding root **MEMOR-** is more commonly used in everyday English, where it shows up in words such as "memorial" and "memorabilia." The commonly used medical and scientific root for "memory" is **MNEMON-**, which shows up in terms such as mnemonic. Derived from the Greek word for memory *mneme*, the suffix used for "memory" and "memory disorders" is **-MNESIA**. Thus, a distorted or abnormal memory is termed **paramnesia**; false memories are associated with **pseudomnesia**; and a recalling of a memory is **anamnesia** (or **anamnesis**). A loss of short-term or long-term memory is **amnesia**. The other term for amnesia used in medicine is **lethe**, which comes from the Greek words for "oblivion" and "forgetfulness." In Greek mythology, wisdom and mental activities are often personified as female deities (e.g. Metis = Counsel, Athena = Wisdom, Themis = divine law, custom). Memory was personified by the goddess Mnemosyne, who was a daughter of Ouranos (Heaven). Her offspring were the Mousai (Muses), which were the goddesses of poetry and other forms of literature. The antithesis of memory was also personified as a goddess. In the Myth of Er in Plato's *Republic*, Lethe appears as an underworld river that the souls drink to forget their past lives before they are reincarnated into a human or animal. The form Lethe was altered in Late Latin to form the term *lethalis*, which is when the root **LETH-** took on the meaning of "fatal." (Fig. 10.11)

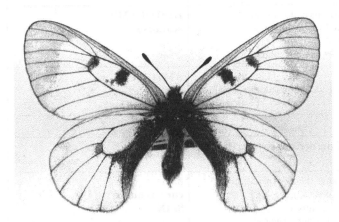

Fig. 10.11 Image of the butterfly known as the *Parnassius mnemosyne*, which is named after the Greek goddess of memory, modified image and extracted from *Europas bekannteste Schmetterlinge. Beschreibung der wichtigsten Arten und Anleitung zur Kenntnis und zum Sammeln der Schmetterlinge und Raupen* (1895), F. Nemos, Oestergaard. *Source:* Dr. F. Nemos / Wikimedia Commons / Public domain.

Sensation – Taber's defines sensation as "an awareness of conditions inside or outside the body resulting from the stimulation of sensory receptors." The English word "sensation" comes from the Latin verb *sentire*, "to perceive by the senses." The roots **SENS-**, **SENT-**, and **SENSOR-** carry this meaning and are commonly used in everyday English (e.g. sentient, sensory, sense). Derived from the Greek word *aisthesis* "feeling"/"sensation," the commonly used roots for "sensation" are **ESTHET-** and **ESTHESI-**. Likewise, the suffix commonly used for "sensation" is **-ESTHESIA**. Thus, an abnormal sensation is termed a **paresthesia.** Excessive sensitivity to stimuli is **hyperesthesia**, and diminished sensitivity to stimuli is hypesthesia. A lack of sensation of motion would be akinesthesia. Perception of stimulus in the limb that is opposite to the one that is stimulated is called allesthesia. The suffix **-ALGIA** is used for a "painful sensation." Hence, an abnormal sensation of pain is a **paralgia**. A painful sensation of cold is a **psychralgia**. A painful burning sensation is called **causalgia**. Pain in the back is called **notalgia** or **dorsalgia**. The technical term for a "headache" is cephalgia.

Gnosia – Gnosia is defined by Taber as "the perceptive faculty of recognizing persons, things, and forms." An awareness of sensations is one thing, but the understanding of what these sensations indicate is quite another. The processing of sensations takes "knowledge" or "understanding," which is why the root **GNOST-** and the suffixes **-GNOSIA** and **-GNOSIS** are often used for "knowledge" of sensations. A **topagnosis** is the loss of the ability to know the site of a tactile sensation. The root **TOP-** means "place," "spot," or "region." **Astereognosis** is the inability to distinguish the shape of objects by a sense of touch. The root **STERE-** means "solid" or "three-dimensional." In ancient Greek literature, the Greek word *gnosis* was used for "knowledge." These authors differed as to what kind of knowledge the term *gnosis* and its derivatives referred to. When drawing a distinction between theoretical knowledge and practical knowledge, Plato used the term *gnostikos* in reference to theoretical knowledge. Among Hellenistic religions and the Gnostic cults, *gnosis* was often used to denote a type of spiritual knowledge found within a person. Today, this religious connotation is somewhat preserved in the term agnostic, which refers to the inability to prove/know for certain the existence of God.

Movement

Kinesis (also Cinesis) – Kinesis is the loan word used for movement. Likewise, the roots **KINESI-** and **KINE-**, as well as the suffix -**KINESIA** are used for "movement." A wide array of faulty movements or movement disorders fall under the term **dyskinesia**. The slow movement that is characteristic of Parkinson's Disease and some other pathologies is termed **bradykinesia**.

Motor – The loan word **motor** and its root **MOT-** means "motion/movement."

Ataxia – A movement disorder in which there is a lack of coordination is called **ataxia**. The root **TAX-** is used for "order" and "coordination" in a large number of terms.

Apraxia – The root **PRAX-** and the suffixes -**PRAXIS** and -**PRAXIA** are used for "activity," "doing," and "practice." The inability to perform an activity/purposeful movement is called **apraxia**.

Athetosis – Athetosis is derived from the Greek word *athetos*, "not fixed, without position or place, set aside." Athetosis is a condition of constant involuntary movements that are slow, irregular, twisting, and snakelike that primarily occur in the upper extremities.

Chorea – The Greek root **CHORE-** literally means "dance," but with respect to the nervous system and movement disorders, it is used for "involuntary dancing, writhing, or jerking movement." The loan word **chorea** is used for disorders that produce such movements. Huntington's chorea is a neurodegenerative, autosomal dominant disease of the CNS marked by **choreoathetosis**. The first thorough description of this hereditary disease was made by an American physician, George Huntington, in 1872. Sydenham's chorea, which is named after the famous British physician Thomas Sydenham (1624–1689), is a neurological syndrome associated with acute rheumatic fever that is associated with chorea of the face and limbs. This type of chorea is also called Saint Vitus' dance in reference to Saint Vitus, who was considered the patron saint of dance (Fig. 10.12).

Fig. 10.12 An 1818 image of a boy with Sydenham's chorea, which is called Danse de Saint-Guy (St. Vitus' Dance). *Source:* Unknown author / Wikimedia Commons / Public domain.

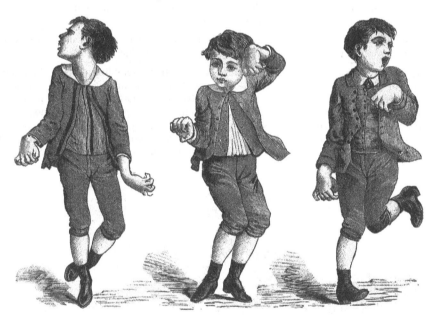

DANSE DE SAINT-GUY.

Speech and reading

Speech pathologies – Disorders of speech are used to recognize the presence of disorders of the nervous system. Although they have different specific usages, the roots **PHAS-**, **LAL-**, **PHRAS-**, and **LOG-** all can refer to "speech." The **LAL-** strictly means "speech." Hence, the combining form in laloplegia reveals that this is a paralysis of speech. As a suffix -**LALIA** is used for specific speech disorders. For instance, echolalia is a disorder in which there is a repetition of the words spoken by others. Based on its root **PHAS-**, dysphasia is an inability or difficulty with speech. Often dysphasia and aphasia are used with disorders of the CNS, particularly strokes. The root **PHRAS-** means "speech" and "phrase." **Bradyphrasia** would be literally a condition of slow speech. The inability to speak or understand phrases is dysphrasia. The root **LOG-** means "speech," "reason," or "word." Any disorder of speech that is derived from a derangement of the CNS is termed a **logopathy**, and **logorrhea** is continuous and excessive speech associated with intoxication. However, **logomania** is an excessive fascination with words, and the suffix -**LOGY** and words such as logic denote study and reason.

Reading disorders – The root **LEX-** means "reading," "word," and sometimes "speech." Most commonly it appears with words for reading disorders, such as dyslexia and bradylexia, which literally mean "difficulty reading" and "slow reading" respectively. **Dyslexia** is defined by Taber's as "difficulty reading and interpreting written forms of communication by a person whose vision and general intelligence are otherwise unimpaired."

Consciousness, awareness

Coma – Derived from the Greek word for "deep sleep," a state of unconsciousness from which one cannot be aroused is termed a coma, and the root used for this state is **COMAT-**.

Syncope – An acute, transient loss of consciousness is commonly termed "fainting." The technical term for fainting is syncope, which is a loan word from the Greek word "cut short." In ancient Greek medicine, syncope was used differently. For example, Galen used *synkope* for a "sudden loss of strength." The word "faint" is derived from a French word for "vapors" since fainting used to be associated with the medieval notion of vapors from the stomach and other organs affecting the brain, causing a person to faint or have hysteria.

Sopor – Based on its use of the root **SOPOR-**, a soporific medication produces sleep. The loan word for "sleep," **sopor**, is naturally from the Latin word for "sleep."

Insomnia – *Somnus* was another Latin word for "sleep." Based on the root **SOMN-**, **insomnia** is the inability to sleep.

Narcolepsy – The combining form **NARC/O** in narcolepsy indicates that this disorder is marked by uncontrollable seizures of "sleep." **NARC-** also has the meaning of "stupor" as in the case of narcotics.

Stupor – Stupor is defined in Taber's as "a state of altered mental status, of decreased responsiveness to one's environment." It is a Latin loan word that means "senselessness, amazement."

Lethargic – The term lethargic is used for a state of mental sluggishness and drowsiness. The root for this word is **LETHARG-**. It is derived from the Greek word, *lethargos*, which means "drowsiness."

Hypnosis – According to Taber's, "hypnosis is a condition resembling sleep in which the objective manifestations of the mind are more or less inactive." The root **HYPN-** is used for "hypnosis" and "sleep." Thus, "the inducing of sleep" or "something induced by sleep" is termed hypnagogic. The suffixes **-AGOGIC** and **-AGOGUE** are derived from the Greek word *agogos*, which means "leading" or "inducing." In Greek mythology, Hypnos was the god of sleep. Hypnos was often paired with his twin brother Thanatos (Peaceful Death). In some respects, this pairing makes sense, given how a sleeping body looks dead. The Greek god Hypnos is also associated with the Oneiroi (Dreams), who were said to be either his brothers or sons. Today, we use the roots **THANAT-** for "death" and **ONEIR-** for "dreams." The Greek god Hypnos was known by the Latin name Somnus or Sopor in Roman mythology (Fig. 10.13).

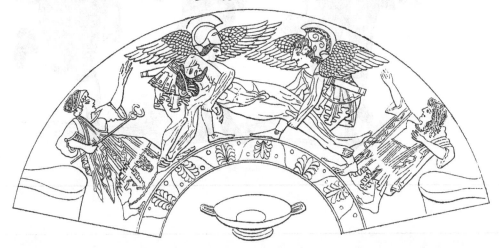

Fig. 10.13 In Greek artwork, Hypnos and Thanatos are commonly depicted as winged deities, which may speak to the volatile nature of death. In Book XVI of the *Iliad*, Hypnos and Thanatos carry the body of the hero Sarpedon, which is the event of this 6th-century-BC image on a red-Fig. kylix is commonly interpreted as representing. *Source:* Wilhelm Heinrich Roscher, (1894)./B. G. Teubner/Public Domain.

Muscle health

Tone – In respect to muscles, tone is a state of slight contraction of muscles that contributes to posture and function. The root **TON-** means "tension" and "stretching." Thus, **hypertonicity** manifests in excessive tension in the muscles and **hypotonicity** is too little tension in the muscles.

Dystonia is a term used for movement disorders characterized by involuntary muscle contractions affecting movement. **Atony** is the lack of normal muscle tone or strength. **Opisthotonos** is the condition of increased tone and spasms of the back muscles causing one to bend backwards. It is a sign of severe tetanus. The root **OPISTH-** means "backward" or "behind." (Fig. 10.14)

Fig. 10.14 Line drawing showing opisthotonos in a patient suffering from tetanus, by Sir Charles Bell, 1829. *Source:* Charles Bell/Wellcome Collection/Public domain.

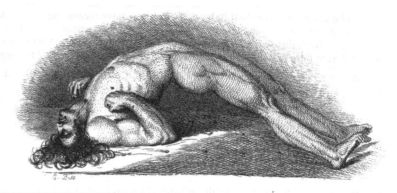

Spasm and **Spasticity** – Derived from the Greek word for "a wrenching" *spasmos*, a sudden involuntary muscle contraction is called a spasm. Spasticity is a movement disorder in which an abnormal increase in muscle tone interferes with movement. The roots for "spasm" are **SPASM-** and **SPAST-**.

Tremor – Tremors are another type of movement disorder that is from the Latin word *tremor*, "a shaking." A tremor is an involuntary shaking or trembling of a body part that can appear at rest or with movement. The roots for "tremor" or any type of "shaking" are **TREM-** and **TREMUL-**.

Atrophy – A decrease in size of muscle is termed atrophy. Atrophy can be a sign of a nervous system disorder. Thus, a characteristic feature of **amyotrophic lateral sclerosis (ALS)** is the loss of muscle size due to the deterioration of motor nerve cells. ALS ultimately leads to a loss of voluntary muscle control, which is why ALS is termed a motor neuron disease.

Strength – The root **STHEN-** means "strength." The suffix **-ASTHENIA** means a condition where there is a lack of strength. Hence, the autoimmune disease that affects the receptors at the neuromuscular synapses causing a rapid loss of strength is termed **myasthenia gravis**.

Paralysis

Paralysis – Derived from the Greek verb meaning "to disable at the side" *paralyein*, **paralysis** is a loss or impairment of motor function or sensation caused by injuries to peripheral nerves or to the CNS. The roots **PLEG-**, **PLECT-**, and the suffixes **-PLEXY** and **-PLEGIA** are all used for "paralysis." For instance, **apoplexy** and its adjective **apoplectic** are used as the term for a "stroke" because of the paralysis caused by a stroke (Fig. 10.15).

Fig. 10.15 Illustration of some of the common types of paralysis. *Source:* DP/Alamy Stock Photo.

Paralysis types illustration

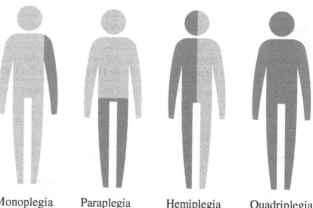

Monoplegia   Paraplegia   Hemiplegia   Quadriplegia

Stroke – A stroke, which is also called a cerebrovascular accident (CVA), is an infarct of the brain due to the disruption of blood flow. It often causes paralysis of half the body, which is termed **hemiplegia**.

Spinal Cord Injury – A lower spinal cord injury can cause paralysis of the legs, which is termed **paraplegia**. A higher spinal cord injury can cause paralysis of the arms and legs (all four limbs), which is termed **quadriplegia**.

Palsy – The word palsy as in **Bell Palsy** and **Cerebral Palsy** means "paralysis." As defined in Taber's, cerebral palsy (CP) is an "umbrella term for a group of nonprogressive but frequently changing motor impairment syndromes secondary to lesions or anomalies of the brain arising in the early stages of its development." Due to the location of the lesions and its varied etiologies, CP can manifest in rather unique forms of paralysis such as **monoplegia** and **triplegia**.

Paresis – The loan word paresis is used for "partial or incomplete paralysis." It often appears as a suffix for terms denoting a partial paralysis of a specific position or part, such as **vasoparesis**.

Seizures

Seizure – A convulsion or transient disturbance of the brain's function caused by abnormal discharge of electrical activity in the brain is termed a seizure. The loan word **ictus** is used for a sudden attack of neurological symptoms/signs, such as with a seizure or stroke. Its root is **ICT-**. Thus, the period after a seizure can be referred to as the **postictal period**. Like the terms seizure and stroke, which speak to grabbing or hitting of something, the Latin word *ictus* meant a physical "strike" or "blow."

Tonic–Clonic Seizure – A grand mal seizure, which is French for "great bad," manifests in convulsions and spasms referred to as tonic–clonic or clonicotonic seizure. Derived from the Greek word for a "confused motion, turmoil," **Clonus** is a spasmodic alteration of muscle contractions between antagonist muscles. Thus, **tonic–clonic seizure** is characterized by the presence of hypertonicity in some parts and spasmodic alterations of muscle contractions in other parts. Seizures that are localized and are without convulsions and spasms are typically called **petit mal (little bad) seizures**.

Epilepsy – Epilepsy is a disorder that is characterized by seizures. Derived from the Greek word for "a taking, seizing" *lepsis*, the roots **LEPS-** and **LEPT-**, as well as the suffix **-LEPSY** are used for "seizure." There is a variety of causes for seizures. A febrile seizure is caused by a fever. The etymology of the term "epilepsy" reveals a similar connotation since it is derived from the Greek verb *epilambanein*, which means "to seize, take hold of, and to attack." Seizures, as well as other conditions that suddenly come upon a person causing convulsions and paralysis, were commonly described as being caused by a god or gods grabbing or striking a person. In ancient Greek literature, seizure disorders were referred to as the sacred disease, which spoke to the belief that the gods and spirits of heroes could assault a person causing a wide variety of seizure-like signs and symptoms. The Hippocratic work entitled *On the Sacred Disease* (*De morbo sacro*) is the earliest medical text to use a natural explanation to account for such dramatic phenomena. The author of *On the Sacred Disease* uses the humor phlegm to provide a natural causality for the signs of seizures, and consequently, he is able to offer a natural pathway to treatment that differs from the therapies of incantations and magic that he attacks at the beginning of this work.

Swelling, infection, and inflammation

Meningitis – An inflammation of the membranes of the brain and spinal cord. Meningitis is usually caused by a bacterial or viral infection. The term is derived from the root for "membrane," **MENING-**, and the suffix for inflammation, **-ITIS**.

Encephalitis – An inflammation of the brain. The term is derived from the root for "brain," **ENCEPHAL-**, and the suffix for inflammation, **-ITIS**.

Hydrocephalus – According to Taber's, hydrocephalus is the accumulation of excessive amounts of CSF within the ventricles of the brain. The term was formed from the Greek **HYDR-** "water" + **CEPHAL-** "head."

Radiculitis – An inflammation of a nerve root. The term is derived from the root for "nerve root" and "root," **RADICUL-**, and the suffix for inflammation, **-ITIS**.

Myelitis – An inflammation of the spinal cord. The term is derived from the root for "bone marrow" and "spinal cord," **MYEL-**, and the suffix for inflammation, **-ITIS**.

Poliomyelitis – A viral infection causing inflammation of the brain and spinal cord is called encephalomyelitis. The root for "gray" and "gray matter" is **POLI-**. Thus, an inflammation of the gray matter of the spinal cord is poliomyelitis. The term **Polio** refers to an acute viral attack of the anterior horns of the spinal cord, known specifically as **acute anterior poliomyelitis**. The term poliomyelitis was coined by the German physician Adolph Kussmaul in 1874. Just prior to this, the disease was called infantile paralysis (1843) (Fig. 10.16).

Fig. 10.16 Image of a quarantine sign during the Polio epidemic of the early 1900s. Polio was once one of the most dreaded diseases, but the discovery of two distinct vaccines, that were developed by Dr. Jonas Salk and Dr. Albert Sabin, led to Polio being eliminated in the Americas by 1994. *Source:* Courtesy of the National Library of Medicine. Images from the History of Medicine (IHM).

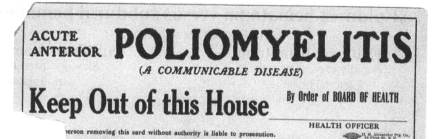

Tumors and cancer

Neuroma – A tumor of a nerve is called a neuroma. The term is formed from the root for "nerve," **NEUR-**, and the suffix for tumor, **-OMA.**

Neurofibroma – A fibrous tumor originating in the fibrous tissue of a nerve sheath is called a neurofibroma. The term is formed from the combining form for "nerve," **NEUR/O**, the root for "fiber" or "filament," **FIBR-**, and the suffix for "tumor," **-OMA.**

Meningioma – A tumor of a membrane of the brain and spinal cord is a meningioma. The term is derived from the root for "membrane," **MENING-**, and the suffix for "tumor," **-OMA.**

Encephaloma – A tumor of the brain is called an encephaloma. The term is derived from the root for "brain," **ENCEPHAL-**, and the suffix for "tumor," **-OMA**.

Glioma – A neoplasm or tumor composed of neuroglial cells, glue cells, is called a glioma. The term is formed from the root for "glue" or "glue cells," **GLI-**, and the suffix for "tumor," **-OMA**. The plural of glioma is **gliomata**. The types of gliomata include **astrocytoma, ependymoma**, and **oligodendroglioma**. An astrocytoma is a tumor of the brain or spinal cord composed of astrocytes. Astrocytoma is formed from the combining form for "star," **ASTR/O**, the root for "cell," **CYT-**, and the suffix for "tumor," **-OMA**. An ependymoma is a tumor of the brain and spinal cord that arises from ependymal cells, which are the CSF-producing cells that line the ventricles and spinal cord. The term is formed from the root **EPENDYM-**, which is derived from a Greek word for "an upper garment." **Oligodendroglioma** is a tumor of the oligodendrocytes, which are glial cells found along axon tracts that myelinate axons in the CNS. The term for these cells is derived from the combining form for "few" or "scanty," **OLIG/O**, and the root for "tree" or "tree-like," **DENDR-** (Fig. 10.17).

Fig. 10.17 Gliomata of right temporosphenoidal lobe of the cerebrum. Image modified form original found in Archibald Church, *Nervous and Mental Disease*, 1911. *Source:* Internet Archive Book Images / Wikimedia Commons / Public domain.

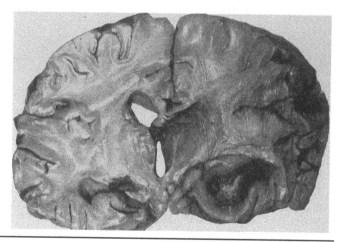

Traumatic brain injuries

Traumatic brain injury – According to Taber's, a traumatic brain injury (TBI) is "any injury involving direct trauma to the head, accompanied by alterations in mental status or consciousness."

Concussion – A cerebral concussion is a common TBI that often results in a loss of consciousness and/or function due to the impact of an object. The term is derived from the Latin word for "a shaking," *concussio*. This general meaning can be observed in the emblematic Latin phrase, *Concussus surgo*, which means "though shaken, I rise."

Hematoma – TBI can cause a swelling of blood in the cranium known as a hematoma. A **subdural hematoma** is located under the dura mater, and it is typically venous. An **epidural hematoma** is located upon the dura mater, and it is most often cause by disruption of an artery. In addition to medications, sometimes a craniotomy is performed to relieve the pressure caused by the blood pooling in the confined space under the cranium (Fig. 10.18).

Epidural hematoma versus subdural hematoma

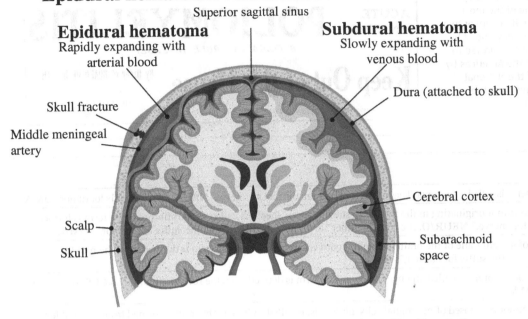

Epidural hematoma
Rapidly expanding with
arterial blood

Superior sagittal sinus

Subdural hematoma
Slowly expanding with
venous blood

Dura (attached to skull)

Skull fracture

Middle meningeal
artery

Cerebral cortex

Scalp

Subarachnoid
space

Skull

Fig. 10.18 Image of the differences between a subdural hematoma and an epidural hematoma.

Greek or Latin word element	Current usage	Etymology	Examples
ESTHESI/O (ĕs-thē-zē-ō) **ESTHET/O** (ĕs-thĕt-ō) **-ESTHESIA** (es-thē-zh-ē-ă)	Sensation, perception	Gr. *aisthesis*, feeling, sensation	Par**esthesia**, an**esthet**ic, **esthesi**ology
GNOST/O (gnos-tō) **-GNOSIA** (gnō-sē-ă) **-GNOSIS** (-gnō-sĭs)	Knowledge	Gr. *gnosis*, a knowing, knowledge	Pro**gnost**icate, a**gnosia**, atopo**gnosis**
MNEMON/O (nē-mŏn-ō) **-MNESIA** (mnē-zhă)	Memory	Gr. *mneme*, memory	**A**mnesia, **mnemon**ic, hyper**mnesia**
LETH/O (lē-thō)	Forgetfulness	Gr. *lethe*, oblivion, forgetfulness	**Leth**ologica, **leth**al Loan word: **Lethe** (lē′thē)
LETHARG/O (lĕth-ăr-gō)	Mental sluggishness, drowsiness	Gr. *lethargos*, drowsiness	**Letharg**ic, **letharg**y
TOP/O (tō-pō)	Place, spot, region	Gr. *topos*, place, spot	**Top**algia, **top**ography, ec**top**ic
STERE/O (ster-ē-ō)	Solid, three-dimensional	Gr. *stereos*, solid	A**stere**ognosis, **stere**oplasm, **stere**oscopic

Greek or Latin word element	Current usage	Etymology	Examples
KINESI/O (kĭ-nē-sē-ō) **KINE/O** (kin-ĕ-ō) **-KINESIA** (kī-nē-zhē-ă)	Movement	Gr. *kineein*, to move	**Kinesi**ology, **Kine**sthesia, Hyper**kinesia**, Loan word: **Kinesis** (kĭ-nē′sĭs)
MOT/O (mōt-ō)	Movement	L. *movere*, *motum*, to move	**Mot**oneuron, **mot**or, **mot**ile
PRAXI/O (prăk-sē-ō) **-PRAXIA** (prak-sē-ă) **-PRAXIS** (prăk-sĭs)	Activity, doing, practice	Gr. *praxis*, a doing	**Praxi**ology, A**praxia**, Actino**praxis** Loan word: **Praxis** (prăk′sĭs) pl. **Praxes** (prăk′sēz″)
TAX/O (tak-sō)	Coordination, order	Gr. *taxis*, order, arrangement	A**taxia**, **tax**onomy, rhizo**taxis** Loan word: **Taxis** (tak′sĭs) pl. **Taxes** (tak′sēz″)
TON/O (ton-ō)	Tension, stretching, tone (esp. in muscles)	Gr. *tonos*, that which is stretched, cord, rope	Hyper**ton**icity, mono**tone**, opitho**ton**os
SPASM/O (spaz-mō) **SPAST/O** (spas-tō)	Spasm (a sudden involuntary muscle contraction)	L. *spasmus*, -*i*, m. spasm fr. Gr. *spasmos*, a wrenching	**Spast**ic, Chiro**spasm**, **spast**icity Loan word: **Spasmus** (spaz′mŭs)
LEPS/O (lep-sō) **LEPT/O** (lĕp-tō) **-LEPSY** (lep-sē)	Seizure	Gr. *lepsis*, a taking, seizing	Pro**leps**is, Cata**lept**ic, Narco**lepsy**
ICT/O (ik-tō) **-ICTAL** (ik-tăl)	Seizure, stroke (CVA), Blow	L. *ictus*, -*us*, m. a strike, blow	Post**ictal**, **ict**ometer Loan word: **Ictus** (ĭk′tŭs)
PYKN/O (pĭk-nō) **PYCN/O** (pĭk-nō)	Thick, dense, frequent	Gr. *pyknos*, thick, dense	**Pykn**ocyte, **pykn**emia, **pykn**olepsy
PLEG/O (plĕg-ō) **-PLEGIA** (plē-jē-ă) **PLECT/O** (plĕk-tō) **-PLEXY** (plĕks-ē)	Paralysis, stroke	Gr. *plessein*, to strike, hit, smite	Hemi**pleg**ic, Mono**plegia**, Apo**plect**ic, Cata**plexy**

Greek or Latin word element	Current usage	Etymology	Examples
PALSY (pal-zē)	Paralysis	Gr. *paralysis*, loosening, disabling by the side	**Palsy**
-PARESIS (pă-rē-sĭs)	Partial paralysis	Gr. *paresis*, a letting go	Hemi**paresis** Loan word: **Paresis** (pă-rē′sĭs)
STHEN/O (sthĕ-nō)	Strength	Gr. *sthenos*, strength	Mya**sthen**ia, hyper**sthen**ic, **sthen**ometer
CLON/O (klŏ-nō)	Clonus (i.e. spasmodic alteration of muscle contractions)	Gr. *klonos*, a confused motion, turmoil	**Clon**ospasm, myo**clon**ia Loan word: **Clonus** (klŏ′nŭs)
CHORE/O (kŏ-rē-ō)	Chorea (i.e. involuntary dancing/writhing movement), dance	Gr. *choreia*, dancing	**Chore**oathetosis, **chore**ography Loan word: **Chorea** (kŏ-rē′ă)
NARC/O (nar-kō)	Stupor, sleep	Gr. *narke*, numbness, deadness	**Narc**olepsy, **narc**otic
HYPN/O (hip-nō)	Sleep	Gr. *hypnos*, sleep	**Hypn**agogue, **hypn**osis
SOMN/O (som-nō)	Sleep	L. *somnus, -i*, m. sleep	In**somn**ia, **somn**ambulism
SOPOR/O (sō-pŏ-rō)	Sleep	L. *sopor, soporis*, m. sleep	**Sopor**ific, **sopor**ous Loan word: **Sopor** (sō′pŏr)
COMAT/O (kŏ-mă-tō) **-COMA** (kŏ-mă)	Coma (i.e. state of unconsciousness that cannot be aroused from)	Gr. *koma, kamatos*, deep sleep	**Comat**ose, pseudo**coma** Loan word: **Coma** (kŏ′mă)
LAL/O (lăl-ō) **-LALIA** (lă-lē-ă)	Speech	Gr. *lalein*, to talk, speak	**Lal**oplegia, tachy**lalia**, echo**lalia**
PHAS/O (fă-zō) **-PHASIS** (f-ă-sĭs) **-PHASIA** (fă-z-ē-ă)	Speech	Gr. *phasis*, speech fr. Gr. *phanai*, to speak	A**phas**iac, allo**phasis**, a**phasia**
PHRAS/O (fră-zō) **-PHRASIA** (fră-zē-ă)	Speech, phrase	Gr. *phrasis*, speech, expression	Para**phras**e, a**phrasia**
LEX/O (lek-sō)	Word, speech, reading	Gr. *lexis*, speaking, diction	Dys**lex**ia, **lex**icon, brady**lex**ia
LOG/O (log-ō) **-LOGY** (l-ŏ-jē)	Speech, reason, word (-logy: body of knowledge, study of)	Gr. *logos*, reason, word, speech	**Log**orrhea, psycho**logy**, **log**ic

Greek or Latin word element	Current usage	Etymology	Examples
PHAG/O (făg-ō) **-PHAGIA** (fă′jē-ă)	Eat, swallow	Gr. *phagein*, to eat, swallow	**Phag**ocytosis, a**phagia**
VERT/O (věr-tō) **VERS/O** (věr-sō)	Turning	L. *vertere*, *versum*, to turn	**Vert**igo, in**vers**ion
TREM/O (tre-mō) **TREMUL/O** (trěm-ū-lō)	Shaking, trembling	L. *tremor*, *-oris*, m. a shaking	**Trem**ophobia, **tremul**ous Loan word: **Tremor** (trem′ŏr)
OPISTHO- (ō-pĭs-thō)	Backward, behind	Gr. *opisthen*, behind, at the back, backward	**Opisth**otonos, **opisth**oglossal, **opisth**ocoelus
ONEIR/O (ō-nī-rō)	Dream	Gr. *oneiros*, dream	**Oneir**ic, **oneir**ology

Review	Answers
Based on its root **PHAG-**, dysphagia is an inability or difficulty with _____ or _____.	**eating, swallowing**
Based on its root **PHAS-**, dysphasia is an inability or difficulty with _____.	**speech**
The root **VERT-** in vertigo suggests that this condition involves a sensation of _____.	**turning**
The combining form in laloplegia reveals that this is a paralysis of _____.	**speech**
The root PHRAS- means _____ and _____. Bradyphrasia would be literally a condition of _____ speech. The inability to speak or understand phrases is _____.	**speech, phrase** **slow** **aphrasia**
The root LOG- means _____, _____, or _____. Any disorder of speech that is derived from a derangement of the central nervous system is termed _____.	**speech, reason, word** **logopathy**
The root meaning "reading," "word," and sometimes "speech" is _____. Most commonly it appears with words for reading disorders, such as dyslexia and bradylexia, which literally mean _____ reading and _____ reading, respectively.	**LEX-** **faulty, slow**
The loan word for "involuntary dancing/writhing movement" is _____. The root CHORE- literally means _____.	**chorea** **dance**
The combining form _____ in narcolepsy indicates that this disorder is marked by uncontrollable seizures of _____. NARC/O also has the meaning of _____ as in the case of narcotics. Stupor is defined as "A state of altered mental status, of decreased responsiveness to one's environment."	**NARC/O, sleep** **stupor**
Based on its root _____, a soporific medication produces _____. The loan word for sleep that is derived from this word is _____.	**SOPOR-, sleep** **sopor**
Based on the root _____, insomnia is the inability to _____.	**SOMN-, sleep**
HYPN- is used for "hypnosis" and "_____." Thus, the inducing of sleep or something induced by sleep is termed hypnagogic. The -AGOGIC and -AGOGUE are derived from the Greek word *agogos*, which means "leading" or "inducing."	**sleep**
A state of unconsciousness from which one cannot be aroused is termed a _____. The root used for this state is _____.	**coma, COMAT-**

Review	Answers
Fainting, which is characterized as a sudden loss of consciousness and inability to maintain an upright position, is called _____.	**syncope**
The term _____ is used for a state of mental sluggishness and drowsiness. The root for this word is _____.	**lethargic, LETHARG-**
Pain occurring along the course of a nerve is called _____ algia.	**neur**
A convulsion or transient disturbance of the brain's function caused by abnormal discharge of electrical activity in the brain is termed a seizure. _____ is a disorder that is characterized by seizures. The Greek roots _____ and _____, as well as the suffix _____ are used for "seizure."	**Epilepsy** **LEPT-, LEPS-, -LEPSY**
The roots _____ and _____ mean "thick," "dense," and "frequent." For the term pyknolepsy is used for very frequent seizures.	**PYKN-, PYCN-**
The loan word _____ is used for a sudden attack of neurological symptoms/signs, such as with a seizure or stroke.	**ictus**
The suffix typically used for partial paralysis is _____.	**-PARESIS**
The word palsy as in Bell Palsy and Cerebral Palsy means _____.	**paralysis**
A stroke, also called a cerebrovascular accident, often causes paralysis of half the body, which is termed _____. A lower spinal cord injury can cause paralysis of the legs which is termed _____. A higher spinal cord injury can cause paralysis of the arms and legs (all four limbs), which is termed _____.	**hemiplegia** **paraplegia** **quadriplegia**
The root STHEN- means _____. The suffix -ASTHENIA means a condition of _____. Hence, the autoimmune disease causing a rapid loss of strength is called myasthenia gravis.	**strength** **weakness**
The suffix used for "movement" is _____. Based on this suffix, faulty movement would be _____, and slow movement is termed _____.	**-KINESIA** **dyskinesia, bradykinesia**
The suffix used for "sensation" is _____. Thus, an abnormal sensation is termed a _____. Excessive sensitivity to stimuli is _____, and diminished sensitivity to stimuli is _____.	**-ESTHESIA** **paresthesia** **hyperesthesia, hypesthesia**
The suffix used for "memory" is _____. The loss of memory is _____. Distorted or abnormal memory is _____.	**-MNESIA** **amnesia** **paramnesia**
The root used for "forgetfulness" is _____. That said, it is more commonly used for "fatal."	**LETH-**
The suffixes used for "knowledge" are _____ and _____. A topagnosis is the loss of the ability to know the site of a tactile sensation. The root TOP- means _____, _____, or _____. Astereognosis is the inability to distinguish the shape of objects by the sense of touch. The root STERE- means _____ or _____.	**-GNOSIA, -GNOSIS** **place, spot, region** **solid, three-dimensional**
TON- means _____, _____, and _____. Muscular tone is a state of slight contraction that contributes to posture and function. Excessive tone is called _____. Low tone is called _____.	**tension, stretching, tone** **hypertonicity** **hypotonicity**
A sudden involuntary muscle contraction is called a _____. _____ is a movement disorder in which an abnormal increase in muscle tone interferes with movement.	**spasm or spasmus** **spasticity**
_____ is a spasmodic alteration of muscle contractions between antagonist muscles. A tonic–clonic seizure, also known as a grand mal (big bad) seizure is characterized by the presence of hypertonicity and spasmodic alterations of muscle contractions.	**Clonus**
An involuntary shaking or trembling of a body part is called a _____.	**tremor**
The root _____ is used for "order" and "coordination." A movement disorder in which there is a lack of coordination is called _____.	**TAX-** **ataxia**
The root _____ is used for "activity," "doing," and "practice." The inability to perform an activity/purposeful movement is called _____.	**PRAX-** **apraxia**

Review	Answers
_____ is used for water or watery substances, such as cerebrospinal fluid. Thus, the excessive accumulation of cerebrospinal fluid in the ventricles is called _____, which literally means "water head."	**HYDR-** **hydrocephalus**
An inflammation of the membranes of the brain and spinal cord is called _____, usually caused by a bacterial or viral infection. An inflammation of the brain is called _____. An inflammation of many nerves is called _____. An inflammation of the spinal cord is called _____.	**meningitis** **encephalitis** **polyneuritis** **myelitis**
The root for "gray" and "gray matter" is _____. Inflammation of the gray matter of the spinal cord is _____. Polio refers to an acute viral attack of the anterior horns of the spinal cord and acute anterior poliomyelitis.	**POLI-** **poliomyelitis**
A neoplasm or tumor composed of neuroglial cells is called a _____. A tumor of a nerve is a _____. A fibrous tumor originating in the fibrous tissue of a nerve sheath is called a _____. A tumor of a membrane of the brain and spinal cord is a _____. A tumor of the brain is called an _____.	**glioma** **neuroma** **neurofibroma** **meningioma** **encephaloma**
A radiculopathy is any disease affecting a nerve _____.	**root**
The suffix -ALGIA is used for a painful condition, which often is due to disorders of the nervous system. Thus, an abnormal sensation of pain is a _____algia. A painful sensation of cold is a _____algia. A painful burning sensation is called causalgia. Pain in the back is called _____algia or _____algia. The technical term for a "headache" is _____algia.	**par** **psychr** **not, dors** **cephal**
A decrease in size of muscle is termed _____. Thus, a characteristic feature of amyotrophic lateral sclerosis (ALS) is the loss of muscle size due to the deterioration of motor nerve cells, which ultimately leads to a loss of voluntary muscle control. ALS is termed a motor neuron disease. The loan word "motor" means _____.	**atrophy** **motion**
A cerebral _____ (L. *concussio*, a shaking) is a common traumatic brain injury (TBI). According to Taber's, a TBI is "any injury involving direct trauma to the head, accompanied by alterations in mental status or consciousness." Such trauma can cause swelling of blood in the cranium known as a _____. A subdural hematoma is located _____ the dura mater. An epidural hematoma is located _____ the dura mater.	**concussion** **hematoma** **under** **upon**

Lessons from History: Mental Illness in Ancient Greek Medicine

Food for Thought as You Read:

In what ways did ancient Greek concepts of the "mind" and its relationship to the body (psyche-soma) affect their understanding of mental illness?
In what ways do modern concepts of the "mind" and its relationship to the body (psyche-soma) affect our understanding of mental illness?

In modern medicine, **psychology** is the study of normal and abnormal mental processes. **Psychiatry** is the medical treatment of mental illnesses. **Psychotherapy** is the use of verbal or nonverbal techniques or mental exercises (e.g. behavioral therapy and cognitive therapy) to treat mental illness, and it is the approach of treatment used by psychologists. Psychiatrists are physicians who specialize in mental disorders. In addition to psychotherapy, psychiatry also entails the use of medications such as anxiolytics, antidepressants, sedatives, neuroleptics, and other psychotropic drugs. **Psychology** and **Psychiatry** are both derived from the root commonly used for the "mind," **PSYCH-**, and likewise, the loan word **"psyche"** is used in modern medicine to mean the "mind" and "mental processes." However, the array of meanings that the ancient Greek word *psyche* carried (e.g. "breath," "spirit," "life," "soul," "mind," "understanding," and "ghost") make it a very difficult word to accurately translate into modern English. Most of this difficulty is due to modern connotations of the terms "mind" and "soul," particularly as they relate to the human body. In modern English, the "soul" has religious connotations of an individual's eternal and immaterial self. As for the term "mind," theorists vacillate between immaterial and material explanations as to its nature and faculties. Whether the mind is understood as being purely the chemical and electrical activities of the brain or if it is conceptualized as being something more than the body is not purely a matter of philosophical speculation; it has a direct effect on how medicine approaches mental health and illness. In the following discussion, we will look at how ancient Greek medicine's understanding of the psyche impacted physicians' approaches to mental illnesses.

The Greek word *psyche*, and its correlative *pneuma*, were closely linked to "breath," particularly as it relates to the life of an organism. In contrast to modern notions of the "psyche," Greek philosophy and medicine understood the function of the *psyche* as being more than the mental faculties and emotions; the *psyche* was linked to bodily functions and physical impulses. This, perhaps, explains why ancient medicine generally did not categorize diseases that affected the mental faculties as "mental illnesses." For the most part, diseases that adversely affected consciousness, cognition, and behaviors were construed as being caused by disturbances within the body, and therefore, what we term "mental illness" often would have been considered just another type of *nosos* (disease) of the body. In the introduction to *Mental Illness in Ancient Medicine*, Chiara Thumiger and Peter Singer point out that Celsus' use of the Latin term *insania* (literally "unhealthy") in *De medicina* provides some evidence as to a "starting point" for mental illness being considered somewhat of a "discrete concept." Celsus categorizes *insania* as being not localized to a specific body part, and therefore, affecting the person as a whole. Using medical terms for diseases that affect the mental faculties, Celsus states there are three types of *insania*: "acute" (*acuta*) for which *phrenitis* is an example, "longer" (*spatium longius recipit*) which is typified by the disease *melancholia*, and the "longest" (*longissimum*) for which *mania* is his example. The distinction of the duration is clearly his criteria for each type of *insania*. It also should be noted that the ancient medical explanations for the causes of his three examples are purely somatic, being closely linked with humoral and pneumatic pathological models.

A philosophical–ethical conception of mental health is evident in Galen's descriptions of conditions caused by the *psyche*. Pulling from philosophical conceptions of emotions and reason, Galen describes how a *pathos* (affection) of the *psyche* is an irrational impulse in us that is not amenable to reason, such as excessive desire, anger, fear, and envy. Thus, these emotional affections can affect one's behavior as well as one's bodily health if they are not tempered. In his work *Affections of the Soul* (*De proprium animi cuiuslibet affectuum dignotione et curatione*), Galen prescribes therapeutic measures that resemble in some respects a "talk therapy" approach found in modern psychology. For instance, he claims that awareness of the problem is the beginning of controlling such impulses, and then he recommends finding a suitable mentor and self-monitoring so that one can tame the irrational force on the spirited part of the soul. In *Errors of the Soul* (*De animi cuius libet peccatorum dignotione et curatione*), Galen speaks to another issue with the *psyche*, one that would not fall neatly into our own categories of "mental health." He describes how an "error" (*hamartia*) of the *psyche* is different from a "affection" (*pathos*) of the *psyche*. He uses the term *hamartia* to speak to errors in reason or false opinion, which is rather different from the meaning of *hamartia* = "sin" found in Christian literature of this time. For Galen, a person's inability to reason effectively was a serious matter in that it left one without the means to make good choices, and he recommends that one gain a more solid grasp of formal logic, therefore improving the rational faculties of one's soul. That said, Galenic works such as the *Faculties of the Soul are Dependent on the Mixtures of the Body* (*Quod animi mores corporis temperamenta sequuntur*), a work in which he suggests emotion and intelligence are dependent on the health of the body, reveal that Galen's understating of the mental faculties was often decidedly somatic.

The humoral concepts of mental diseases are evident in much of our modern terminology, particularly the humor "black bile" (*melaina chole*). The term *melancholia* (a pathological condition of black bile), which is often translated "melancholy," became a prominent explanation for a wide variety of mental illnesses in medical literature. The concept of melancholy also interested philosophers because of its relevance to the relationship between the mind and the body. This can be observed in the Aristotelian *Problemata XXX.1*, which asks, "why the most prominent people are melancholic (*melancholikoi*)?" After discussing how the dual qualities (i.e. hot and cold) of melancholy can respectively produce both manic and depressive states in an individual, he notes how a temporary balance between these two polar opposites can produce a preternatural genius in the same individual. The explanation offered in *Problemata XXX.1* seems to point not only to an ancient notion of bipolar depression but also to the modern concept of "melancholic genius." Melancholy's growing importance can be observed in medical texts being devoted to this humor and its effects on the body. Rufus of Ephesus' *On Melancholy* is a medical work written in probably the 1st century AD that is dedicated to conditions associated with black bile. In this work, one finds Rufus using the concept of melancholy to explain symptoms such as excessive fear, anxiety, and hallucinations caused by this humor, and quite interestingly, he also notes how lovesickness and over devotion to math can lead to physical complaints that resemble melancholy. Rufus' psychological explanation predates Galen's conception of an affection of the soul, pointing to a potential medical origin for some of Galen's theories. The plasticity of the concept of melancholy allowed it to be shaped to fit a wide variety of conditions that would be deemed neurotic or psychotic in modern psychology. A condition such as **lycanthropy**, which in modern terms is a rare form of psychosis in which one believes he or she is a wolf, was attributed to black bile by Paulus of Aegina in the 7th century AD. Likewise, our term **hypochondriasis (hypochondria)**, which is used for an anxiety disorder in which there is a false belief that one is suffering from some disease(s) despite medical reassurance to the contrary, has its origins in ancient medical theories of melancholy. The term hypochondriasis, which literally means "under the cartilage," speaks to the spleen's location in the body and the belief that this organ was associated with the production of black bile (Fig. 10.19). Today **melancholy** and **melancholia** are used in a much more restricted sense; according to Taber's Cyclopedic Medical Dictionary, melancholy is an "extreme depression, esp. when complicated by frequent crying, anhedonia, and fearfulness."

Ancient concepts of bodily humor seem to address, albeit in a deterministic and decidedly somatic way, some of the questions of personality found in modern psychology. This can be observed in the etymologies of some of our modern psychological and medical terms. For instance, the etymology of the term **temperament**, which is defined in Taber's as "the combination of intellectual, emotional, ethical, and physical characteristics of a specific individual," reveals that it is derived from the Latin word *temperamentum*, which meant "the proper proportion of things mixed together." Beginning with the 5th century BC, the mixture

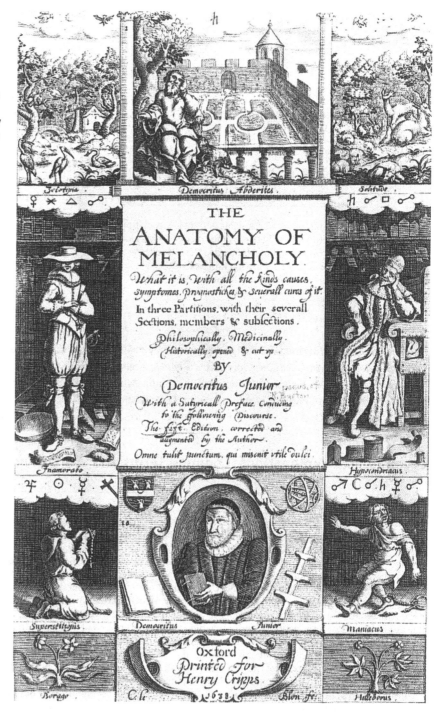

Fig. 10.19 The frontispiece for the 1638 edition of *The Anatomy of Melancholy*. The text is written by self-avowed melancholic, Robert Burton. The top middle box represents Democritus, who is an ancient Greek philosopher that supposedly suffered from melancholy. The boxes left and right to this top middle box represent symptoms Burton associated with melancholy: jealousy and solitariness. The middle four boxes have forms of melancholy. The box to the left is "inamorato," which is associated with lovesickness; the box to the right marked "hypochondriacus" is associated with hypochondriasis; the lower left box marked "superstitiosus" reveals a man who suffers from a religious madness; and the middle bottom right is "maniacus," whom Burton describes as a "madman." Above each of these figures are astrological signs that indicate the origin and nature of these melancholic figures. *Source:* Robert Burton/Wikimedia Commons/Public domain.

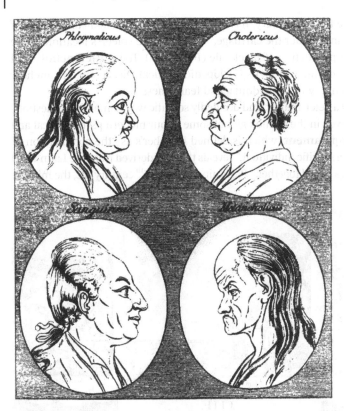

of bodily humor was thought to have a deterministic effect on a person's health, appearance, and character. Thus, if one were born with an excessive amount of black bile, he or she would be said to be melancholic. This humoral concept of innate constitutions became typified by the four humors and closely associated with the four seasons. Because the seasons were associated with engendering specific humors due to their respective qualities (e.g. autumn is cold and dry – black bile is cold and dry), the season of one's birth became an explanation for an individual's personality traits. This seasonal approach to humoral constitutions naturally gave rise to astronomical concepts of the stars' relationship to one's health and personality since the constellations were used as seasonal markers. Thus, a person's particular constitution could be linked to the stars, moon, and planets that were present at birth. While astronomical conceptions of personality types today are delimited to the pseudoscience of horoscopes, the ideas of distinct constitutions and their corresponding personalities are still evident in medical terms and their modern usages: **choleric** (irritable and quick-tempered), **phlegmatic** (sluggish or dull), **sanguine** (optimistic and cheerful), and **melancholic** (depressed and sad) (Fig. 10.20).

Fig. 10.20 Image of the four temperaments and their association with physiognomic features. Modified image form original woodcut from *Physiognomische Fragmente zur Beförderung der Menschenkenntnis und Menschenliebe* (1775–1778) by Johann Kaspar Lavater. *Source:* Thomas Holloway / Wikimedia Commons / Public domain.

Suggested Readings

Galen Psychological Writings, Edited and translated by Peter N Singer. Cambridge: Cambridge University Press, 2013.
Mental Illness in Ancient Medicine: From Celsus to Paul of Aegina. Edited by Chiara Thumiger and Peter N. Singer. Leiden: Brill, 2018.
Psyche and Soma: Physicians and Metaphysicians on the Mind-body Problem from Antiquity to Enlightenment. Edited by John P. Wright and Paul Potter. Oxford: Clarendon Press, 2000.
Rufus of Ephesus. *On Melancholy*. Edited by Peter E. Porman, Tübingen: Mohr Siebeck, 2008.

Etymological Explanations: Common Terms and Word Elements for Psychological Terms

Psychological terms

Neurosis and **Psychosis** – The etymologies of two major classifications of mental illnesses, neurosis and psychosis, are unfortunately not that useful. A neurosis is a maladaptive psychological disorder that affects personality, mood, or some behaviors, without a radical loss of contact with reality. Neurosis was coined by the Scottish doctor William Cullen in 1769 to describe movement and sense disorders caused by an affection of the nervous system. Therefore, the root **NEUR-** in neurosis refers to the nervous system, but generally the root **NEUR-** means strictly "nerve." Neurosis is the category currently used for mood disorders (e.g. depression, dysthymia, bipolar disorder, seasonal affect disorder), anxiety disorders (e.g. panic disorder, phobia, post-traumatic stress disorder (PTSD), obsessive compulsive disorder (OCD), and hypochondriasis), histrionic personality disorders, and dissociative disorders. Psychosis is a mental disorder in which there is severe loss of contact with reality, often accompanied by hallucinations, delusions, impaired reasoning, and catatonic behavior. The term "psychosis" was first introduced into psychiatric literature by Carl Canstatt in 1841. Neurosis was already introduced for nervous system related disorders, and therefore, he used psychosis and psychotic neurosis to emphasize the psychic manifestation of a disease in the brain. The root **PSYCH-** in psychosis means "mind." **Schizophrenia** is a type of psychosis that can manifest in a variety of ways such as delusions, hallucinations, disorganized speech, paranoia, and catatonic behavior. The root **PHREN-** in this term means "mind," but in other contexts, it can refer to the "diaphragm," such as the nerve that innervates the diaphragm being called the "phrenic" nerve. The connection between the diaphragm and the mind is due to the ancient Greek concept of the midriff being the seat of emotion and mental activities.

Neuroticism – Although derived from the same root, neurosis should not be confused with neuroticism. In psychology, neuroticism is considered one of the "Big Five" personality traits: openness to experience, conscientiousness, extraversion, agreeableness, and neuroticism. Neuroticism is a strong tendency to experience negative emotions, such as anger, anxiety, or depression.

Depression – Coming from the Latin verb *deprimere* (to press down), depression is used for mood disorders that are associated with a loss of interest or pleasure in living. Clinical depression, manic depression, and dysthymia fall under the broad umbrella of depression. **Dysthymia** is used for a mild form of chronic depression or dysphoric mood. The root **THYM-** means "emotion" or "state of mind." In ancient Greek thought, the *thumos* was a term used for the "soul" and the "breath of life," and *thumos* was commonly used in Greek literature to describe the depth of a character's emotions. Achilles' *thumos* was where his pain and rage manifested, and therefore, the *thumos* was linked to the spiritedness of a hero.

Dysmorphia – Body image disorders fall under the term dysmorphia. Anorexia nervosa and bulimia nervosa are two eating disorders whose cause is typically ascribed to abnormal perceptions of one's body weight. The term "nervosa" is used in terms such as anorexia nervosa and bulimia nervosa to signify that these disorders are psychosomatic in origin. The term bulimia means "ravenous hunger." **Bulimia nervosa** is characterized by binge eating followed by severe purging. The root **OREX-** means "appetite." **OREX-** is used in a wide variety of eating disorders. **Anorexia nervosa** is characterized by a fear of becoming fat and a subsequent refusal to eat despite having a bodyweight that is well-below normal.

Complexes – Derived from a Latin word meaning "woven together," in Freudian and Jungian psychology, a complex is a collection of emotionally significant ideas that are repressed causing mental conflict and abnormal behaviors. Often Greek mythological figures are used to signify the ideas associated with a complex. **Oedipus complex** is defined as child's abnormally intense love for the parent of the opposite sex that often manifests as jealously toward the parent of the same sex. The term is derived from Freud's reception of *Oedipus Rex*, the ancient Greek tragedy that portrays the horrible ramifications of Oedipus unwittingly killing his father and marrying his mother. Since much of Freud's ideas centered on male sexual experience, the term **Electra complex** was created for a group of symptoms due to the suppressed sexual love of a daughter for her father. In Greek mythology, Electra helped her brother Orestes kill their mother, Clytemnestra, supposedly because of Electra's love for her father, whom Clytemnestra had murdered. Similarly, Narcissistic personality disorder (NPD) is understood through a figure in Greek mythology. Based on the mythological figure Narcissus, who fell in love with an image of himself causing his ultimate demise, the root **NARCISS-** means "self-love." NPD is characterized by an individual's over-inflated sense of self-importance and a need for excessive admiration (Fig. 10.21).

Fig. 10.21 Fresco of Narcissus staring at his reflection from Pompeii. *Source:* Unknown author/Wikimedia Commons/ CC0 1.0.

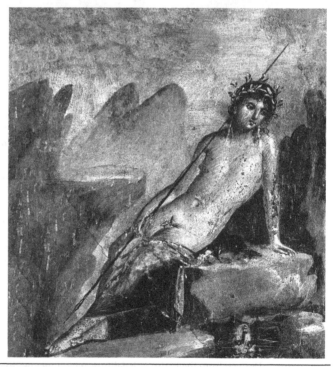

Affect – The term affect is used to describe the mood or emotional reaction associated with a situation or experience. Hence, a flat affect is an absence of emotional response to a situation or experience that typically warrants a reaction. Affect is derived from the Latin *affectus*, which literally means "acted up" and was used for "a mood or state of mind produced by some external influence."

Apathy – Apathy is characterized by a generalized lack of emotion or state of indifference. The root **PATH-** in this term means "feeling," which is similar to its use in "empathy" and "sympathy." In other contexts, **PATH-** can mean "disease." The connection between "feeling" and "disease" in this root's modern usage stems from the ancient Greek meaning of the word *pathos*. In ancient Greek a *pathos* was "what one has suffered, one's experience," which in other words is an "affection." In ancient Greek medicine, the term *pathos* of the soul was used for a strong emotion that could affect the body.

Dysphoria and **Euphoria** – Dysphoria is a long-lasting mood disorder that is marked by feelings of restlessness, general dissatisfaction, discomfort, and unhappiness without an apparent cause. **Euphoria** is an exaggerated feeling of well-being or elation without an apparent cause. Derived from the Greek root for "bearing" and "carrying," the root **PHOR-** in these terms is related "to bear" oneself.

Anhedonia – Formed from the root for "pleasure," **HEDON-**, anhedonia is the lack of pleasure with experiences that are normally pleasurable.

Mania – In the context of mood disorders, such as bipolar disorder, **mania** is a state of excessive excitement, elation, impulsivity, and restlessness. When used as a suffix, **-MANIA** refers to "a compulsion or excessive fascination with something." Hence, **pyromania** is an excessive fascination with fire, **thanatomania** is a fascination with homicidal or suicidal subjects, and **egomania** is literally an excessive fascination with oneself. The suffix **-MANIA** and its root **MANI-** ultimately come from the Greek verb *mainomai*, which meant "to be raving, frenzied." Consequently, the female followers of the Greek god of wine, Dionysus, were called the Mainads, or Maenads, which meant "raving ones." The title is descriptive because in their worship of Dionysus, the Mainads were said to enter into ecstatic states of frenzy resulting in abnormal behaviors, such as *sparagmos* (tearing apart animals and eating them). Whether or not the actual female worshipers of Dionysus participated in *sparagmos* is debatable. That said, entering into an ecstatic state of mind was a fundamental part of the religious practices of both the mythological and the real Mainads of the ancient Greek world (Fig. 10.22).

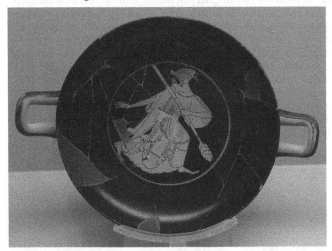

Fig. 10.22 Red-figure Kylix illustrating a Maenad with thyrsus, 510–500 BC. Ancient Agora Museum at Athens. Modified from original image by Dorieo. *Source:* Jerónimo Roure Pérez / Wikimedia Commons/CC BY-SA 4.0.

Catatonia – Catatonia is a state of unresponsiveness to one's environment that manifests in a lack movement and communication. This term is derived from the Greek prefix **KATA-** (downward) and the Greek word *tonos* (tension, tone). It was coined by Karl Kahlbaum in 1874, appearing in the title of his book *Die Katatonie oder das Spannungsirresein* (Catatonia or Tension Insanity). The Greek root **TON-** was, therefore, associated with the lack of movement and rigidity of this condition.

Hallucination – Derived from the Latin verb *alucinor* (to dream, wonder in mind), a hallucination is a false perception of the senses (i.e. sight, taste, touch, hearing, smelling) that has no relationship to reality. Hence a hallucinogen is a drug that grossly affects one's sensory perceptions.

Delusion – Derived from the Latin verb *deludere* (to fool, trick), a delusion is a persistent thought or belief that has no relationship to reality. A **delusion of grandeur** involves the euphoric mental assessment of one's power or importance. A **delusion of persecution** is the erroneous belief that a person, people, or agency is seeking to injure or harass an individual. **Paranoia** is a condition in which there is persistent persecutory delusions or delusional jealousy. The root **NO-** in paranoia means "mind" and "thought." Hence, **NO-** is used in noetic therapy, which is treatment based on deep beliefs or thoughts, and **noesis** is a loan word used for the "act of thinking."

Dementia – Dementia is a progressive impairment of the mental faculties characterized by a loss of reasoning, memory, confusion, and disorientation. Derived from the Latin word for "mind" (*mens, mentis*), the root **MENT-** in dementia means "mind." In Classical Latin, *demens* and *dementia* meant being out of one's mind, insane. This connotation is still prevalent in modern terms such as "demented."

Delirium – Derived from the Latin verb *delirare*, which means "to go off the furrow" (i.e. to be mad), the term delirium is a temporary state of mental confusion that manifests in disorientation and confusion. The association of madness and not plowing in a straight line can be observed in the myth associated with Odysseus' recruitment for the Trojan War. Palamedes was charged with summoning Odysseus to participate in the recovery of Helen, which was the premise for the Trojan War. When Palamedes arrived in Ithaca, he found Odysseus pretending to be insane by plowing erratically and sowing salt in the ground. Palamedes recognized that Odysseus was feigning madness, so he put Odysseus' infant son, Telemachus, in front of the plow. Unwilling to kill his own son, Odysseus stopped plowing and, therefore, Odysseus was forced to join the Greek army's expedition to Troy.

Deviant behaviors – Deviant behaviors are those activities that are considered to be at variance from an accepted norm. The etymology of the term deviant reveals it to be similar to delirium. Deviant comes from the Latin *devius* (DE-, from + VIA-, road), which literally meant "out of the way" in Classical Latin, but it also could mean "erroneous" and "unreasonable." Some sexual behaviors are considered to be deviant in medicine and psychology. The suffixes **-PHILIA** and **-LAGNIA** are often used for sexual deviant behaviors. Thus, **necrophilia** is a sexual arousal to dead bodies; **zoolagnia** is a sexual desire for animals; and **pedophilia** is an adult sexual attraction to children. That said, the suffix **-PHILIA** can be used for simply "attraction," such as lipophilia being defined as a chemical affinity toward fats or fatty acids.

Anxiety – Anxiety is an excessive and persistent worry, agitation, restlessness, or fear about everyday situations and uncertainties. It is commonly associated with phobias and panic attacks. It is derived from the Latin word *anxius*, which means "troubled, distressed." The modern psychological use of the term anxiety dates back to 1904.

Phobia – The root **PHOB-** is used for "fear." A phobia is an anxiety disorder in which there is an unreasonable fear or avoidance of something. Likewise, **-PHOBIA** is often used as a suffix indicating an unreasonable fear of something. For instance, **acrophobia** is the fear of high places. **Arachnophobia** is the fear of spiders. Derived from the Greek word for the marketplace, *agora*, **agoraphobia** is the avoidance of crowds or crowded places. In Greek mythology, Phobos was the child of the Greek god of war, Ares. And thus, Phobos was a personification of panic, flight, and rout in war. Typically, his appearance is that of a young man, but in some ancient iconography, he is given the face of a lion. The connection between the Roman god Mars and the Greek god Ares is why one of the moons of Mars is named Phobos.

Panic Attack – From the Greek *panikos* (pertaining to the god Pan), sudden feelings of fear and anxiety that cause physical symptoms such as heart palpitations, sweating, trembling, shortness of breath, feelings of choking, and chest pain are associated with the term panic attack. Pan was the Greek god of shepherds and hunters, and having goat legs, he was one of the only theriomorphic Olympian gods. In Greek literature, he is associated with instilling fear and confusion in those he desired to attack. Herodotus relates how before the Battle of Marathon, Pan approached Pheidippides, promising to terrify the Persians if the Athenians would worship him. Pheidippides is associated with the modern marathon race because it is said this Athenian messenger ran from Marathon to Athens to deliver the news of the victory at the Battle of Marathon (Fig. 10.23).

Fig. 10.23 Woodcut engraving of the Greek god Pan from "*Der Olymp oder die Mythologie der Griechen und Römer (The Olympus or the Mythology of the Greeks and Romans)*," 1878, 18th edition. *Source:* Engravings on Wood./Wikimedia Commons/ Public domain.

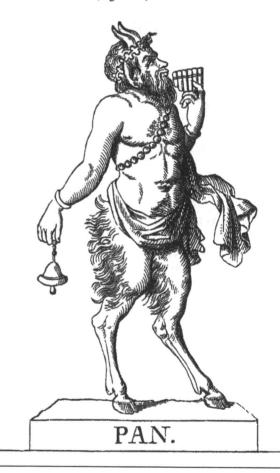

Greek or Latin word element	Current usage	Etymology	Examples
PSYCH/O (sī-kō)	Mind, soul	Gr. *psyche*, spirit, soul, breath of life	**Psych**osis, **psych**ology, **psych**osomatic Loan word: **Psyche** (sī'kē)
PHREN/O (frĕ-nō)	Mind, diaphragm, phrenic nerve	Gr. *phren*, midriff, mind, diaphragm	Schizo**phren**ia, **phren**optosis
MENT/O (men-tō)	Mind	L. *mens, mentis*, f. mind	De**ment**ia, **ment**al Loan word: **Mens** (mĕnz)
NO/O (nō-ō)	Mind, thought	Gr. *noos*, mind; Gr. *noesis*, thought	Para**no**ia, **no**opsyche, dia**no**etic Loan word: **Noesis** (nō-ē'sĭs)
THYM/O (thī-mō)	Emotion, state of mind	Gr. *thymos*, spirit, soul, mind, anger, strong feeling	Dys**thym**ia, amphi**thym**ia
PATH/O (pă-thō) **-PATHY** (pă'-thē)	Feeling, disease	Gr. *pathos*, feeling, suffering, disease	**Path**omimesis, a**pathy**, sym**pathy**
PHOR/O (fo-rō) **-PHORIA** (for-ē-ă)	Bearing (*in psychology, a mental state in respect to emotional well-being), carrying, bringing	Gr. *phoros*, bearing, carrying, bringing	Eu**phor**ic, dys**phor**ia
HEDON/O (hē-dō-nō)	Pleasure	Gr. *hedone*, pleasure	An**hedon**ia, **hedon**ism
MANI/O (mā-nē-ō) **-MANIA** (mā-nē-ă)	Frenzy, madness	Gr. *mania*, madness, frenzy	**Mani**ac, pyro**mania** Loan word: **Mania** (mā'nē-ă)
HALLUCIN/O (hă-loo-sĭ-nō)	A false sensory perception	L. *alucinari*, to wander in mind, to dream	**Hallucin**ogen, **hallucin**otic
PHANT/O (fan-tō) **PHANTASM/O** (fan-taz-mō)	Illusion, hallucination	Gr. *phantasma*, image, vision	**Phant**ogeusia, **phantasm**agoria Derivative: **Phantasm** (fan'tazm)
PHANER/O (făn-ĕr-ō)	Evident, visible	Gr. *phaneros*, visible	**Phaner**ogenic, **phaner**osis
PHOB/O (fō-bō) **-PHOBIA** (fō-bē-ă)	Fear, avoidance	Gr. *phobos*, fear	**Phob**ophobia, agora**phobia** Derivative: **Phobia** (fō'bē-ă)
PANIC (pan-ik)	Panic	Gr. *panikos*, of or for Pan, the goat-legged Greek god of shepherds	**Panic**
NARCISS/O (nar-sĭ-sō)	Self-love	Gr. *Narkissos*, a Greek mythological character who fell in love with his reflection	**Narciss**ism, **narciss**istic

Greek or Latin word element	Current usage	Etymology	Examples
PHIL/O (fĭ-lō) **-PHILIA** (fil-ē-ă)	Attraction, love (*in psychology, the suffix PHILIA means sexual arousal)	Gr. *philia*, love, affection	Homo**phile**, necro**philia**
-LAGNIA (lăg-nē-ă)	Lust, sexual arousal	Gr. *lagneia*, lust	Algo**lagnia**, **lagn**olalia
ORECT/O (ŏ-rek-tō) **OREX/O** (or-ek- sō)	Appetite	Gr. *orexis*, appetite	An**orect**ic, an**orex**ia, **orex**in

Review	Answers
Based on the mythological figure Narcissus, who fell in love with an image of himself according to Ovid's *Metamorphoses*, the root NARCISS- means _____.	**Self-love**
From the Greek *panikos* (pertaining to the god Pan), sudden feelings of fear and anxiety that cause physical symptoms such as heart palpitations, sweating, trembling, shortness of breath, feelings of choking, and chest pain are called a _____ attack.	**panic**
The root _____ is used for "fear." A _____ is an anxiety disorder in which there is an unreasonable fear or avoidance of something.	**PHOB- phobia**
The root _____ is used for "attraction" and "love." In psychology, the suffixes _____ and _____ are used for "sexual arousal."	**PHIL- -PHILIA, -LAGNIA**
Paranoia is a condition in which there is persistent persecutory delusions or delusional jealousy. The root NO- in paranoia means _____ and _____.	**mind, thought**
Dementia is a progressive impairment of the mental faculties characterized by a loss of memory, confusion, and disorientation. The root MENT- in dementia means _____.	**mind**
Psychosis is a mental disorder in which there is severe loss of contact with reality, often accompanied by hallucinations, delusions, impaired reasoning, and catatonic behavior. The root PSYCH- in psychosis means _____.	**mind**
A neurosis is a maladaptive psychological disorder that affects personality, mood, or some behaviors, without a radical loss of contact with reality. The root NEUR- in neurosis refers to the _____, but generally the term means _____.	**nervous system, nerve**
_____ is an anxiety disorder in which there is a false belief that one is suffering from some disease or diseases despite medical reassurance to the contrary.	**hypochondria (hypochondriasis)**
_____ is a type of psychosis that can manifest in a variety of ways such as delusions, hallucinations, and disorganized speech, paranoia, and catatonic behavior. The root PHREN- in this term means _____.	**Schizophrenia mind**
_____ is a long-lasting mood disorder that is marked by feelings of restlessness, general dissatisfaction, discomfort, and unhappiness without an apparent cause. _____ is an exaggerated feeling of well-being or elation without an apparent cause. The root PHOR- in these terms is related to _____ oneself.	**Dysphoria Euphoria bearing**
_____ is characterized by a lack of emotion or state of indifference. The root PATH- in this term means _____.	**Apathy feeling**
In psychology, _____ is used to describe the mood or emotional reaction associated with a situation or experience.	**affect**
_____ is the lack of pleasure with experiences that are normally pleasurable.	**Anhedonia**
_____ is a state of unresponsiveness to one's environment that manifests in a lack of movement and communication, in which a person appears to be in a state of stupor.	**Catatonia**

Review	Answers
In the context of mood disorders, such as bipolar disorder, _____ is the state of excessive excitement, elation, impulsivity, and restlessness. When used as a suffix, _____, refers to a compulsion or excessive fascination with something.	**Mania** **-MANIA**
_____ is used for a mild form of chronic depression or dysphoric mood. The root THYM- means _____ or _____.	**Dysthymia** **mood, state of mind**
Derived from the Latin verb *alucinor* (to dream, wonder in mind), a _____ is a false perception of the senses (i.e. sight, taste, touch, hearing, smelling) that has no relationship to reality.	**hallucination**
Derived from the Latin verb *deludere* (to fool, trick), a _____ is a persistent thought or belief that has no relationship to reality.	**delusion**
Derived from the Latin verb that meant "to go off the furrow" (i.e. to be mad), the term _____ is a temporary state of mental confusion that manifests in disorientation and confusion.	**delirium**
The term "nervosa" is used in terms such as anorexia nervosa and bulimia nervosa to signify that these disorders are _____ somatic in origin. The term bulimia means _____. The root OREX- means _____. OREX- is used in a wide variety of eating disorders.	**psycho** **ravenous hunger** **appetite**
Body image disorders fall under the term _____.	**Dysmorphia**
Coming from the Latin verb *deprimere* (to press down), _____ is used for mood disorders that are associated with a loss of interest or pleasure in living.	**depression**
Derived from the verb *angere* (to distress, torment), _____ is characterized by intense feelings of discomfort or dread (e.g. obsessive compulsive disorder [OCD] and post-traumatic stress disorder [PTSD]).	**anxiety**
Based on the humoral notion of temperaments, today we still use the terms _____ for irritable and quick-tempered, _____ for sluggish or dull, _____ for optimistic and cheerful, and _____ for depressed and sad.	**choleric, phlegmatic, sanguine, melancholic**
According to Taber's, _____ is a medical term used for "extreme depression, esp. when complicated by frequent crying, anhedonia, and fearfulness."	**melancholia**
Derived from a Latin word meaning "woven together," in Freudian and Jungian psychology, a _____ is a collection of emotionally significant ideas that are repressed, causing mental conflict and abnormal behaviors.	**complex**
Formed from the Greek word for "self," _____ is the term used for developmental disorders that produce difficulties with verbal and non-verbal communication resulting in an inability to socially interact with others. It is often accompanied by repetitive movements, particularly of the hands.	**autism**

11

Eye, Ear, and Special Senses

CHAPTER LEARNING OBJECTIVES

1) You will learn the word elements, loan words, and key terms associated with the organs of sense.
2) You will become familiar with some of the historical concepts associated with sensation, vision, and hearing.

Lessons from History: Aristotle's Hierarchy of Senses

Food for Thought as You Read:

To what extent are Aristotle's evaluations of the senses derived from sociocultural influences? How does this affect his assessment of the senses?

What sociocultural factors affect our own valuation of the different senses? Does such a belief have any effect on the practice of medicine?

A recent study (2015) at the Max Planck Institute for Psycholinguistics in Nijmegen examined the terms used for the 5 senses in 13 different languages around the world. The results of this study revealed that all of these languages had a greater frequency of usage of terms for "vision," but after vision, there was no fixed hierarchy of the senses in these speakers' linguistic usages. While terms for hearing often ranked second, in certain languages, particularly those of hunter-gather peoples, olfactory terms were second. After hearing, there was a greater variation as to the usages of words for the other senses in these languages. The conclusion of this study was that the hierarchy of the senses is shaped by both biological predispositions and cultural influences. In regards to medicine, the question of the hierarchy of the senses comes into play in both practical and ethical questions. For example, which senses are relevant and/or reliable to use in making a diagnosis? Are we overly relying on our sense of sight in our approach to medicine? Which sense should receive the most attention in the development of new therapies and medical procedures?

The five senses and their relationship to the soul are taken up by Aristotle in *On the Soul* (*De anima*), and he revisits this subject in many of his "biological" works, such as *On Sense and the Sensibilia* (*De sensu et sensili*). Aristotle theorized that the organs of the five senses have the power of sensation because they can become potentially similar to what the sensible objects actually are. For example, the eye "sees" an orange because the sense organ becomes like the sensible aspect of the orange, namely its color. Sight, hearing, and the sense of smell each have sense organs that only work with mediums specific to each of them. The medium for sight is called the visible/clear, the medium for hearing is air, and the mediums of the sense of smell are water and air. However, for Aristotle, touch and taste seem to differ from the other three senses in that they do not require a special medium. Instead, the sense organs of touch or taste are changed by coming into contact with the special object of sense that is germane to them. Aristotle recognizes that the senses' synergistic function allows for our ability to perceive objects more fully. Thus, Aristotle also speaks of a *koine aisthesis*, which is commonly translated "common sense," by which he seems to be speaking of a higher-order perceptual capacity that unifies the special senses' ability to perceive the properties of objects, such as size, shape, number, and motion. The organs of sensation provide a somatic explanation to Aristotle's understanding of sensation, but it is important to recognize that the form and capacity of these organs follow the

Greek and Latin Roots of Medical and Scientific Terminologies, First Edition. Todd A. Curtis.
© 2025 John Wiley & Sons, Inc. Published 2025 by John Wiley & Sons, Inc.
Companion website: www.wiley.com/go/Curtis

nature of the soul. The senses provide "a gateway to reality" that can be understood via imagination, memory, and intellect of the soul. While all animals have senses and, therefore, a perceptual part of the soul, and while some animals have the capacity for imagination and memory, only humans have an intellectual part of the soul that enables cognition and the acquisition of true knowledge.

The relationship between cognitive abilities and the five senses is one of the principles by which Aristotle puts forward a hierarchy of senses. His evaluation of these senses reflects his culture's appreciation for the intellectual pursuits and cognitive abilities of mankind. On account of its association with perceptiveness, Aristotle gives the sense of sight the nod as the most important sense. While sight is most important to perceptiveness, Aristotle highly esteems the sense of hearing, claiming that it is most important to the development of human cognitive abilities/intelligence (*phronesis*). Aristotle gives us some idea as to vision and hearing's respective values in the following passage from *Sense and Sensibilia* (437a):

> Of the two last mentioned, seeing, regarded as a supply for the primary wants of life is in its own right the superior sense; but for developing thought, hearing incidentally takes precedence. The faculty of seeing, thanks to the fact that all bodies are colored, brings tidings of multitudes of distinctive qualities of all sorts; whence it is through this sense especially we perceive common sensibles, viz. figure, magnitude, motion, number; while hearing announces only the distinctive qualities of sound, and, to some few animals, those also of voice. Incidentally, however, it is hearing that contributes most to the growth of intelligence. For rational discourse is a cause of instruction in virtue of its being audible, which it is, not in its own right, but incidentally; since it is composed of words, and each word is a symbol. Accordingly, of people destitute from birth of either sense, the blind are more intelligent than the deaf.

Translation in Barnes, J. ed. *The Complete Words of Aristotle.*
vol. 1 and 2. Princeton: Princeton University Press, 1995.

For Aristotle, vision is superior to hearing because, of all the senses, it makes known the greatest number of distinctions between things; in other words, we inherently gain more information about the world around us from vision. However, for Aristotle, hearing is clearly fundamental to learning. The reason for this can be found in his statement that "rational discourse" is a cause of instruction and is audible. While reading was indeed an important means of learning in the 5th- and 4th century BC, rhetorical and philosophical discourse were the fundamental means for the exchange of ideas and instruction, which seems to explain Aristotle's notion that hearing is the sense fundamental to intelligence. Perhaps, if Aristotle lived in our society, which arguably relies more heavily on visual methods of instruction, he would not have esteemed hearing as being fundamental to intelligence.

Aristotle's hierarchy of the senses also corresponds to their perceived contributions to human ethics. In Aristotle's *Nicomachean Ethics*, the senses are said to provide pleasures. A sensory pleasure can intensify or promote a corresponding activity, and pleasures that promote one activity can deter a person from pursing another activity. For Aristotle, not all human activities are of equal merit, and therefore, some sensory pleasures are better than others. In respect to the best of the senses, Aristotle places vision at the top, which he claims is superior "in purity" to touch. He also states that hearing and smell are superior to taste (*Nicomachean Ethics* 1176a). Aristotle's belief that touch and taste are inferior to the other senses appears to be derived from his devaluation of bodily activities versus mental activities. Aristotle argues that the problem with the pleasures of touch and taste is that they produce appetites for bodily activities (*Nicomachean Ethics* 1150a), which can distract one from the pleasures of cognition. His examples of gluttony and sexual indulgence suggest that strong bodily appetites tend to produce senseless behaviors in a human. In contrast, the pleasures of vision and hearing are associated with activities of the mind, and therefore, they are laudable and good. The belief that bodily pleasures detract from the contemplative life and, therefore, should be avoided/controlled is a reoccurring theme in both ancient philosophical and religious literature. Perhaps Aristotle's and Plato's depreciation of bodily desires in some ways reflects the persistent and erroneous belief among segments of educated society that their intellectual pursuits are of greater value to society when compared to those engaged in manual labor.

Aristotle's hierarchy of senses also comes into play in his classification of animals. In Aristotle's biological classification of the senses, all animals have sensation, which means they all have the capacity for pleasure and pain. Thus, sensation is fundamental to the survival of an animal in that it shows the animal what is particularly pleasant to it for life itself (*On the Soul*, 414b). For Aristotle, the sense of touch appears to be the most primitive of senses in that all animals possess this. The reason he gives for this is that an animal is a body with a soul in it, and a body is tangible (i.e. it is perceptible by touch); therefore, if an animal is to survive, its body must have the tactile sense to avoid that which is unpleasant and not conducive to life (*On the Soul*, 434b). Aristotle lumps the sense of taste and touch together in that he sees both as bodily sensations since neither requires an external medium. He notes that taste serves the function of nutrition, and, therefore, all animals seem to possess this sense as well. In *Sense and Sensibilia* (436b), he supports this by claiming "it is by taste that one distinguishes in food the pleasant and the unpleasant, so as to flee from the latter and pursue the former." He goes on to say that "the senses which operate through external media (i.e. smelling, hearing, and seeing) are only found in animals that possess the faculty of locomotion." He explains that these animals need such senses to anticipate danger, as well as to find food, prior to coming into contact with it. Aristotle seems to think that animals with locomotion should have all five senses, "for even the mole is observed to have eyes beneath its skin," and therefore, "not having one of these senses is a sign of imperfection or mutilation (*On the Soul* 425a)." It is quite clear that Aristotle's approach to the senses in animals is delimited to the five senses that humans also possess, which as modern biology has shown, is an incomplete list of sensations that animals use to survive and procreate.

Aristotle uses a wide variety of criteria to justify why humans are the most intelligent of all animals; for example upright stance, supple tongue, bloody lungs, and our large brain are all anatomical features that indicate humans possess intelligence. Likewise, human sensation is observed as being superior to that of animals. That said, Aristotle recognizes that animals vary in the scope and acuity of their sensory abilities, and human beings are not superior to all animals in these regards. He notes that humans, which have good capacity for vision, have relatively poor sense of smell. His reason for this is that the sense of smell is less important to what should be feared or avoided than it is for animals with poor vision due to their hard eyes (*On the Soul*, 421a). Thus, Aristotle's suggests that the relative ability of one sense can have an effect on the strength of another sense. Given that Aristotle associates vision and hearing with human intelligence and cognitive development, it should come as no surprise that he tends to speak of the human sense of hearing and vision as being very well developed. However, in *On the Soul*, Aristotle claims that some animals have a superior sense of vision and hearing, particularly in respect to how far away they can see or hear something. Given Aristotle's depreciation of the value of touch, it is quite surprising that Aristotle claims human beings excel over all other animals with respect to our sense of touch. When stating that man is the most intelligent of all animals, he supports this claim by pointing to mankind's highly developed sense of touch. At face value, such a statement seems to contradict the high value he places on vision and hearing in regard to the intellectual activities of humans. However, the fact that we have such a well-developed sense of touch, a sensation that is quite universal and primitive among animals, for Aristotle, is the best evidence for humans being superior to animals with respect to all the sensations because humans are the best at discriminating sensations. Unlike animals, whose sensations are delimited to appetitive behaviors and the avoidance of what is unpleasant, Aristotle suggests that human beings experience a wider range of sensations, and therefore, they can better assess the "aesthetic" pleasures that these sensations produce. Supposedly, our supple skin is designed for greater discriminatory powers, which leads in turn to a greater capacity for intelligence. The suppleness of the organs of sense leads to greater discriminative ability, which is why he claims "men whose flesh is hard are ill-endowed with intellect, and men whose flesh is soft are well-endowed (*On the Soul*, 421a)." For Aristotle, it is neither the scope of senses that humans possess nor the acuity of their vision and hearing that makes our senses superior to animals; it is the human capacity to discriminate a wider variety of sensory information from a given sense that makes human sensation compatible with the intellectual part of our souls. Aristotle's anthropocentric understanding of sensation blinded him to the fact that some animals have more than five senses and that humans' discriminative abilities are far inferior to a litany of other creatures, but these are lofty expectations to place upon a philosopher who did not have the benefit of two millennia of biological research and whose society was quite different from our own.

As to hierarchy of the senses in medicine, much like today, ancient Greek medicine hierarchy focused primarily on the treatment of vision and hearing. After discussing the treatments for a variety of eye diseases, Celsus writes in *De medicina* (VI.7.1), "So much, then, for those classes of eye disease, for which medicaments are most successful; and now we pass to the ears, the use of which comes next to eyesight as Nature's gift to us." While Celsus does mention treating lesions of the nose and tongue, none of these treatments are in the context of the restoration of the senses. Perhaps this is because these senses were not appreciated as being that valuable in the 1st century AD. If that is the case, then it is somewhat consistent with a survey study by Rachel Herz and Martha Bajec of the value of olfaction, which was published in *Brain Science*. The study revealed that olfaction is not perceived as very valuable in American culture as evidence by "one-quarter of the college student respondents would give up their sense of smell in order to keep their phone and nearly half of all women would give up their sense of smell to keep their hair."

Some Suggested Readings

Barnes, Jonathan, ed. *The Cambridge Companion to Aristotle.* Cambridge: Cambridge University Press, 1995.

Barnes, Jonathan, ed. *The Complete Words of Aristotle.* Volume 1 and 2. Princeton: Princeton University Press, 1995.

Freeland, Cynthia. "*Aristotle on the Sense of Touch.*" In *Essays on Aristotle's de Anima.* Edited by Martha Nussbaum and Am'elie Oksenberg Rorty, 227–248. Oxford: Oxford University Press, 1995.

Herz, Rachel S., and Martha R Bajec. "Your Money or Your Sense of Smell? A Comparative Analysis of the Sensory and Psychological Value of Olfaction." *Brain Sciences* 12, no. 3 (2022): 299.

Majid, Asifa, et al. "Differential Coding of Perception in the World's Languages." *Proceedings of the National Academy of Sciences* 115, no. 45 (2018): 11369–11376.

Toivanen, Juhana, ed. *Forms of Representation in the Aristotelian Tradition. Volume 1: Sense Perception.* Leiden: Brill, 2022.

Etymological Explanations: Common Terms and Word Elements for the Five Senses

Five senses

Receptors – In respect to modern understanding of the five senses (i.e. sight, taste, touch, hearing, and smelling), the sensation is understood as "receiving" information from the world around us. Thus, the senses are linked to receptors (L. *receptor*, a receiver), which are sensory nerve endings, cells, or sense organs that produce afferent-sensory impulses to the brain. The receptors of the five senses are collectively called **exteroceptors**, which delineates them from the **interoceptors** that respond to internal stimuli of the body. The exteroceptors are classified with respect to the nature of the stimuli that they respond to. Thus, **photoreceptors** (rods and cones of the eye) respond to light (**PHOT-**, light), **chemoreceptors** (taste buds and olfactory cells) respond to chemicals (**CHEM-**, chemical), **tactile receptors** (Meissner corpuscles) respond to touch (**TACT-**, touch), and **auditory receptors** (hair cells in the organ of Corti in the cochlea) respond to sound (**AUDIT-**, hearing). The root **CEPT-** and its corresponding root **CAPT-** come from the Latin verb *capere, captum,* which means to "take," "seize," or "grasp."

Touch – **HAPT-**, **TACT-**, **TAG-**, and **TANG-** are roots for the sense of "touch." **HAPT-** has the additional meaning of "to seize." Despite its similarity, the dance called the "tango" does not come from the Latin *tangere* (to touch); it appears to be derived from a Niger-Congo word for an African drum dance.

Smell – The roots used for the sense of "smell" are **OSM-**, **OLFACT-**, and **OSPHRESI-**, and their corresponding suffixes are **-OSMIA** and **-OSPHRESIS**. **OSM-** is a homograph that can mean "smell" (Gr. *osme*, smell), as well as "pushing" and "osmosis" (Gr. *osmos*, thrusting, pushing), for example: osmesthesia (sensation of smell) and osmology (study of osmosis).

Taste – The roots used for the sense of "taste" are **GUST-**, **GUSTAT-**, and **GEUS-**, and the corresponding suffix is **-GEUSIA**.

Vision – The roots used for the sense of "vision" or "sight" are **OPT-**, **OPTIC-**, **OP-**, **OPS-**, **BLEPS-**, and **VIS-**, and their corresponding suffixes are **-OPIA**, **-OPSIA**, **-OPSIS**, **-BLEPSIA**, and **-BLEPSIS**. **OPS-** is a homograph that can also mean "face" (Gr. *ops*, face, eye), "late" (Gr. *opse*, late), and "food" (Gr. *opson*, food), for example: triceratops (three-horned face), opsigamy (late-age marriage), and opsophagy (eating food).

Hearing – The roots used for the sense of "hearing" are **AUDIT-**, **AUD-**, **ACUST-**, and **ACOUST-**, and their corresponding suffixes are **-ACUSIS** and **-ACOUSIA**.

Greek or Latin word element	Current usage	Etymology	Examples
VIS/O (vĭ-zō)	Seeing, sense of sight	L. *videre, visum,* to see	**Vis**ible, **vis**or, tele**vis**ion
OPT/O (ŏp-tō) OPTIC/O (ŏptĭ-kō)	Seeing, sense of sight	Gr. *optos,* seen, visible; Gr. *optikos,* pertaining to vision	**Opt**ometry, **optic**ociliary, orth**optic**
OP/O (ŏp/ō) -OPIA (ō-pē-ă)	Seeing, sense of sight	Gr. *ops, opos,* eye, face; Gr. *opsis,* a sight, vision; Gr.	Ambly**opia**, stere**opsis**, my**opic**, xanth**opsia**

Greek or Latin word element	Current usage	Etymology	Examples
OPS/O (ŏp-sō) **-OPSIA** (op-sē-ă) **-OPSIS** (op-sĭs)			
BLEPS/O (blep-sō) **-BLEPSIA** (blep-sē-ă) **-BLEPSIS** (blep-sĭs)	Sense of sight	Gr. *blepsis*, sight	**Ablepsia**, para**blepsis**, oxy**bleps**ia
OLFACT/O (ol-fak-tō)	Smelling, sense of smell	L. *olfactare*, to smell	**Olfact**ion, **olfact**ory
OSM/O (oz-mō) **-OSMIA** (oz-mē-ă)	Smelling, sense of smell	Gr. *osme*, smell, sense of smell	Cac**osmia**, **osm**esthesia Loan word: **Osmesis** (ŏz-mē′sĭs)
OSPHRESI/O (ŏs-frē-zē-ō) **-OSPHRESIS** (ŏs-frē-sĭs)	Smelling, sense of smell	Gr. *osphresis*, smell, sense of smell	Oxy**osphresi**a, **osphresi**omter Loan word: **Osphresis** (ŏs-frē′sĭs)
GUST/O (gŭs-tō) **GUSTAT/O** (gŭs-tă-tō)	Tasting, sense of taste	L. *gustare*, *gustatum*, to taste	**Gustat**ory, **gust**ometry, **gustat**ion
GEUS/O (gŭs-ō) **-GEUSIA** (gŭ-zē-ă)	Tasting, sense of taste	Gr. *geusis*, taste	Oxy**geusia**, dys**geusia**,
TACT/O (tak-tō) **TAG/O** (tag-gō) **TANG/O** (tang-gō)	Touching, sense of touch	L. *tangere*, *tactum*, to touch	**Tact**ometer, **tang**oreceptor, con**tag**ion
HAPT/O (hăp-tō)	Touching, sense of touch, to seize	Gr. *haptein*, to touch, to seize	**Hapt**ic, **hapt**in
AUDIT/O (od-ĭ-tō) **AUDI/O** (od-ē-ō)	Listening, sense of hearing	L. *audire*, *auditum*, to hear	**Audi**ometry, **audit**ory

Greek or Latin word element	Current usage	Etymology	Examples
ACUST/O (ă-koos-tō) ACOUST/O (ă-koos-tō) -ACUSIS (a-kū-sĭs) -ACOUSIA (ă-kū-sē-ă)	Listening, sense of hearing	Gr. *akouein*, to hear	Para**cusis**, a**coust**ic, presby**acousia**

Review	Answers
The roots used for the sense of "touch" are _____, _____, _____, and _____.	HAPT-, TACT-, TAG-, TANG-
The roots used for the sense of "smell" are _____, _____, and _____.	OSM-, OLFACT-, OSPHRESI-
The roots used for the sense of "sight" are _____, _____, _____, _____, _____, and _____.	OPT-, OPTIC-, OP-, OPS-, BLEPS-, VIS-
The roots used for the sense of "hearing" are _____, _____, _____, and _____.	AUDIT-, AUD-, ACUST-, ACOUST-
The roots used for the sense of "taste" are _____, _____, and _____.	GUST-, GUSTAT-, GEUS-

Etymological Explanations: Common Terms and Word Elements for the Anatomy of the Eye

In the following discussion of the anatomical terms associated with the eye, the nominative and genitive singular forms of the anatomical Latin term are provided in parenthesis. The Greek and Latin roots are formatted in all caps and emboldened.

Adnexa of the eye

Adnexa – Derived from the Latin verb *adnectere* (to attach), the word adnexa is used in anatomical terminology for accessory structures to an organ. The eyelids, eyebrows, and the lacrimal apparatus are the protective adnexa for the eye.

Eyelid (L. *palpebra, -ae*) – The palpebrae are the moveable protective folds that cover the eye, which are commonly referred to as eyelids. **Palpebra** is the anatomical Latin term for eyelid. The roots for the "eyelid" are **PALPEBR-** and **BLEPHAR-**, which are derived from the Latin (*palpebra*) and Greek (*blepharon*) terms for this anatomical part. **Blepharon** is used as a loan word for "eyelid." The suffix **-BLEPHARON** is currently used in a variety of medical terms, such as **corneoblepharon** (an adhesion of the eyelid to the cornea) and **varicoblepharon** (varices associated with eyelid).

Eyelash (L. *cilium, -i*) and Eyebrow (L. *supercilium, -i*) – At the margin of the eyelids are the eyelashes. These hairs are the first line of defense keeping dirt and debris from the eye. The anatomical Latin term and loan word for an eyelash is **cilium**, and consequently, an eyebrow hair is called a **supercilium**. The root **CILI-** is used extensively in medicine and science for hair-like projections. With respect to the eye, **CILI-** can refer to the "eyelash" or to the "ciliary body." The **ciliary body** is a ring of tissue behind the iris that is composed of ciliary muscle and ciliary processes.

Fig. 11.1 Anatomical Latin terms for the lacrimal apparatus. *Source:* Drawing by Chloe Kim.

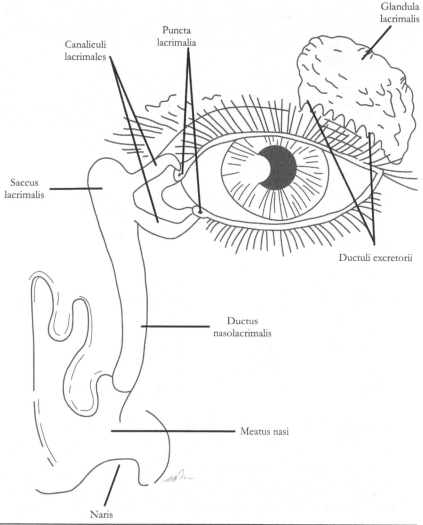

Conjunctiva (L. *conjunctiva, -ae*) – The mucous membrane that lines the eyelids and reflects back onto the eyeball is called conjunctiva, and its root is **CONJUNCTIV-**. It's etymological meaning of "joining together" reflects the role of this membrane in that it "conjoins" the eyelids to the eyeball. The root **JUNCT-** in conjunctiva is derived from the Latin verb *jungere* (to join), and therefore, **JUNCT-**, as well as **JUG-**, are commonly used word elements that indicate "a joining, or connecting of things." For example, the anatomical term **jugum**, which is also the Latin term for a yoke, refers to a depression that connects two parts.

Lacrimal Apparatus (L. *apparatus lacrimalis*) – The roots for "tear" and by extension, the anatomical structures associated with tears are **DACRY-** (Gr. *dacryon*) and **LACRIM-** (L. *lacrima*). The root for the tear gland is **DACRYOADEN-**, and the common root for the lacrimal sac is **DACRYOCYST-**. Tears produced by the lacrimal gland serve a number of important functions. Most importantly, they clean the eye and keep the cornea moist. The tears pass through to the surface eye via the lacrimal points (*puncta lacrimalia*) in the lacrimal canals (*canaliculi lacrimales*). From there, they go to the lacrimal sac, and then from there into the nasolacrimal duct (*ductus nasolacrimalis*) and out the nasal opening termed the *meatus nasi*, which ultimately leads to the wonderful phenomenon of having a snotty nose when we cry (Fig. 11.1).

Anatomical parts of the eye

Eye (L. *oculus, -i*) – The eye, also known as the **oculus**, is collectively the organ of sight. The roots used for the "eye" are **OCUL-** (L. *oculus*) and **OPHTHALM-** (Gr. *ophthalmos*). The observable external structures of the eye are the iris, pupil, sclera, and cornea (Fig. 11.2).

Iris (L. *iris, iridis*) – The colorful circle of the human eye is called the iris. The iris contracts and dilates the hole in its center to regulate the amount of light that enters the eye. The roots for this colorful part of the human eye are **IR-** and **IRID-**. Outside of its use with the eye, these roots also mean "rainbow" and "rainbow-like." The anatomical Latin term is derived from the Greek word iris, which was used, according to Liddell and Scott, for "any brightly colored circle," such as the "round the eyes of a peacock's tail." In Greek mythology, Iris was the goddess of the rainbow, and like Hermes, she was a messenger for the Olympian gods. The modern iris flower's name is from this ancient Greek word, which is evident in Dioscorides' description of its medicinal usages in *De materia medica*. Dioscorides described how it could be used for menstrual flow, sciatica, fistulae, and applied as an eye salve with honey to draw out particles.

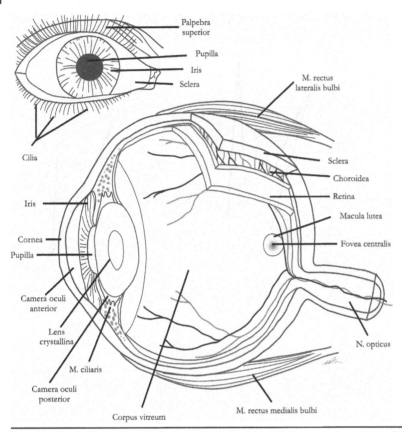

Fig. 11.2 Anatomical Latin terms for the eye. *Source:* Drawing by Chloe Kim.

Pupil (L. *pupilla*, *-ae*) – The hole in the iris by which light enters the eye is called the **pupil** or **pupilla**. The roots for this dark hole in the center of the iris are **PUPILL-** and **COR-**. These roots are derived from Latin and Greek words (L. *pupilla*, Gr. *kore*) that have a connotation of a "young girl," and both words were used for the anatomical part of the eye known as the pupil. The supposed connection between these very different meanings has to do with the phenomenon in which one can observe a little image of oneself in the pupil of another person. The Latin word *pupilla* is a diminutive of the Latin word *pupa* (doll, child). **Pupa** is used today as a loan word for the developmental stage of an insect after the larva stage. The most famous Kore in Greek myth is the young daughter of Demeter, Persephone, who was abducted by Hades to be his new bride. In the *Homeric Hymn to Demeter*, the goddess Iris was said to have been sent by Zeus to implore Demeter to relent from causing humans to die by famine since Demeter had caused the crops to no longer grow in order to recover Kore from Hades.

Ciliary body (L. *corpus ciliare*) – As noted, **CILI-** is a root used for the ciliary body. The ciliary body is a ring of tissue behind the iris that is composed of ciliary muscle and ciliary processes. The ciliary muscle contracts, helping to focus the lens. The ciliary processes secrete the aqueous humor that fills the anterior chamber of the eye. Owing to its circular shape, the common root used for the "ciliary body" of the eye is **CYCL-**, which in other contexts means "circle" or "wheel."

Sclera (L. *sclera*, *-ae*) – The iris stands out much more in the human eye than in most animals because it is surrounded by the "white of our eyes," which is called the sclera. Consequently, the root for the "white of the eye" is **SCLER-**, which in other contexts means "hard." This tough, fibrous layer of the eye was originally known in Greek as the *chiton scleros* (χιτὼν σκληρός), the "hard tunic" of the eye. Galen called the next two inner layers of the eye the *chiton choroeides* (χιτὼν χοροειδής), which means "lambskin-like tunic," and the *amphiblestroeides* (ἀμφιβληστροειδής), which means "net-like." The modern terms for the middle and inner layers of the eye (i.e. choroid and retina) are derived from these Greek anatomical terms. The anatomical Latin term **sclera** came into use in 1886.

Choroid (L. *choroidea*, *-ae*) and Retina (L. *retina*, *-ae*) – The **choroid** is the middle vascular layer of the eyeball. The term choroid is formed from the Greek word for lambskin, *chorion*, which is commonly used for the outer membrane surrounding the fetus. The root for this layer of the eye is **CHOROID-**. The **retina** is the innermost layer of the eye that contains the photoceptors known as the rod and cone cells, which are highly specialized, light-sensitive cells. The **retina** and its root **RETIN-** come from the Latin word for "net," *rete*. As we have seen in earlier chapters, the root **RET-** shows up in numerous terms that have to do with nets and net-like structures. This is also true in Classical Latin. For instance, the type of gladiator that fought with a net and spear/trident was called a *retiarius* ("net-thrower"). The strength of this type of gladiator's armament was commonly opposed by a gladiator who carried a shield and sword called a *secutor* ("purser"), the idea being that each gladiator's weapons and armor had particular strengths and weaknesses (Fig. 11.3).

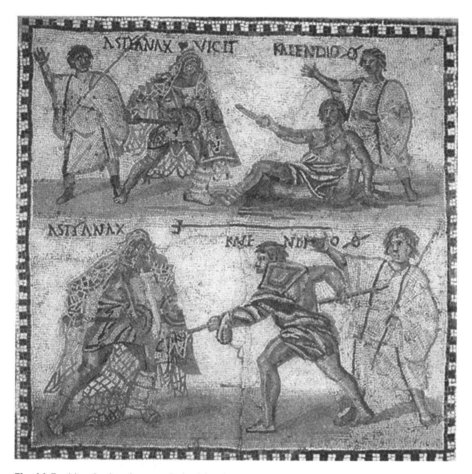

Fig. 11.3 Mosaic showing a *retiarius* (right) named Kalendio fighting a *secutor* (left) named Astyanax. The bottom image depicts the *secutor* covered in the *retiarius's* net. The "theta nigra" by Kalendio's name indicates that he was killed in combat. *Source:* Unknown author/Wikimedia Commons/Public domain.

Cornea (L. *cornea, -ae*) – The transparent anterior continuation of the sclera that is convex anteriorly is called the cornea. The roots used for the "cornea" of the eye are **CORNE-** and **KERAT-** (which is also spelled **CERAT-**). Derived from Greek and Latin words for "horn" and "horn-like," these roots also can mean "horn," "horn-like," and "hard." In many respects, the cornea is the "window of the eye" because it is the first structure through which light enters the eye. The cornea refracts the light to focus the visual image. This refracted light travels through the **anterior camera** (*camera anterior oculi*) of the eye. The anterior camera is the space between the lens and the cornea. The **posterior camera** of the eye (*camera posterior oculi*) lies between the iris and the lens. The term **camera** and its root **CAMER-** literally mean "chamber" or "cavity."

Lens (L. *lens, lentis*) – Via the pupil, the light refracted by the cornea enters the transparent structure known as the crystalline lens (*lens, lentis*). This biconvex structure of the eye is truly a lenticular structure in that it resembles a lentil. In fact, the roots for the lens of the eye, **LENT-** and **PHAK-** (or **PHAC-**), are derived from Latin and Greek words for this type of edible legume.

Aqueous humor (L. *humor aquosus*) – The anterior camera is filled with a watery fluid called the aqueous humor. Derived from the Latin word for "water," *aqua*, the roots **AQU-** and **AQUE-** mean "water" and "water-like."

Vitreous humor (L. *humor vitreus*) – Focused light travels through the *corpus vitreum* (glassy body), which derives its name from the presence of a glass-like semisolid humor known as the vitreous humor. The roots used for the vitreous humor are **VITR-**, **VITRE-**, and **HYAL-**. These roots can also mean "glass" or "glass-like" since they come from Greek and Latin words for "glass." The vitreous humor helps to create the shape of the eye.

Macula lutea (L. *macula lutea*) – The light that has been refracted by the cornea and lens comes to a focal point at the central yellow spot on the posterior wall of the retina known as the macula lutea (*lutea*, yellow). The root **MACUL-** is used for the macula lutea in the context of the eye; in other contexts, it means "spot" or "spotted." At the center of the macula lutea is a depression known as the **fovea centralis**, which means "central pit" (L. *fovea*, pit). The macula lutea contains the majority of the cone cells. Together, this area of the eye is responsible for central vision, fine visual detail, and color vision. Proximal to the macula lutea lies the **optic disc** (L. *discus nervi optici*), which is where the **optic nerve** (L. *nervus opticus*) enters the eye.

Greek or Latin word element	Current usage	Etymology	Examples
OCUL/O (ŏk-ū-lō)	Eye	L. *oculus, -i,* m. eye	**Ocul**omotor, intra**ocul**ar, **sinistr**ocular Loan word: **Oculus** (ŏk′ū-lŭs) pl. **Oculi** (ŏk′ū-lī)
OPHTHALM/O (ŏf-thăl-mō)	Eye	Gr. *ophthalmos,* eye	Xer**ophthalm**ia, **ophthalm**ologist
CAMER/O (kăm-ĕr-ō)	Chamber, cavity	L. *camera, -ae,* f. camera, chamber fr. Gr. *kamara,* anything with an arched cover	Bi**camer**al, tri**camer**al Loan word: **Camera** (kăm′ĕr-ă) pl. **Camerae** (kăm′ĕr-ē″)
AQU/O (ak-wō) **AQUE/O** (ak-wē-ō)	Water, water-like	L. *aqua, -ae,* f. water	**Aqu**eous, **aqu**ifer, **aqu**aphobia Loan word: **Aqua** (ak′wă) pl. **Aquae** (ak′wē″)
VITRE/O (vi-trē-ō) **VITR/O** (vi-trō)	Glass, glass-like (*vitreous humor of the eye)	L. *vitrum, -i,* n. glass	**Vitre**itis, **vitr**iform, de**vitr**ification
HYAL/O (hī-ă-lō)	Glass, glass-like (*vitreous humor of the eye)	Gr. *hyalos,* glass	**Hyal**itis, **hyal**ine, **hyal**omere
RETIN/O (rĕt-ĭ-nō)	Retina (*innermost tunic of the eye)	L. *retina, -ae,* f. retina fr. L. *rete, retis,* n. net, network	**Retin**oschisis, sub**retin**al, **retin**oschisis Loan word: **Retina** (rĕt′ĭ-nă) pl. **Retinae** (rĕt′ĭ-nē″)
CHOROID/O (kō-roy-dō)	Choroid (*middle tunic of the eye)	L. *choroidea, -ae,* f. choroid fr. Gr. *chorion,* lambskin	**Choroid**itis, supra**choroid**, peri**choroid**al Loan word: **Choroid** (kō′royd)
MACUL/O (mak-yŭ-lō)	Spot, macule (*macula lutea retinae* of the eye)	L. *macula, -ae,* f. spot, stain	**Macul**opathy, **macul**ar, **macul**ose Loan word: **Macula** (mak′yŭ-lă) pl. **Maculae** (mak′yŭ-lē″)
CORNE/O (kor-nē-ō)	Cornea, hard, horn-like	L. *cornea, -ae,* f. cornea fr. L. *cornu, cornus,* n. horn	**Corne**oblepharon, **corne**oscleral, **corne**ous Loan word: **Cornea** (kor′nē-ă) pl. **Corneae** (kor′nē-ē″)
KERAT/O (kĕr-ăt-ō) **CERAT/O** (sĕr-ăt-ō)	Cornea, horn, hard, horn-like	Gr. *keras, keratos,* horn	**Kerat**ocele, **cerat**ocele, tri**cerat**ops, **kerat**ocentesis

Greek or Latin word element	Current usage	Etymology	Examples
LENT/O (lĕn-tō) **LENTICUL/O** (lĕn-tĭk-ū-lō)	Lens, lentil, lentil-shaped	L. *lens, lentis*, f. lentil; L. *lenticula, -ae*, f. lentil-shaped	**Lenticul**ar, **lent**iform, **lent**iconus Loan word: **Lens** (lenz) pl. **Lentes** (len'tēz″)
PHAC/O (făk-ō) **PHAK/O** (făk-ō)	Lens, lentil	Gr. *phakos*, lentil	**Phak**olysis, **phac**ocele, **phac**oma
CYCL/O (sī-klō)	Ciliary body of the eye, circle, wheel	Gr. *kyklos*, circle, wheel, ring	**Cycl**oplegia, bi**cycl**e, **cycl**othymic
CILI/O (sil-ē-ō)	Ciliary body, eyelash, hair-like process	L. *cilium, -i*, n. eyelash	**Cili**ectomy, **cili**ograde, naso**cili**ary Loan words: **Cilium** (sil'ē-ŭm) pl. **Cilia** (sil'ē-ă) **Supercilium** (soo″pĕr-sĭl'ē-ŭm) pl. **Supercilia** (soo″pĕr-sil'ē-ă)
SCLER/O (sklĕ-rō)	Sclera of the eye, hard	L. *sclera, -ae*, f. sclera fr. Gr. *skleros*, hard	**Scler**itis, **scler**osis, acro**scler**oderma, **scler**otomy Loan word: **Sclera** (sklĕr'ă) pl. **Sclerae** (sklĕr'ē″)
IR/O (ī-rō) **IRID/O** (ir-ĭ-dō)	Iris of the eye, rainbow, rainbow-like	L. *iris, iridis*, f. iris fr. Gr. *iris, iridos*, rainbow	**Irid**oplegia, **irid**ic, **ir**itis Loan word: **Iris** (ī'rĭs) pl. **Irides** (ī'rĭ-dēz″)
PUPILL/O (pū-pĭl-ō)	Pupil of the eye	L. *pupilla, -ae*, f. pupil of the eye fr. L. *pupa, -ae*, doll, child	**Pupill**ometer, **pupill**ary Loan word: **Pupilla** (pū-pĭl'ă) pl. **Pupillae** (pū-pĭl'ē″)
PUP/O (pū-pō)	Pupa (developmental stage after a larva)	L. *pupa, -ae*, f. doll, child	Pre**pupa**, **pup**ate, **pup**iparous Loan word: **Pupa** (pū'pă) **Pupae** (pū'pē″)
COR/O (kor-ō) **-CORIA** (kŏr-ē-ă)	Pupil of the eye	Gr. *kore*, maiden, doll	**Cor**eplasty, aniso**coria**, steno**cor**iasis
PALPEBR/O (pal-pĕ-brō)	Eyelid	L. *palpebra, -ae*, f. eyelid	Inter**palpebr**al, **palpebr**ation Loan word: **Palpebra** (pal'pĕ-bră) pl. **Palpebrae** (pal'pĕ-brē″)
BLEPHAR/O (blĕf-ă-rō)	Eyelid	Gr. *blepharon*, eyelid	**Blephar**itis, corneo**blephar**on, pachy**blephar**osis

Greek or Latin word element	Current usage	Etymology	Examples
CONJUNCTIV/O (kŏn-jŭnk-tĭ-vō)	Conjunctiva	L. *conjunctiva, -ae,* f. conjunctiva	**Conjunctiv**itis, **conjunctiv**al Loan word: **Conjunctiva** (kon″jŭngk-tī′vă) pl. **Conjunctivae** (kon″jŭngk-tī′vē″)
JUNCT/O (junk-tō) **JUG/O** (joo-gō)	To join, joined	L. *jungere, junctum,* to join	Dis**junct**ion, **jug**al, ad**junct**
LACRIM/O (lak-rĭ-mō)	Tear	L. *lacrima, -ae,* tear	**Lacrim**onasal, de**lacrim**ation, naso**lacrim**al Loan word: **Lacrima** (lak′rĭ-mă) pl. **Lacrimae** (lak′rĭ-mē″)
DACRY/O (dak-rē-ŏ)	Tear	Gr. *dakryon,* tear	**Dacry**oadenalgia, **dacry**ocystitis, **dacry**adenalgia
MITT/O (mĭt-tō) **MISS/O** (mĭs-sō)	To send, let go	L. *mittere, missum,* to send, let go	Intro**mitt**ent, e**miss**ion, ad**miss**ion

Review	Answers
The root for the "white of the eye" is _____, which in other contexts means "hard."	**SCLER-**
The roots used for the vitreous humor are _____, and _____. Both of these roots can also mean _____ or _____.	**HYAL-, VITRE-** glass, glass-like
The anterior chamber is filled with the aqueous humor. The root AQUE- means _____ and _____.	**water, water-like**
The root used for the "chambers" of the eye is _____.	**CAMER-**
The roots used for the "eye" are _____ and_____.	**OCUL-, OPHTHALM-**
The root for the innermost coat/layer of the eye is _____.	**RETIN-**
The lentil shape structure of the eye is called the lens. The roots for the lens are _____ and _____ (also spelled _____).	**LENT-, PHAK-, PHAC-**
The root for the ciliary body of the eye is _____, which in other contexts means _____ or _____.	**CYCL-, circle, wheel**
The root _____ means "ciliary body" or a "hair-like process." The loan word for the "eyelash" is _____. The loan word for the "eyebrow" is _____.	**CILI-** cilium supercilium
The roots used for the cornea of the eye are _____ and _____ (which is also spelled _____). In other contexts, these roots also can mean _____, _____, and _____.	**CORNE-,KERAT-,CERAT-** horn, horn-like, hard
The roots for the colorful part of the human eye are _____ and _____. In other contexts, these roots also mean _____ and _____.	**IR-, IRID-** rainbow, rainbow-like
The roots for "tear" and by extension, the anatomical structures associated with tears are _____ and_____.	**LACRIM-, DACRY-**
The roots for the "eyelid" are _____ and _____.	**PALPEBR-, BLEPHAR-**
The roots for the dark hole in the center of the iris are _____ and _____.	**COR-, PUPILL-**
_____ is the root for the membrane that lines the eyelids and reflects back onto the eyeball.	**CONJUNCTIV-**
The word macula in *macula lutea retinae* indicates that this is a yellow_____ on the retina.	**spot**

Etymological Explanations: Common Terms and Word Elements for the Pathologies of the Eye

Problems with vision

Vision – As noted earlier, the roots used for the sense of "sight" are **OPT-**, **OPTIC-**, **OP-**, **OPS-**, **BLEPS-**, and **VIS-**, and their corresponding suffixes are **-OPIA**, **-OPSIA**, **-OPSIS**, **-BLEPSIA**, and **-BLEPSIS**. Hence, an abnormality of vision, such as hallucinations, is termed **parablepsis**.

Amblyopia – Based on its root **AMBLY-**, which means "dull," the literal meaning of amblyopia is "dull vision." In Taber's, it is defined as a unilateral or bilateral decrease of best corrected vision in an otherwise healthy eye.

Presbyopia – In Taber's, presbyopia is the permanent loss of accommodation of the crystalline lens of the eye that occurs when people are in their 40s. The root **PRESBY-** comes from the Greek word for "an older person," *presbys*. Thus, presbyopia is literally the vision of an old person. An elder in the ancient Jewish Sanhedrin was also called a *presbys*, which is where we get the terms presbyter and presbyterian.

Asthenopia – The compound root **ASTHEN-** means "weak," and therefore, the term for "weak" vision is asthenopia, which is defined in Taber's as weakness or tiring of the eyes.

Photopia – Based on its root **PHOT-**, which means "light," the literal meaning of photopia is "light vision." In Taber's, photopia is the adjustment of the eye for vision in bright light.

Scotopia – The root **SCOT-** means "dark, darkness." Thus, scotopia literally means "dark vision." Scotopia is defined in Taber's as the adjustment of the eye for vision in dim light.

Diplopia – **DIPL-** means "double." Thus, "double vision" is diplopia, which is defined in Taber's as two images of an object seen at the same time.

Anisopia – Based on its compound root **ANIS-**, which means "unequal," anisopia is "unequal vision." In Taber's, anisopia is a condition where visual power of the eyes is unequal.

Scotoma – A dark spot or an area of diminished acuity in the visual field is termed a scotoma. It is a loan word that was used in an ancient Greek medicine for "dizziness, vertigo."

Blindness – **Anopia** is the term for blindness or "lack of vision." Based on the word element **HEMI-**, blindness in one-half field of vision is **hemianopia**. Based on the root meaning "first," **PROT-**, a lack of "primary" vision (red color blindness) is **protanopia**. Based on the root meaning "second," **DEUTER-**, a lack of "secondary" vision (green color blindness) is **deuteranopia**. Derived from the Greek root for night **NYCT-**, night blindness is called **nyctalopia**.

Refractive error – A refractive error of vision is due to the light refractive powers of the eye not being appropriate for clear vision. Among other things, these can be caused by an irregularly shaped cornea, lens, or eyeball. Refractive errors of vision are termed **ametropia**, which, based on its compound root **AMETR-** (lack of measure), literally means "disproportionate" or "lack of measure" vision.

Hyperopia – The term for "farsightedness" is hyperopia. Farsightedness is a type of refractive error that allows one to see at a distance but not close up (Fig. 11.4).

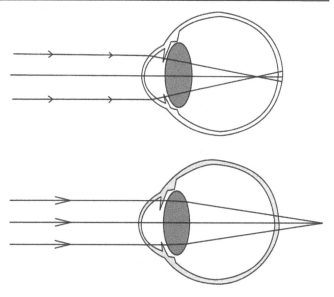

Fig. 11.4 Image of hyperopia (inferior) and myopia (superior).

Myopia – The term for "nearsightedness" is myopia. Nearsightedness is a type of refractive error that allows one to see close up but not at a distance. The etymology of myopia is somewhat debatable. Typically, it is said to have been derived from the Greek verb *myein* "to shut," owing to the belief that people with this refractive error often squint to see objects.

Astigmatism – The form of ametropia in which the refraction of rays is spread over a wide area rather than coming to focal point on the retina is an astigmatism (Fig. 11.5). The root **STIGMAT-** means "point," "spot," and "shame/disgrace." In regard to the meaning of "shame," this was acquired during the 16th century when the Greek word *stigma* was used for a mark made on the skin by burning it with a hot iron, which was typically pointed. That said, stigmata on the skin were not always considered shameful. The plural stigmata have been used in the Roman Catholic tradition for the marks of Jesus Christ's crucifixion that saints were said to have received in their hands, feet, and sides due to their devotion.

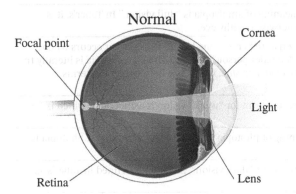

Fig. 11.5 Image of the distorted focal points associated with astigmatism.

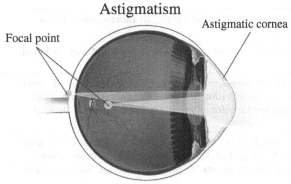

Astigmatic cornea distorts the focal point of light in front of and/or behind the retina

Cataract – Named after the Latin word for a "waterfall," *cataracta*, the opacity of a lens leading to a loss of vision and photophobia (an aversion to bright light), is called a cataract in modern medical terminology. While the root, **CATARACT-**, does not appear too often in English terms, the derivative "cataract" is quite prevalent, and in addition to its medical definition, it is still used as a term for "a waterfall" today.

Glaucoma – Glaucoma is an intraocular disease of the eye characterized by increased intraocular pressure due to the overaccumulation of the aqueous humor. In other contexts, the root **GLAUC-** means "silver," "gray," or "bluish-green." In antiquity there was no terminological distinction made between the conditions we call glaucoma and cataract; perhaps this is because the terms simply spoke to a "blurring of vision" that appears silvery like a waterfall. Among the many epithets that the Greek goddess of wisdom, Athena, received, one finds that she is commonly referred to as *glaukopis* in Homeric poetry and elsewhere. *Glaukopis* is typically translated "bright-eyed." The name *Glaukopis* is related to the Greek word for an owl, *glaux*, which is the animal closely associated with Athena. The owl seems to be called a *glaux* due to its bright, glaring eyes. Perhaps the notion of "light" and "keen vision" being associated with wisdom is the reason for this connection.

Position and movement of the eye

Strabismus – Derived from the Greek word for "squinting," strabismus is used for disorders of the eye in which the optic axes cannot be directed to the same object (Fig. 11.6). **STRABISM-** is the root used for this condition. The term **heterotropia** is a synonym for strabismus. The root **HETER-** has the meaning "opposite" in this term. The compound suffix **-TROPIA**, which literally means "a condition of turning" is used to denote which direction an eye is deviating. An inward deviation (**ESO-** inward) is called **esotropia**. An outward deviation (**EXO-** outward, without) is called **exotropia**.

Fig. 11.6 Image of the different types of strabismus. *Source:* myUpchar/Wikimedia Commons/CC BY-SA 4.0.

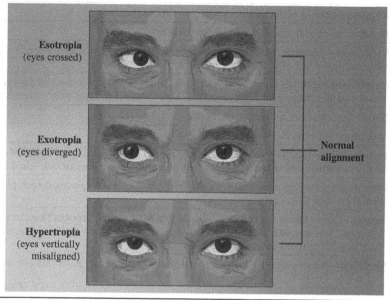

Nystagmus – Derived from the Greek word for "nodding," nystagmus is an involuntary back-and-forth movement of the eyes. Consequently, **NYSTAGM-** is the root of this movement. Nystagmus may be caused by damage or lesions to the inner ear, cerebellum, or brainstem, as well as drug intoxications.

Paralysis – Paralysis of the sphincter muscles of the iris resulting in a dilated pupil is called **iridoplegia**. As mentioned earlier, **CYCL-** is used for the "ciliary body," and therefore, paralysis of the ciliary body resulting in a loss of accommodation is called **cycloplegia**. Paralysis of the ocular muscles that move the eyeball is termed **ophthalmoplegia**.

Pathologies of the anatomical parts of the eye

Ophthalmia – Ophthalmia is used for severe inflammation of the eye.

Endophthalmitis – Endophthalmitis is an inflammation of the internal eye that may occur in the anterior or posterior camera of the eye.

Exophthalmos (or exophthalmia) – Exophthalmos is an abnormal anterior protrusion of the eyeball.

Scleritis – Scleritis is an inflammation of the sclera.

Conjunctivitis – Conjunctivitis is an inflammation of the conjunctiva, also known as "pinkeye."

Trachoma – Trachoma is a chronic conjunctivitis caused by the bacteria *Chlamydia trachomatis*. Its root **TRACH-** is used to describe the "rough" appearance of its lesions.

Pterygium – Pterygium is a triangular or "wing-like" thickening of the conjunctiva extending onto the eye (Fig. 11.7). The root **PTERYG-**, as well as the root **PTER-** and suffix **-PTERYX**, are commonly used in a variety of contexts meaning "wing" or "wing-like." For instance, the term "helicopter" literally means "helix/circular wing."

Fig. 11.7 Photo of an eye with pterygium. *Source:* Jmvaras/ Wikimedia Commons/CC BY-SA 4.0.

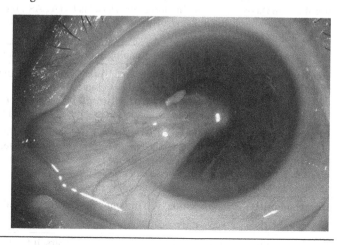

Keratitis – Keratitis is an inflammation of the cornea.

Keratorrhexis – Keratorrhexis is a rupture of the cornea.

Keratocele – Keratocele is a corneal protrusion.

Keratoncus – Literally meaning tumor (**-ONCUS**) of the cornea, a keratoncus is a type of hereditary corneal dystrophy resulting in a conical protrusion of the central part of the cornea.

Keratoconjunctivitis sicca – Keratoconjunctivitis sicca is also known as dry eye syndrome. This is a pathological Latin term that uses the Latin adjective for "dry," *siccus, -a, -um*. As was noted in earlier chapters the roots for "dry" are **SICC-** and **XER-**.

Iritis – Iritis is an inflammation of the iris.

Aniridia – Aniridia is the absence of all or part of the iris.

Heterochromia iridis – Formed from the roots **HETER-** (other) and **CHROM-** (color), heterochromia iridis is a congenital disorder in which one iris is a different color than the other iris in an individual.

Corectopia – Formed from the prefix **EC-** (outside) root **TOP-** (place), corectopia is a congenital defect where the pupil is not in its normal position (Fig. 11.8).

Miosis – Formed from the root **MI-** (also spelled **MEI-**), which means "less," miosis is a condition in which the pupil is "smaller" or "lessened." The root **MI-** (**MEI-**) shows up in a number of terms. For instance, **meiosis** is the process of cell division resulting in the "lessening" of chromosomes into haploids.

Mydriasis – Mydriasis is a condition in which the pupil is enlarged or dilated (Fig. 11.8).

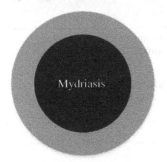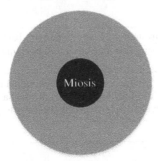

Fig. 11.8 Image of miosis and mydriasis of the pupil.

Retinitis – Retinitis is an inflammation of the retina of the eye.

Photoretinitis – Photoretinitis is an inflammation of the retina caused by bright light. As mentioned earlier in this textbook, **PHOT-** and **LUMIN-** mean "light," which is why "a unit of energy of a light ray" is called a "photon" (a lumen is a term for "a unit of light"), and why "luminiferous" means "pertaining to the bearing of light."

Retinoschisis – Retinoschisis is the pathological splitting of the retina.

Maculopathy – Maculopathy is a term for a collection of retinal pathologies affecting the macula of the eye.

Entropion and Ectropion – The root **TROP-** means "turning," "changing," and "stimulating." An outward turning of an eyelid is called **ectropion**. An inward turning of an eyelid is called **entropion**.

Trichiasis – Entropion is often accompanied by trichiasis. Formed by the root for "hair," **TRICH-**, trichiasis is a condition in which an eyelash rubs on the conjunctiva or the cornea.

Blepharitis – Inflammation of an eyelid is called blepharitis.

Blepharochalasis – The root for "loose" or "slack" is **CHALAS-**. It often appears as the suffix **-CHALASIS**, denoting the weakness of a sphincter muscle or similar structure. The loss of elasticity of the skin of the upper eyelid with old age that causes it to become slack is called blepharochalasis.

Blepharoptosis – Blepharoptosis is a drooping or downward displacement of an eyelid.

Hordeolum – Derived from the Latin term for a "barley cord," hordeolum is the technical term for a stye. A stye is an infection of the glands of the border of the eyelid. *Hordeolum* is used by Celsus in *De medicina*: *"A very small tumor forms in the same upper eyelid, above the line of the eyelashes, which from its resemblance to a barleycorn (hordeolum) is termed by the Greeks krithe (barleycorn)."* (Celsus 7.7) Translation in Celsus. *De medicina*. W. G. Spencer. Cambridge, Massachusetts. Harvard University Press. 1971 (republication of the 1935 edition).

Chalazion – Derived from the Greek word for "a hailstone," a swelling in the middle part of the eyelid that is formed by a distention of a meibomian gland is called a chalazion. Celsus reveals that this term also has its origin in ancient Greek medicine for the eye: *"Other tumors also, not unlike these, form on the eyelids; but they are not quite the same shape and are mobile, so that they can be pushed about with the finger; and so the Greeks call them chalazia, ..."* (Celsus 7.7) Translation in Celsus. *De medicina*. W. G. Spencer. Cambridge, Massachusetts. Harvard University Press. 1971 (Republication of the 1935 edition).

Dacryoadenitis – Dacryoadenitis is an inflammation of the lacrimal gland.

Dacryocystitis – Dacryocystitis, an inflammation of the tear sac.

Epiphora – Epiphora is an abnormal excessive flow of tears. It is a loan from the ancient Greek medical term for the same condition. Outside of ancient Greek medicine, the Greek word *epiphora* was used as a term for "a donation" or "a bringing to."

Greek or Latin word element	Current usage	Etymology	Examples
AMBLY/O (am-blē-ō)	Dull	Gr. *amblys*, blunt, dull	**Ambly**opia, **ambly**acousia, **ambly**chromasia
PRESBY/O (prĕz-bē-ō)	Old age	Gr. *presbys*, an old man, elder	**Presby**acusia, **presby**opia, **presby**cardia
DIPL/O (dĭp-lō)	Double	Gr *diploos*, twofold, double	**Dipl**opia, **dipl**oid, **diplo**bacterium
DEUTER/O (doo-tĕr-ō)	Second, secondary (*in vision, green blindness i.e. secondary color)	Gr. *deuteros*, 2nd	**Deuter**anopia, **deuter**oplasm, **deuter**ium
PROT/O (prō-tō)	First, primary (*in vision, red blindness i.e. primary color)	Gr. *protos*, 1st	**Prot**anopia, **prot**otype, **proto**biology
METR/O (mĕ-trō) **-METER** (mĕt-ĕr)	Measure, measuring (*METER, device for measure)	Gr. *metron*, a measure	A**metr**opia, ophthalmo**meter**
STIGMAT/O (stĭg-măt-ō)	Spot, point, shame/disgrace	Gr. *stigma, stigmatos*, a mark of a pointed instrument, brand, tattoo-mark	A**stigmat**ism, **stigmat**ical Loan word: **Stigma** (stĭg'mă)
PHOT/O (fō-tō)	Light	Gr. *phos, photos*, light	**Phot**ophobia, **phot**on, **photo**graph, **photo**retinitis
LUMIN/O (loo-mĭ-nō)	Light, lumen (unit of light)	L. *lumen, luminis*, n. light	Trans**lumin**al, il**lumin**ate Loan word: **Lumen** (loo'mĕn) pl. **Lumina** (loo'mĭ-nă)
SCOT/O (skō-tō)	Darkness	Gr. *skotos*, darkness	**Scot**oma, **scot**ophobia, **scot**opia
NYCT/O (nik-tō)	Night	Gr. *nyx, nyktos*, night	**Nyct**alopia, **nyct**amblyopia, epi**nyct**al
NOCT/O (nok-tō)	Night	L. *nox, noctis*, f. night	**Noct**ilucent, **noct**urnal
TROP/O (trō-pō) **-TROPIA** (trō-pē-ă) **-TROPION** (trō-pē-ŏn)	Turning, change, stimulating (*TROPIA, deviation of eyes from the visual axis; *TROPION, turning the edge or margin, particularly of the eyelid)	Gr. *trope*, turning, change; stimulating	Eso**tropia**, en**tropion**, geo**trop**ism, en**trop**y
STRABISM/O (stră-biz-mō)	Strabismus (*disorder of the eye in respect to the optic axis)	L. *strabismus, -i,* m. strabismus fr. Gr. *strabismus*, a squinting	**Strabism**ometer, **strabism**al Loan word: **Strabismus** (stră-biz'mŭs)
NYSTAGM/O (nis-tag-mō)	Nystagmus (*disorder involving involuntary movement of the eye)	L. *nystagmus, -i,* m. nystagmus fr. Gr. *nystagmus*, nodding, drowsiness	**Nystagm**ograph, **nystagm**iform Loan word: **Nystagmus** (nis-tag'mŭs)

Greek or Latin word element	Current usage	Etymology	Examples
SCHIST/O (skĭs-tō) SCHIZ/O (skĭz-ō) -SCHISIS (skĭ-sĭs)	Split, cleft	Gr. *schizein*, to split, cleave; Gr. *schistos*, cleft	Retino**schisis**, **schiz**oblepharia, **schist**ocoelia
CHALAS/O (kăl-ă-sō) -CHALASIS (kăl'ă-sĭs)	Loose, slack	Gr. *chalaein*, to loosen, relax	Blepharo**chalasis**, **chalas**ia, arthro**chalas**ia
PTERYG/O (ter-ĭ-gō) PTER/O (ter-ō) -PTERYX (ter-iks)	Wing, wing-like	Gr. *pteryx, pterygos*, wing; Gr. *pteron*, wing	**Pteryg**ium, **pter**ion, archaeo**pteryx**
GLAUC/O (glaw-kō)	Silver, gray, or bluish green	Gr. *glaukos*, gleaming, gray	**Glauc**oma, **glauc**odot, **glauc**onite
CATARACT/O (kăt-ă-răk-tō)	Cataract	L. *cataracta, -ae*, f. waterfall	**Cataract**ogenic Derivative: **Cataract** (kat'ă-rakt″)
MI/O (mī-ō) MEI/O (mī-ō)	Less, smaller	L. *meion*, less, smaller	**Mi**osis, **mei**osis, **mi**ocardia
MYDRIAT- (mĭ-drī-ă-tō)	Enlargement of the pupil	Gr. *mydriasis*, enlargement of the pupil	**Mydriat**ic Loan word **Mydriasis** (mĭ-drī'ă-sĭs)

Review	Answers
The root OPT- in optometrist means _____. The root OPHTHALM- in ophthalmologist means _____.	**vision** **eye**
Refractive errors of vision are termed _____ opia, which literally means "disproportionate" or "lack of measure" vision. The term for farsightedness is _____ opia. The term for nearsightedness is _____ opia, which has a somewhat debatable etymology. The form of ametropia in which the refraction of rays is spread over a wide area rather than coming to point on the retina is an _____. The root STIGMAT- means _____, _____, and _____.	**ametr** **hyper** **my** **astigmatism** **point, spot, shame/ disgrace**
The term for "dull" vision is _____ opia. The term for "old-age" vision is _____ opia. The term for "weak" vision is _____ opia. The term for "light" vision is _____ opia. The term for "darkness" vision is _____ opia. "Double" vision is _____ opia. "Equal" vision is _____ opia.	**ambly** **presby** **asthen** **phot** **scot** **dipl** **is**

Review	Answers
Blindness or "no vision" is _____ opia. Blindness in one-half field of vision is _____ opia. A lack of "primary" vision (red color blindness) is _____ opia. A lack of "secondary" vision (green color blindness) is _____ opia. Night blindness is called _____ opia.	**an** **hemian** **protan** **deuteran** **nyctal**
Inflammation of an eyelid is called _____itis. Inflammation of a lacrimal gland is called _____itis. Inflammation of the tear sac is called _____itis. Inflammation of the conjunctiva, also known as pinkeye, is called _____itis. Inflammation of the sclera is called _____itis. Inflammation of the retina of the eye is called _____itis. Inflammation of the cornea is called _____itis. Inflammation of the iris is called _____itis.	**blephar** **dacryoaden** **dacryocyst** **conjunctiv** **scler** **retin** **kerat** **ir**
Abnormal anterior protrusion of the eyeball is called _____.	**Exophthalmia** **(exophthalmos)**
The absence of the lens of the eye is called _____.	**aphakia**
The root for loose" or "slack" is _____. The loss of elasticity of the skin of the upper eyelid that causes it to become slack is called blepharo _____. This differs from a dropping or downward displacement of an eyelid, which is called blepharo _____.	**CHALAS-** **chalasis** **ptosis**
Named after the Latin word for a waterfall, the opacity of a lens is called a _____.	**cataract**
_____ is a disease of the eye characterized by increased intraocular pressure due to the overaccumulation of the aqueous humor. The root GLAUC- means _____, _____, or _____.	**glaucoma** **silver, gray, blue-green**
A condition in which the pupil is "smaller" or "lessened" is called _____. A condition in which the pupil is enlarged or dilated is called_____.	**miosis** **mydriasis**
A dark spot in one's field of vision is called a _____.	**scotoma**
An aversion to light _____phobia.	**photo**
The loan word used for a unit of light is _____.	**lumen**
Paralysis of the sphincter muscles of the iris resulting in a dilated pupil is called _____plegia. Paralysis of the ciliary body resulting in a loss of accommodation is _____plegia. Paralysis of the ocular muscles is _____plegia.	**irido** **cyclo** **ophthalmo**
The pathological splitting of the retina is called retino _____.	**schisis**
A ruptured cornea is called kerato _____.	**rrhexis**
The root _____ means "turning," "changing," and "stimulating." An inward turning of an eyelid is called _____. An outward turning of an eyelid is called _____.	**TROP-** **entropion** **ectropion**
_____ is a condition in which an eyelash rubs on the conjunctiva or the cornea.	**trichiasis**
Derived from the Greek word for "squinting," the term _____ is used for disorders of the eye in which the optic axes cannot be directed to the same object. The term _____ is a synonym for strabismus. The root HETER- means _____ in this term. The compound suffix _____, which literally means "a condition of turning" is used to denote which direction an eye is deviating. An inward deviation (i.e. medial) is called _____ tropia. An outward deviation (i.e. lateral) is called _____ tropia.	**strabismus** **heterotropia** **opposite** **-TROPIA** **eso** **exo**
Derived from the Greek word for "nodding," _____ is an involuntary back-and-forth movement of the eyes that is observed with tracking tests.	**nystagmus**
A sty or stye is an infection of the glands of the border of the eyelid. Derived from the term for a "barley cord," _____ is the technical term for a stye.	**hordeolum**
Derived from the word for a hailstone, a swelling in the middle part of the eyelid that is formed by a distention of a meibomian gland is called a _____.	**chalazion**
A triangular or "wing-like" thickening of the conjunctiva extending onto the eye is called _____. The root PTERYG- means _____ or _____.	**Pterygium** **wing, winglike**
An abnormal excessive flow of tears is called _____.	**epiphora**

Etymological Explanations: Common Terms and Word Elements for the Anatomy of the Ear

In the following discussion of the anatomical terms associated with the ear, the nominative and genitive singular forms of the anatomical Latin term are provided in parenthesis. The Greek and Latin roots are formatted in all caps and emboldened (Fig. 11.9).

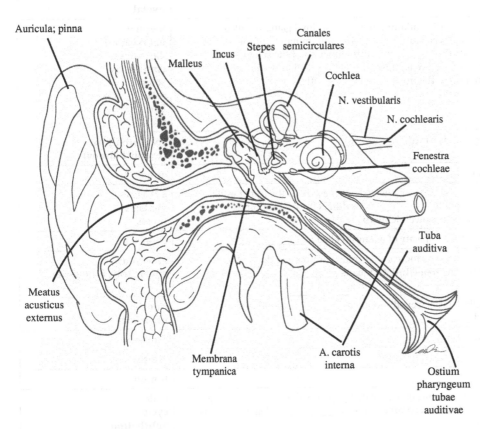

Fig. 11.9 Anatomical Latin terms for the ear. *Source:* Drawing by Chloe Kim.

Labels in figure: Auricula; pinna — Malleus — Incus — Stepes — Canales semicirculares — Cochlea — N. vestibularis — N. cochlearis — Fenestra cochleae — Tuba auditiva — A. carotis interna — Ostium pharyngeum tubae auditivae — Membrana tympanica — Meatus acusticus externus

---

Anatomical parts of the ear

Ear (L. *auris*, *-is*) – The anatomical Latin term for the "ear" is the **auris**. The Latin and Greek roots **AUR-** and **OT-** are used for the "ear." Hence, a specialist in ear diseases is called an otologist, and a device for looking into the ear is called an otoscope. The ear is divided into three anatomical areas: **the external ear (L. *auris externa*)**, which extends from the eardrum outward; **the middle ear (L. *auris media*)**, which is located between the eardrum and the oval window; and **the inner ear (L. *auris interna*)**, which extends inward from the oval window.

Auricle (L. *auricula*, *-ae*) – The *auris externa* is comprised of the conspicuous "ear flap" at the side of the head called the auricle, the external auditory canal, also known as the external auditory meatus, and the eardrum. The external ear's structure is designed to funnel sound inward. The loan words for the "visible external ear" are **auricula (L. *auricula*, *-ae*), pinna (L. *pinna*, *-ae*)**, and **concha (L. *concha*, *-ae*)**. Their corresponding roots **PINN-, PENN-, AURICUL-**, and **CONCH-** can be used for the visible external ear that sits on the sides of our heads. In other contexts, the root **CONCH-** can mean "shell" or "shell-like." In addition to the external ear, the roots **PINN-** and **PENN-** can mean "feather," "fin," and "wing."

Auditory meatus (L. *Meatus acusticus*) – The external opening of the auditory canal is called the meatus (*meatus*, *-us*) and by extension, the external auditory canal is known as the external auditory meatus. This pathway conducts sound, and it contains numerous glands that produce earwax. In Classical Latin, a *meatus* was a "way" or "path." In anatomical Latin, a meatus is typically a pathway to the outside of the body. Thus, the root **MEAT-** means "opening" or "passageway."

Eardrum (L. *tympanum*, *-i*) – The loan words for the "eardrum" are **tympanum** and **myringa (L. *myringa*, *-ae*)**. The roots for the "eardrum" are correspondingly **TYMPAN-** and **MYRING-**. In contexts other than the ear, **TYMPAN-** can be used for "drum," and **MYRING-** can mean "membrane." The Latin term tympanum comes from the Greek word for a type of kettledrum, *tympanon*, that was used in the worship of the Cybele.

Ossicles (L. *ossicula auditus*) – The *auris media* is comprised of the eardrum, the three auditory bones called the ossicles, the oval window, and its openings to the mastoid and eustachian tube. The three ossicles of the ear are known as the "hammer," "anvil," and "stirrup." The loan words for these are respectively the **malleus** (**L. *malleus, -i***), **incus** (**L. *incus, incudis***), and stapes (**L. *stapes, stapedis***). The root for the "hammer" is **MALLE-**; the root for the "anvil" is **INCUD-**; and the root for the "stirrup" is **STAPED-**. At one end, the malleus is attached to the eardrum, and at the other end, the stapes is attached to the oval window.

Eustachian Tube (L. *tuba auditiva*) – There are two openings in the middle ear. One pathway leads to sinuses located in the mastoid process, which is a bony projection behind the ear. The other pathway leads to the Eustachian tube, which derives its name from the Italian physician Bartolomeo Eustachio (d.1574), who discovered this passage from the ears to the throat. The Eustachian tube regulates the air in the middle ear to accommodate for atmospheric pressure. The tube is typically closed, but it opens with swallowing and yawing, which is why it is commonly recommended to do both when a plane is ascending or descending. The Eustachian tube is also called the salpinx (**L. *salpinx, salpingis***), and its corresponding root is **SALPING-**. This loan word and its root also refer to the Fallopian (uterine) tubes. In the ancient Greek world, a salpinx was a type of horn that had a long bronze tube attached to a small bell at the end of this horn. It is typically depicted in the hands of a soldier because it was used in battle to signal troops, which is why it is frequently described as the "piercing sound" of war in ancient Greek literature. Based on the shape of this ancient horn, the root **SALPING-** is used for any very long tubular structure (Fig. 11.10).

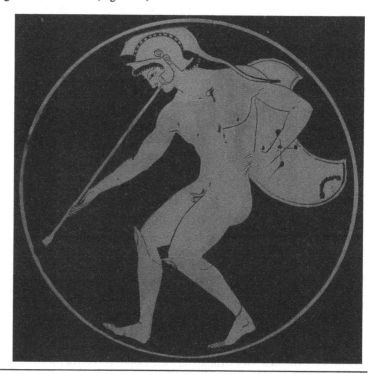

Fig. 11.10 Soldier blowing on a salpinx, image on a 5th-century-BC kylix (drinking cup). *Source:* Unknown Greek painter, circa 500 B.C./Wikimedia Commons/ CC0 1.0.

Oval window (L. *fenestra vestibuli*) – The oval window is also known as the *fenestra vestibuli* (window of the vestibule). The oval window transmits vibrations to the cochlea for hearing. In anatomy, a **fenestra** is a term used for an aperture often closed by a membrane. Derived from this Latin word for a "window," the root **FENESTR-** refers to an "opening" or "window." In the Roman world, a fenestra was originally a small opening in a house that was well above ground level. Roman windows were typically covered with lattice work to keep poisonous animals out. Later, windows were covered with a transparent stone, called *lapis specularis*. By the time of the early emperors, Roman windows began to be covered with glass called *vitrum*.

Labyrinth (L. *labyrinthus, -i*) – The *auris interna* is comprised of the oval window and the labyrinth. The labyrinth consists of the bony and the membranous labyrinths. The labyrinth of the ear is comprised of three parts: the semicircular canals, vestibule, and the cochlea. This complicated structure derives its name from the ancient Greek word for a maze, *labyrinthos*. The term is especially associated with the mythological structure built by the Athenian Daedalus to hold the Minotaur. The bull-headed monster lived in the twisting maze of the labyrinth where it was offered a regular sacrifice of youths and maidens. The beast was eventually slain by the Athenian hero, Theseus, with the help of the Cretan princess, Ariadne. As to the origins of this monster, Apollodorus *Bibliotheca* (3. 8–11) provides the following disturbing myth: "Minos aspired to the throne [of Crete], but was rebuffed. He claimed, however, that he had received the sovereignty from the gods, and to prove it he said that whatever he prayed for would come about. So while sacrificing to Poseidon, he prayed for a bull to appear from the depths of the sea, and promised to sacrifice it upon its appearance. And Poseidon did send up to him a splendid bull. Thus, Minos received the rule, but he sent the bull to his herds and sacrificed another .... Poseidon was angry that the bull was not sacrificed, and turned it wild. He also devised that Pasiphae should develop a lust for it. In her passion for the bull she took on as her accomplice an architect named Daidalos (Daedalus) .... He built a wooden cow on wheels, ... skinned a real cow, and sewed the contraption into the skin, and then, after placing Pasiphae inside, set it in a meadow where the bull normally grazed. The bull came up and had intercourse with it, as if with a real cow. Pasiphae gave birth to Asterios (Asterius), who was called Minotauros (Minotaur). He had the face of a bull, but was otherwise human. Minos, following certain oracular instructions, kept him confined and under guard in the labyrinth. This labyrinth, which Daidalos built, was a 'cage with convoluted flexions (Fig. 11.11).'"

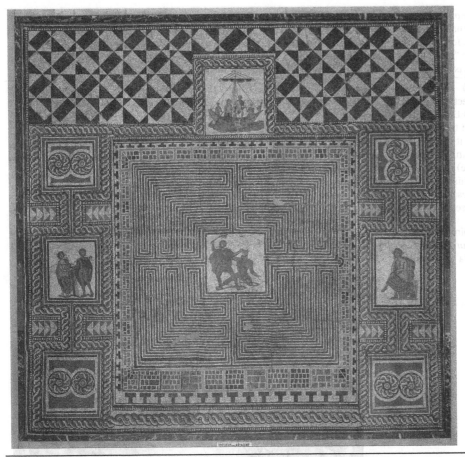

Fig. 11.11 4th-century-AD Roman mosaic of a labyrinth with Theseus killing the Minotaur in the center. This mosaic is in a Roman villa near Salzburg, Austria. *Source:* Unknown author/Wikimedia Commons/Public domain.

Vestibule (L. *vestibulum, -i*) – The vestibule connects the cochlea and semicircular canals and assists in their function. The root **VESTIBUL-** is used for this middle part of the inner ear. In Classical Latin, a *vestibulum* was a "forecourt" or "entrance" to a building. In anatomical terminology, a *vestibulum* is a cavity forming the entryway to another cavity. The vestibule contains two sacks called the **utricle** (*utriculus, -i*) and **saccule** (*saccus, -i*). The loan word for the larger of the two sacks of the vestibule is the **utriculus**. The loan word for the smaller of the two sacks of the vestibule is the **sacculus**. The roots **UTRICUL-** and **SACCUL-** are used respectively for these structures of the vestibule, and elsewhere, they have the meaning of a "bag" or "sac." The endolymph is a clear fluid that is inside the membranous labyrinth, connecting all three parts via a series of ducts. This liquid connection explains why hearing loss is accompanied with a loss of balance in some disorders.

Cochlea (L. *cochlea, -ae*) – The spiral snail-shaped portion of the inner ear responsible for hearing is called the cochlea. The cochlea is the area of the labyrinth associated with hearing. The root for this part of the inner ear, as well as for the spiral shell-like structures, is **COCHLE-**. When sound waves enter the ear through external auditory meatus, they cause the eardrum to vibrate, which in turn causes the ossicles to vibrate at the same frequency. The vibration of the stapes on the oval window disturbs the endolymph, which in turn moves the hair cells of the organ of Corti. These tactile receptors send impulses to the brain via the auditory nerve, which the brain, particularly the temporal lobe, interprets.

Greek or Latin word element	Current usage	Etymology	Examples
AUR/O (or-ō)	Ear	L. *auris, auris*, f. ear	**Aur**icle, post**aur**al, **aur**ophore Loan word: **Auris** (ow′ris) pl. **Aures** (ow′rēz″)
AURICUL/O (or-ik-yŭ-lō)	Auricle (visible external ear)	L. *auricula, -ae*, f. auricle, little ear	**Auricul**ar, **auricul**ate **Auricula** (or-ik′yŭ-lă) pl. **Auriculae** (or-ik′yŭ-lē″)

Greek or Latin word element	Current usage	Etymology	Examples
PINN/O **(pin-ō)** **PENN/O** **(pen-ō)**	Auricle (visible external ear), feather, fin, wing	L. *pinna, -ae*, f. feather, fin, wing,	**Pinn**aplasty, **penn**iform Loan word: **Pinna** (pin′ă) pl. **Pinnae** (pin′ē″)
CONCH/O **(kŏng-kō)**	Auricle (visible external ear), shell, shell-like	L. *concha, -ae*, f. concha fr. Gr. *konche*, shell, cockle	**Conch**oscope, **chonch**iform Loan word: **Concha** (kŏng′kă) pl. **Conchae** (kŏng′kē″)
OT/O **(ō-tō)** **-OTIA** **(ō-shē-ă)**	Ear	Gr. *ous, otos*, ear	Mac**rotia**, **ot**orrhea, **ot**algia
MALLE/O **(mal-ē-ō)**	Malleus (one of the ossicles of the ear), hammer	L. *malleus, -i*, m. hammer	**Malle**oincudal, supra**malle**olar Loan word: **Malleus** (mal′ē-ŭs) pl. **Mallei** (mal′ē-ī″)
INCUD/O **(ing-kyŭ-dō)**	Incus (one of the ossicles of the ear), anvil	L. *incus, incudis*, f. anvil	**Incud**ectomy, **incud**iform Loan word: **Incus** (ing′kŭs) pl. **Incudes** (ing-kūd′ēz″)
STAPED/O **(stă-pēd-ō)**	Stapes (one of the ossicles of the ear), stirrup	L. *stapes, stapedis*, m. stirrup	**Staped**ectomy, medio**staped**ial Loan word: **Stapes** (stā′pēz″) pl. **Stapedes** (stă-pē′dēz″)
LABYRINTH/O **(lab-ĭ-rin-thō)**	Labyrinth of the ear, maze	L. *labyrinthus, -i*, m. labyrinth fr. Gr. *labyrinthos*, a maze	**Labyrinth**itis, **labyrinth**ectomy Loan word: **Labyrinthus** (lab″ĭ-rin′thŭs) pl. **Labyrinthi** (lab″ĭ-rin′thī″)
VESTIBUL/O **(vĕs-tĭb-ū-lō)**	Vestibule of the inner ear, an entrance	L. *vestibulum, -i*, n. an entrance-court, entrance to a place	**Vestibul**odynia, **vestibul**ar Loan word: **Vestibulum** (vĕs-tĭb′ū-lŭm) pl. **Vestibula** (vĕs-tĭb′ū-la)
UTRICUL/O **(ū-trik-yŭ-lō)**	Utricle of the inner ear, bag, sack	L. *utriculus, -i*, m. utricle fr. L. *uter, utris*, m. a bag or bottle	**Utricul**itis, **utricul**ar Loan word: **Utriculus** (ū-trik′yŭ-lŭs) pl. **Utriculi** (ū-trik′yŭ-lī″)
SACCUL/O **(sak-yŭ-lō)**	Saccule of the inner ear, bag, sack	L. *sacculus, -i*, m. saccule fr. L. *saccus, -i*, m. sack, bag	Utriculo**saccul**ar, **saccul**ation Loan word: **Sacculus** (sak′yŭ-lŭs) pl. **Sacculi** (sak′yŭ-lī″)

Greek or Latin word element	Current usage	Etymology	Examples
COCHLE/O (kok-lē-ō)	Cochlea of the inner ear, spiral shell	L. *cochlea, -ae*, f. cochlea fr. Gr. *kochlias*, snail with a spiral shell	**Cochle**ar, gyro**cochle**a Loan word: **Cochlea** (kok′lē-ă) pl. **Cochleae** (kok′lē-ē″)
MEAT/O (mē-ă-tō)	Opening, passageway	L. *meatus, -us*, m. a path or course	**Meat**ometer, **meat**itis Loan word: **Meatus** (mē-āt′ŭs)
FENESTR/O (fĕ-nes-trō)	Opening, window	L. *fenestra, -ae*, f. window	**Fenestr**ated, **fenestr**ule Loan word: **Fenestra** (fĕ-nes′tră) pl. **Fenestrae** (fĕ-nes′trē″)
SALPING/O (săl-pĭng-gō) **-SALPINX** (sal-pingks)	Eustachian tube, or Fallopian (Uterine), a long tubular structure	L. *salpinx, salpingis*, f. eustachian tube fr. Gr. *salpinx, salpingos*, long tubed trumpet	**Salping**oscope, **salping**ectomy Loan word: **Salpinx** (sal′pingks) pl. **Salpinges** (sal-pin′jēz″)
TYMPAN/O (tĭm-pă-nō)	Eardrum, drum	L. *tympanum, -i*, n. tympanum fr. Gr. *tympanon*, a drum	**Tympan**itis, **tymp**anic Loan word: **Tympanum** (tĭm′păn-ŭm) pl. **Tympana** (tĭm′păn-a)
MYRING/O (mĭ-ring-gō)	Eardrum, membrane	Gr. *myrinx, myringos*, a membrane	**Myring**otomy, **myring**itis Loan word: **Myringa** (mĭ-ring′gă)

Review	Answers
The loan words for the "visible external ear" are _____, _____, and _____. In other contexts, the root CONCH- can mean _____ or _____. In addition to the external ear, the roots PINN- and PENN- can mean _____, _____, and _____.	**auricula, pinna, concha shell, shell-like feather, fin, wing**
The roots _____ and _____ are used for the "ear."	**AUR-, OT-**
The three ossicles of the ear are called the hammer, anvil, and stirrup. The loan words for these are respectively the _____, _____, and _____. The root for the "hammer" is _____. The root for the "anvil" is _____. The root for the "stirrup" is _____.	**malleus, incus, stapes** **MALLE-** **INCUD-** **STAPED-**
The root for the Eustachian tube is _____.	**SALPING-**
The loan words for the "eardrum" are _____ and _____.	**tympanum, myringa**
The root _____ is used for the middle part of the inner ear, behind the cochlea, in front of the semicircular canals, which contains the utricle and saccule. The loan word for the larger of the two sacks of the vestibule is the _____. The loan word for the smaller of the two sacks of the vestibule is the _____.	**VESTIBUL-** **utriculus** **sacculus**
The _____ is the maze-like structure of the inner ear that is comprised of the semicircular canals, vestibule, and cochlea.	**labyrinth**
The spiral snail-shaped portion of the inner ear responsible for hearing is called the _____. The root for this part of the inner ear, as well as for spiral shell-like structures, is _____.	**Cochlea** **COCHLE-**

Review	Answers
The external opening of the ear is called the auditory _____.	**meatus**
The root _____ is used for the "oval window," which is the anatomical boundary between the middle and inner ear.	**FENESTR-**

Etymological Explanations: Common Terms and Word Elements for the Pathologies of the Ear

Disorders of hearing

Hearing – The roots used for the sense of "hearing" are **AUDIT-**, **AUD-**, **ACUST-**, and **ACOUST-**, and their corresponding suffixes are **-ACUSIS** and **-ACOUSIA**. Hence, a professional who specializes in the study of hearing impairments is called an **audiologist**.

Presbyacusis – A hearing impairment of old age is called presbyacusis.

Brayacusis – Based on its root **BRADY-**, bradyacusis literally means "slow hearing." According to Taber's, bradyacusis is abnormally diminished hearing acuity.

Amblyacousia – Dullness of hearing is termed amblyacousia.

Hyperacusis or **Oxyacusis** – "Excessive" or "keen" hearing is termed hyperacusis. Derived from the root for "sharp," OXY-, it is also called oxyacusis.

Anacusia or **Anacusus** – Anacusia and anacusis are used for total deafness.

Sound – The roots that are used for "a sound" are **PHON-**, **SON-**, and **ACOUSMAT-**. The loan word/derivative for a single speech sound is **phone**. The loan word/derivative for a unit of sound is **sone**. The loan word for an auditory hallucination of a simple nonverbal character is **acousma**.

Tinnitus (L. *tinnitus, -us*) – An abnormal ringing or buzzing sound in the ear is called tinnitus. Given this is a 4th declension Latin noun, the plural form in English is **tinnituses**. This loan word's root **TINNIT-** does not appear in medical terminology. The term **syrigmus**, which is derived from the Greek word for "whistle," is sometimes used as a synonym for tinnitus.

Pathologies of the anatomical parts of the ear

Otalgia or **Otodynia** – An earache is termed otalgia or otodynia.

Otorrhagia – A rupture causing bleeding from the ear is otorrhagia.

Otomycosis – Derived from the root for "fungus" **MYC-**, a fungus of the ear, is called otomycosis.

Conditions of the auricle – The compound suffix -OTIA is used for conditions of the ear, particularly those involving the auricle. Thus, the condition of abnormally small ears is called **microtia**. A condition of abnormally large ears is called **macrotia**. Having more than two ears is called **polyotia**. **Anotia** is the absence of the ears.

Otitis – Inflammation of the ear is called otitis. An inflammation of the middle ear caused by changes in atmospheric pressure is termed aerotitis or barotitis. The root **AER-** means "air." The roots **BAR-** and **BARY-** mean "pressure," "weight," and "heavy." The roots **BATH-** and **BATHY-** mean "depth" and "deep." Although they look similar, the modern English terms "bath" and "bathing" do not come from the Greek root **BATH-**. They are derived from an old English word for "immersing oneself." A bath in the Greek world was termed a *loutron* and in the Roman world, it was a *balineum*.

Myringitis or **Tympanitis** – An inflammation of the eardrum is called myringitis or tympanitis.

Labyrinthitis – Inflammation of the maze-like structure of the inner ear is termed labyrinthitis.

Mastoiditis – Mastoiditis is an inflammation of the mastoid sinuses due to an infection from acute otitis media. Derived from the root for "a breast," **MAST-**, the mastoid sinus derives its name from its supposed "breast-like" shape.

Ceruminosis – Ceruminosis is a condition in which there is an excessive amount of earwax being produced. The root used for "earwax" is **CERUMIN-**, and the loan word for "earwax" is cerumen (*cerumen, ceruminis*). Owing to their etymological relationship, the root for earwax is easily confused with the root for "wax," which is **CER-**.

Aural atresia – The external auditory meatus is the visible hole in the external ear. If this hole is covered with flesh, it is called atresia. The root **TRET**- means "perforated" or "bored."

Salpingemphraxis – Derived from the compound suffix for "obstruction," -**EMPHRAXIS**, an obstruction of the eustachian tube, is called a salpingemphraxis.

Otosclerosis – Otosclerosis is the progressive loss of hearing due to the formation of bone around the oval window. The surgical creation of a new window in the labyrinth to treat deafness associated with otosclerosis is termed fenestration. The surgical removal of the stirrup due to otosclerosis is called a **stapedectomy**.

Greek or Latin word element	Current usage	Etymology	Examples
SON/O (sō-nō)	Sound	L. *sonus, -i,* m. sound	Ultra**son**ic, **son**ogram, **son**olucent Loan word: **Sone** (sōn)
PHON/O (fŏ-nō)	Sound, voice	Gr. *phone,* sound, voice	**Phon**ometer, **phon**ograph, tele**phone** Loan word: **Phone** (fōn)
ACOUSMAT/O (ă-kooz-măt-ō)	Sound	Gr. *akousma, akousmatos,* a thing heard	**Acousmat**amnesia, **acousmat**agnosis Loan word: **Acousma** (ă-kooz-mä)
BAR/O (bar-ō) BARY/O (bar-ē-ō)	Weight, pressure, heavy	Gr. *barys,* heavy Gr. *baros, bareos,* weight, pressure	**Bar**otitis, **Bary**phonia, **bar**iatric
BATH/O (băth-ō) BATHY/O (băth-ē-ō)	Depth, deep	Gr. *bathys,* deep, inner; *bathos,* depth	**Bathy**anesthesia, **bath**olite, **bath**ometer
TRET/O (trē-tō) -TRESIA (trē-zē-ă)	Perforated, bored	Gr. *tresis,* perforation; Gr. *tretos,* bored, perforated	A**tresia**, a**tret**ic, a**tresia**plasty
MASTOID/O (mas-toyd-ō)	Mastoid (process of the temporal bone)	Gr. *mastoeides,* like a breast	**Mastoid**itis, **mastoid**ectomy Loan word: **Mastoid** (mas′toyd″)
TINNIT/O (tĭn-ī-tō)	A ringing, buzzing, hissing sound in the ear	L. *tinnitus, -us,* m. a ringing	Loan word: **Tinnitus** (tĭn-ī′tŭs)
CERUMIN/O (sĕ-roo-mĭ-nō)	Earwax	L. *cerumen, ceruminis,* n. earwax	**Cerumin**olysis, **cerumin**osis Loan word: **Cerumen** (sĕ-roo′mĕn)
CER/O (sē-rō) -CERE (sēr)	Wax	L. *cera, -ae,* wax	Adipo**cere**, **cer**oplasty Loan word: **Cera** (sē′ră)

Greek or Latin word element	Current usage	Etymology	Examples
AUDIT/O (od-ĭ-tō) **AUDI/O** (od-ē-ō)	Listening, sense of hearing	L. *audire*, *auditum*, to hear	**Audi**ometry, **audit**ory
ACUST/O (ă-koos-tō) **ACOUST/O** (ă-koos-tō) **-ACUSIS** (a-kū-sĭs) **-ACOUSIA** (ă-kū-sē-ă)	Listening, sense of hearing	Gr. *akouein*, to hear	Par**acusi**a, **acoust**ic, an**acousis**

Review	Answers
The compound suffix -OTIA is used for conditions of the ear. Thus, the condition of abnormally small ears is called _____ otia. A condition of abnormally large ears is called _____ otia. Having more than two ears is called _____ otia.	**micr** **mac** **poly**
The suffixes -ACOUSIA and -ACUSIS are used for the sense of _____. Thus, hearing impairment of old age is called _____ acusis. "Slow" hearing is _____ acusis. "Excessive" hearing is _____ acusis. "Dullness" of hearing is _____ acousia.	**hearing** **presby** **brady** **hyper** **ambly**
The auditory nerve is also called the _____ nerve. A tumor of this cranial nerve is called a _____ _____.	**acoustic** **acoustic neuroma**
An inflammation of the eardrum is called _____ or _____.	**tympanitis, myringitis**
A ringing or buzzing of the ear is called _____.	**tinnitus**
Inflammation of the ear is called _____. An inflammation of the middle ear cause by changes in atmospheric pressure is termed _____ or _____. The root AER- means "air." The roots BAR- and BARY- mean _____, _____, and _____. The roots BATH- and BATHY- mean _____ and _____.	**otitis** **aerotitis, barotitis** **pressure, weight, heavy** **depth, deep**
An earache is termed _____ or _____. A discharge from the ear is called _____. A rupture causing bleeding from the ear is _____. A fungus of the ear is _____.	**otalgia, otodynia** **otorrhea** **otorrhagia** **otomycosis**
_____ is a condition in which there is an excessive amount of earwax being produced. The root used for "earwax" is _____, and the loan word for "earwax" is _____. Owing to their etymological relationship, the root for earwax is easily confused with the root for "wax," which is _____.	**Ceruminosis** **CERUMIN-** **cerumen** **CER-**
The roots that are used for "a sound" are _____, _____, and _____. The loan word/derivative for a single speech sound is _____. The loan word/derivative for a unit of sound is _____. The loan word for an auditory hallucination of a simple nonverbal character is _____.	**PHON-, SON-, ACOUSMAT-** **phone** **sone** **acousma**
The external auditory _____ is the visible hole in the external ear. If this hole is covered with flesh, it is called _____.	**meatus, atresia**
_____itis is an inflammation of the mastoid sinuses due to an infection from acute otitis media.	**Mastoid**

Review	Answers
A professional who specializes in the study of hearing impairments is an _____ logist. A specialist in ear diseases is called an _____ logist.	**audio** **oto**
A device for looking into the ear is called an _____.	**otoscope**
The surgical removal of the stirrup due to otosclerosis is called a _____. The surgical repair of the eardrum is called a _____. Surgical repair of the external ear is called _____.	**stapedectomy** **tympanoplasty** **otoplasty**
Inflammation of the maze-like structure of the inner ear is termed _____.	**labyrinthitis**
An obstruction of the Eustachian tube is called a _____.	**salpingemphraxis**

12

Endocrine System

CHAPTER LEARNING OBJECTIVES

1) You will learn the word elements, loan words, and key terms associated with the endocrine system and glands.
2) You will become familiar with the historical concepts associated with ancient Greek notions of glands.

Lessons from History: Paradigm, Perception, and the Pineal Gland

Food for Thought as You Read:

In what ways does the history of the pineal gland suggest that science and scientific discovery can also be construed as a social operation?
Is Galen's approach to the pineal gland more or less scientific? Why?

The pineal gland is a small, highly vascularized, cone-shaped structure located behind the 3rd cerebral ventricle (Fig. 12.1). In ancient Greek medicine, the pineal gland was known as the *konarion* on account of its resemblance to the shape of a pine cone (*konos*). This resemblance also explains why in anatomical Latin, it came to be referred to as the *glandula pinealis* ("pine-like gland"), and why it is simply called the "pineal gland" in English. Due to its distinctive shape and central location in the brain, for over two millennia, this rather small appendage has received an enormous amount of speculation as to its function. Most of this speculation has centered on the pineal gland's relationship to the soul and mental faculties in humans. In ancient Greek medicine, the pineal gland was considered by some to be a structure that regulated the movement of psychic pneuma between the ventricles, and thus, it played a role in the mental faculties of the human brain. This ventricular explanation of the pineal gland's relationship to the mental faculties is also evident in Medieval Islamic medicine. In his *On the Difference Between Spirit and Soul*, the Syrian Melkite Christian, Qusta ibn Luqa (864–923), proposed that the pineal gland played a role in the retrieval of memories by opening a passage between the middle and posterior ventricles.

Perhaps the most famous theory of the pineal gland's mental functions is found in René Descartes' (1596–1650) *Dioptrics* and his *Treatise of Man*. Descartes argued that the pineal gland functions as the seat of the soul, which he made to be the physical point of connection between the human soul and the body (Fig. 12.2). Shortly after his death, Descartes' theory was criticized by Thomas Willis (1621–1675), the English physician and anatomist for whom the Circle of Willis of the brain is named. He noted animals that clearly lack cognition and reason also have well-developed pineal glands, and therefore, it is unlikely that this anatomical organ functions as the seat of the human soul. In the 19th century, the pineal gland tended to be considered a vestigial part of the brain, and research tended to look at its neurological connection to the eye in animals. The discovery of hormones in the early 20th century led to a radical reconceptualization of the pineal gland. In 1958, the hormone melatonin was isolated by Aaron Lerner, which led to the pineal gland being understood as a neuroendocrine gland whose primary function is to maintain circadian rhythm through the secretion of this hormone. Research into the pineal gland's function as a neuroendocrine gland is still

Greek and Latin Roots of Medical and Scientific Terminologies, First Edition. Todd A. Curtis.
© 2025 John Wiley & Sons, Inc. Published 2025 by John Wiley & Sons, Inc.
Companion website: www.wiley.com/go/Curtis

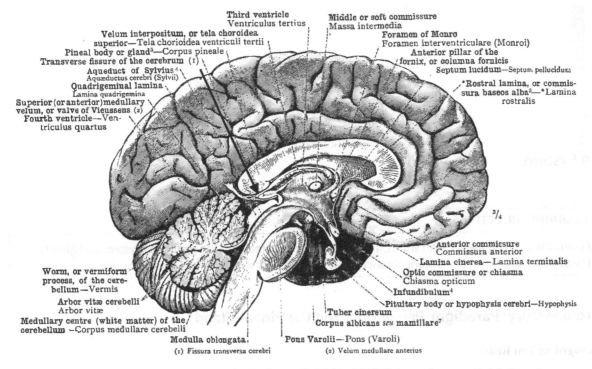

Fig. 12.1 Location of the pineal gland in the brain. *Source:* Carl Toldt, (1919)/Rebman Company/Public Domain.

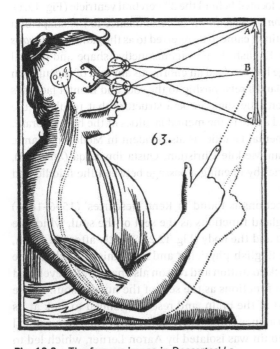

Fig. 12.2 The famous image in Descartes' *La Dioptrique* (Dioptrics) published in 1637. The image depicts the passage of sensory impulses from the eye to the pineal gland, which in turn, allows the soul/mind to control the muscles of the arm. *Source:* René Descartes / Wikimedia Commons / Public domain.

ongoing, but this new approach to the pineal gland has led to a holistic change in the way we understand this cone-shaped appendage of the brain.

In the 2nd century AD, long before Lerner's discovery, Galen claimed that the pineal gland was an *aden* (gland), which, at first glance, seems to suggest that Galen's approach to the pineal gland was more scientific than, for example, Descartes' seat of the soul because it seems to comport with our current understanding of the pineal gland. While it would be tempting to contextualize Galen's claim as being more scientific and to describe how it is an important progression toward a true understanding of the pineal gland, such an approach to the history of medicine is rather myopic in that it fails to see how science is a social operation that is paradigmatic in respect to culture and historical context. In the following discussion, we will evaluate Galen's theory with respect to the concept of scientific paradigms and how such paradigms lead to different perceptions of the pineal gland's anatomy and function.

The word "paradigm" is commonly used today, and therefore, it has taken on a constellation of meanings, which requires clarifying what is meant by this term in the history of science. The term "paradigm" is derived from the Greek word for "a pattern, model, example," *paradeigma*. Beginning in the 15th century, it began to appear in Late Latin as *paradigma*. Prior to the 20th century, it was infrequently used in English literature. "Paradigm" became a frequently used word in modern English after it took on a more philosophical meaning, which is one of the definitions for this term found in Merriam-Webster's Dictionary: "A philosophical or theoretical framework of a scientific school or discipline with which theories, laws, and generalizations and the experiments performed in support of them are formulated." The popularity of this philosophical meaning can be traced to Thomas Kuhn's extremely influential text on the philosophy of science, *The Structure of Scientific Revolutions* (1962). In this text, Kuhn sees science as a social operation that has historically specific practices, theories, instruments, and assumptions. Kuhn suggests that "the practices that define a scientific discipline at a certain point in time" can be understood as a scientific paradigm. Thus, a paradigm is formed by a scientific discipline's adoption of a collection of key theories, values, and assumptions. He suggests a scientific paradigm often can be traced to an exemplary instance of scientific research (e.g. Aristotle's analysis of motion, Ptolemy's computations of planetary positions, Lavoisier's application of the balance). A scientific paradigm is not permanent, since the paradigm may change in a scientific revolution. For Kuhn, a mature science has alternating periods of what he termed "normal science" and "revolutions," which are also called "paradigm shifts." Normal science is a period of time in which "questions" and "puzzles" are solved via widespread or partial consensus to a particular paradigm. During this period of normal science, a theory is evaluated by comparing it to the prevailing paradigmatic science. As would be expected, anomalies will arise that cannot be explained by the prevailing scientific paradigm. A revolution occurs when such anomalies create a crisis in a scientific discipline requiring extraordinary research that pushes the boundaries of normal science. Kuhn describes this stage of scientific revolution as "the proliferation of competing articulations, the willingness to try anything, the expression of explicit discontent, the recourse to philosophy and to debate over fundamentals." The result of such a revolution is that a new paradigm is adopted by a scientific discipline, leading to another phase of "normal science" during which new theories and their explanation of evidence are evaluated on the basis of the current paradigmatic view. Thus, the building upon and challenging paradigms is a social operation of science that relies on the consensus of the members of a discipline and it trains its members to perceive what is scientifically acceptable.

In *The Structure of Scientific Revolutions*, Kuhn uses the Gestalt duck–rabbit image as a metaphor for the radical change in perception that occurs with a scientific revolution (Fig. 12.3). He states that "what were ducks in the scientist's world before the revolution are rabbits afterwards." His point being that the source of stimuli is unchanged; the lines that make the rabbit and the duck remain the same. What changes is the scientist's perception of the stimuli. Kuhn explains this stating, "though the world does not change with a change in paradigm, the scientist afterwards works in a different world." Thus, a paradigm shift creates a radical and holistic transformation of scientific perception, not a partial change.

As noted, one of the first ancient Greek descriptions of the pineal gland and its perceived functions can be found in Galen's 8th book of *On the Usefulness of the Parts* (K. III.674–683; May 1968, vol. 1, pp. 418–423). In this passage, Galen refutes the position held by a collection of

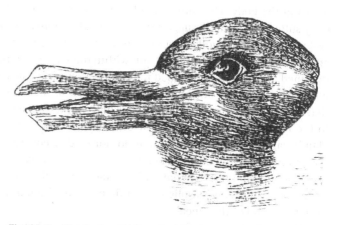

Fig. 12.3 The duck–rabbit optical illusion that was made famous by Wittgenstein and was later used by Kuhn to illustrate scientific paradigms and perception. *Source:* Unknown author / Wikimedia Commons / Public domain.

unnamed theorists that the function of the pineal gland is to regulate the flow of psychic pneuma between the middle and posterior ventricles of the brain, similar to how the pylorus controls the movement of food from the stomach to the intestines. The basis for Galen's rejection of this theoretical position is as follows: Firstly, Galen correctly recognizes that the body and apex of the penial gland lie outside of the ventricles, and therefore, he concludes that its anatomical position does not suggest that the pineal gland can regulate the flow of the psychic pneuma in a way similar to the pylorus. Secondly, he notes that the pineal gland cannot move on its own, and therefore, it cannot act in such a way as to restrict or permit the flow of psychic pneuma. In some respects, Galen's rejection of the aforementioned theory is striking since such a view of the pineal gland's function would be consistent with the ventricular model that Galen espouses in his anatomical works. However, Galen's rejection of the pineal gland as a conduit of the soul is consistent with the normal science of his community of anatomists in that the anatomical appearances of a part (e.g. location, nature, size, shape, etc.) served as a fundamental means by which this scientific discipline understood the physiology of the human body.

Galen notes that the blood vessels that lie in close proximity to this pine-cone-shaped anatomical structure reveal that the pineal gland's true function is that of an *aden* (gland). Thus, rather than viewing the pineal gland as a conduit of the soul, Galen claims that the pineal gland functions like an *aden* (gland), which makes him the first to recognize this anatomical structure as a "gland." While Galen's claim that the pineal gland is an *aden* is novel, his understanding of an *aden* is influenced by the humoral theories found in the "Hippocratic" work entitled *On Glands*, a work that was composed in the 4th century BC by an unknown author. Galen's use of the term *aden* does not comport with our modern understanding of the basic function of a gland, namely the secretion of material. What constitutes an *aden* in ancient Greek medicine is understood from the following passage in *On Glands*:

> On glands (*peri adenōn*) as a whole, this is the situation. Their character is spongy; they are fine and fatty; they are neither fleshy parts like the rest of the body, nor anything else similar to the body; but they are loose-textured and have numerous vessels ... they do not suffer much trouble, but when they do suffer, they make the rest of the body suffer through their own ailment.
>
> Hippocrates, *On Glands*, trans. Elizabeth Craik in *The Hippocratic Treatise on Glands*.

In *On Glands*, an *aden* is a recognizable anatomical part whose spongy character is linked to its primary role, which is to assist in regulating fluid in the moist areas of the body. An *aden* was likened to a sponge since its apparent purpose was to absorb excess fluid. From the description of the nature, function, and pathology of an *aden*, it appears that the author's understanding of an *aden* is built upon a misconception of the function of lymph nodes. This becomes apparent by his statement: "when they do suffer, they make the rest of the body suffer through their own ailment." While a wide variety of anatomical structures could be said to do this, his description of their presence being in the moistest parts of the body, which he claims to be the groin, armpits, neck, and abdomen, corresponds roughly to the location of the lymph nodes in the body. The connection between a pathologically swollen gland, which he calls a *boubon*, and the "whole body suffering" seems to suggest that he is inadvertently speaking to the kinds of infectious diseases that tax the immune system and lead to swollen lymph nodes. This connection is also apparent when he states, "and if the stream is copious and diseased, the glands become taut within themselves. In this way, fever is kindled and the glands become swollen and inflamed." As is well understood today, infections that cause a **bubo** (i.e. a swollen lymph node) will often be accompanied by the presence of a fever. Another data point that supports this interpretation of what is an *aden* in *On Glands* is that the author claims that these glands have numerous vessels associated with them, by which he seems to be speaking to the lymphatic vessels that connect the lymph nodes to the body. This author presents an amalgam of places that glands can appear in the body that do not readily correspond to the location of lymph nodes in modern anatomical descriptions and the parts he claims to be glands or gland-like, such as the tonsils and the glands of the breasts, are clearly not lymph nodes. What makes something a gland or gland-like is that its perceived function is to regulate fluids and that it can become swollen and inflamed. This humoral model of glandular function influenced Galen's perception of the function of the pineal gland.

Although Galen is the first to perceive the pineal gland as a "gland," his theory is not revolutionary. This is certainly true with respect to its effect on subsequent approaches to the function of the pineal gland. As noted, the pineal gland's association with the regulation of the psychic pneuma, particularly in the context of ventricular theory, became the common way in which the pineal gland was understood and researched well into the Renaissance and slightly beyond. Even if Galen's theory of the pineal gland's function had ultimately won out in the competition of ideas, his theory would not meet the criteria of a paradigm shift with respect to Kuhn's criteria of a scientific revolution because it is not a radical departure from the science of his time in that it did not push the boundaries of normal science. While he did reach a different conclusion as to the function of the pineal gland, with respect to his reliance on humoral theory and the kind of assumptions that he makes from anatomical dissections, Galen's perception of the pineal gland's function is consistent with the paradigm of his scientific discipline in that it reflects the key theories, values, and assumptions of his scientific culture. Thus, with respect to duck–rabbit metaphor, Galen was trained by this community to perceive the pineal gland as a duck, which is why he saw a duck, albeit a slightly different type of duck, not a rabbit.

As noted, in 1958, the pineal gland was recognized as an endocrine gland thanks to Lerner's discovery that it secretes the hormone known as melatonin. This discovery has led to the reconceptualization of the pineal gland and a new line of research. However, Lerner's discovery is not a revolutionary. Lerner's perception that the pineal is an endocrine gland is consistent with the normal science of his time frame, which recognized that certain glands were capable of secreting hormones that had powerful effects on the body. Again, with respect to the duck–rabbit metaphor, Lerner was trained by his scientific community to perceive the pineal gland and its vasculature as being indicative of a rabbit, which is why he saw a rabbit, rather than Galen's duck.

The reason that Lerner saw a rabbit rather than a duck is due to a revolution/paradigm shift that was brought about by the discovery of hormones and the conceptualization of the endocrine system. Ernest Starling (1866–1927) and William Bayliss (1860–1924), an English physician and physiologist respectively, discovered the first hormone in 1902 via their experimentations on anesthetized dogs. At this time, it was understood that enzymes from the pancreas were stimulated by the presence of food in the intestines; Pavlov thought that the origin of this stimulation was a neural reflex. To determine if this was a neural response or not, Bayliss and Starling removed the nerves from the small intestine and then stimulated it. By doing this, they were able to produce the pancreatic enzymes. This helped them to isolate a chemical substance that they later called "secretin" as the causal factor. When they introduced the concept of chemical regulation of bodily functions, Starling used the Greek word *hormon* "that which sets in motion or impels" to denote this class of chemical stimulants of the body. The participle *hormon*, which is derived from the Greek verb *horman* "to impel, urge on," was first used in the 5th century BC by the author of the Hippocratic work *On Epidemics*. In this text and in other places in the Hippocratic Corpus, it is used to denote a faculty or vital principle, rather than a chemical reflex. The root for our modern understanding of a hormone is naturally **HORMON**-. Starling's and Bayliss' discovery is revolutionary in that it radically and holistically changed the way in which science viewed the excretions of glands; it caused a reconceptualization of the systems of the body; it introduced a specific vocabulary that embodied this physiological discovery; and it led to a new discipline of research and methodologies. The concept of hormones and the endocrine system also has changed the way in which society views human pathologies, such as dwarfism, gigantism, goiters, and hirsutism, that were once thought to be biological anomalies and regrettably the subjects of "freak shows."

The point of this discussion is not to depreciate scientific theories that are not revolutionary because they did not create a paradigm shift. Likewise, we should not delimit our assessment of figures in the history of science to whether or not their theories reflect a progression toward our modern scientific understandings of human physiology. It is important to consider how these figures reflect the goals and assumptions of their specific scientific culture. Such an approach leads to recognizing how medical science can also be understood as a social operation rather than strictly a historical progression toward a correct understanding of the human body.

Some Suggested Readings

Galen. *On the Usefulness of the Parts of the Body*. Translated by Margaret T. May. Ithaca: Cornell University Press, 1968.

Hippocrates. *The Hippocratic Treatise on Glands*. Translated and edited Elizabeth M. Craik. Leiden: Brill, 2009.

Kuhn, Thomas. *The Structure of Scientific Revolutions*. Second Edition, with postscript. Chicago: University of Chicago Press, 1970.

Lloyd, Geoffrey E. R. *The Revolutions of Wisdom: Studies in the Claims and Practice of Ancient Greek Science*. Berkeley: University of California Press, 1987.

Lokhorst, Gert-Jan. "Descartes and the Pineal Gland." *The Stanford Encyclopedia of Philosophy* (Winter 2021 Edition), Edited by Edward N. Zalta, URL = https://plato.stanford.edu/archives/win2021/entries/pineal-gland/.

Etymological Explanations: Common Terms and Word Elements for the Anatomy and Physiology of Glands

Types of Glands and Secretions

In the following discussion of the anatomical terms associated with glands, the nominative and genitive singular forms of the anatomical Latin term are provided in parenthesis. The Greek and Latin roots are formatted in all caps and emboldened.

Types of glands and secretions

Gland – The roots meaning "gland" and "glandule" are **ADEN-** and **GLANDUL-**. The loan word for "glandule" is glandula (L. *glandula, -ae*), and the loan word for "gland" is glans (L. *glans, glandis*). When anatomists were looking for Latin terms to describe the size and shape of a gland, they turned to words meaning "nut." The terms *glans* and *glandula* in Classical Latin meant "acorn" and "little acorn," respectively. It is only via the French *glande* that it took on its current meaning of "gland." This acorn-like shape is certainly similar to the structures of the lymphatic system (i.e. lymph nodes and tonsils), but with respect to the numerous types of glands in the body (e.g. sebaceous, sudoriferous, salivary, adrenal, etc.), this is a less appropriate analogy. The specific names for the glands that make up the endocrine system are derived from ancient Greek terms that denoted their shape and their hypothesized functions.

Secretion – Our understanding of what defines a gland is built on the concept of "secretion." Derived from the Greek verb "to separate," *krinein*, we currently use the suffix **-CRINE** and the root **CRIN-** for "secretion" and "to secrete." In respect to glands, there are three basic types of secretions: holocrine, merocrine, and apocrine (Fig. 12.4). In addition to what makes up their secretions, glands are also differentiated by whether they have a duct or not (i.e. exocrine and endocrine glands).

(a) Merocrine secretion

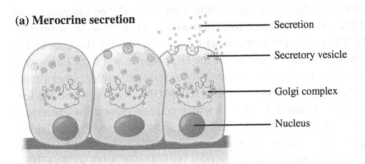

— Secretion

— Secretory vesicle

— Golgi complex

— Nucleus

Fig. 12.4 Modes of secretions. *Source:* OpenStax College/Wikimedia Commons/CC by 3.0.

(b) Apocrine secretion

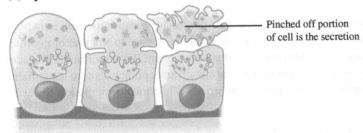

— Pinched off portion
of cell is the secretion

(c) Holocrine secretion

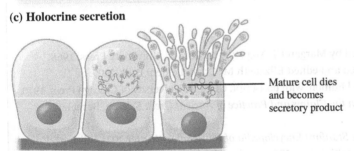

— Mature cell dies
and becomes
secretory product

Holocrine gland – A gland whose altered cells make up the product of its secretion is termed a holocrine gland (e.g. sebaceous gland). The root **HOL-** means "whole" or "complete."

Merocrine gland – A gland whose secretory products are released without resulting in any damage to the cell (e.g. salivary gland). The root **MER-** means "part" or "partial."

Apocrine gland – A gland whose apical portion of the cell becomes a part of the secretion is called an apocrine gland (e.g. mammary glands). The combining form **APIC-** means "tip," "summit," or "end."

Exocrine gland – A gland that secretes its products outside the gland via a duct is called an exocrine gland (e.g. sweat and sebaceous glands).

Endocrine gland – A gland that secretes its products into the blood vessels inside of the gland is called an endocrine gland. Hormones are associated with endocrine glands, and therefore, a physician who specializes in hormones and the glands that produce them is called an endocrinologist.

Endocrine Glands

In the following discussion of the anatomical terms associated with the endocrine system, the nominative and genitive singular forms of the anatomical Latin term are provided in parenthesis. The Greek and Latin roots are formatted in all caps and emboldened (Fig. 12.5).

Fig. 12.5 Anatomical Latin terms for the glands of the endocrine system. *Source:* Drawing by Chloe Kim.

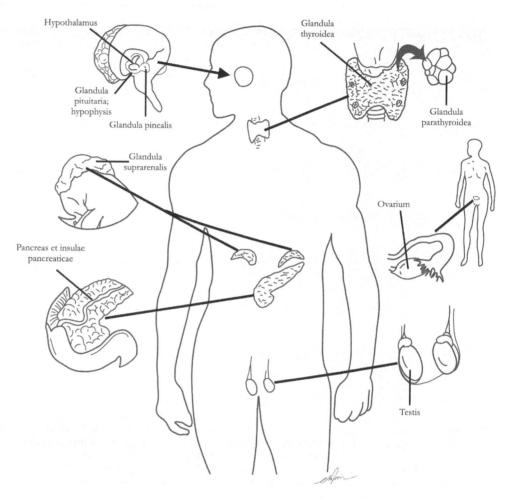

Endocrine glands

Pineal gland (L. *glandula pinealis*) – The pineal gland is a cone-shaped gland located in the corpus callosum of the brain. The pineal gland was recognized by ancient Greek anatomists and physicians, and owing to its shape, was originally called the *konarion*, which meant "small pine cone-like." The roots **PINEAL-** and **PINE-**, which are used for the "pineal gland" and the "pine cone," are derived from the Latin noun *pineus* (pine) and its corresponding adjective *pinealis*, which reflects the tradition of naming this gland according to its shape.

Pituitary gland (L. *glandula pituitaria*) – The pituitary is a pea-sized endocrine gland located at the base of the brain under the hypothalamus. The pituitary gland is also called the hypophysis. The roots for the pituitary gland are **PITUI-**, **PITUITAR-**, and **HYPOPHYS-**. In ancient Greek, a hypophysis is an "outgrowth," which is why the anatomist Samuel Sömmerring (1755–1830) used this term to denote the appendage-like appearance of the pituitary gland. The Latin adjective *pituitarius* means "phlegm-producing," which speaks to the supposed function of the pituitary gland in ancient Greek medicine. In *On the Use of the Parts*, Galen describes the pituitary gland as the draining route and receptacle for phlegm passing from the brain to the nose. The pituitary gland is the master gland of the endocrine system in that it is responsible for stimulating the secretions of a number of endocrine glands: thyroid stimulating hormone (TSH) stimulates secretions from the thyroid gland; adrenocorticotropic hormone (ACTH) stimulates the adrenal cortex; follicle-stimulating hormone (FSH) stimulates the secretion of estrogen in females and sperm production in males; and luteinizing hormone (LH) stimulates the secretion of progesterone by the corpus luteum and causes the secretion of testosterone in the testes. The pituitary gland also affects skin pigmentation via melanocyte-stimulating hormone (MSH), influences the growth of the body via growth hormone (GH), and stimulates milk production in the breasts during pregnancy via prolactin. All of the aforementioned hormones are associated with the **anterior pituitary gland**, also known as the **adenohypophysis**. The **posterior pituitary gland**, which is called the **neurohypophysis**, produces antidiuretic hormone (ADH), which influences the absorption of water by the kidney. The neurohypophysis also releases oxytocin, which influences uterine contractions.

Thyroid glands (L. *glandulae thyroideae*) and parathyroid glands (L. *glandulae parathyroideae*) – The thyroid glands are located on the anterior neck and the parathyroid glands are found on the posterior aspect of the thyroid gland. The roots for the thyroid gland are **THYR-** and **THYROID-**. The root of the parathyroid gland is **PARATHYROID-**. The thyroid hormones, thyroxine and triiodothyronine, regulate metabolism, particularly iodine. The thyroid, via calcitonin, regulates calcium in the blood. The parathyroid glands maintain the right balance of calcium in the body via parathyroid hormone (PTH). The etymology of thyroid reveals that it was named after an oval-shaped shield called a *thureos*, which was carried by Hellenistic soldiers, such as the Macedonian armies (Fig. 12.6).

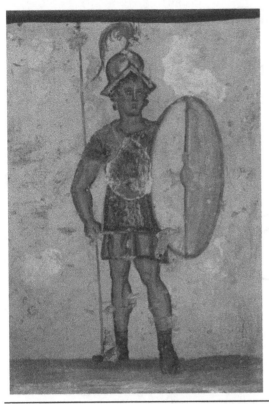

Fig. 12.6 Fresco of an ancient Macedonian soldier bearing a *thureos* shield, 3rd century BC, Archeological Museum in Istanbul. *Source:* DeFly94 / Wikimedia Commons / Public domain.

Thymus (L. *thymus, -i*) – The thymus is located in the mediastinal cavity above the heart. The root for the thymus gland is **THYM-**. The **THYM-** is a homomorph, in that it is derived from two different Greek words, whose only discernable difference is the vowel that is stressed in their respective pronunciations (Gr. θύμος, a warty excrescence vs. θυμός, soul, seat of emotion). Thus, **THYM-** can be used for the "thymus gland," "emotion," and "state of mind." **THYM-** is also the root for the herb thyme, which in Greek was called θύμος and θύμον. While it might be tempting to assume that the thymus gland is etymologically related to thyme, this connection is not found in the writings of Rufus of Ephesus (c. 70–110 AD) and Galen. When discussing the name of the thymus gland, both authors associate its appearance with the warty excrescences, particularly those found at the anus and genitalia. The thymosins are six hormones from the thymus that participate in regulating the immune system.

Adrenal glands (or suprarenal glands) (L. *glandulae suprarenales*) – The adrenal glands are small triangular-shaped glands that sit on top of the kidneys. Formed from the root for "kidney," **REN-**, the roots **ADREN-** and **SUPRAREN-** refer to these two lobulated glands. As with organs, the outside part of the adrenal gland is called the **cortex**, and its root is **CORTIC-**. The inner part is called the **medulla**, and its root is **MEDULL-**. Five classes of steroid hormones are associated with the adrenal cortex: glucocorticoids, mineralocorticoids, progestins, androgens, and estrogens. Of these five, the glucocorticoids and mineralocorticoids are almost exclusively produced in the adrenal cortex. The glucocorticoids regulate carbohydrate metabolism and modulate the immune system. The mineralocorticoids regulate mineral and water balance. The main hormones secreted by the adrenal medulla include epinephrine (adrenaline) and norepinephrine (noradrenaline), which affect the sympathetic nervous system in a response to stress.

Pancreatic glands (L. *glandulae pancreaticae*) – Located behind the stomach, the pancreas (*pancreas, pancreatis*) has pancreatic glands on it called the islets of Langerhans. The islets of Langerhans produce insulin and glucagon, which are fundamental to carbohydrate/sugar metabolism. The root for the pancreas is **PANCREAT-**. The term pancreas (Gr. *pan*, all + *kreas*, flesh) was used by ancient Greek physicians, such as Rufus and Galen. Why the word pancreas was chosen for this organ is uncertain.

Gonads (L. *gonas*) – The term gonad can refer to an ovary or a testicle, and consequently, the root for the ovaries and the testes is **GONAD-**. The term gonad comes from the Greek *gone*, which meant "seed" and "offspring." In addition to their role in reproduction, the male and female gonads create male and female sex characteristics via hormones. The hormone testosterone that is produced by the testicles is said to be an androgenic hormone because it produces male characteristics. Likewise, the hormone estrogen is a gynogenic hormone because it produces female characteristics. The roots specific to the ovary are **OVARI-** and **OOPHOR-**, and the roots specific to testes are **TEST-**, **TESTICUL-**, **ORCHID-**, and **ORCH-**.

Greek or Latin word element	Current usage	Etymology	Examples
GLANDUL/O (glan-jŭ-lō)	Glandule, gland	L. *glandula, -ae*, f. little acorn; gland fr. L. *glans, glandis*, f. acorn; gland	**Glandul**ose, **glandul**ar Loan words: **Glandula** (glan'jŭ-lă) Pl. **Glandulae** (glan'jŭ-lē") **Glans** (glanz) pl. **Glandes** (glan'dēz")
ADEN/O (ad-ĕn-ō)	Gland	Gr. *aden, adenos*, gland	Thyro**aden**itis, **aden**opathy, lymph**aden**itis
CRIN/O (krĭn-ō) -CRINE (krĭn)	To secrete	Gr. *krinein*, to separate; to secrete	**Crin**ogenic, exo**crine**, endo**crine**
APIC/O (ap-I-kō)	Tip, summit, end	L. *apex, apices*, m. tip, summit, end	**Apic**es, **apic**al Loan word: **Apex** (ā'peks") pl. **Apices** (ā'pĭ-sēz")
HOL/O (hŏl-ō)	Whole, entire	Gr. *holos*, whole, entire	**Hol**ocrine, **hol**ogram
MER/O (mer-ō)	Partial, part	Gr. *meros*, part, segment; partial	**Mer**ocrine, **mer**oblastic
PINE/O (pĭn-ē-ō) PINEAL/O (pĭn-ē-ăl-ō)	Pineal gland, pine cone	L. *pineus; pinealis*, of a pine cone; pineal gland	**Pine**oblastoma, **pineal**ectomy
THYR/O (thĭ-rō) THYROID/O (thĭ-royd-ō)	Thyroid gland	Gr. *thyreos*, shield in the shape of door; thyroid gland	**Thyr**otoxin, **thyroid**itis
PARATHYROID/O (par-ă-thĭ-royd-ō)	Parathyroid gland	Parathyroid gland	**Parathyroid**ocyte, hyper**parathyroid**ism
PITUI/O (pĭ-too-ō) PITUITAR/O (pĭ-tū-ĭt-ă-rō)	Pituitary gland, hypophysis	L. *pituita, pituitaries*, phlegm, mucus; pituitary gland	**Pitui**cyte, hypo**pituitar**ism
HYPOPHYS/O (hĭ-pō-fĭz-ō)	An undergrowth, pituitary gland	Gr. *hypo + physis*, undergrowth; pituitary gland	**Hypophys**itis, **hypophys**eal Loan word: **Hypophysis** (hĭ-pof'ĭ-sĭs)
PANCREAT/O (păn-krē-ă-tō)	Pancreas	L. *pancreas, pancreatis*, n. pancreas fr. Gr. *pankreas, pankreatos*, all flesh; pancreas	**Pancreat**algia, **pancreat**ic Loan word: **Pancreas** (pang'krē-ăs) pl. **Pancreata** (pan-krē'ăt-ă)
THYM/O (thĭ-mō)	Thymus gland	L. *thymus, -i*, m. thymus fr. Gr. *thymos*, warty excrescence; thymus gland	**Thym**ectomy, **thym**oma Loan word: **Thymus** (thĭ'mŭs)

Greek or Latin word element	Current usage	Etymology	Examples
OVARI/O (ō-vă-rē-ō)	Ovary	L. *ovarium, -i,* n. egg holder; ovary	**Ovari**otomy, **ovari**oprival Loan word: **Ovarium** (ō-vă′rē-ŭm) pl. **Ovaria** (ō-vă′rē-a)
OOPHOR/O (ō-ŏf-ō-rō)	Ovary	Gr. *oophoron,* egg carrier	**Oophor**ocystosis
TEST/O (tĕs-tō) **TESTICUL/O** (tĕs-tĭk-ū-lō)	Testicle, testis, witness	L. *testis, is,* m. witness L. *testiculus, -i,* m. testicle	**Test**algia, **testicul**ar Loan word: **Testis** (tes′tĭs) pl. **Testes** (tes′tēz″)
ORCH/O (or-kō) **ORCHID/O** (or-kĭ-dō)	Testicle; orchid (the flower)	Gr. *orchis, orchios,* testicle, Gr. *orchidion*	An**orch**ism, **orch**itis, crypt**orchid**ism
GONAD/O (gŏn-ă-dō)	Testicle or ovary	L. *gonas, gonadis,* f. gonad fr. Gr. *gone,* seed	**Gonad**opathy, hypo**gonad**ism
ADREN/O (ă-drē-nō)	Adrenal gland, suprarenal gland	L. *ad-* + L. *ren,* kidney = adren-, adrenal gland	**Adren**ocortical, **adren**olytic
SUPRAREN/O (soo-pră-rē-nō)	Suprarenal gland, adrenal gland	L. *supra* + L. *ren,* kidney = supraren-, adrenal gland	**Supraren**al
CORTIC/O (kor-tĭ-kō)	Cortex, outer surface of organ or gland, bark	L. *cortex, corticis,* m. bark, outer layer	**Cortic**osteroid, adreno**cortic**al Loan word: **Cortex** (kor′teks″) pl. **Cortices** (kort′ĭ-sēz″)
MEDULL/O (mĕ-dŭl-ō)	Medulla, marrow, inner part of an organ	L. *medulla, -ae,* f. marrow, pith	**Medull**ectomy, adreno**medull**in Loan word: **Medulla** (mĕ-dŭl′ă) pl. **Medullae** (mĕ-dŭl′ē″)

Review	Answers
The roots for any gland and glandule are _____ and _____. The loan word for "glandule" is _____, and the loan word for "gland" is _____.	**ADEN-, GLANDUL-** **glandula, glans**
The suffix _____ and the root _____ are used for "to secrete." A gland that secretes its products outside the gland via a duct is called an _____ gland. A gland that secretes its products inside the gland via blood vessels is called an _____ gland.	**-CRINE, CRIN-** **exocrine** **endocrine**
A gland whose altered cells are part of the secretions is termed a holocrine (e.g. sebaceous gland). The combining form HOL/O means _____ or _____. A gland whose secretory products are released without resulting in any damage to the cell is called a merocrine gland (e.g. salivary gland). The combining form MER/O means _____ or _____. A gland whose apical surface becomes part of the secretion is called an apocrine gland (e.g. mammary glands). The combining form APIC/O means _____, _____, or _____.	**whole, complete** **part, partial** **tip, summit, end**
The roots PINEAL- and PINE- are used for _____ and _____.	**pineal, pine cone**
The roots for the pituitary gland are _____, _____, and _____.	**PITUI-, PITUITAR-, HYPOPHYS-**
The roots for the thyroid gland are _____ and _____. The root for the parathyroid gland is _____.	**THYR-, THYROID-** **PARATHYROID-**

Review	Answers
The root for the thymus gland is _____.	**THYM-**
Formed from the root for "kidney," REN-, the roots _____ and _____ refer to the two lobulated glands which sit atop each kidney. As with organs, the outside part of the adrenal gland is called the _____, and its root is _____. The inner part is called the _____, and its root is _____.	**ADREN-, SUPRARENA-** **cortex, CORTIC-** **medulla, MEDULL-**
The root for the pancreas is _____.	**PANCREAT-**
The root for the female ovaries and the male testes is _____.	**GONAD-**
The roots specific to the ovary are _____ and _____.	**OVARI-, OOPHOR-**
The roots specific to testes are _____, _____, _____, and _____.	**TEST-, TESTICUL-, ORCH-, ORCHID-**

Etymological Explanations: Common Terms and Word Elements for Hormones

The suffixes **-IN** and **-INE** are commonly used for hormones and chemical substances. They are often combined with specific roots to denote a particular action of the hormone or chemical substance. That said, other suffixes are also used for hormones as well. The following is a list of common roots and suffixes used with hormones:

Actions of hormones

-TROPIN – Hormones that exert their effect on nonendocrine target tissues are called "nontropic hormones." Derived from the Greek word for "a turn," *trope*, hormones that stimulate another endocrine gland are called "tropic hormones." Consequently, their names often have the root **TROP-** in them. With respect to hormones, the root **TROP-** means "stimulating," but in other contexts, it can mean a "turn," "turning," and "change." An example of a hormonal term with this root would be **adrenocorticotropin**, which is a hormone that stimulates secretion from the adrenal cortex.

-TROPHIN – A growth hormone is called a **somatotrophin**. The root **TROPH-** in this word literally means "growth" or "stimulating" in the context of hormones. In other contexts, this root means "nourishment." It is derived from the Greek word for nourishment, *trophe*.

-LIBERIN – A hormone or chemical that releases something, such as another hormone, will have the compound suffix **-LIBERIN**.

-STATIN – A hormone or chemical that inhibits or stops something will use the compound suffix. **-STATIN**. For example, a **folliculostatin** inhibits the secretion of follicle-stimulating hormone. The root comes from the Latin verb *stare, statum*, "to stand."

-KININ – A protein hormone or chemical that stimulates activity or the movement of something will have the compound suffix **-KININ**. For example, **cholecystokinin** is a hormone secreted by the small intestine that stimulates the contraction of the gallbladder and pancreatic secretions. The root is derived from the Greek verb *kineein*, "to move."

-POIETIN – The compound suffix **-POIETIN** is used for a hormone or chemical substance that stimulates the "making" or "producing" of something. For example, **erythropoietin** stimulates the production of red blood cells. In general, the suffix **-POIESIS** and the root **POIET-** are used in numerous contexts with the meanings of "making or producing" something. The root comes from the Greek verb *poieein*, "to make, produce."

-TONIN – The hormones **serotonin, melatonin,** and **calcitonin** share the root **TON-**, which means "tension" or "tone." Thus, a chemical or a hormone that uses the suffix **-TONIN** produces a healthy tension/strength" of something. **-TONIN** is derived from the use of the word "**tonic**," which was a term used for anything (mostly liquids) having the property of restoring health, hence the phrase "gin and tonic." Calcitonin regulates calcium and phosphorus metabolism. The term serotonin is derived from the root for "serum," **SER-**, assumedly because of its association with blood clotting and vasoconstriction. The term melatonin is derived from the roots for "black," **MELA-/MELAN-**, assumedly because daylight inhibits its production.

-AGOGUE – The suffix **-AGOGUE** is used for a hormone that promotes something (e.g. **lactagogue**). The root **AGOG-** comes from the Greek noun *agogos* "a leading forth," and it is used for a "duct" (e.g. dacryagogatresia). The root **AG-** comes from the Greek verb *agein*, "to lead forth." The root **AG-** appears in the term glucagon. Derived from the root for "sugar" **GLUC-** (or **GLYC-**), glucagon is pancreatic hormone that increases the glucose in the blood by stimulating the liver to change stored glycogen to glucose.

Insulin – Along with glucagon, insulin helps to control the amount of sugar in the blood. Insulin derives its name from its association with the islets of Langerhans, which are island-like tissue on the pancreas that produce this hormone. In addition to insulin, the root **INSUL-** literally means "island." Therefore, this root is used for structures that resemble an island, and the Latin loan word **insula** is also used in this way. The word peninsula is derived from this Latin word (L. *paene* = "nearly, almost").

-GESTIN – In pharmacology and with hormones, the root **GEST-** and the suffix **-GESTIN** are used to designate a **progestin** (also called **progesterone, progestogen**), which is a hormone that prepares the endometrium for implantation of the fertilized ovum. The roots **GEST-** and **GER-** and the suffix **-GER** have the meanings "to carry, produce, or bear." The prefix **PRO-** in the aforementioned terms indicates that it acts "before" gestation.

-TOCIN – **Oxytocin** is a hormone that increases labor by influencing uterine contractions. Derived from the Greek word for "childbirth," *tokos*, the root **TOC-** is commonly used for "labor"/"parturition."

-GEN – A hormone or chemical that produces something will have the suffix **-GEN**. A **gynogen** produces female sex characteristics and an **androgen** produces male sex characteristics. The root **ANDR-** in androgen means "male." The root **GYN-** in gynogen means "female." Testosterone is an androgenic hormone. Estrogen is a gynecogenic hormone.

Estrogen – Estrogen is a steroid that produces female sex characteristics. The etymology of estrogen reveals it to be somewhat of a misnomer. The root **ESTR-** in estrogen refers to the estrus cycle, which in mammals is the period of time when the female feels the urge to mate. The term "estrus" is derived from the Greek word for a "gadfly," *oistros*. The word *oistros* has a variety of meanings. At its core, *oistros* refers to the stinging fly that torments livestock and thereby goads them to move. Much like the use of estrus today, *oistros* was also used for sexual impulses in animals. This can be observed in the following quote from Herodotus' (484–425 BC) *Histories* (2.93.1): "Fish that go in schools are seldom born in rivers; they are raised in the lakes, and this is how they behave: when the desire to conceive (*oistros kuiskesthai*) comes on them, they swim out to sea in schools, the males leading, and throwing out their milt, while the females come after and swallow and conceive from it." That said, in modern philosophy, the term "gadfly" represents a person who interferes with the status quo of a society. For instance, in Plato's (428–348 BC) *Apology*, Socrates states, "I am the gadfly of the Athenian people, given to them by god, and they will never have another, if they kill me ... For if you kill me you will not easily find a successor to me, who, if I may use such a ludicrous figure of speech, am a sort of gadfly, given to the state by god; and the state is a great and noble steed who is tardy in his motions owing to his very size, and requires to be stirred into life." One can surmise from this quote and from the character of Socrates in Plato's dialogues that Socrates sees himself as an annoying gadfly whose stinging philosophical inquiries impel the people of Athens toward true knowledge.

Testosterone – Testosterone is a steroid that produces male sex characteristics, as well as spermatogenesis, and fertility. The term appears to be formed from the root for "testicle," **TEST-**, + the root for "sterol," **STER-**, + chemical ending **-ONE**. Sterol was first used with the term cholesterol, which is formed from the Greek roots **CHOLE-** (bile) + **STER-** (solid) + the chemical suffix for alcohol, **-OL**.

Greek or Latin word element	Current usage	Etymology	Examples
HORMON/O (hor-mō-nō)	Hormone	Gr. *hormon, hormonos,* stimulating, arousing; hormone	**Hormon**agogue, **hormon**opoiesis
-IN (ĭn) **-INE** (ĭn)	Hormone or chemical substance	Suffix often used for hormones and chemical substances	Secret**in**, norepineph**rine**
TROP/O (trŏ-pō)	Hormone that stimulates something; a turn, turning, change	Gr. *trope,* turning, change; stimulating	Cortico**trop**in, gonado**trop**in, **trop**ism
TROPH/O (trŏf-ō)	Nourishment, growth	Gr. *trophe,* nourishment	Somato**troph**in, a**troph**y
AG/O (ăg-ō) **AGOG/O** (ă-gŏg-ō) **-AGOGUE** (ă-gŏg)	Hormone that promotes something; leading forth, duct	Gr. *agein* to lead forth, convey Gr. *agogos,* leading forth; promoting flow, expelling	An**agog**ic, galact**agogue**, dacry**agog**atresia, gluc**ag**on

Greek or Latin word element	Current usage	Etymology	Examples
GEST/O (jĕs-tō) **GER/O** (jĕr-ō) **-GER** (jĕr)	Hormone that helps with bearing (progestin); to carry, produce, bear	L. *gerere, gestum,* to carry, produce, bear; progestin	Pro**gest**in, lacti**ger**ous, penni**ger**, **gest**ation
POIET/O (poy-ē-tō) **-POIESIS** (poy-ē-sĭs)	Hormone that stimulates the production/making of something (-poietin); to make or produce	Gr. *poieein,* to make, produce	Erythro**poiet**in, thrombo**poiesis**
STAT/O (stat-ō)	Hormone that inhibits/stops something (-statin); to stand or stop	L. *stare, statum,* to stand; stop	Corti**statin**, **statin**, ortho**static**
GEN/O (jĕn-ō) **-GEN** (jĕn)	hormone that produces something (-gen), become, produced, born	Gr. *-genes,* to be born, become; hormone that produces something	Andro**gen**, **gen**oblast
KIN/O (kĭ-nō) **CIN/O** (sĭ-nō) **-KINESIS** (kĭ-nē-sĭs) **-CINESIS** (sĭ-nē-sĭs)	Hormone or chemical that stimulates activity, movement (-kinin), action	Gr. *kineein,* to movement, action; hormone that stimulates activity	Cholecysto**kin**in, acro**cin**esis
GYNEC/O (gī-nĕ-kō) **GYN/O** (gī-nō)	Female, woman, pistil of a flower	Gr. *gyne, gynaikos,* woman	**Gynec**omastia, **gynec**ogenic
ANDR/O (an-drō)	Male, man, stamen of a flower	Gr. *aner, andros,* a man, male	**Andr**ogen, **andr**oblastoma
LIBER/O (lĭ-buh-rō)	A hormone or chemical that releases another hormone (-liberin), to free	L. *liberare,* to free	**Liber**in, **liber**ation
ESTR/O (ĕs-trō)	Estrogen, estrus cycle (breeding period), sexual desire	Gr. *oistros,* gadfly; sexual desire, breeding period	**Estr**ogen, **estr**one Loan word: **Estrus** (es′trŭs)
INSUL/O (in-sŭ-lō)	Insulin, island	L. *insula, -ae,* f. island; insulin	**Insul**in, **insul**ar Loan word: **Insula** (in′sū-lă) pl. **Insulae** (in′sū-lē″)
GLUC/O (gloo-kō) **GLYC/O** (glī-kō)	Sugar, glucose	Gr. *glykys,* sweet; sugar, glucose	**Glyc**ogenic, **gluc**ogenesis

Greek or Latin word element	Current usage	Etymology	Examples
TON/O (ton-ō)	A hormone that produces a healthy strength or tension (-tonin) of something; tension, stretching, tone (esp. in muscles)	Gr. *tonos*, that which is stretched, cord, rope	Sera**ton**in, hyper**ton**icity, **ton**ometer
TOC/O (tō-kō)	Labor, parturition	Gr. *tokos*, childbirth	Oxy**toc**in, **toc**ograph

Review	Answers
The root for hormone is _____. The suffixes _____ and _____ are commonly used for hormones and chemical substances.	**HORMON-** **-IN, -INE**
Hormones that exert their effect on nonendocrine target tissues are called "nontropic hormones." Hormones that stimulate another endocrine gland are called "tropic hormones." Consequently, their names often have the root TROP- in them. In the respect to hormones, the root TROP- means _____, but in other contexts, it can mean _____, _____, and _____.	**Stimulating, turn, turning, change**
A growth hormone is also called a somatotrophin. The root TROPH- in this word means _____, but in other contexts, this root can mean _____.	**growth, nourishment**
Glucagon is a pancreatic hormone that increases the glucose in the blood by stimulating the liver to change stored glycogen to glucose. The roots _____ and _____ mean a "leading forth." The suffix _____ is used for a hormone that promotes something (e.g. lactagogue), but in other contexts, this suffix is used for a _____.	**AGOG-, AG-** **-AGOGUE, duct**
Insulin derives its name from its association with the islets of Langerhans. In addition to insulin, the root INSUL- literally means _____.	**island**
The root _____ and the suffix _____ have the meanings "to carry," "produce," or "bear." In pharmacology and with hormones, the root _____ and the suffix _____ are used to designate a progestin.	**GER-, -GER** **GEST-, -GEST**
The compound suffix -POIETIN is used for a hormone or chemical substance that stimulates the _____ or _____ of something. In general, the suffix _____ and the root _____ are used for "making" or "producing" something.	**production, making** **-POIESIS, POIET-**
A hormone or chemical that inhibits or stops something will use the compound suffix _____.	**-STATIN**
A hormone or chemical that stimulates activity or the movement of something will have the compound suffix _____.	**-KININ**
A hormone or chemical that produces something will have the suffix _____. A gynogen produces female sex characteristics and an androgen produces male sex characteristics. The root ANDR- in androgen means _____. The root GYN- in gynogen means _____. Estrogen is a gynecogenic hormone. The root _____ is used for the estrus cycle, which is associated with sexual desire, particularly in female animals.	**-GEN** **male** **female** **ESTR-**
A hormone or chemical that releases something, such as another hormone, will have the compound suffix_____.	**-LIBERIN**
Oxytocin is a hormone that increases labor by influencing uterine contractions. The root _____ means "labor"/"parturition."	**TOC-**
The hormones serotonin, melatonin, and calcitonin share the root _____ which means "tension" or "tone." Thus, a chemical or a hormone that uses the suffix -TONIN produces a "healthy tension/strength" of something.	**TON-**

Etymological Explanations: Common Terms and Word Elements for the Physiology and Pathophysiology of the Endocrine System

The correct amount and timing of hormone secretion are pivotal to health. Pathological changes are evident both with **hyposecretion** and **hypersecretion** of a hormone. Thus, the prefixes **HYPER-** and **HYPO-** are commonly attached to the name of a gland or hormone to indicate these conditions (e.g. hyperparathyroidism and hypoparathyroidism). Naturally, the removal of an endocrine gland would also lead to sequela of potentially pathological changes. The root **PRIV-** and the suffix **-PRIVIA** are used in medicine to denote the corresponding effects caused by a gland's dysfunction or its removal from the body. In Classical Latin, the verb *privare* means "to deprive of." The following pathological signs and diseases are grouped according to endocrine gland.

Thyroid and parathyroid

Hyperthyroidism – Hyperthyroidism is associated with excessive secretion from the thyroid gland. The characteristic signs of this are a rapid heart rate (tachycardia) and protrusion of the eyeballs (exophthalmus/exophthalmos).

Hypothyroidism – Hypothyroidism is associated with diminished secretion from the thyroid gland. The characteristic signs of this are a slow heart rate (bradycardia), sluggishness (lethargy), and obesity.

Hyperorexia and Hyporexia – Hyperorexia (i.e. a marked increase in appetite) is another sign of hyperthyroidism. Hyporexia (i.e. a marked decrease in appetite) is also a sign of hypothyroidism. The root **OREX-** means "appetite" or "hunger."

Goiter – A goiter is an enlargement of the thyroid gland. Goiters can be present with hyperthyroidism and hypothyroidism. Goiter is from the French word *goitre* which comes from the Latin word for throat, *guttur*. Today the loan word **guttur** and the root **GUTTUR-** are used for "throat" (Fig. 12.7).

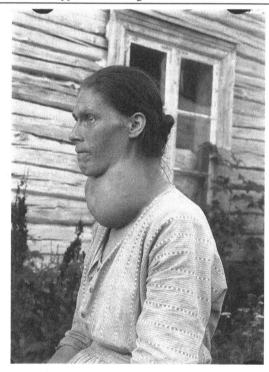

Fig. 12.7 Picture of a woman with a large goiter. *Source:* Martin Finborud / Wikimedia Commons / Public domain.

Myxedema – Myxedema is a clinical manifestation of hypothyroidism characterized by the infiltration of the subcutaneous layers of the skin by mucopolysaccharides, which causes the skin **to swell** and the underlying tissues to have a waxy consistency. The Greek word *myxa* meant "slime." The root **MYX-** is used today for "mucus."

Cretinism – Cretinism is a form of congenital hypothyroidism in children that produces dwarfism and arrests mental development. The term cretin, which has been used in English for a "stupid person," appears to have come from *crestin*, which is a word from an Alpine French dialect that was used for people who appear to have suffered from cretinism. Beyond this, the root **CRETIN-** is of uncertain origins. Some etymologists believe the term is derived from a Vulgar Latin word for "a Christian," *christianus*, which appears to have been used as a generic term for "a person" since most Europeans identified themselves as Christians during this period of time.

Hypercalcemia – Hypercalcemia (excessive calcium in the blood) can be caused by excessive secretion of parathyroid hormone. Derived from the Latin word for limestone, calx, **CALC-** is used today for "calcium."

Pancreas

Diabetes mellitus – Diabetes mellitus (DM) is the general term for metabolic diseases that exhibit excessive urination and elevated blood sugars. Type I (DM 1) is called insulin-dependent diabetes. Type 2 (DM 2) is insulin-resistant diabetes, which means these patients are not dependent on taking insulin to regulate their blood sugars. Derived from the Greek word *diabainein* "to pass through," **diabetes** is a general term for diseases marked by excessive urination. The **mellitus**, in diabetes mellitus, indicates that the urine is "honey-sweet." This is due to the presence of glucose in the urine. The root **MELIT-** (also spelled **MELLIT-** and **MELITT-**) and **MEL-** are used for "sugar and honey." These roots are also used for honey bees. **MEL-** is a homograph that also can mean "cheek" (Gr. *melon*) and "limb" (Gr. *melos*).

Polydipsia – A common sign associated with diabetes is "excessive thirst," which is called polydipsia. Formed from the Greek word for "thirst," *dipsa*, the root **DIPS-** means "thirst."

Polyuria – A common sign associated with diabetes is polyuria, which is the technical term for "excessive urination." Derived from the Greek word for "urine," *ouron*, **UR-** is the common root for "urine."

Glucosuria or glycosuria – Glucose in the urine is called glucosuria or glycosuria, which is the cardinal sign of diabetes mellitus. The roots **GLUC-** and **GLYC-** are used for "sugar" and "glucose."

Hyperglycemia and Hypoglycemia – Hyperglycemia and hypoglycemia are respectively "excessive glucose in the blood" and "abnormally diminished glucose in the blood." Both hyperglycemia and hypoglycemia are associated with diabetes mellitus.

Pituitary

Diabetes insipidus – Inadequate secretion of the **pituitary antidiuretic hormone** causes diabetes insipidus, which literally means "tasteless diabetes." The term **diuretic** comes from the word for "urination," **diuresis**, which is derived from the Greek *diourein*, "to urinate." *Insipidus* is a Late Latin adjective that means "tasteless," which comes from the Classical Latin verb, *sapere* "to taste." The term *Homo sapiens* ("wise human") is derived from this verb. The connection between taste and wisdom is found in the notion of being "sensible" or "discerning." Hence, an "insipid" person is used for a person who lacks culture and is therefore dull.

Pituitary gigantism – Pituitary gigantism is caused by hypersecretion of growth hormone from childhood. The term gigantism is derived from the Greek word for "giant," *gigas* (pl. *gigantes)*. The root **GIGANT-** primarily means "large." Also derived from the Greek *gigas*, **GIGA-** is a prefix meaning "a billion" (10^9).

In Greek myth, the Gigantes were a race of large, monstrous beings, who were said to be the sons of Gaia and Uranus. The most famous of the giants were the Thracian Gigantes, who waged war on the Olympian gods in the gigantomachy (*gigantes*, giants + *mache*, battle). This war was not the same as the Titanomachy which was a battle between the Olympian gods and the previous generation of gods, named the Titans (Fig. 12.8).

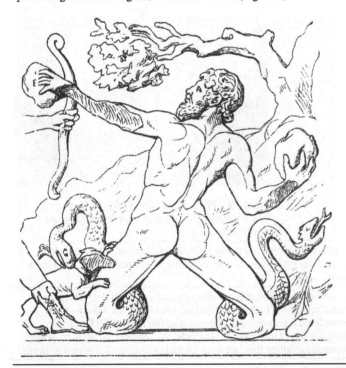

Fig. 12.8 Line drawing of a relief in the Vatican Museum depicting a giant fighting against the Olympian goddess, Artemis, in the Gigantomachy. During the Hellenistic period, the *Gigantes* began to be depicted with snake legs and as more bestial to reflect their association with Gaia and uncivilized peoples. *Source:* Meyers Konversations-Lexikon/ Bibliographisches Institute / Public Domain.

Pituitary dwarfism – Pituitary dwarfism is caused by hyposecretion of growth hormone from childhood. The term "dwarf" comes from Germanic mythology. In Germanic myth, dwarves were a race of humanoid creatures of diminished size that dwelt in the hills and rocks. Dwarves are associated with being skilled smiths and craftsmen. Another term for dwarfism is **nanism**. The root **NAN-** means "dwarf" and "very small." **NAN-** is also used as an SI unit for "one billionth" (10^{-9}). The most common cause of short-limbed dwarfism is **achondroplasia**, which inhibits the growth plates in the long bones. Derived from the root meaning "limb" **MEL-**, the term for short-limbed dwarfism is **nanomelic**.

Adrenal

Adrenal virilism – Adrenal virilism (L. *virilis*, masculine) is caused by the hypersecretion of androgen hormones in a female, which manifests in the absence of menstruation, deepening voice, and **hirsutism** (i.e. excessive growth of hair in abnormal places). Derived from the Latin word for "hairy," *hirsutus*, the root **HIRSUT-** is likewise used for "hairy."

Hypernatremia – Hypernatremia (excessive sodium in the blood) can be caused by aldosterone and glucocorticoids. Derived from the Latin word for "salt," natrium, **NATR-** is a root used for "sodium."

Hyperkalemia – Hyperkalemia (excessive potassium in the blood) can be caused by a deficiency of the hormone aldosterone. Derived from the Latin word for "potash," **KAL-** is a root used for "potassium."

Greek or Latin word element	Current usage	Etymology	Examples
GIGANT/O (jī-găn-tō)	Giant, large; SI), GIGA- is a prefix meaning a *billion* (10^9).	Gr. *gigas, gigantos*, giant	**Gigant**ism, **gigant**ic, **giga**watt
MEG/O (meg-ō) **MEGAL/O** (meg-ă-lō) **-MEGALY** (meg-ă-lē)	Large, enlargement	Gr. *megas, megalou*, large	**Megal**ops, acro**megaly**
NAN/O (nă-nō) **NANN/O** (nă-nō)	Dwarf, very small, one billionth	Gr. *nanos*, dwarf; one billionth	**Nan**ism, **nan**ometer
CRETIN/O (krĕt-ĭn-ō)	Cretinism	Supposedly from French crétin (18th century)	**Cretin**ism, **cretin**oid
MEL/O (mel-ō)	Limb	Gr. *melos*, limb	Campto**mel**ic, nano**mel**ic
MELIT/O (mel-ĭ-tō) **MEL/O** (mel-ō)	Honey, sugar, bees	Gr. *meli, melitos*, honey; sugar	**Melit**uria, **melitt**ology
UR/O (ū-rō) **-URIA** (ū-rē-ă)	Urine	Gr. *ouron*, urine	Gluco**suria**, **ur**obilinemia
OREX/I (or-ek-sĭ) **-OREXIA** (ŏ-rek-sē-ă)	Appetite	Gr. *orexis*, desire for; appetite	An**orexia**, **orex**igen

Greek or Latin word element	Current usage	Etymology	Examples
DIPS/O (dip-sō)	Thirst	Gr. *dipsa*, thirst	Poly**dips**ia, **dips**ophobia
HIRSUT/O (hĭr-sŭ-tō)	Hairy	L. *hirsutus, -a, -um*, hairy, shaggy	**Hirsut**ism, **hirsut**e
MYX/O (mĭks-ō)	Mucus, slime	Gr. *myxa*, slime; mucus	**Myx**edema, **myx**adenoma
PRIV/O (prĭv-ō)	Deprived of	L. *privare*, to strip, deprive of	Thymo**privic**, calci**privia**
-PRIVIA (prĭv-ē-ă)			

Review	Answers
The root _____ and the suffix _____ are used in medicine to denote the corresponding effects of a gland's dysfunction or removal from the body.	**PRIV-, -PRIVIA**
Hyperthyroidism is associated with excessive secretion from the thyroid gland. The characteristic signs of this are a rapid heart rate (_____), protrusion of the eyeballs (_____), and enlargement of the thyroid gland (_____). _____ (i.e. a marked increase in appetite) is another sign of hyperthyroidism.	**tachycardia, exophthalmos, goiter hyperorexia**
Hypothyroidism is associated with diminished secretion from the thyroid gland. The characteristic signs of this are a slow heart rate (_____), sluggishness (_____), and obesity. _____ (i.e. a marked decrease in appetite) is a sign of hypothyroidism.	**bradycardia, lethargy hyporexia**
_____ is a clinical manifestation of hypothyroidism characterized by the infiltration of the subcutaneous layers of the skin by mucopolysaccharides, which causes swelling of the skin and underlying tissues to have a waxy consistency.	**Myxedema**
_____ is a form of congenital hypothyroidism in children that produces dwarfism and arrested mental development.	**Cretinism**
Pituitary _____ is caused by hypersecretion of growth hormone from childhood. Pituitary _____ is caused by hyposecretion of growth hormone from childhood. Another term for dwarfism is _____.	**Gigantism Dwarfism nanism**
_____ is characterized by an increase in the size of the hands and/or feet, and is caused by hypersecretion of growth hormone in adulthood.	**Acromegaly**
Adrenal virilism (L. *virilis*, masculine) is caused by the hypersecretion of androgen hormones in a female, which manifests in the absence of menstruation, deepening voice, and _____ (i.e. excessive growth of hair in abnormal places).	**hirsutism**
Derived from the Greek word *diabainein* "to pass through," diabetes is a general term for diseases marked by _____ (i.e. excessive urination). The other common sign associated with diabetes is excessive thirst, which is called _____. The mellitus, in diabetes mellitus indicates that the urine is "honey-sweet." This is due to the presence of glucose in the urine, which is called _____ or _____. Another sign of diabetes mellitus is excessive sugar in the blood, which is called _____. Diabetes mellitus is often due to issues with insulin deficiencies. Inadequate secretion of the pituitary antidiuretic hormone causes diabetes _____, which literally means "tasteless diabetes."	**polyuria polydipsia glucosuria, glycosuria hyperglycemia insipidus**
_____ (excessive potassium in the blood) can be caused by a deficiency of the hormone aldosterone.	**Hyperkalemia**
_____ (excessive calcium in the blood) can be caused by excessive secretion of the parathyroid hormone.	**Hypercalcemia**
_____ (excessive sodium in the blood) can be caused by aldosterone and glucocorticoids.	**Hypernatremia**

13

Gastrointestinal System

CHAPTER LEARNING OBJECTIVES
1) You will learn the word elements, loan words, and key terms associated with the gastrointestinal system.
2) You will become familiar with the historical concepts associated with ancient Greek concepts of the parts of the digestive system, digestion, and food.

Lessons from History: The Gastrointestinal System and Figures of Speech

Food for Thought as You Read:

What are some of the socio-cultural reasons that we use the innards of our abdominal cavity in figures of speech? To what extent does science come into play in these figures of speech? Do metaphors have a place in medicine?

It is common for parts of the human body to be used as figures of speech in everyday English. In the following discussion, we will look at some of the abstract meanings that parts of the digestive system and the abdomen have conveyed in both the Modern and the Classical worlds. The fact that the origins of these figures of speech are not widely understood reveals that they have become dead metaphors. A dead metaphor is a figure of speech that has lost the original imagery of its meaning over time through frequent, popular usage. That said, the presence of such figures of speech in English also reveals the influence of the Classical world on Western thought and language, as well as the experiences human beings have shared over the centuries.

The internal organs of the body, particularly those of the abdominal cavity, commonly appear as figures of speech to convey strong emotions in the English language. The English word "gut" meaning entrails, the inner organs of the abdomen of the body, is used in contexts of deep emotions. For instance, one says he or she is "gutted" when feeling extremely disappointed. The root from the Latin word for the entrails/inner organs of the abdomen, viscera, is also used to convey strong emotions. When experiencing a deep feeling about something, one may say that one is having a "visceral reaction to X." The internal organs of the abdomen are also used in figures of speech about one's courage or lack thereof. We describe someone as being "gutless" because they lack courage due to fear. Going back to Shakespeare, the idiom "X has not stomach for" has been used to describe someone who lacks the courage and the determination to do something. Conversely, we speak of the "intestinal fortitude" of people with courage and determination to do something. The innards of others can be the target of our emotions as well. We say that we "hate someone's guts" to express an intense hatred for someone, and "to hate someone's intestines" was used as a figure of speech during the early 20th century to express this emotion as well. Likewise, "I can't stand your guts" speaks to hating everything about someone. The origins of some of these phrases can be associated with the physiological reactions of humans when experiencing strong emotions. For instance, when someone is said to be "gutless" or "lacking the stomach to do something," the figure of speech appears to be derived from the human experience of nausea and vomiting due to intense fear. Likewise, one can experience discomfort under the stress of a great loss, and therefore, it makes sense to claim that you have been "gutted" by this event. However, this physiological link does

Greek and Latin Roots of Medical and Scientific Terminologies, First Edition. Todd A. Curtis.
© 2025 John Wiley & Sons, Inc. Published 2025 by John Wiley & Sons, Inc.
Companion website: www.wiley.com/go/Curtis

not seem to explain why the innards of another are the target of our hatred. Some have argued that this figure of speech is linked to the practice of eviscerating, removing the innards, of one's enemy in battle or in punishment, which is a dark part of human history. That said, these figures of speech do not suggest that one is doing actual harm to another's innards. Another explanation would be that the innards of a human being in some way signify the internal emotional being of a person, something akin to a person's soul.

In some respects, the use of the Greek word *phrenes* in Homeric literature of the 8th century BC carries similar meanings to "guts" and "viscera." On one hand, the *phrenes* can refer to the physical innards of a human in that they express positional relationships without the body. For instance, in *Iliad* XVI.481, Sarpedon is said to be struck in battle where the *phrenes* are set around the heart. Likewise, in *Odyssey* IX.301, Odysseus considers killing the cyclops with a sword blow where the *phrenes* hold the liver. On account of this, later Homeric commentators interpreted *phrenes* to refer to the diaphragm. Such explanations are somewhat anachronistic given the level of anatomical knowledge in the 8th century BC and the lack of detailed descriptions. It would suffice to say that the *phrenes* was used less specifically, similarly to how "innards" and "guts" are used today. The *phrenes* are also associated with situations that correlate to a wide variety of human emotions in the *Iliad*. Agamemnon's reaction to the prophet Calchas' advice to return Chryseis to her father in *Iliad* I.103f is that of intense anger, which is described by his *phrenes* becoming darkened. In *Iliad* 15.16f, Zeus sends Apollo to arouse Hector to battle because distress has weakened the *phrenes* of Hector. In some respects, this suggests that distress of the *phrenes* can weaken one's resolve to fight. In *Iliad* 24.514f, Achilles' deep sorrow over Patroclus and his father is associated with his *phrenes*. Thus, the *phrenes* is often described by translators as the seat of emotions, which is why in all three instances, the word "heart" is most often used for *phrenes* since in modern metaphorical language the heart is understood in these terms. However, in other places within the *Iliad*, particularly with verbs of thinking, *phrenes* is translated as "mind." In Iliad 9.189, when Phoenix is closing his exhortation to Achilles to return to battle, he concludes his speech: "as for you (Achilles), don't go on thinking (*noein*) in your mind (*phrenes*) such things." While cognition is located in the mind in modern English, in some of these instances, thinking with one's heart would have been an acceptable translation as well, considering that strong emotions are involved in many of these instances. In some cases, the phrenes appear to be associated with the internal emotional being of a person, and therefore, phrenes could be translated as "heart" or "mind": "Hateful (*echthros*) to me like the gates of Hades is the man who says one thing while he hides another thing in his *phrenes* (*Iliad* 9.307)." While it is impossible to be certain how literally or metaphorically *phrenes* can be understood in passages to do with emotion and thought, particularly in instances relaying thought and emotions, it is quite clear that the *phrenes* can both occupy a physical location in the body and be linked to a variety of strong emotions.

The innards are sometimes associated with intuition and revelation, which can be observed in English figures of speech, such as "having a gut feeling" and asking someone to "spill their guts." The origins of these expressions are not entirely clear. Interestingly, in the ancient Greek and Romans worlds, the innards of animals, particularly the liver, were believed to hold prophetic value. The Greek loan word **splanchna** is a synonym for **viscera** in modern medical terminology because both the Greek and Latin words refer to the innards of a body. There was a religious or prophetic understanding of the term *splanchna* in Greek culture, which can be observed in the meanings of the Greek verb *splanchneuein*: (i) to eat the innards of a sacrificed animal and (ii) to prophesy from the innards of an animal. As to the second meaning, the viscera were used as a means of determining the will of the gods in ancient Greek and Roman culture. This practice was not limited to the Greeks and Romans; many of the neighboring Mediterranean cultures also practiced this form of prophetic activity. In Latin, this practice was called *haruspicium* and the practitioner of this form of prophetic activity was called a *haruspex*, if male, or a *haruspica*, if female. The term *haruspicium* is derived from the Latin *hira* (gut, intestines) and the Latin verb "to look, behold" *specere*. Haruspicy originated with the Etruscans and was introduced into Roman society during the Republican era. Evidence of some of the elements of this practice can be observed in the famous Piacenza Liver, which is an Etruscan artifact found in Rome that has the parts of a sheep's liver labeled according to specific Etruscan gods (Fig. 13.1). The liver appears to be one of the more common organs to be used. The reading of the gods' messages through specific parts of the liver is known by the terms **hepatoscopy** and **hepatomancy**.

As would be expected, ancient Greek medical theory has also had an influence on modern figures of speech. The idioms "lily-livered" and "white-livered" have been used since the 17th century to speak to the cowardly nature of an individual. The white color of the liver in both of these idioms conveys that the liver is unhealthy because a healthy liver is bloody. Due to the reception of Greek medicine, particularly Galenic medicine, the liver was associated with the production of blood, and the hepatic ducts in the liver were supposed to be the active agents in extracting bile from the blood. In the context of the four temperaments, bile (chole) was commonly associated with a quick-tempered, irritable nature, and blood was associated with a cheerful, optimistic nature. Thus, a person with a pathological liver lacked the appropriate humors and temperament necessary for bravery.

Fig. 13.1 Diagram of the inscriptions with the names of Etruscan gods on the bronze liver of Piacenza. *Source:* Wilhelm Deecke, 1880/ Public Domain.

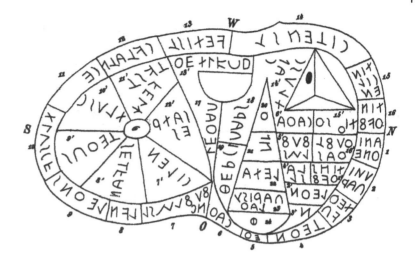

Given that our understanding of the physiologies of the parts of the abdominal cavity is quite different from the theories of antiquity, one should be careful not to assume that apparent similarities in the usages of such figures of speech indicate an analogous understanding of these parts and their functions. That said, the similar usages of these innards in figures of speech perhaps reveal that mankind's perception of the human body is driven by more than our scientific understanding.

Some Suggested Readings

Casarett, David, et al. "Can Metaphors and Analogies Improve Communication with Seriously Ill Patients?" *Journal of Palliative Medicine* 13, no. 3 (2010): 255–260.

Ireland, S. and Steel, F. L. "Phrenes as an Anatomical Organ in the Works of Homer." *Glotta* 53 (1975): 183–195.

Etymological Explanations: Common Terms and Word Elements for the Anatomy of the Gastrointestinal System

In the following discussion of the anatomical terms associated with the gastrointestinal system, the nominative and genitive singular forms of the anatomical Latin term are provided in parenthesis. The Greek and Latin roots are formatted in all caps and emboldened.

Oral cavity, mouth, and throat

Oral cavity (L. *cavitas oris*) – The oral cavity is the first portion of the digestive tract and is where the digestive process begins (Fig. 13.2).

Mouth (L. *os, oris*) – The opening to the oral cavity is termed the "mouth." The roots used for the "mouth" are **STOM-**, **STOMAT-**, and **OR-**. The anatomical Latin term for the mouth is os (*os, oris*). The Greek loan word **stoma** can be used for an anatomical or surgical "opening" or "mouth."

Lip (L. *labium, -i*) – The lips form the external boundary of the mouth. The roots for "lip" are **LABI-**, **CHIL-**, and **CHEIL-**. The anatomical Latin term for a "lip" is **labium**.

Jaw – The jaw forms the bony superior and inferior boundaries of the mouth. The root for the "whole jaw" is **GNATH-**. The root for the top part of the jaw bone is **MAXILL-**. The root for the bottom part of the jaw bone is **MANDIBUL-**. The corresponding anatomical terms for these bones are **maxilla (L. *maxilla, -ae*)** and **mandibula (L. *mandibula, -ae*)**.

Cheek (L. *bucca, -ae*) – The soft lateral borders of the oral cavity are called the cheeks. The roots for "cheek" are **BUCC-** and **MEL-**. The anatomical term for a "cheek" is **bucca**.

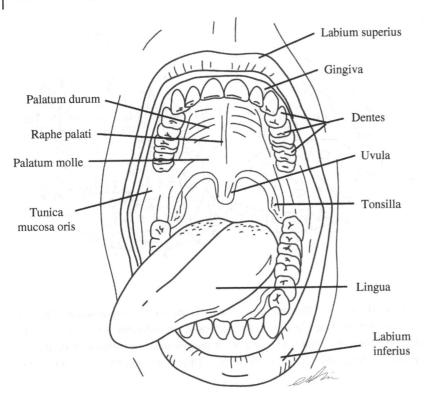

Fig. 13.2 Anatomical Latin terms for the oral cavity. *Source:* Drawing by Chloe Kim.

Labium superius

Gingiva

Palatum durum

Dentes

Raphe palati

Palatum molle

Uvula

Tunica mucosa oris

Tonsilla

Lingua

Labium inferius

Palate (L. *palatum, -i*) – The palate forms the top portion of the oral cavity, which is commonly called the "roof of the mouth." The root for the palate of the oral cavity is **PALAT-**. The anatomical Latin term is palatum. The anterior part of the palate is called the **hard palate (L. *palatum durum*)**, and the posterior part of the palate is called the **soft palate (L. *palatum molle*)**. The crease or seam of the palate is called the rhaphe. The palate has been long associated with the sense of taste. Ancient Roman poets such as Ovid, Vergil, Horace, and Juvenal commonly refer to the *palatum* as the organ of taste. On account of this, the *palatum* was used as a metaphor for judgement by Cicero (*De natura rerum* 2.49): *Epicurus dum palato quid sit optimum iudicat* ("...while Epicurus judges with the palate what is best..."). It is worthy to note that this belief is not entirely wrong. While the palate is not the primary area of taste, modern studies have shown that it does in fact contribute to the sense of taste, albeit a much smaller amount in comparison to the tongue.

Tongue (L. *lingua, -ae*) – Thanks in part to the numerous taste buds in the papillae on the tongue's surface, the tongue is the primary organ of taste. The roots for "tongue" are **LINGU-**, **GLOSS-**, and **GLOTT-**. The anatomical Latin term for a "tongue" is **lingua**.

Tooth (L. *dens, dentis*) – The teeth are the instruments of mastication. The roots for "tooth" are **DENT-** and **ODONT-**. The anatomical Latin term for a "tooth" is **dens**; the plural is **dentes**. **DENTIN-** is the root used for dentine, which makes the teeth hard.

Gum (L. *gingiva, -ae*) – The teeth are situated in the gums, which is the mucosal tissue covering the margins of the alveoli of the mandible and maxilla. The roots for "gum" of the mouth are **GINGIV-** and **OUL-**. The anatomical Latin term for a "gum" is **gingiva**.

Salivary gland (L. *glandula salivaria*) – The salivary glands produce saliva that contains **ptyalin**, which is a digestive enzyme that breaks down starches. As was discussed in the previous chapters, **PTYAL-** is one of the Greek roots for "saliva," the other being **SIAL-**. Hence, the compound root for the salivary glands is **SIALOADEN-**. The different salivary glands are named according to their location: **parotid** (para- + *ous, otos*, ear), **submandibular**, and **sublingual**.

Throat (L. *fauces, faucium*) – As was noted earlier in Chapter 9, the **pharynx** and its root **PHARYNG-** are common anatomical terms for the "throat." However, the narrow passage at the posterior aspect of the oral cavity that leads to the oropharynx is called the **fauces**. The term is the plural form of the Latin word for the "gullet," *faux*. Hence, the root for the anatomical part is **FAUC-**.

Tonsil (L. *tonsilla, -ae*) – The term tonsil and its root **TONSILL-** are from the Latin word meaning "almond." The tonsils provide an immune response to pathogens that enter the body through the mouth. The other root for tonsil, albeit occurring less often, is **AMYGDAL-**, and this term also means "almond."

Uvula (L. *uvula, -ae*) – The uvula hangs from the soft palate at the back of the oral cavity. This little fleshy ball helps to prevent food from going into the nasal cavity when one is swallowing. The roots for the uvula of the oral cavity are **UVUL-** and **STAPHYL-**. Owing to their etymological association with grapes, both roots can be used for grape-like structures.

Abdominal cavity

Abdomen (L. *abdomen, abdominis*) – The roots for the abdomen are **CELI-**, **LAPAR-**, and **ABDOMIN-**. The anatomical Latin term is abdomen (Fig. 13.3). The abdomen is divided into nine regions (Fig. 13.4): right and left **hypochondrium**, right and left **lumbar** (also called the **iliac** or **lateral flank**), right and left **inguinal**, **epigastric**, **umbilical**, and the **hypogastric** (also called the **pubic region**). The center region is called the **umbilical region** after the bellybutton or navel. The loan words for the navel are **umbilicus** and **omphalos**, and their corresponding roots **UMBILIC-** and **OMPHAL-** refer to this anatomical feature.

Peritoneum (L. *peritoneum, -i*) – The abdominal cavity (*cavitas abdominis*) is lined with a serous membrane called the peritoneum; the roots for the peritoneum are **PERITONE-** and **PERITON-**. Similar to the pleura of the thoracic cavity, the peritoneum is divided into **visceral** and **parietal peritoneum**. As was discussed in the chapter on the respiratory system, the adjective visceral means "pertaining to the organ/organs." The roots for internal organs, particularly of the abdominal cavity, are **SPLANCHN-** and **VISCER-**. The loan word **splanchna** is a synonym for **viscera** (Fig. 13.5).

Esophagus and stomach

Esophagus (L. *esophagus, -i*) – Leaving the oral cavity, the digestive tract proceeds from the pharynx into the **esophagus**. The root for the esophagus is **ESOPHAG-**. The anatomical Latin term is **oesophagus**, which is also spelled esophagus (Fig. 13.5). The former spelling preserves the Greek etymology of this anatomical structure. The Greek *oisophagos* literally means "what carries and eats."

Hiatus of the Diaphragm (L. *hiatus, -us*) – The esophagus leaves the thoracic cavity and enters the abdomen through an opening in the diaphragm called the hiatus. The root for the "gap" or "opening" in the diaphragm into which the esophagus passes through is **HIAT-**. Hence, when people are taking a long break from work, they are said to be on "hiatus."

Stomach (L. *gaster, gastris*) – Once the esophagus passes through the diaphragm, it joins the stomach, which is the 1ˢᵗ organ of digestion in the abdominal cavity. The root for the stomach is **GASTR-**. The suffix is **-GASTER**. The anatomical Latin term is **gaster**. The widest part of an organ is called the **fundus**, which for the stomach is the superior part. The gastric folds in the stomach walls are called **rugae**. As was noted in an earlier chapter, the root **RUG-** is used for "wrinkle" or "fold." The walls of the stomach pour out gastric juices that break down the food into **chyme**, which is a mixture of partly digested food and digestive secretions. The superior sphincter of the stomach prevents the digestive juices from flowing back up (i.e. reflux), and the inferior sphincter ensures that food properly turns into chyme before it enters the intestines. The **omentum** (L. *omentum, -i*) is a fold of peritoneum that attaches to the stomach with certain of the abdominal viscera. The root for this anatomical part is **OMENT-**.

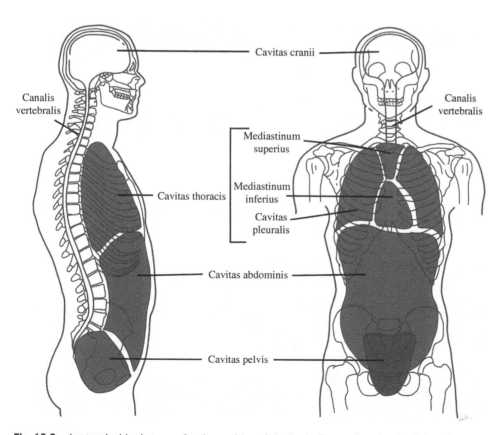

Fig. 13.3 Anatomical Latin terms for the cavities of the body. *Source:* Drawing by Chloe Kim.

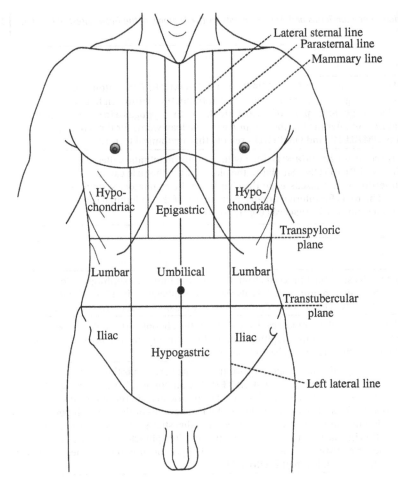

Fig. 13.4 Image of the nine regions of the abdominal cavity from Gray's *Anatomy of the Human Body (1858)*. Note that during Gray's time, the lumbar region was called the iliac region. *Source:* Henry Gray's, (1858)/ The Royal College of Surgeons of England/ Public Domain.

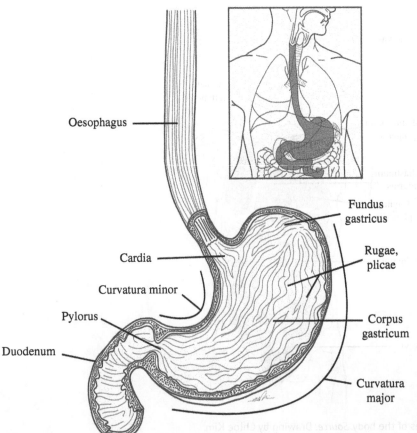

Fig. 13.5 Anatomical Latin terms for the esophagus and stomach. *Source: Image by Chloe Kim.*

Sphincters of the Stomach – The root for sphincter is **SPHINCTER-**. The anatomical Latin term is **sphincter (L. *sphincter, sphincteris*)**. The sphincter superior to the stomach is called the cardiac sphincter, and therefore, the root for this sphincter is **CARDI-**. The inferior sphincter is called the pyloric sphincter. The root **PYLOR-** is used for the pylorus (L. *pylorus, -i*), which is the area of the digestive tract prior to this sphincter. The term pylorus comes from the Greek word *pyloros*, which means gate-keeper, as this is the portion of stomach that empties into the duodenum. As to the etymology of the term sphincter, it appears to be derived from the Greek verb, *sphingein* "to squeeze, bind," which is appropriate, given the sphincter muscles constrict to close off an opening of a tubular structure. Via the verb *sphingein*, sphincter appears to share an etymology with "Sphinx," which is a Greek mythological monster having a winged lion's body and a woman's torso. In the Greek myths associated with Thebes, the sphinx attacked travelers around Thebes. It would appear that the Sphinx's name literally meant, "the strangler." The Sphinx was defeated by the Greek hero, Oedipus, who solved the so-called "Riddle of the Sphinx": "What goes on four legs in the morning, two legs in the afternoon, and three legs in the evening?" The answer to this question was "Man": "Man, who crawls on all fours as a baby, then walks on two legs, and finally needs a cane in old age." Upon hearing this, the Sphinx killed herself by plunging off a cliff to her death (Figs. 13.6).

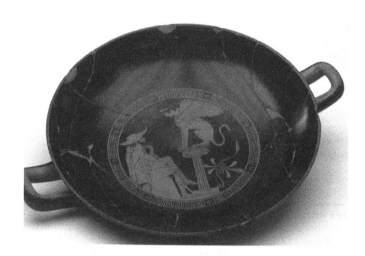

Fig. 13.6 Image on red-figured kylix (480–470 BC), depicting Oedipus and the Sphinx of Thebes. *Source:* Todd A Curtis (Book author).

Intestines

Intestines (L. *intestinum, -i*) – After leaving the stomach via the pylorus, the next structures of the gastrointestinal tract are the intestines (Fig. 13.7). The roots for intestine are **INTESTIN-** and **ENTER-**. Hence, the study of the digestive organs is called **gastroenterology**. The anatomical Latin term is **intestinum** and **enteron** is the loan word for "the alimentary canal." The connective tissue between the intestines is called **mesentery**. The root for mesentery is **MESENTER-**. The anatomical Latin term is **mesenterium**.

Small intestine (L. *intestinum tenue*) – The small intestine, which in anatomical Latin is called the *intestinum tenue* (= thin intestine), is the first major part of the intestines. The small intestine is broken down into three areas, from superior to inferior: the **duodenum**, the **jejunum**, and the **ileum**.

Duodenum (L. *duodenum, -i*) – The root for the first part of the small intestine is **DUODEN-**. The anatomical Latin term is **duodenum**. The 3rd-century-BC anatomist, Herophilus, appears to be responsible for the names of the parts of the small intestines. The term duodenum is the short form of the medieval Latin term *intestinum duodenum digitorum*, which is derived from the Greek name for this section of the small intestine, *dodekadaktylos* ("12 fingers long"), that Herophilus used to describe the length of this part of the small intestine.

Jejunum (L. *jejunum, -i*) – The root for the second part of the small intestine is **JEJUN-**. The anatomical Latin term is **jejunum**. Perhaps because it was empty when Herophilus examined it, this part of the small intestine was called the "fasting intestine," which is why the Latin *jejunum* ("empty, hungry, fasting") was used for this second part of the small intestine.

Ileum (L. *ileum, -i*) – The root for the third part of the small intestine is **ILE-**. The anatomical Latin term is **ileum**. The term ileum is a derivative of the Latin *ile*, which meant "guts" and "loin." The latter meaning is why the upper portion of the pelvic bone (**ilium**) and this lowest part of the intestine (**ileum**) share a similar etymology. That said, the root **ILI-** is used for the ilium, and **ILE-** is used for the ileum.

Fig. 13.7 Anatomical Latin terms for the parts of the lower GI. *Source:* Drawing by Chloe Kim.

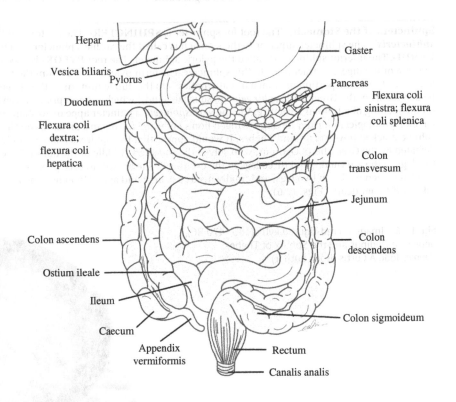

Large intestine (L. *intestinum crassum*) – The ileocecal junction is where the small intestine turns into the large intestine (*intestinum crassum* = "dense intestine"). The whole large intestine is called the **colon (L. *colon, -i*)**. The roots for the large intestine are **COL-** and **COLON-**. There are three parts to the colon: the ascending colon, the transverse colon, and the descending colon. The bends in the colon are called **flexurae (singular *flexura*)**.

Cecum (L. *caecum, -i*) – The portion of the large intestine that appears to be going the opposite direction of the flow of the large intestine is called the **cecum**. The roots for the cecum are **CEC-** and **TYPHL-**. These roots come from Latin and Greek words that mean blind, assumedly because this part of the large intestine is going in the wrong direction. Consequently, the root **TYPHL-** is used for being visually blind in some contexts.

Appendix (L. *appendix, appendicis*) – At the end of the cecum is an appendix that is called the vermiform appendix because it looks like a worm. The **vermiform appendix** is one of many appendices of the body. The etymology of appendix reveals that anything that hangs on a body could be called an appendix (e.g. the appendix of a book, the appendages of the body). The roots for the appendix are **APPEND-** and **APPENDIC-**.

Sigmoid colon (L. *colon sigmoideum*) – The descending colon gives way to an S-shaped part of the large intestine called the sigmoid colon. It derives its name from being shaped like the Greek letter sigma. The root for the S-shaped part of the large intestine is **SIGMOID-**.

Rectum (L. *rectum, -i*) – The next portion of the intestine is straight, which is why its full anatomical Latin name is *intestinum rectum*, but this anatomical Latin term is often shortened to **rectum** in medical terminology. Therefore, it is important to bear in mind that the root **RECT-** is used for the "rectum," as well as anything that is "straight."

Anus (L. *anus, -i*) – The anus is the last sphincter of the gastrointestinal tract and the passageway out of the body. The root for the anus is **AN-**. The anus is derived from the Latin word for a "ring," which explains why its diminutive form, **ANUL-**, is used for ring-like structures. In Classical Latin, an *anus (anus, -us)* was the term for an old woman, which could be a rather unfortunate similarity between these two words when they are in the nominative singular. However, pronunciation forms the important point of distinction when these terms are in their nominative singular form: ănus (old woman) and ānus (anus/ring). The root referring to the rectum and the anus is **PROCT-**, which is why a physician who specializes in the lower intestine is called a **proctologist**.

Pancreas, gallbladder, and liver

Pancreas (L. *pancreas, pancreatis*) – The pancreas, liver, and gallbladder are three important organs of digestion (Fig. 13.8). Located behind the stomach, the pancreas secretes enzymes that digest all three major kinds of foods (i.e. proteins, carbohydrates, and fats). The pancreas secretes these enzymes through the pancreatic duct into the duodenum. The root for the pancreas is **PANCREAT-**.

Fig. 13.8 Anatomical Latin terms for the liver, gallbladder, and pancreas. *Source:* Drawing by Chloe Kim.

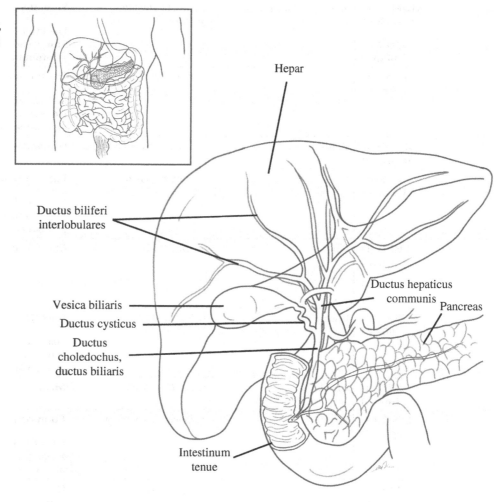

Liver (L. *hepar, hepatis*) – The liver secretes bile (also known as gall), which is a fluid that contains enzymes and bile salts that contribute to emulsifying fat. The roots for bile are **CHOLE-** and **BIL-**. Bile is stored in the gall bladder that sits under the liver. When stimulated, both structures send bile into the duodenum via the common bile duct. The roots for the liver are **HEPAR-** and **HEPAT-**. The anatomical Latin term is **hepar**.

Gallbladder (L. *vesica biliaris*) – Bile is stored in the gallbladder located under the liver. When stimulated, both the gall bladder and liver send bile into the duodenum via the common bile duct. The roots for a bladder are **CYST-** and **VESIC-**. The root commonly used for the gallbladder is **CHOLECYST-**. The anatomical Latin term for the "bladder" is **vesica (L. *vesica, -ae*)**, which is why the anatomical Latin term for the gallbladder is ***vesica biliaris***.

Bile duct (L. *ductus biliaris*) – The roots for a duct are **DOCH-** and **DUCT-**. **DOCH-** coming from the Greek word *doche*, which meant "a receptacle." **DUCT-** ultimately comes from the verb *ducere, ductus* (to lead, draw, and convey), which is why this root carries the meaning of "leading" and "drawing," as well as "duct." That said, **ANGI-** and **-AGOGUE** are also used for anatomical structures referred to as ducts, as well as vessels. Thus, the compound roots commonly used for bile vessels and ducts are **CHOLANGI-** and **CHOLEDOCH-**.

Greek or Latin word element	Current usage	Etymology	Examples
OR/O (ō-rō)	Mouth	L. *os, oris*, n. mouth	Ab**or**ad, **or**opharynx, **or**ofacial Loan word: **Os** (ōs) pl. **Ora** (ōr′ă)
STOMAT/O (stō-măt-ō) STOM/O (stō-mō)	Mouth, outlet, opening	Gr. *stoma, stomatos*, mouth	**Stomat**ocyte, **stomat**itis Loan word: **Stoma** (stō′mă) pl. **Stomata** (stō′măt-ă)
DENT/O (děn-tō)	Tooth	L. *dens, dentis*, m. tooth	**Dent**in, **dent**ist, **dent**oalveolar Loan word: **Dens** (denz) pl. **Dentes** (den′tēz″)
ODONT/O (ō-don-tō)	Tooth	Gr. *odous, ondontos*, tooth	Orth**odont**ist, **odont**oblast
LABI/O (lā-bē-ō)	Lip	L. *labium, -i*, n. lip	**Labi**oclination, **labi**oglossolaryngeal Loan word: **Labium** (lā′bē-ŭm) pl. **Labia** (lā′bē-ă)
CHEIL/O (kī-lō) CHIL/O (kī-lō)	Lip	Gr. *cheilos*, lip	**Cheil**itis, **chil**ophagia, **chil**oplasty
BUCC/O (bŭk-ō)	Cheek	L. *bucca, -ae*, f. cheek	**Bucc**oclination, retro**bucc**al, **bucc**inator Loan word: **Bucca** (bŭk′ă) pl. **Buccae** (bŭk′ē″)
MEL/O (měl-ō)	Cheek	Gr. *melon*, cheek	**Mel**itis, **mel**oncus, **mel**oschisis
LINGU/O (lĭng-gwō)	Tongue	L. *lingua, -ae*, f. tongue	**Lingu**odental, **lingu**omesial Loan word: **Lingua** (ling′gwă) pl. **Linguae** (ling′gwē″)
GLOSS/O (glos-ō) GLOTT/O (glŏ-tō) -GLOT (glŏt)	Tongue	Gr. *glossa; glotta*, tongue	**Gloss**opharyngeal, **glott**ology, anthropo**glot**
GINGIV/O (jĭn-jĭ-vō)	Gum	L. *gingiva, -ae*, f. the gum	**Gingiv**itis, **gingiv**oglossitis Loan word: **Gingiva** (jin′jĭ-vă) pl. **Gingivae** (jin′jĭ-vē″)
OUL/O (oo-lō)	Gum	Gr. *oulon*, the gum	**Oul**orrhagia, **oul**itis
GNATH/O (năth-ō)	Jaw	Gr. *gnathos*, jaw	**Gnath**algia, **gnath**oplasty

Greek or Latin word element	Current usage	Etymology	Examples
MAXILL/O **(mak-sil-ō)**	Maxilla	L. *maxilla, -ae*, f. upper bone of jaw, maxilla	**Maxill**ofacial, **maxill**otomy Loan word: **Maxilla** (mak-sil′ă) pl. **Maxillae** (mak-sil′ē″)
MANDIBUL/O **(man-dib-yŭ-lō)**	Mandible	L. *mandibula, -ae*, f. lower bone of jaw, mandible	**Mandibul**opharyngeal, **mandibul**otomy˙ Loan word: **Mandibula** (man-dib′yŭ-lă) pl. **Mandibulae** (man-dib′yŭ-lē″)
PALAT/O **(păl-ă-tŏ)**	Palate	L. *palatum, -i*, n. palate, upper part of the mouth	**Palat**oschisis, **palat**orrhaphy Loan word: **Palatum** (pă-lat′ŭm) pl. **Palata** (pă-lat′ă)
UVUL/O **(ū-vyŭ-lō)**	Uvula	L. *uvula, -ae*, f. small grape, uvula fr. L. *uva*, grape	**Uvul**itis, **uvul**aptosis Loan word: **Uvula** (ū′vyŭ-lă) pl. **Uvulae** (ū′vyŭ-lē)
STAPHYL/O **(staf-ĭ-lō)**	Uvula, staphlycoccus bacteria, grape-like	Gr. *staphyle*, bunch of grapes, uvula	**Staphyl**ectomy, **staphyl**ine, peri**staphyl**itis
TONSILL/O **(tŏn-sĭl-ō)**	Tonsil	L. *tonsilla, -ae*, f. tonsil, almond	**Tonsill**itis, **tonsill**ectomy, supra**tonsil**ar Loan word: **Tonsilla** (tŏn-sĭl′ă) pl. **Tonsillae** (tŏn-sĭ-lē)
SPLANCHN/O **(splangk-nō)**	Viscera (internal organs enclosed in a cavity, particularly the abdominal cavity)	Gr. *splanchna*, innards, viscera	**Splanchn**otomy, **splanchn**ectopia, **splanchn**ocoel Loan word: **Splanchna** (splangk′nă)
ESOPHAG/O **(ĕ-sof-ă-gō)**	Esophagus	L. *esophagus, -i*, m. esophagus fr. Gr. *oisophagos*, esophagus, gullet	**Esophag**algia, **esophag**itis, pharyngo**esophag**eal Loan word: **Esophagus** (ē-sof′ă-gŭs) pl. **Esophagi** (ē-sof′ă-jī″)
GASTR/O **(gas-trŏ)** **-GASTER** **(găs-tĕr)**	Stomach, belly	L. *gaster, gastris*, f. stomach fr. Gr. *gaster, gastros*, belly, stomach	**Gastr**ectasis, proto**gaster**, **gastr**ocele Loan word: **Gaster** (gas′tĕr) pl. **Gastres** (gas′trēz″)
ABDOMIN/O **(ab-dom-i-nō)**	Abdomen	L. *abdomen, abdominis*, n. abdomen	**Abdomin**ocentesis, **abdomin**al, post**abdomen** Loan word: **Abdomen** (ab-dō′mĕn) pl. **Abdomina** (ab-dom′I-nă)
LAPAR/O **(lap-ă-rō)**	Abdomen	Gr. *lapara*, loins; abdomen	**Lapar**oscopy, **lapar**ocolostomy, hystero**lapar**otomy

Greek or Latin word element	Current usage	Etymology	Examples
COEL/O (sē-lō) **KOIL/O** (koy-lō) **CEL/O** (sē-lō) **CELI/O** (sē-lē-ō) **-COELE** (sēl) **-CELE** (sēl)	Abdomen, cavity, hollow	Gr. *koilia*, cavity, hollow, belly; abdomen	**Celi**ac, **celi**oenterotomy, **celi**ectasia, **koil**onychia, **coel**osperm, hemo**cel**om
OMPHAL/O (om-fă-lō)	Navel, umbilicus, center	Gr. *omphalos*, the navel, center	**Omphal**ocele, **omphal**omesenteric, par**omphal**ocelic Loan word: **Omphalos** (om′fă-lŏs)
UMBILIC/O (ŭm-bil-ĭ-kō)	Navel, umbilical cord	L. *umbilicus, -i,* m. the navel	**Umbilic**ocpubic, peri**umbilic**al Loan word: **Umbilicus** (ŭm-bĭ-lī′kŭs) pl. **Umbilici** (ŭm-bĭ-lī′sī)
HEPAT/O (hĕp-ă-tō) **HEPAR/O** (hep-ă-rō)	Liver **** HEPATIC/O** = pertaining to the liver; hepatic vessels	L. *hepar, hepatis,* n. liver fr. Gr. *hepar, hepatos,* liver	**Hepat**itis, **Hepar**in, **hepat**algia Loan word: **Hepar** (hē′par″) pl. **Hepatia** (hē-pat′ē-a)
DOCH/O (dō-kō)	Duct, receptacle ****CHOLEDOCH/O** = bile duct	Gr. *doche,* a receptacle, receiver	Sialo**doch**otomy, chole**doch**ectomy
DUCT/O (dŭk-tō)	Duct, to draw, lead, or convey	L. *ductus, -us,* m. a duct fr. L. *ducere, ductus,* to lead, draw, convey	**Duct**ogram, **duct**ile, ad**duct**or Loan word: **Ductus** (dŭk′tŭs) pl. **Ductus** (dŭk′tūs)
VESIC/O (vĕ-sĭ-kō) **VESICUL/O** (vĕ-sĭk-ū-lō)	bladder, blister small blister, vesicle	L. *vesica, -ae,* f. bladder *vesicula, -ae,* f. little bladder	**Vesic**ant, **vesic**ospinal, **vesicul**oform Loan word: **Vesica** (vĕ-sī′kă) pl. **Vesicae** (vĕ-sī′kē″) **Vesicula** (vĕ-sĭk′ū-lă) pl. **Vesiculae** (vĕ-sĭk′ū-ē″)
CYST/O (sĭs-tō)	Bladder, cyst, sac ****CHOLECYST/O** = gall bladder	Gr. *kystis,* bladder, cyst, sac	Chole**cyst**ectomy, chole**cyst**ogram, **cyst**olithectomy
PANCREAT/O (păn-krē-ă-tō)	Pancreas	L. *pancreas, pancreatis,* n. pancreas fr. Gr. *pankreas, pankreatos,* all flesh; pancreas	**Pancreat**algia, **pancreat**ic Loan word: **Pancreas** (pang′krē-ăs) **Pancreata** (pan-krē′ăt-ă)
HIAT/O (hī-ăt-ō)	An opening, gap (hiatus of the diaphragm)	L. *hiatus, -us,* m. an opening, gap	**Hiat**al, Loan word: **Hiatus** (hī-ăt′ŭs) pl. **Hiatus** (hī-ăt′ūs)

Greek or Latin word element	Current usage	Etymology	Examples
ENTER/O (ent-ĕ-rō)	Intestine (usually the small intestine)	Gr. *enteron*, that within, intestine	Gastro**enter**itis, my**enter**on, **enter**olith Loan word: **Enteron** (ĕn′tĕr-ŏn)
INTESTIN/O (in-tes-tĭn-ō)	Intestine	L. *intestinum*, *-i*, n. internal, intestine	Gastro**intestin**al, **intestin**iform Loan word: **Intestinum** (in″tĕs-tī′nŭm) pl. **Intestina** (in″tĕs-tī′nă)
DUODEN/O (dū-ō-dē-nō)	Duodenum (first part of the small intestine)	L. *duodenum*, *-i*, n. duodenum (1ˢᵗ part of the small intestine) fr. Medieval Latin *duodenum digitorum* "space of twelve digits"	**Duoden**ojejunostomy, **duoden**al Loan word: **Duodenum** (doo″ŏ-dē′nŭm) pl. **Duodena** (doo″ŏ-dē′nă)
JEJUN/O (jĕ-joon-ō)	Jejunum (second portion of the small intestine)	L. *jejunum*, *-i*, n. the jejunum, fr. Latin adjective for "empty"	**Jejun**oileal, **jejun**o**jejun**ostomy Loan word: **Jejunum** (jē-joon′ŭm) pl. **Jejuna** (jē-joon′ă)
ILE/O (il-ē-ō)	Ileum (third portion of the small intestine)	L. *ileum*, *-i*, n. the ileum	**Ile**ectomy, **Ile**ojejunostomy Loan word: **Ileum** (il′ē-ŭm) pl. **Ilea** (il′ē-ă)
CEC/O (sē-kō)	Cecum (caecum)	L. *caecum*, *-i*, n. cecum fr. Latin adjective for "blind"	Ileo**cec**al, **cec**opexy Loan word: **Cecum** (sē′kŭm) pl. **Ceca** (sē′kă)
TYPHL/O (tĭf-lō)	Cecum (caecum), blindness	Gr. *typhlos*, blind; the cecum	**Typhl**enteritis, **typhl**ectomy, nycto**typhl**osis
APPEND/O (ap-ĕn-dō) **APPENDIC/O** (ă-pen-dĭ-kō)	Appendix (something hanging onto another part/body)	L. *appendix*, *appendicis*, f. hung to, appendage; appendix fr. L. *pendere*, *pensum*, to hang	**Append**ectomy, **appendic**itis Loan word: **Appendix** (ă-pen′diks) pl. **Appendices** (ă-pen′dĭ-sēz)
COL/O (kŏ-lō) **COLON/O** (kō-lŏ-nō)	Colon	L. *colon*, *-i*, n. colon fr. Gr. *kolon*, colon	Entero**col**itis, **colon**oscopy, **col**ostomy Loan word: **Colon** (kō′lŏn) pl. **Cola** (kō′lă)
SIGMOID/O (sĭg-moyd-ō)	Sigmoid colon	Gr. *sigmoeides*, shaped like the capital sigma Σ; sigmoid colon	**Sigmoid**ectomy, **sigmoid**oproctostomy Loan word: **Sigmoid** (sĭg′moyd)
PROCT/O (prok-tol-ō)	Anus and rectum	Gr. *proktos*, anus; the rectum and anus	**Proct**ologist, **proct**itis
AN/O (ā-nō)	Anus	L. *anus*, *-i*, m. a ring, the anus	**An**ococcygeal, pre**an**al, **an**ovesical Loan word: **Anus** (ā′nŭs) pl. **Ani** (ā′nī)
RECT/O (rek-tō)	Straight, rectum (the straight terminal part of the colon, *intestinum rectum* "straight intestine")	L. *rectum*, *-i*, n. rectum fr. L. *rectus*, *-a*, *-um*, straight	**Rect**ocele, ano**rect**al, **rect**olabial Loan word: **Rectum** (rek′tŭm) pl. **Recta** (rek′tă)

Greek or Latin word element	Current usage	Etymology	Examples
SPHINCTER/O (sfĭngk-tĕr-ō)	Sphincter (ringlike muscle of an orifice)	L. *sphincter, sphincteris,* m. sphincter fr. Gr. *sphinkter,* that which binds; the sphincter	**Sphincter**algia, **sphincter**oplasty Loan word: **Sphincter** (sfingk'tĕr) pl. **Sphincteres** (sfingk'tĕr-ēz″)
PYL/O (pī-lō)	Orifice, portal vein	Gr. *pyle,* gait; orifice esp. portal vein	**Pyl**emphraxis, **pyl**ephlebectasis, **pyl**ephlebitis
PYLOR/O (pī-lor-ō)	Pylorus (portion of stomach that empties into the duodenum)	L. *pylorus, -i,* m. pylorus fr. Gr. *pyloros,* gatekeeper; the pylorus	**Pylor**omytomy, **pylor**ic, gastro**pylor**ectomy Loan word: **Pylorus** (pī-lor'ŭs) pl. **Pylori** (pī-lor'ī)
CARDI/O (kard-ē-ō)	The cardiac sphincter, heart	Gr. *kardia,* heart,**the cardiac sphincter of the stomach	**Cardi**ectomy, **cardi**ac
MESENTER/O (mĕs-ĕn-tĕr-ō)	Mesentery	L. *mesenterium, -i,* n. the mesentery	**Mesenter**itis, **mesenter**ectomy Derivative: **Mesentery** (mes'ĕn-ter″ē)
PERITONE/O (per-it-ŏ-nē-ō) **PERITON/O** (per-it-ŏ-nō)	Peritoneum	L. *peritoneum, -i,* n. peritoneum fr. Gr. *peritonaion,* stretched around; peritoneum	**Periten**eoscopy, **periton**itis Loan word: **Peritoneum** (per″it-ŏ-nē'ŭm) pl. **Peritonea** (per″it-ŏ-nē'ă)
OMENT/O (ō-mĕn'tō)	Omentum	L. *omentum, -i,* n. fat skin, caul, omentum	**Oment**otomy, **oment**ovolvulus Loan word: **Omentum** (ō-ment'ŭm) **Omenta** (ō-ment'ă)

Review	Answers
The roots used for the "mouth" are _____, _____, and _____. The anatomical Latin term for the mouth is _____. The Greek loan word _____ can be used for an "opening" or "a mouth."	**OR-, STOMAT-, STOM-** os **stoma**
The roots for "tooth" are _____ and _____. The anatomical Latin term for a "tooth" is _____.	**DENT-, ODONT-** **dens**
The roots for "lip" are _____, _____, and _____. The anatomical Latin term for a "lip" is _____.	**LABI-, CHEIL-, CHIL-** **labium**
The roots for "cheek" are _____ and _____. The anatomical Latin term for a "cheek" is _____.	**BUCC-. MEL-** **bucca**
The roots for "tongue" are _____, _____, and _____. The anatomical Latin term for a "tongue" is _____.	**GLOTT-, GLOSS-, LINGU-** **lingua**
The roots for "gum" of the mouth are _____ and _____. The anatomical Latin term for a "gum" is _____.	**GINGIV-, OUL-** **gingiva**
The root for the "whole jaw" is _____. The root for the top part of the jaw bone is _____. The root for the bottom part of the jaw bone is _____.	**GNATH-** **MAXILL-** **MANDIBUL-**
The root for the hard and soft palate of the oral cavity is _____. The anatomical Latin term is _____.	**PALAT-** **palatum**
The roots for the uvula of the oral cavity are _____ and _____. The anatomical Latin term is _____.	**UVUL-, STAPHYL-** **Uvula**
The root for the tonsil is _____. The anatomical Latin term is _____.	**TONSILL-** **tonsilla**

Review	Answers
The roots for internal organs, particularly of the abdominal cavity, are _____ and _____.	**SPLANCHN-, VISCER-**
The root for the esophagus is _____. The anatomical Latin term is _____.	**ESOPHAG-** **esophagus (oesophagus)**
The root for the stomach is _____. The suffix is _____. The anatomical Latin term is _____.	**GASTR-** **-GASTER** **gaster**
The root for sphincter is _____. The anatomical Latin term is _____.	**SPHINCTER-** **sphincter**
The root for the superior sphincter of the stomach is _____.	**CARDI-**
The root for the inferior sphincter associated with stomach is _____. The anatomical Latin term is _____.	**PYLOR-** **pylorus**
The roots for the abdomen are _____, _____, and _____. The anatomical Latin term is _____.	**ABDOMIN-, LAPAR-, CELI-** **abdomen**
The root for the serous membrane that lines the abdominal cavity is _____ and _____. The anatomical Latin term for this membrane is _____.	**PERITONE-, PERITON-** **peritoneum**
The root for the "navel"/"bellybutton" are _____ and _____. The anatomical Latin for the "navel" is _____. The loan word also meaning umbilicus is _____.	**OMPHAL-, UMBILIC-** **umbilicus** **omphalos**
The roots of the liver are _____ and _____. The anatomical Latin term is _____.	**HEPAT-, HEPAR-** **hepar**
The root for the portal vein or an orifice is _____.	**PYL-**
The roots for a duct are _____ and _____. The root for the common bile duct is _____.	**DOCH-, DUCT-** **CHOLEDOCH-**
The roots for a bladder are _____ and _____. The root of the gall bladder is _____. The anatomical Latin term for the bladder is _____.	**CYST-, VESIC-** **CHOLECYST-** **vesica**
The root for the "gap" or "opening" in the diaphragm into which the esophagus pass through is _____. The anatomical Latin term for this opening is _____.	**HIAT-** **hiatus**
The roots for the intestine are _____ and _____. The anatomical Latin term is _____.	**ENTER-, INTESTIN-** **intestinum**
The root for mesentery is _____. The anatomical Latin term is _____.	**MESENTER-** **mesenterium**
The root for the first part of the small intestine is _____. The anatomical Latin term is _____.	**DUODEN-** **duodenum**
The root for the second part of the small intestine is _____. The anatomical Latin term is _____.	**JEJUN-** **jejunum**
The root for the third part of the small intestine is _____. The anatomical Latin term is _____.	**ILE-** **ileum**
The roots for the cecum are _____ and _____. The anatomical Latin term is _____.	**CEC-, TYPHL-** **cecum**
The roots for the appendix are _____ and _____. The anatomical Latin term is _____.	**APPEND-, APPENDIC-** **appendix**
The roots for the large intestine are _____ and _____. The anatomical Latin term is _____.	**COLON-, COL-** **colon**
The root for the S-shaped part of the large intestine is _____.	**SIGMOID-**
The root for the straight part of the large intestine is _____.	**RECT-**
The root for the anus is _____. The anatomical Latin is _____.	**AN-** **Anus**
The root meaning the rectum and anus is _____.	**PROCT-**

Lessons from History: Digestion and Diet in Hippocratic and Modern Medicine

Food for Thought as You Read:

What makes diet less important to modern medicine?
How and why was diet important to Hippocratic medicine?
To what extent does the use of diet in medicine affect the patient–practitioner relationship?

The plethora of books, videos, and programs on the kinds of food one should eat attests to the high-value modern society places on a diet as a means to obtain health and wellness. However, when it comes to the treatment of disease, the use of diet to treat disease, particularly the reliance on a therapeutic diet, is often met with a high level of skepticism. This is because therapeutic diets are considered to be less effective, and therefore, ancillary at best to treating disease. The use of diet as the primary means of treating disease is often viewed as being somewhat outside of the practices of modern medicine, which, at this time, tends to rely more on surgical and chemical interventions to treat diseases. There are people who hold a strong belief in the therapeutic value of diets, but they tend to promote their methods as being natural or holistic rather than medical approaches to disease. Given that modern medicine traces its origins back to Hippocrates, we will consider the role of diet in modern and Hippocratic medicine and what potential effects the use of diet in medicine has had on patient–practitioner interactions.

The modern term **digestion** is ultimately derived from the Latin verb *digerere*, "to separate, divide, arrange." In modern medicine, the purpose of digestion is understood as the "breaking down" or "dissolving" of ingested food into nutritious components that the body can absorb. Digestion is understood as a complex mechanical and chemical process that occurs in the organs of the gastrointestinal tract (esophagus, stomach, and small and large intestines) with the assistance of the accessory digestive organs (liver, gallbladder, and pancreas). Mastication (fr. L. *masticare*, to chew), which is the chewing of food, and peristalsis (fr. *peri-* around + Gr. *stalsis*, contraction), which is the wavelike movement of the digestive tract, are the mechanical processes of digestion. Hormones, enzymes, and bile provide the chemical means by which food is broken down into smaller and absorbable molecules. The value of food is that it contains water, starches, fats, proteins, vitamins, and minerals, which are understood as the basic nutritious components that the body needs for growth and physical well-being. This modern understanding of digestion and nutrition provides the foundation for medical interventions that do not rely on dietary interventions. Thus, in modern medicine, issues with digestion are often recognized as tangible, observable, and measurable changes in the structure, as well as the chemical and mechanical functions of a digestive organ, and therefore, these problems are typically addressed by the restoration or preservation of the function of the digestive organs (i.e. esophagus, stomach, intestines, liver, bile ducts, pancreas, and gallbladder) via surgery or medication. The medical use of **hyperalimentation**, which is the enteral and parenteral infusion of solutions that contain the necessary nutritious elements for life that are not being absorbed by the patient's body due to issues with his or her GI tract, reveals that the nutritional status of the patient is determined by the standard levels of water, starches, fats, proteins, vitamins, and minerals that a human being needs.

Modern medicine uses the term **diet** in reference to a prescribed regimen of food for a particular state of health or disease. The value of food is that it contains water, starches, fats, proteins, vitamins, and minerals, which are understood as the basic nutritious components that the body needs for growth and physical well-being. Thanks in part to public education, it is almost common knowledge in western civilization that foods vary in their makeup of the nutritious components, and therefore, it is necessary to seek or avoid foods based on standard amounts needed for optimum health. In the practice of medicine, the nutritional status of a patient is determined by evaluating the levels of the nutritious components present in the patient's body, which are then compared with the scientifically established levels necessary for health. While most doctors consider diet important to health, as noted, therapeutic diets are not the primary methods that physicians use to treat diseases. Instead, a therapeutic diet is generally considered an ancillary part of the treatment of some medical conditions and diseases. Thus, when a doctor gives a recommendation for a particular diet, most often, the dietary advice consists of telling the patient what type of food should be avoided based on a particular condition or disease. For example, physicians may tell their patients to avoid fatty foods if they have been diagnosed with cholelithiasis. Sometimes, a physician will encourage a patient to eat a particular type of food in response to a disease. With hyperhomocysteinemia, the medical recommendation is to increase one's intake of folates and vitamin B_{12}. The use of dietary advice in medicine, therefore, consists of general recommendations that are linked to specific diagnoses, and these diets are prescribed mostly in the context of prevention, rather than treatment. Naturally, part of the reason for this limited use of medicine is the success of modern surgery and chemical interventions in the treatment of disease. The other reason is the limited amount of education medical students receive on nutrition and dietary recommendations. Medical students on average receive only around 11 hours of training on nutrition during the 130–180 weeks of their formal education. The learning objectives of first-year fellows in gastroenterology, the field of medicine that specializes in the treatment of GI diseases, reveal that their training focuses on diagnosing and treating diseases of digestive organs, and their primary forms of intervention are surgery, medications, and hyperalimentation. In other words, there is not a specialty in medical school that focuses on diet as a form of treatment. Recently, there have been programs established, such as Cleveland Clinic's Nutrition Fellowship Program and National Board of Physician Nutrition Specialists, that have attempted to fill this void by educating and certifying physicians in nutrition and dietary interventions. Nevertheless, it is the registered dietitian nutritionist, rather than the physician, that is recognized as the expert in diets since his or her primary job is to assess, educate, and manage patients with special nutritional needs. Therefore, while dietary advice is a part of modern medicine, it is not central to the practices that identify one as a physician.

Although our term "diet" is derived from the ancient Greek term *diaita*, there are important differences in their meanings. Similar to the modern definition of diet, *diaita* commonly refers to the habitual food and drink of a person or group of people. However, in addition to an alimentary diet, *diaita* could refer to the regular activities of a person (e.g. exercise, sleep, clothing, fasting, bathing, massage, sex, etc.). What holds all of these together is the belief that food and the aforementioned activities of life have qualitative effects on the body (e.g. drying, heating, cooling, moistening, thickening, and thinning), which explains why some Hippocratic authors extended the technical meaning of *diaita* to nonalimentary habits. Thus, in the Hippocratic Corpus, *diaita*, which is often translated as "regimen," was a common technical term that broadly meant "a way of life, or habitual behavior." Ancient physicians' use of *diaita*, therefore, required them to be highly involved in almost every aspect of a patient's life, which may also explain the emphasis on patient confidentiality in the original Hippocratic Oath. Therefore, the Hippocratic use of *diaita* shaped the nature of the patient–physician relationship.

Diaita was understood as being central to the practice and identity of ancient Greek physicians because it was their primary form of medical intervention, appearing frequently in their discussions of the treatment of diseases. There is also a collection of works in the Hippocratic Corpus, such as *On Regimen, On Nutrition, Regimen in Acute Diseases*, and *Regimen in Health,* that are dedicated to the use of *diaita* to treat a wide variety of pathological conditions and to preserve the health of people with different constitutions. In the first book of the four books that make up *On Regimen*, the author claims that a physician must not only know the nature of human body, but also the nature of different foods and exercises to recognize and treat the unhealthy constitution of a patient. Book II of *On Regimen* discusses knowledge of the external environment, particularly the winds and the corresponding qualities they bring, that will have an effect on the human body. For example, he claims the following: "the southern countries are hotter and drier than the northern; because they are very near the sun. The races of men and plants in these countries must of necessity be drier, hotter and stronger than those which are in the opposite countries." This information allows the physician to choose the right *diaita* for a group of people based on their environment. In many respects, the advice in *Regimen II* resembles the advice given in the famous Hippocratic work *Airs, Waters, and Places*. The author of *Airs, Waters, and Places* advises physicians who plan to travel to a new area to treat patients to pay attention to the prevailing winds, changes in weather, and water in order to recognize the physical constitution of the people. In addition to the nature of the external environment where people live, the author of *Airs, Waters, and Places* recommends that a physician must consider the *diaita* of people:

> The mode of life (*diaita*), too, that the inhabitants prefer, whether they are given to drink, they take lunch, and they are adverse to exertion, or they like exercise and effort, they eat heartily, and they drink little.
> L. 2.13 trans. Paul Potter in Loeb edition of *Airs, Waters, and Places*, 2022.

In what follows in *Airs, Waters, and Places*, it becomes quite evident that the alimentary diets of different groups of people appear to correspond to the environments in which they live, and therefore, knowledge of society's *diaita* allows a physician to anticipate the kinds of diseases groups of peoples are prone to suffer.

The title and subject matter of *Regimen in Acute Diseases* and *Regimen in Health* reveal that *diaita*, particularly alimentary diets, could and should be modified to meet the individual needs of patients in different states of health and disease. Acute diseases, such as pleurisy, pneumonia, phrenitis, and fevers, have their own unique requirements, particularly because these types of diseases are often fatal in antiquity and there is a limited window of opportunity to treat them. In addition to providing advice on the use of foods such as barley gruel, hydromel, and oxymel, the author stresses to avoid making radical changes to the patient's diet with acute disease because this will adversely affect the patient. Thus, ancient physicians perceived food as having the power to make quick and significant changes to the human body. The recommendations made in the Hippocratic *On Regimen in Health*, which is a work some have argued is actually a part of *On the Nature of Man*, demonstrate that a broad range of activities, such as walks, baths, emetics, and enemas, were part of the regimen used to preserve a patient's health. The author of *On Regimen in Health* advises that one should consider factors such as the individual's constitution, age, sex, normal activity, and the season before creating a healthy regimen for a patient. As with many other discussions of therapeutic regimens in the Hippocratic Corpus, the physicians' recommendations were based on the patient's individual needs, which the physician should be trained to recognize.

Theoretical conceptions of digestion provided the basis for ancient Greek medicine's use of alimentary cures for disease. The word *pepsis* is one of the words used by ancient Greek authors to describe what happens to ingested food in the abdomen. In everyday Greek, *pepsis* literally meant "softening or ripening by means of heat," "cooking," and "boiling"; *pepsis* is rendered as "digestion" or "coction" in modern translations of ancient Greek medical texts. Cognates of the Greek verb *sepein* (to ferment, putrefy), from which we get our pathological term **sepsis**, is the other commonly used term for digestion in Greek medical texts. For instance, the author of the Hippocratic work *On Anatomy* refers to the stomach as the "septic cavity" (*septike koilia*). Given that heat is often an accompanying factor in the putrefaction of food, it seems that with the use of either word, *sepein* or *pepsis*, ancient Greek physicians likened human digestion to the observable effects that heat has on food. As to the source of this heat, according to Ps. Soranus *Medical Questions* 61, Hippocrates and Diocles disagreed as to whether digestion was derived from putrefaction/fermentation of the food in the abdomen or whether an innate heat of the body altered the food. According to the humoral physiologies found in Hippocratic texts, the purpose of digestion was to soften the food into humors that the body needed for nourishment, health, and growth. If the food was not properly digested, it was said to overpower the body and be a source of a wide variety of diseases. Thus, simply changing the thickness of the food in response to the patient's illness is one of the ways a physician was said to modify the food to meet the body's ability to digest. Owing to this concept of digestion, it is not surprising that ancient Greek medicine paid enormous attention to the food that patients ate. What is somewhat surprising, at least to many modern readers, is that the Hippocratic author of *On Ancient Medicine* argues that the origin of medicine itself is based on the art of modifying foods for people who are sick:

> The art of medicine would neither have been discovered, nor even looked for – as there would have been no need for medicine – if sick people had benefited by the same mode of living and regimen as the food, drink and mode of living used by people in health, and if there had been no other things better for the sick than these. But in fact, it was sheer necessity that caused humans to seek and to discover medicine, because the sick did not, and do not, benefit by the same regimen as the healthy."
>
> Trans. Paul Potter in Loeb edition of *Ancient Medicine*, p. 13, 2022.

Greek medicine's belief in food as the primary treatment of disease perhaps influenced this author's history of medicine. Nevertheless, such a history of medicine reflects the public face of Greek medicine in that the physician's primary role was to recognize the nature of food and the alimentary needs of his patient.

As to what is considered nutritious, the author of the Hippocratic work *On Nutrition* provides a collection of aphorisms on nutrition (*trophe*) that point to the theoretical principles behind the use of food in medicine. It should be noted that the ancient Greek medical definition of *trophe* differs from our modern understanding of nutrition. Firstly, the substances of *trophe* in this text are more than liquid and dry food; breath is *trophe* to the lungs, and pus is said to be *trophe* to wounds. *Trophe* can produce fluids that are fundamental to life; human milk and blood, which are derived from the digestion of food, are said to be created from the surplus of *trophe* (36). A substance must have a power/faculty (*dynamis*) to be considered *trophe* (21). Via its faculties, *trophe* is said to affect the whole body (7). Some of the broad qualitative characteristics of the faculties of *trophe* are that they strengthen, augment, attenuate, assimilate, or dissimilate according to the nature of the part of the body (2). There are various natures of the *dynamis* of *trophe* (13); heating and cooling, as well as other qualities, fall under the author's definition of a *dynamis*. The author explains that whatever *trophe* comes upon and overpowers, it will make similar to the *trophe*'s nature (*physis*) and faculty (*dynamis*) (3). Thus, depending on the part of the body, the *dynamis* of warming could be good or bad (12). In regards to food, some foods are suitable to certain people but not to others (33). For example, one should consider what foods a person is accustomed to (33), and the age of the person (41). When selecting food for a patient, one should consider how easily it is changed and therefore how easily it will be digested (49), as well as the speed of the effects of the food (50).

Regimen II provides a wealth of information on the kinds of foods used in *diaita*. It lists in order the properties of grains, beans, animals, eggs, cheese, water, honey, vegetables, and fruits before it moves to the non-alimentary parts of regimen. By discussing the medicinal value of eating scorpion fish, fox, and hedgehog, one can appreciate how varied the diets of Greeks living in different regions may have been. The author begins his discussion of food and drink by making the following remark: "The power (*dynamis*) of each food and drink, what they are by nature and what by art, it is necessary to discern." Again, the fundamental concept of each food is that it has a particular faculty/power that is derived from its basic nature and from the medical art of modifying food for its therapeutic effect on the body. Some of these descriptions are longer than others; the following description of Cyceon is a good example of the nature of these entries:

> Cyceon made with barley only added to water cools and nourishes, with wine it heats, nourishes and is astringent. With honey it heats and nourishes less, but is more laxative unless the honey be unmixed; with unmixed honey it is astringent. With milk all cyceons are nourishing; made with sheep's milk they are astringent, with goats' milk they are more laxative, with cows' milk less, but with mares' or asses' milk they are more laxative.
>
> Trans. W. H. Jones in Loeb edition of *Regimen II*, p. 311, 1931.

Cyceon was a beverage in ancient Greece that usually consisted of barley and some liquid, typically water. The medicinal value of Cyceon is closely connected to its faculties, which in turn are modified by the addition of water, wine, honey, and various types of milk. Modification of cyceon by adding water or wine can change it from being cold or being hot, but in both cases, it retains its nourishing quality. The faculties of hot and cold are part of its therapeutic value, which one can deduce has to do with the theory of opposites, namely that diseases of a particular quality are treated with *diaita* of an opposing quality (hot versus cold, wet versus dry, etc.). The other faculties discussed are "nourishing" and "laxative." Their therapeutic value has to do with the movement of the food in the body; nourishing equates to the thickening of the body and laxative equates to the thinning of the body. What is interesting about this account is that there is no mention of specific diseases for which *cyceon* is said to be therapeutic. Rather, it appears that the physician's art is to deduce not only which alimentary *diaita* by innate faculty and by the art of modifying food best addresses the nature of the disease and the patient. While such qualitative faculties of foods seem foreign to our own understanding of the nutritive value of food, the notion that unseen elements of food are what make them healthy or unhealthy is somewhat similar to our understanding. Likewise, both ancient Greek medicine and modern medicine recognize that adding ingredients or modifying a basic ingredient can have an effect on a food's value to the body. Unlike their modern counterparts, ancient Greek physicians were not only expected to be able to speak about the medicinal value of a wide variety of foods, but they were also supposed to know how to modify foods for their patients.

From this discussion, one can recognize that diet played a central role in the practice of Hippocratic medicine. The practice of *diaita* in ancient Greek medicine put the physician in control of much of a patient's day-to-day life. It can also be understood that a patient's expectations of a physician's knowledge of foods were much different than they are today. In some regards, medicine's technical treatment of this subject may have helped to promote a widespread belief in the effectiveness of *diaita* in the treatment of disease and thereby establish an orthodox view of the therapeutic value of food in ancient Greek society.

Some Suggested Readings

Hippocrates. *Nature of Man. Regimen in Health. Humours. Aphorisms. Regimen 1-3. Dreams*. Translated by W. H. S. Jones. Loeb Classical Library 150. Cambridge, MA: Harvard University Press, 1931.

Hippocrates. *Ancient Medicine. Airs, Waters, Places. Epidemics 1 and 3. The Oath. Precepts. Nutriment*. Edited and translated by Paul Potter. Loeb Classical Library 147. Cambridge, MA: Harvard University Press, 2022.

Jouanna, Jacques. "*Dietetics in Hippocratic Medicine: Definition, Main Problems, Discussion*." In *Greek Medicine from Hippocrates to Galen: Selected Papers*. Trans. N. Allies and ed. P. J. van der Eijk. 137–154. Leiden: Brill, 2012.

Scarborough, John. "*Eating, Digestion, and Elimination*." In *Medical and Biological Terminologies*. Norman: University of Oklahoma Press, 1992.

Etymological Explanations: Common Terms and Word Elements for Aliment, Digestion, and Defecation

Aliment

Aliment – Derived from the Latin *alimentum*, **aliment** means food or nourishment. *Alimentum* comes from the Latin verb *alere*, "to nourish, support." This also is the origin of the adjective used in Alma Mater, which means "nourishing mother." The gastrointestinal tract is also called the alimentary tract because of its association with the digestion of food. The Greek and Latin roots used for "food" are **ALIMENT-**, **CIB-**, and **SIT-**. The root **CIB-** also carries the meaning of "meal," which is evident in the medical abbreviations a.c. (*ante cibum*) and p.c. (*post cibum*) used in prescriptions for "before meal" and "after meal." The root **SIT-** is derived from the Greek word for "grain," and in some instances, its meaning is delimited to "grain." That said, grain was tantamount to food in antiquity since the vast majority of most Greek and Roman diets involved eating grains. This is evident in the Greek terms for a human being. For example, in Book 2.168, Herodotus uses *siton edontes* (σῖτον ἔδοντες), which means "eaters of grain/bread" as a general epithet for human beings as opposed to beasts. This notion of what one eats defines who they are is also evident in Greek myth. For instance, in the *Odyssey*, Odysseus' journeys take him to the land of the "lotus-eaters" (*lotophagi*), whose name alone reveals they are not like other humans. Their diet of lotus led to lethargy, forgetfulness, and apathy. SIT- is also the root used in the term "parasite." In ancient Greek, a *parasitos* was "one who eats at another one's table," in other words, one who lives at another's expense. Hence, in the 2nd century AD, Lucian wrote a work called *The Parasitic Art*, which is a satirical explanation of how to sponge off others.

Fat – Fat is the macronutrient that is oxidized into carbon dioxide and water to produce energy. The primary roots used for "fat" are **LIP-**, **ADIP-**, and **STEAT-**.

Protein – Protein is the macronutrient essential for the growth of new tissue or the repair of damaged tissue. The term is derived from the Greek word *proteios*, which means "first" or "primary," because it was believed to be a constituent of food essential to life. The roots used for "protein" are **PROTE-** and **ALBUMIN-**. Derived from the Latin word for egg whites, *albumen*, **albumin** refers to groups of simple proteins found in both plant and animal tissues.

Carbohydrate – Carbohydrates are the macronutrient used as a basic source of energy for the body. They are stored in the body as glycogen. Starch is carbohydrate found in grains, fruits, and vegetables that is broken down into disaccharides. The root used for "starch" is **AMYL-**. Carbohydrates are further broken down for absorption by the body. Carbohydrates are absorbed as **glucose**, **galactose**, or **fructose**. In respect to food, the suffix commonly used for "carbohydrates" is **-OSE** (e.g. fructose, glucose, dextrose, levulose, sucrose, galactose, and lactose), in other contexts **-OSE** means "of the nature" and "relating to" (e.g. adenose). On account of its root meaning "fruit," fructose is known as "fruit sugar." In addition to **FRUCT-**, the roots for "fruit" are **MEL-** and **CARP-**. The root in glucose means "sugar" and "sweet." Similarly, the root in sucrose means "sugar." The chemical distinction between these two is that glucose is a monosaccharide and sucrose is a disaccharide. In addition to **SUCR-**, the roots that can be used for "sugar" are **GLUC-**, **GLYC-**, and **SACCHAR-**, and **MELIT-**. Glucose is also called **dextrose** and fructose is called **levulose**. Since both fructose and glucose share the same empirical formula $C_6H_{12}O_6$, the different chemical chirality is being expressed in these terms: **dextrose** being "right-handed" and **levulose** being "left-handed" in chirality. **Galactose** is an isomer of glucose. Lactose is a disaccharide whose hydrolysis leads to glucose and galactose. In ancient Greek, both **GALACT-** and **LACT-** meant "milk." While both roots are used today for "milk," **GALACT-** also has the meaning of "galaxy." This meaning extends back to the ancient Greeks calling "the Milky Way" the *galaxias kyklos* (milky circle). According to Hyginus' *Astronomica* (2.43), the Milky Way was formed from the milk of the breast of Hera. This occurred when Zeus tried to place the infant Heracles at the breast of Hera while she was asleep (Hera was not at all fond of Heracles since he was the son of Zeus and a mortal, Alcmene). The goddess woke from her sleep and pushed Heracles away in disgust, and the milk that flowed forth formed the Milky Way.

Gluten – Gluten is a protein found in some grains including wheat, barley, and rye that acts like a binder. Intolerance to gluten is associated with celiac disease. Derived from the Latin word for "glue," the root **GLUTIN-** means "gluten," as well a "sticky" and "adhesive." Thus, in Classical Latin, a *glutinator* was someone who glued together books.

Digestion

Digestion – Digestion is the process by which food is broken down mechanically and chemically in the gastrointestinal tract for use by the body. The word "digestion" comes from the Latin verb *digerere, digestum*, to separate. While our notions of digestion are quite different from ancient Greek physicians', the suffix (**-PEPSIA**) and roots (**PEPT-** and **PEPS-**) that we use for "digestion" are derived from the Greek word, *pepsis*. For example, the technical term for indigestion is **dyspepsia** and a **peptic ulcer** is a lesion found in the digestive tract.

Metabolism – Formed from the Greek word for "change," *metabole*, Metabolism is the process of changing food into energy. Metabolism involves the two processes of **anabolism** (constructive metabolism) and **catabolism** (destructive metabolism).

Mastication – The act of mechanically breaking food down via chewing is called **mastication**. The term comes from the Greek verb *massein*, "to knead" or "massage." The Greek word *masesis* means "chewing," and it appears as a suffix **-MASESIS** in words such as **dysmasesis**. Hence, the Greek term *maseter* means chewer, which is why the muscle of the jaw is called the **masseter**.

Saliva – Digestion begins in the oral cavity, where food is broken down by chewing (i.e. mastication) and the effects of saliva's chemical enzymes. In addition to **PTYAL-**, the roots for saliva are **SALIV-** and **SIAL-**. After the food has been masticated in the mouth, it forms a mass called a **bolus**, which is then swallowed. The roots used for "eating" and "swallowing" are **PHAG-** and **VOR-**. The aforementioned bolus moves down the esophagus into the stomach, where it is further broken down with enzymes.

Enzymes – Carbohydrates, proteins, and fats are broken down by enzymes into their basic units: carbohydrates into sugars, proteins into amino acids, fats into fatty acids, and glycerol. The root used for "enzyme" is **ZYM-**. The suffixes for enzyme are **-ASE** and **-ZYME**, the former being used most commonly. **Lipase**, which is created in the pancreas, breaks down fats. **Protease**, which is formed in pancreas, breaks down proteins. **Amylase**, which is formed in the mouth and pancreas, breaks down complex carbohydrates, also known as starches.

Chyme and Chyle – The aforementioned bolus moves down the esophagus into the stomach, where it is further broken down with enzymes. Having been broken down, it leaves the stomach as a semisolid fluid. This thick semifluid mass of partly digested food and enzymes in the intestines is called **chyme**, and its root is **CHYM-**. The term chyme is easily confused with the other fluid of the digestive track, **chyle**. Lymphatic fluid with emulsified fats in it is called chyle, and its root is **CHYL-**. In ancient Greek *chymos* and *chylos* were indistinct, meaning simply "a humor."

Bile – Duodenal digestion of chyme involves biliary and pancreatic secretions. Bile/gall is a thick, bitter-tasting fluid that is secreted by the liver and stored in the gall bladder. Through the common bile duct, bile enters into the duodenum, where it emulsifies fats. The roots for "bile" are **BIL-** and **CHOL-**. After the nutriments of the chyme have been absorbed in the intestines, the remnant material moves into the colon, which has the primary role to gradually dehydrate this content until it becomes the consistency of normal feces.

Defecation

Defecation – Defecation is the evacuation of bowels of fecal material. The suffix for defecation is **-CHEZIA**.

Feces – Feces is the bodily waste discharged from the bowels. The Greek and Latin roots for fecal material are **SCAT-**, **COPR-**, **FEC-**, **STERC-**, and **STERCOR-**. Quite a number of euphemisms form the loan words that we use for fecal material: feces, excrement, excreta, dejecta, and stool. **Feces** is derived from the Latin *faeces*, which meant "sediment" or "dregs." In other words, *faeces* originally referred to the solid remnants of wine that were not suitable for consumption. **Excrement** and **excreta** come from the Latin verb *excernere*, which means "to separate, sift, or sort." Thus, the agrarian metaphor is such that the excreta represents the inedible chaff that is separated from grain at a threshing floor. **Dejecta** simply means "what is thrown out." The term "**stool**" comes from the Old English word stol "seat for one person." Thus, the seat one sat on to defecate became the name for the product of defecation.

Greek or Latin word element	Current usage	Etymology	Examples
ALIMENT/O (al-ĭ-měnt-ō)	Food	L. *alimentum, -i,* n. nourishment, food	**Aliment**ary, **aliment**otherapy Derivative: **Aliment** (al'ĭ-měnt)
CIB/O (sī-bō)	Food, meal	L. *cibus, -i,* food	**Cib**ophobia, post**cib**al
SIT/O (sī-tō)	Food, grain	Gr. *sitos,* grain; food	**Sit**ology, para**site**
FRUCT/O (frŭk-tō)	Fruit, fructose	L. *fructus, -us,* m. fruit	**Fruct**okinase, **fruct**ose
CARP/O (kăr-pō)	Fruit	Gr. *karpos,* fruit, seed	A**carp**ous, allo**carp**y
LACT/O (lak-tō)	Milk, lactose	L. *lac, lactis,* n. milk*	**Lact**igerous, **lact**ose
GALACT/O (gă-lăk-tō)	Milk, galactose, galaxy	Gr. *gala, galaktos,* milk, Milk Way	**Galact**ocele, **galact**ose
GLUC/O (gloo-kō) **GLYC/O** (glī-kō)	Sugar, glucose	Gr. *glykys,* sweet; sugar, glucose	**Glyc**ogenic, **gluc**ogenesis
SACCHAR/O (sak-ă-rō)	Sugar	Gr. *sakcharon,* sugar	**Sacchar**olytic, di**sacchar**ide

Greek or Latin word element	Current usage	Etymology	Examples
MELIT/O (mel-ĭ-tō)	Honey, sugar, bees	Gr. *meli, melitos*, honey; sugar	**Melit**uria, **melit**emia
AMYL/O (am-ĭ-lō)	Starch	Gr. *amylon*, starch	**Amyl**odyspepsia, **amyl**ase
PROTE/O (prōt-ē-ō)	Protein, first, primary	Gr. *proteios*, first; protein	**Prote**ase, **prote**opepsis
ALBUMIN/O (al-bū-mĭ-nō)	Albumin, protein	L. *albumen, albuminis*, n. egg white; albumen protein	**Albumin**ocholia, **albumin**uria Derivative: **Albumin** (al-bū′mĭn)
LIP/O (lĭp-ō)	Fat	Gr. *lipos*, fat	**Lip**oblast, **lip**oma
STEAT/O (stē-ă-tō)	Fat, sebum	Gr. *stear, steatos*, fat, oil; sebum	**Steat**orrhea, hypo**steat**olysis
GLUTIN/O (gloo-tĭn-ō)	Sticky, adhesive, gluten	L. *gluten, glutinis*, n. glue	**Glutin**ous, ag**glutin**ation, con**glutin**ant Loan word: **Gluten** (gloot′ĕn)
ZYM/O (zī-mō) **-ZYME** (zīm)	Enzyme, fermentation	Gr. *zyme*, ferment; enzyme	**Zym**ogen, allo**zyme**
-ASE (ās)	Enzyme	Suffix used for "enzyme"	Amyl**ase**, lip**ase**
-OSE (ōs)	Carbohydrate	Suffix used for "carbohydrate"	Fruct**ose**, dextr**ose**
PHAG/O (făg-ō)	To swallow, eat	Gr. *phagein*, to swallow	A**phag**ia, **phag**ocyte
VOR/O (vō-rō)	To devour, eat	L. *vorare*, to devour	**Vor**acious, carni**vore**
BOL/O (bō-lō)	Mass of masticated food, lump, mass	Gr. *bolos*, rounded mass, lump, clod	Sphygmo**bolo**gram, pilo**bolus** Loan word: **Bolus** (bō′lŭs)
PEPT/O (pĕp-tō) **PEPS/O** (pĕp-sō)	Digestion	Gr. *peptein*, to cook, digestion	**Pept**ic, dys**peps**ia
CHOL/E (kō-lē)	Bile	Gr. *chole*, bile, gall; bitter anger	**Chol**ecystectomy, **chol**era
BIL/I (bil-ĭ)	Bile	L. *bilis, -is* f. bile	**Bil**igenic, **bil**ification
SIAL/O (sī-al-ō)	Saliva	Gr. *sialon*, saliva	**Sial**oadenitis, glyco**sial**ia
SALIV/O (să-lĭ-vō)	Saliva	L. *saliva, -ae*, f. saliva	**Saliv**ation, **saliv**ator Loan word: **Saliva** (să-lī′vă)
CHYL/O (kī-lō)	Chyle (fluid of the lymph system)	Gr. *chylos*, humor	**Chyl**ocele, **chyl**othorax Derivative: **Chyle** (kīl)

Greek or Latin word element	Current usage	Etymology	Examples
CHYM/O (kī-mō)	Chyme (nearly liquid mass of digested foot)	Gr. *chymos*, humor	**Chym**ase Derivative: **Chyme** (kīm)
STERC/O (stĕr-kō) **STERCOR/O** (stĕr-kō-rō)	Feces	L. *stercus*, *stercoris*, n. feces	**Sterc**olith, **stercor**acious Loan word: **Stercus** (stĕr′kŭs)
COPR/O (kop-rō)	Feces	Gr. *kopros*, feces	**Copr**olalia, **copr**olite
SCAT/O (skă-tō)	Feces	Gr *skor*, *skateos*, feces	**Scat**ology, **scat**ologic
FEC/O (fē-kō)	Feces	L. *faex*, *faecis*, f. dregs of wine; feces	**Fec**al, de**fec**ation Loan word: **Feces** (fē′sēz″)
-CHEZIA (kē-zē-ă)	Defecation	Gr. *chezein*, to defecate	Hemato**chezia**, dys**chezia**
EXCRET- (ĕks-krē-tō)	Defecation	L. *excernere*, to separate	**Excret**ion, **excret**ory Loan word: **Excreta** (ĕks-krē′tă)

Review	Answers
The roots for digestion are_____ and _____.	**PEPT-, PEPS-**
The roots for fecal material are _____, _____, _____, _____, and _____. The suffix for defecation is _____.	**COPR-, SCAT-, FEC-, STERC-, STERCOR-** **-CHEZIA**
Bile/gall is a thick, bitter-tasting fluid that is secreted by the liver and stored in the gall bladder. Through the common bile duct, bile enters into the duodenum, where it emulsifies fats. The roots for "bile" are _____ and _____.	**BIL-, CHOL-**
The roots for "food" are _____, _____, and _____.	**SIT-, CIB-, ALIMENT-**
In addition to MEL-, the roots for "fruit" are _____ and _____.	**FRUCT-, CARP-**
The roots used for "milk" are _____ and _____.	**LACT-, GALACT-**
In addition to SUCR-, the roots used for "sugar" are _____, _____, and _____, and _____.	**GLYC-, GLUC-, SACCHAR-, MELIT-**
The roots used for "protein" are _____ and _____.	**PROTE-, ALBUMIN-**
The root used for "starch" is _____.	**AMYL-**
The roots used for "fat" are _____ and _____.	**LIP-, STEAT-**
The root used of "gluten" is _____.	**GLUTIN-**
The root used for "enzyme" is _____. The suffixes for enzyme are _____ and _____.	**ZYM-** **-ASE, -ZYME**
The suffix commonly used for "carbohydrates" is _____.	**-OSE**
The roots used for "eating" are _____ and _____.	**PHAG-, VOR-**
The root for "appetite" is _____.	**OREX-**
In addition to PTYAL-, which also mean "spit", the roots for saliva are _____ and _____.	**SALIV-, SIAL-**
Lymphatic fluid with emulsified fats in it is called _____, and its root is _____.	**chyle, CHYL-**
The thick semifluid mass of partly digested food and enzymes in the intestines is called _____, and its root is _____.	**chyme, CHYM-**
A soft round mound of masticated food in the upper digestive tract is called a _____.	**bolus**

Etymological Explanations: Common Terms and Word Elements for Pathologies of the Gastrointestinal System

Signs and symptoms of GI pathologies

Dyspepsia – Formed from the prefix for "faulty, painful," **DYS-**, and the compound suffix for "a condition of digestion," -**PEPSIA**, dyspepsia is the technical term for indigestion. Dyspepsia is an upper GI tract discomfort characterized by symptoms as eructation, flatulence, nausea, loss of appetite, or upper abdominal pain.

Dysphagia – Formed from the prefix for "faulty, painful," **DYS-**, and the compound suffix for "a condition of swallowing," -**PHAGIA**, dysphagia is a problem/dysfunction associated with swallowing (eating) food.

Anorexia – Formed from the prefix for "no, not," **AN-**, and the compound suffix for "a condition of appetite," "hunger," -**OREXIA**, anorexia is a lack of appetite.

Eructation – The term for belching. It is derived from the Latin verb *eructare*, which means "to belch forth, throw up, vomit." In medical terms, eructation is delimited to belching.

Emesis – The loan word for vomiting is **emesis**. The suffix -**EMESIS** and the root **EMET-** also means "vomit." Thus, vomiting blood would be called **hematemesis**, and an **antiemetic** is used to stop vomiting.

Nausea – An unpleasant feeling in the throat and/or stomach that may or may not result in vomiting is called nausea. The root **NAUSE-** is used for "nausea." The term nausea originally meant sea-sickness, which is evident from its root **NAUS-**, which meant "ship" in Greek. The root **NAUT-** can mean "ship," "sailor," or "sailing." Hence, an astronaut is a "sailor of the stars."

Flatulence – The passing of gas is called flatulence. The loan word **flatus** and its root **FLAT-** mean "gas in the GI system."

Halitosis – A condition of bad breath. The root **HALIT-** is used for "bad breath." This medical term is derived from the Latin word for "breath, exhalation, and vapor," *halitus*.

Hematochezia – Derived from the Greek root for "blood," **HEMAT-**, and the suffix for defecation, -**CHEZIA**, hematochezia is the discharge of feces with bright red blood.

Melena – Derived from the Greek word for black, *melanos*, the black tarry feces caused by bleeding higher up in the gastrointestinal tract.

Steatorrhea – Derived from the root for "fat," **STEAT-**, and suffix for discharge -**RRHEA**, steatorrhea is a discharge of fatty stool/fecal material.

Diarrhea – The frequent passage of loose, unformed stools is termed diarrhea. As *diarrhoia*, this pathological term first appears in the 5th- and 4th-century-BC medical texts of the Hippocratic Corpus, and it appears to be derived from the Greek verb *diarrhein*, "to flow through."

Peptic ulcers – A peptic ulcer is an ulcer of the digestive tract, typically the stomach. A small ulcer of the mouth, as with thrush, is called an **aphtha**. In addition to **ULCER-**, the root **HELC-** is also used for "ulcer." **APHTH-** is primarily used for mouth ulcers.

Ascites – An accumulation of excess fluid in the peritoneal cavity. **ASC-** is a root that means "sac" and "saclike." It is derived from the Greek word, *askos*, that was used for a large leather bag made from an animal hide (Figs. 13.9 and 13.10).

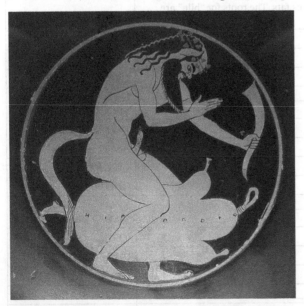

Fig. 13.9 Image of a red-figured kylix (6th century BC), depicting a satyr drinking wine while straddling a large *askos* (wineskin). *Source:* Mark Landon/Wikimedia Commons/Public domain.

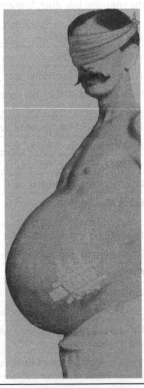

Fig. 13.10 Image of a man with ascites from Hare's *Practical Diagnosis*, 1899. *Source:* Hobart Amory Hare/Wikimedia Commons/Public domain.

Inflammations of the GI system

Somatitis – Inflammation of the mouth.

Cheilitis – Inflammation of the lips.

Sialoadenitis – Inflammation of the salivary gland.

Glossitis – Inflammation of the tongue.

Gingivitis or oulitis – Inflammation of the gums.

Esophagitis – Inflammation of the esophagus.

Gastritis – Inflammation of the stomach.

Gastroenteritis – Inflammation of the stomach and intestines.

Enteritis – Inflammation of the small intestines.

Colitis or colonitis – Inflammation of the large intestine.

Appendicitis – Inflammation of the appendix.

Proctitis – Inflammation of the anus and rectum.

Peritonitis – Inflammation of the peritoneum.

Cholecystitis – Inflammation of the gallbladder.

Cholangitis – Inflammation of the bile duct.

Pancreatitis – Inflammation of the pancreas.

Pathologies of the esophagus

Cardiochalasia – Relaxation of the cardiac sphincter. The compound suffix **-CHALASIA** in this word is derived from the Greek verb *chalaein*, "to slacken, relax." It is commonly used for a sphincter which is unable to close. Conversely, **achalasia** is the failure of a sphincter to open (e.g. **cardiospasm**).

Esophageal varices – Varicose veins located in the lower part of the esophagus. As discussed in the chapter on the cardiovascular system, a **varix** is a swollen, twisted vein. The nominative plural form of varix is **varices**.

Gastroesophageal reflux – Inflammation of the esophagus due to backflow of gastric juices. Derived from the Latin verb *fluere* (to flow), the roots **FLUX-, FLU-, FLUCT-** are commonly used for "flow." Similarly, derived from the Latin word for "river," *fluvius*, the root **FLUVI-** is used for "a river" or "river-like thing" (e.g. fluviomarine, river, and sea).

Pathologies of the intestines

Hernia – A hernia is a protrusion of an anatomical structure, typically an intestine, through the wall that normally contains it. The suffix that can mean "hernia" is **-CELE**, and its root is **HERNI-**. The term hernia is derived from the medieval Latin *hirnia*, which in turn comes from the classical Latin word for "intestine," *hira*. While hernias are generally externally observable or palpable, some hernias are not. The **hiatal hernia** is one in which part of the stomach moves up through the hiatus of the diaphragm into the thoracic cavity (Figs. 13.11 and 13.12).

Fig. 13.11 Image of a paraesophageal hernia; a paraesophageal or hiatal hernia occurs when part of the stomach moves up into the thoracic cavity via the hiatus of the diaphragm. *Source:* Adapted from SMART-Servier Medical Art, part of LaboratoiresServier.

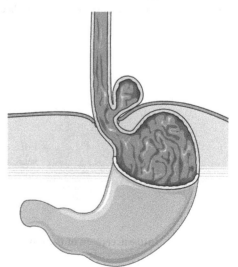

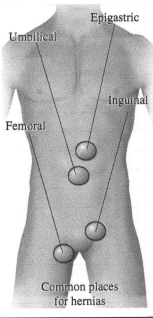

Femoral

Umbilical

Epigastric

Inguinal

Common places
for hernias

Fig. 13.12 Image of some of the common sites of
intestinal hernias. *Source:* Adapted from Blausen.com
staff (2014).

Prolapse – A prolapse is the falling or dropping down of an organ or internal part. The suffix that can mean "prolapse" is -**PTOSIS**.
In Classical Latin, a *lapsus* is a slip, falling, and its root **LAPS-** appears in terms such as collapse and relapse (Fig. 13.13).

(a)   (b)

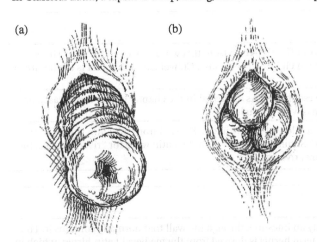

Fig. 13.13 Image (a) depicts a full-thickness external rectal
prolapse, and image (b) depicts a mucosal prolapse.

Intussusception – Formed from the Latin word elements that mean "to receive within," intussusception is the prolapse of an
intestine into another part of the intestine just below it. The outer part of the intestine is designated by the active participle
intussuscipiens (the receiving within part) and the part of the intestine inside of the other is designated with the passive perfect
participle **intussusceptum** (the part having been received in) (Fig. 13.14).

Fig. 13.14 Intussusception of the
colon. *Source:* Adapted from Blausen.
com staff (2014).

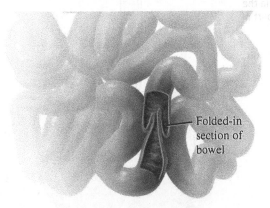

Folded-in
section of
bowel

Intussusception of the bowel

Volvulus – A volvulus is the rolling or twisting of an intestine on itself, which causes an obstruction. Problems with the mesentery, such as a prolapsed mesentery, are often the cause of a volvulus. The root **VOLV-** in volvulus comes from the Latin verb *volvere*, "to roll," and this root carries this meaning in other contexts (e.g. evolve and revolve). Humorously, the name of the car known as the Volvo in Classical Latin means "I roll" (Fig. 13.15).

Fig. 13.15   Intestinal volvulus. *Source:* Adapted from Encyclopædia Britannica (11th ed.), v. 14, (1911).

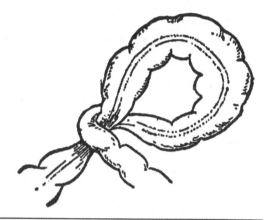

Diverticulitis – Formed from the Latin word meaning a turning out, **diverticulum** is an abnormal side pocket in an intestine. More than one diverticulum would be **diverticula**. The presence of diverticula in the intestines is called **diverticulosis**, and the inflammation of these side pockets is known as **diverticulitis**. As we have learned, the root **VERT-** (and **VERS-**) is from the Latin verb *vertere*, which mean "to turn." Diverticulum appears to be from the classical Latin word, *deverticulum*, which was "a byway on path or road" (Fig. 13.16).

Fig. 13.16   Image of colon with diverticula.

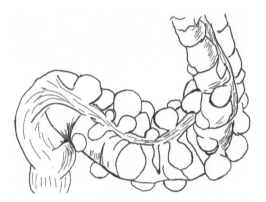

Polyp – A polyp is an abnormal growth (tumor) that emanates from a mucus membrane. They often appear in the colon and nasal mucosa. The term comes from the Greek word for an octopus, *polypous*, which literally means "many feet." Hence, the stalks of these types of growths are likened to a foot. As was previously discussed, the roots **PED-** and **POD-** are commonly used for "foot" or "feet." Likewise, the suffixes **-PUS**, **-POUS**, and **-POD** mean "foot" or "feet" (Fig. 13.17).

Fig. 13.17   Image of polyps in the ascending colon. *Source:* Digestive system/SERVIER MEDICAL ART/ CC by 4.0.

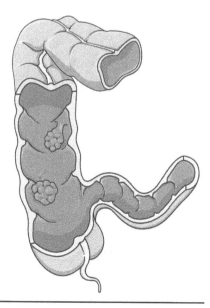

Pathologies of the gallbladder and liver

Hepatitis – Hepatitis is an infectious inflammation of the liver that is caused by the hepatitis A virus (HAV), the hepatitis B virus (HBV), the hepatitis C virus (HCV), the hepatitis D virus (HDV), or the hepatitis E virus (HEV). Acute cases are marked by a yellow appearance of the skin and sclera, known as **jaundice**, which is also called **icterus**, and the enlargement of the liver, which is called **hepatomegaly**.

Cirrhosis – Cirrhosis is a chronic disease of the liver characterized by pathological changes to the tissue of the liver. The term was coined by Rene Laennec in 1827. Laennec used the Greek word *kirrhos* "tawny" supposedly to describe the "yellowish-orange" appearance of the liver.

Cholelithiasis – Derived from the root for "bile," **CHOL**-, and the compound suffix for "condition of stones," -**LITHIASIS**, cholelithiasis is the formation of a gallstone(s) (**cholelith**).

Pathologies of the anus and rectum

Fistula – A fistula is a pathological, tube-like passageway that connects to a normal anatomical cavity or tube. Fistulae commonly occur at the rectum and anus. The roots meaning "fistula" are **FISTUL**- and **SYRING**-. In addition to the loan word "fistula," **syrinx** is another loan word for this pathology. **Syrinx** and **SYRING**- can be used for any "short tubular structure" (e.g. syringe). Syrinx is also the name of panpipe, which is a wind instrument consisting of reed pipes of different lengths tied in a row. In Greek mythology, the syrinx was the god Pan's musical instrument. In Ovid's *Metamorphoses* (1.689), Syrinx was a nymph who escaped Pan by being turned into a clump of reeds from which Pan crafted the pipes for his musical instrument (Figs. 13.18 and 13.19).

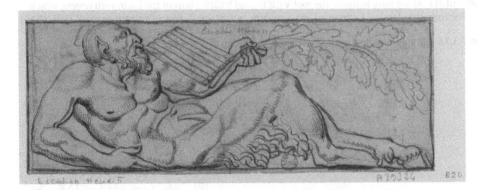

Fig. 13.18 Image of the Greek god Pan playing the syrinx (Pan-flute). *Source:* Drawing by Louis-Pierre Baltard, (1803). *Source:* Louis-Pierre Baltard/Wikimedia Commons/Public domain.

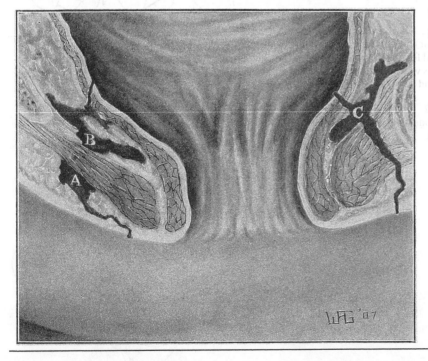

Fig. 13.19 Image of anal fistulae. *Source:* Internet Archive Book Images/ Wikimedia Commons/Public domain.

Hemorrhoid – Formed from the root for "blood," **HEM-**, and the compound suffix meaning "resembling a discharge," **-RRHOID**, the term hemorrhoid refers to a pathologically swollen vein of the rectal plexus, which is also called a **pile**. As the Greek pathological term *haimorrhoides*, this term was in use in the 5th and 4th century BC. Hippocratic author of *On Hemorrhoids* and *On Fistula* claims that hemorrhoids are formed by blood being attracted to the heat produced by peccant bile or phlegm being in the adjacent veins of the rectum, which in turn causes the vessels to swell with blood and later be bruised by the passing of feces. While this humoral explanation is not consistent with modern science, the causes of hemorrhoids are not fully understood to this day (Fig. 13.20).

Fig. 13.20 Image of types of hemorrhoids. *Source:* WikipedianProlific and Mikael Häggström/ wikimedia commons/CC BY-SA 3.0.

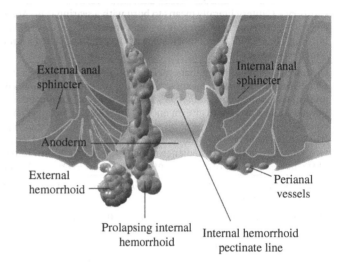

Therapeutic and surgical terms for the GI

Surgical anastomoses – An anastomosis is the union of two vessels. In regards to bowel surgery, the suffix **-STOMY** is used for the surgical creation of an anastomosis (Fig. 13.21). For example, joining of the jejunum to the ileum would be called a **jejunoileostomy**. The hole created by this surgery is called a **stoma**. Thus, the hole in the abdomen made by a colostomy is also called the **stoma**.

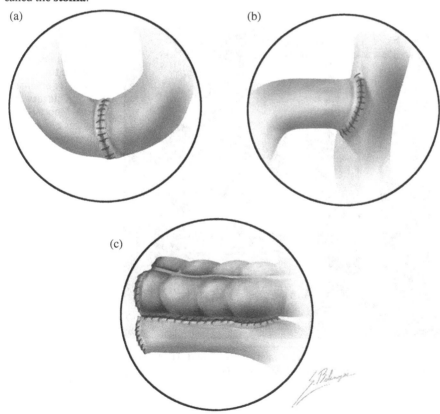

Fig. 13.21 Image of the different types of surgical anastomoses: (a) end-to-end anastomosis between two segments of the small bowel, (b) end-to-side anastomosis between two segments of small bowel, (c) side-to-side anastomosis between small and large bowel. *Source:* Donato Gerardo Terrone/Springer Nature/CC by 2.0.

Plication – The surgical creation of folds or tucks in tissue at an organ's walls to reduce its size. Plication is used in **bariatric surgeries**. The roots **PLIC-** and **PLICAT-** mean "fold." Formed from the root for "pressure" and "weight," **BAR-**, a bariatric surgery is used for weight loss with morbid obesity. This could involve a gastric bypass which is surgery in which most of the stomach is disconnected from the upper GI tract.

Cautery – Cautery literally means to burn with a searing iron. According to Taber's, it is the process of destroying tissue "by electricity, freezing, heat, laser, ultrasound energy, or corrosive chemicals." The roots **CAUS-**, **CAUST-**, and **CAUTER-** refer to "a burning." In ancient Greek medicine, a cautery tile was called a *kauterion* and it was used for a wide variety of conditions, one of which was hemorrhoids.

Cathartic – A medication that evacuates/purges the bowels is called a cathartic. Cathartic is derived from the Greek word *katharsis*, which, broadly speaking, meant a "cleansing" or "purging." That said, in different contexts, the meaning of *katharsis* could vary. In ancient Greek medicine, *katharsis* was the process of purging either the upper or lower cavities of the body. The lower cavities were purged using a **clyster** to give an enema (Fig. 13.22). The upper cavities were purged by causing the patient to vomit. In a religious context, *katharsis* was a type of ceremonial purification or cleansing from guilt of defilement. According to Aristotle, Greek tragedy had a cathartic effect on its audiences, which modern scholars have sometimes interpreted him to mean that the emotive element of Greek tragedy purged the audience of their pent-up emotions. In modern medicine, **catharsis** is used for both the purgative action of the bowels and the release of pent-up thoughts and feelings through psychotherapy.

Laxative – A chemical that loosens the bowels, particularly with constipation, is termed a laxative. This medical term is derived from the Latin verb meaning "to loosen," *laxare*. Thus, words with the root **LAX-** carry the meaning "loosening."

Enema – An introduction of a fluid through the anus into the bowels is called an enema. The etymological origins of this term point to the Greek verb *enienai*, which means "to send in, inject." The use of enemata predates ancient Greek medicine and it was a widespread practice in many cultures of antiquity, particularly the Egyptians. Writing in the 5th century BC, Herodotus claims that for disease prevention, Egyptians purge themselves three days every month, seeking health by both vomiting and enemas because they believe that all diseases in men come from the food that they eat (Herodotus 2.77). Although Herodotus is known to embellish quite a bit in his historical accounts, Egyptian medical papyri confirm that enemata were indeed a part of ancient Egyptian medicine, extending back to 1400 BC.

Clysis – An injection of fluid into the body typically for the purpose of washing/lavage of an internal cavity is termed clysis. It also appears as the suffix **-CLYSIS** when attached to an anatomical root. As noted, the funnel-shaped or syringe-shaped device that ancient Greek physicians used to give enemas was called a *klyster*. The term **clyster** is sometimes used for similar devices in modern medicine (e.g. **coloclyster**). All of these terms are ultimately derived from the Greek verb for "to wash, wash out," *klyzein* (Fig. 13.22).

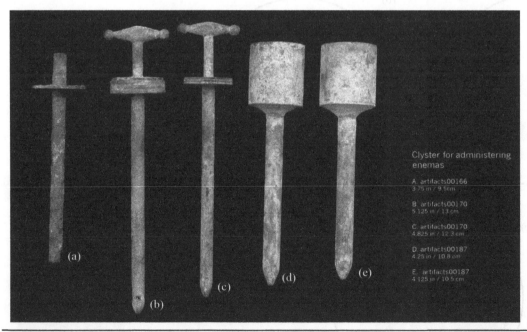

Fig. 13.22 Various clysters used in ancient Greek medicine to administer enemas. *Source:* Courtesy of Claude Moore Health Sciences Library, University of Virginia.

Clyster for administering enemas

A. artifacts00166
3.75 in / 9.5cm

B. artifacts00170
5.125 in / 13 cm

C. artifacts00170
4.825 in / 12.3 cm

D. artifacts00187
4.25 in / 10.8 cm

E. artifacts00187
4.125 in / 10.5 cm

Lavage – According to Taber's, a lavage is the therapeutic washing out of a cavity with a liquid. The term is derived from the Latin verb for "to wash," *lavare*, *lotum*. Derived from this verb, the roots **LUT-**, **LAV-**, and **LOT-** carry the meaning of "a washing."

Greek or Latin word element	Current usage	Etymology	Examples
ASC/O **(as-kō)**	Sac, saclike	Gr. *askos*, leather bag; bladder, sac	**Asc**ites, **asc**omycete Loan word: **Ascus** (as′kŭs) pl. **Asci** (as′(k)ī″)
CHALAS/O **(kă-lă-sĭō)** **-CHALASIS** **(kă-lă-sĭs)**	Relaxation (of a sphincter), slack	Gr. *chalaein*, to slacken, relax	Cardio**chalas**ia, blepharo**chalasis**
EMET/O **(em-ĕ-tō)** **-EMESIS** **(ĕm-ĕ-sĭs)**	Vomiting	Gr. *emetos*, vomit	Anti**emet**ic, copr**emesis** Derivative: **Emesis** (ĕm′ĕ-sĭs)
NAUSE/O **(naw-sĕ-ō)** **NAUT/O** **(naw-tō)**	Nausea, ship, sailor, sailing	Gr. *nausea*, sea sickness Gr. *nautes*, sea sailor	Astro**naut**, **nause**ous Loan word: **Nausea** (naw-zē-ă)
-PTOSIS **(tō-sĭs)**	Prolapse, downward displacement	Gr. *ptosis*, a falling; prolapse	Enter**optosis**, phren**optosis** Loan word: **Ptosis** (tō′sĭs)
FISTUL/O **(fish-chŭ-lō)**	Fistula, tube, pipe-like	L. *fistula*, *-ae*, f. pipe; a fistula	**Fistul**aria, **fistul**ectomy Loan word: **Fistula** (fis′chŭ-lă) pl. **Fistulae** (fis′chŭ-lē″)
SYRING/O **(sĭr-ĭng-ō)** **-SYRINX** **(sir-inks)**	Fistula, short tube, pipe-like	Gr. *syrinx*, *syringos*, pipe; fistula	**Syring**ectomy, dacryo**syrinx** Loan word: **Syrinx** (sir′inks) pl. **Syringes** (sĭ-ring′gēz″)
DIVERTICUL/O **(dī-vĕr-tik-yŭ-lō)**	Diverticulum (an outpouching of a structure, particularly an intestine)	L. *diverticulum*, *-i*, n. turning out; a diverticulum	**Diverticul**itis, **diverticul**ar Loan word: **Diverticulum** (dī″vĕr-tik′yŭ-lŭm) pl. **Diverticula** (dī″vĕr-tik′yŭ-lă)
POLYP/O **(pŏl-ĭ-pō)**	Polyp	Gr. *polypous*, many footed, octopus	**Polyp**ectomy, **polyp**oid Loan word: **Polyp** (pol′ĭp)
-CELE **(sēl)**	Hernia, swelling, tumor	Gr. *kele*, tumor, hernia	Omphalo**cele**, entero**cele**
HERNI/O **(hĕr-nē-ō)**	Hernia	L. *hernia*, rupture	**Herni**otomy, **herni**al Loan word: **Hernia** (hĕr′nē-ă)
CIRRH/O **(sĭ-rō)**	Cirrhosis, yellow	Gr. *kirrhos*, yellow	**Cirrh**osis, **cirrh**otic
ICTER/O **(ĭk-tĕr-ō)**	Jaundice	Gr. *ikteros*, yellow; jaundice	**Icter**ogenic, **icter**oanemia Loan word: **Icterus** (ĭk′tĕr-ŭs)

Greek or Latin word element	Current usage	Etymology	Examples
VOLV/O (vŏl-vō)	To roll	L. *volvere*, to roll	**Volv**ulus, in**volve**
HEMORRHOID/O (hem-ŏ-royd-ō)	Hemorrhoid, pile	Gr. *haimorrhoïdes*, discharging blood	**Hemorrhoid**al, **hemorrhoid**opexy Derivative: **Hemorrhoid** (hem'ŏ-royd")
FLAT/O (flă-tō)	Gas in the GI, to blow	L. *flare, flatum*, to blow	**Flat**ulence, in**flate** Loan word: **Flatus** (flā'tŭs)
HALIT/O (hăl-ĭ-tō)	Bad breath	L. *halare, halitum*, to breath	**Halit**osis, **halit**ophobia
ULCER/O (ŭl-sĕ-rō)	Ulcer	L. *ulcus, ulceris*, n. open sore, ulcer	**Ulcer**ate, **ulcer**ation
APHTH/O (af-thō)	Ulcer of the mouth, thrush	Gr. *aphtha*, thrush, mouth ulcer	**Aphth**osis, **aphth**oid Loan word: **Aphtha** (af'thă) pl. **Aphthae** (af'thē)
-CLYSIS (klī-sĭs)	Washing, lavage	Gr. *klyzein*, to wash or rinse out.	Cysto**clysis**, entero**clysis** Derivative: **Clysis** (klī'sĭs) pl. **Clyses** (klī'sēz")
LAV/O (lă-vō) **LUT/O** (loo-tō) **LOT/O** (lō-tō)	Washing	L. *lavare, lotum*, to wash	**Lot**ion, di**lut**ion, **lav**ation
ENEM/O (en-ĕ-mō)	Enema	Gr. *enema, enematos*, a sending in	**Enem**ator Loan word: **Enema** (en'ĕ-mă)
CATHART/O (kă-thart-ō)	Evacuation (of the bowels)	Gr. *katharis*, evacuation, purification	**Cathart**ic Loan word: **Catharsis** (kă-thar'sĭs) pl. **Catharses** (kă-thar'sēz")
LAX/O (lăk-sō) **LAXAT/O** (lăk-să-tō)	Loosen, relax	L. *laxare*, to loosen	**Lax**ative, **lax**ity
PLIC/O (plĭ-kō) **PLICAT/O** (plĭ-kă-tō)	To fold, a fold	L. *plicare*, to fold	**Plic**ation, **plic**otomy Loan word: **Plica** (plĭ'kă) pl. **Plicae** (plĭ'kē")
CAUS/O (kaw-sō) **CAUST/O** (kaw-stō) **CAUTER/O** (kaw-tĕr-ō)	To burn, burnt	Gr. *kausos*, burning heat; *kaustos*, burnt; *kauterion*, searing-iron	**Caut**ery, **caus**algia, **caus**tic

Review	Answers
The clinical divisions of the abdomen for diagnostic purposes are the right and left inguinal regions, which are located at the _____, the hypogastric region, which is located under the _____, the right and left lumbar regions, which are located at the _____, the umbilical region, which located at the _____, the right and left hypochondriac regions, which are located under the _____ of the ribs, and the epigastric region which is upon the _____.	**groin, stomach, loins, navel, cartilage, stomach**
The technical term for indigestion is _____.	**dyspepsia**
Feces with bright red blood is called _____. Black tarry feces caused by bleeding higher up in the gastrointestinal tract is called _____. A fatty stool/fecal material is called _____. The frequent passage of loose, unformed stools is called _____.	**hematochezia melena steatorrhea diarrhea**
The loan word for vomiting is _____, and its root is _____. Thus, vomiting blood would be called _____.	**emesis, EMET-hematemesis**
The term for belching is _____.	**eructation**
An unpleasant feeling in the throat and/or stomach that may or may not result in vomiting is called _____. In other contexts, the root NAUT- can mean _____, _____, or _____.	**nausea sailor, ship, sailing**
The loan word _____ means gas in the GI system. Thus, the passing of gas is called _____.	**flatus flatulation**
A condition of bad breath is _____.	**halitosis**
Relaxation of the cardiac sphincter is called _____.	**cardiochalasia**
Lack of appetite is called _____.	**anorexia**
Dysphagia is a problem/dysfunction associated with _____.	**swallowing (eating)**
Inflammation of the mouth is called _____. Inflammation of the lips is called _____. Inflammation of the salivary gland is _____. Inflammation of the tongue is _____. Inflammation of the gums is _____ or _____. Inflammation of the esophagus is _____. Inflammation of the stomach _____. Inflammation of the stomach and intestines is _____. Inflammation of the lowest part of the small intestines is _____. Inflammation of the colon is _____. Inflammation of the appendix is _____. Inflammation of the anus and rectum is _____. Inflammation of the peritoneum is _____. Inflammation of the liver is _____. Inflammation of the gallbladder is _____. Inflammation of the bile duct is _____. Inflammation of the pancreas is _____.	**stomatitis cheilitis sialoadenitis glossitis gingivitis, oulitis esophagitis gastritis gastroenteritis ileitis colitis appendicitis proctitis peritonitis hepatitis cholecystitis cholangitis pancreatitis**
Derived from the Greek term for a large bag, an accumulation of excess fluid in the peritoneal cavity is called _____.	**ascites**
A fistula is a pathological, tube-like passageway that connects to a normal anatomical cavity or tube. The roots meaning "fistula" are _____ and _____. In addition to fistula, _____ is another loan word for this pathology.	**SYRING-, FISTUL-syrinx**
A prolapse is the falling or dropping down of an organ or internal part. The suffix that can mean "prolapse" is _____.	**-PTOSIS**
A hernia is a protrusion of an anatomical structure, typically an intestine, through the wall that normally contains it. The suffix that can mean "hernia" is _____.	**-CELE**
Formed from the Latin word elements that mean "to receive within," _____ is the prolapse of an intestine into another part of the intestine just below it.	**intussusception**
Formed from the root meaning "roll," a _____ is the rolling or twisting of an intestine on itself, which causes an obstruction.	**volvulus**
Formed from the Latin word meaning a turning out, _____ is an abnormal side pocket in an intestine.	**diverticulum**

Review	Answers
The term _____ refers to a pathologically swollen vein of the rectal plexus, which is also called a "pile."	**hemorrhoid**
Formed from a Greek word meaning "many feet," a _____ is an abnormal growth (tumor) that emanates from a mucus membrane.	**polyp**
A small ulcer of the mouth, as with thrush, is called an _____.	**aphtha**
A peptic ulcer is an ulcer of the _____ tract.	**digestive**
Hepatitis is an infectious inflammation of the liver that is caused by the hepatitis A virus (HAV), the hepatitis B virus (HBV), the hepatitis C virus (HCV), the hepatitis D virus (HDV), or the hepatitis E virus (HEV). Acute cases are marked by a yellow appearance of the skin and sclera, known as jaundice, which is also called _____, and the enlargement of the liver, which is called _____.	**icterus, hepatomegaly**
_____ is a chronic disease of the liver characterized by pathological changes to the tissue of the liver.	**Cirrhosis**
A _____ is a medication that evacuates/purges the bowels. A _____ is a chemical that loosens the bowels, particularly with constipation. An _____ is the introduction of a fluid through the anus into the bowels. A _____ is an injection of fluid into the body typically for the purpose of washing/lavage of an internal cavity.	**cathartic laxative enema clysis**
Formed from the root for "pressure" and "weight," a _____ surgery is used for weight loss with morbid obesity. This could involve a gastric bypass which is surgery in which most of the stomach is disconnected from the upper GI tract.	**bariatric**
The surgical creation of folds or tucks in tissue at an organ's walls to reduce its size is called _____.	**plication**
An _____ is the union of two vessels. In regards to bowel surgery, the suffix _____ is used for the surgical creation of an anastomosis. The hole created by this surgery is called a _____.	**anastomosis -STOMY stoma**
The roots **CAUS-** and **CAUT-** mean _____ or _____. _____ literally means to burn with a searing iron.	**to burn, burnt Cautery**

14

Urinary System

CHAPTER LEARNING OBJECTIVES

1) You will learn the word elements, loan words, and key terms associated with the urinary system.
2) You will become familiar with the historical concepts associated with the urinary system, particularly the production of urine, uroscopy, and lithotomy.

Lessons from History: Ancient Greek Medical Explanations of the Physiology of the Urinary System

Food for Thought as You Read:

Is a mechanical or materialist approach to the body inherently more scientific than a vitalist approach? Why or why not?

Can a "thought experiment" be considered scientific? Does it have any place in science?

The basic anatomy of the urinary system was well understood by ancient Greek physicians from the 3rd century BC onward. However, knowledge of the anatomy of the urinary system does not easily translate into an understanding of how urine is produced. While it was self-evident that the more fluid one drinks, the more urine the body releases, it was not clear as to how this ingested fluid ends up in the urinary tract, particularly because the anatomy of the gastrointestinal system does not reveal a direct connection to the urinary system. In Book I of *On the Natural Faculties*, Galen discusses the production of urine. He uses this discussion to validate his own theory of the faculties of the parts by demonstrating how the physiological theories of two famous Greek physicians, Erasistratus (c. 3rd century BC) and Asclepiades of Bithynia (c. 1st century BC), are inadequate to explain this function of the body. Galen held that both animal and human bodies had the basic faculties (*dynameis*) of generation, growth, and nutrition, which are in turn supported by lesser faculties of attraction, retention, assimilation, and expulsion. The parts of the body use the lesser faculties to attract, retain, assimilate, or expulse what is particular to their function and necessary for life and growth.

In his discussion of the secretion of urine from the kidneys, Galen notes that Erasistratus believed urine comes from the blood that enters the kidneys. However, Erasistratus makes no attempt to explain this using his "general principles" of the body. Galen notes that one of Erasistratus' general principles of the body is that there is a tendency for fluid to fill an empty space, which in Latin is termed the *horror vacui* (fear of empty spaces). However, as Galen argues, this principle does not provide a sufficient explanation for the separation of urine from blood. Galen notes how the followers of Erasistratus tried to resolve this problem by using another mechanical principle: "Now those near the times of Erasistratus maintain that the parts above the kidneys receive pure blood, whilst the watery residue, being heavy, tends to run downwards." Thus, the heavier fluid (i.e. urine) moves into the kidney, while the lighter blood moves on to fill the void of the vena cava. They support this separation of the heavier from the lighter liquid by observing that "if oil be mixed with water and poured upon the ground, each will take a different route." Galen points out that this heavier watery part would not have the ability to move upward with the blood at any point prior to entering the kidneys. After pointing out the problems with such mechanical explanations, Galen argues that urine comes from the kidneys, and the kidneys have specific natural faculties/powers: one

Greek and Latin Roots of Medical and Scientific Terminologies, First Edition. Todd A. Curtis.
© 2025 John Wiley & Sons, Inc. Published 2025 by John Wiley & Sons, Inc.
Companion website: www.wiley.com/go/Curtis

that attracts watery fluids from the blood and one that excretes urine from the kidneys. Therefore, while both Erasistratus' and Galen's theories are consistent with the gross anatomy of the urinary system, and while both seem to agree that blood is purified of urine at the kidney, they differ on the physiological forces that account for the production of urine. Erasistratus' and his followers' explanations foreshadow the kind of mechanistic approach commonly found in science today. Mechanism holds that the same physical principles that govern nonliving entities are at work in the physiologies of living entities. Hence, the Erasistratean explanations of "filling the void" and the separation of heavier fluids resemble modern principles such as pressure gradients and the specific gravity of fluids. Galen's facultative explanation of kidney function is an example of the sort of vitalistic theory that was used for centuries to explain human physiology. Vitalism is the belief that living organisms are fundamentally different from nonliving entities because they contain certain innate powers that explain their functions. Often, these powers are closely associated with concepts of the soul–body relationship, which partially explains why vitalism has fallen out of favor in modern physiological science. That said, in comparison to Erasistratean theories of the presence of urine in the kidneys, it is tempting to consider Galen's theory of selective attraction as being more scientific because it does a better job of explaining the kidney's removal of urine from the blood.

In his discussion of the kidney's attraction to urine, Galen censures Asclepiades' theory of the production of urine because Asclepiades fails to pay attention to the function of the kidneys and the ureters. When criticizing Asclepiades, Galen states, "one is forced to marvel at the ingenuity of a man who puts aside these broad, clearly visible routes (the ureters), and postulates others, which are narrow, invisible, and indeed, entirely imperceptible." Galen links Asclepiades to atomists, such as Epicurus, who believed that all substances are made of indivisible particles (atoms) that are separated from one another by empty spaces. Asclepiades' theory of urine production, according to Galen, holds that the fluid a person drinks turns into a vapor (assumedly in the stomach). This vapor moves through the invisible channels in the body into the bladder, which Asclepiades likens to a sponge. Once in the bladder, the vapor is condensed, forming urine. Thus, Asclepiades completely bypass the kidneys and the ureters, which Galen notes even butchers would not do since it is obvious that the ureters convey urine to the bladder. He also notes how the bladder of an animal retains air and water if you blow it up and tie off the neck, which disproves that there are invisible channels that run into the bladder. Galen claims to have demonstrated how ureters function by experimenting on a living animal. He claims to have cut the peritoneum of the animal to access the ureters, which he then ligated. Having bandaged the animal, he let it roam off. He then goes on to say that when the external bandages were loosened, the bladder was empty, but the ureters were distended. When the ligature of one of the ureters was removed, the bladder filled with urine. Before the animal urinated, he tied off the urethra at the penis. He notes that if he squeezed the bladder, the urine did not go up the ureters or out of the bladder. Releasing the urethra then allowed the animal to urinate. While it is tempting to say that Galen's anatomical demonstration is an example of the experimental method being used in Greek science, there are a number of features that should give one pause before making such a claim. First, Galen's descriptions of his anatomical demonstrations reveal that they were conducted for the purpose of proving what Galen already believed rather than Galen attempting to discover something new. Second, although Galen's anatomical demonstration appears reasonable based on our understanding of the anatomy of the urinary system, it is quite possible that Galen never actually performed such an experiment. The cause for doubt stems from other Galenic experiments that appear to be simply "thought experiments" that serve to validate his preconceived views. Also, some of the results of this experiment are not reproducible because they appear to be based on what Galen believed would happen rather than what actually occurred. It is unclear if an animal, such as a goat, would survive, much less urinate, given the goat was not anesthetized when its peritoneum was cut open and then bandaged shut. If Galen did not dissect the goat, then both Asclepiades' and Galen's scientific methods are similar in that they relied on physiological premises to see the production of urine. That said, Galen's understanding of the anatomy of the urinary system and its role in urine production is clearly superior to Asclepiades', and therefore, one could argue that Galen's explanation is more scientific than Asclepiades'. However, Asclepiades' physiological principles are more in line with the materialism found in modern science, which holds that nothing exists except matter and its movements. Therefore, one could argue that the "atomic" theory of Asclepiades is similar to modern science because it delimits physiological explanations of matter and its effects on matter.

Some Suggested Readings

Debru, Armelle. "*Physiology*." In *The Cambridge Companion to Galen*, Edited by Robert J. Hankinson, 263–282. Cambridge: Cambridge University Press, 2008.

Duffin, Jacalyn. "*Interrogating Life: History of Physiology*." In *History of Medicine: A Scandously Short Introduction*. Second Edition: Toronto: University of Toronto Press, 2010.

Galen. *On the Natural Faculties*. Translated by A. J. Brock. Loeb Classical Library 71. Cambridge, MA: Harvard University Press, 1916.

Etymological Explanations: Common Terms and Word Elements for the Anatomy of the Urinary System

In the following discussion of the anatomical terms associated with the urinary system, the nominative and genitive singular forms of the anatomical Latin term are provided in parenthesis (Fig. 14.1). The Greek and Latin roots are formatted in all caps and emboldened.

Fig. 14.1 Anatomical Latin terms for the urinary system. *Source:* Drawing by Chloe Kim.

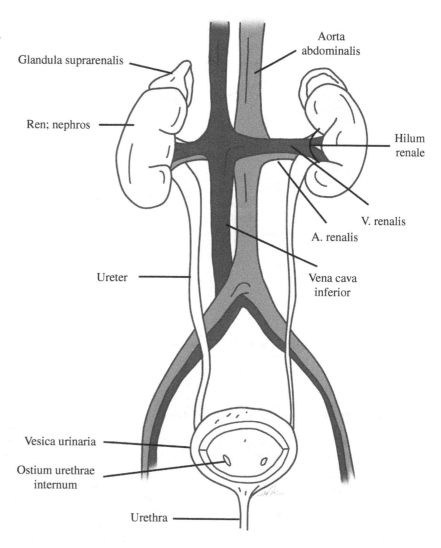

Glandula suprarenalis

Aorta abdominalis

Ren; nephros

Hilum renale

V. renalis

A. renalis

Ureter

Vena cava inferior

Vesica urinaria

Ostium urethrae internum

Urethra

Kidney, ureters, bladder, and urethra

Kidney (L. *ren, renis*) – The urinary system consists of two kidneys that filter the blood and form urine (Fig. 14.2). The loan word for the kidney is **ren** (it is also referred to as the **nephros**). The roots used for "the kidney" are **NEPHR-** and **REN-**. The kidneys are located in the retroperitoneal space, where they are held in place by fat. The outer portion of the kidney is called the **renal capsule (L. *capsula renalis*)**. The renal capsule is composed of layers of fat and fibrous tissue. Under the renal capsule lies the **renal cortex (L. *cortex renalis*)**, which surrounds the soft inner part of the kidney known as the **renal medulla (L. *medulla renalis*)**.

Renal pyramids (L. *pyramides renales*) and renal papillae (L. *papillae renales*) – Each kidney has 7–18 lobes. The number of lobes corresponds to the number of renal pyramids in the kidney's medulla. The nipple-like, pointed tip of each renal pyramid is called the renal papilla. The anatomical Latin term *pyramis, pyramdis* appears to be derived from the Greek word *pyramis*, which is apparently borrowed from the Egyptian word *pimar*, "pyramid." As expected the root **PYRAMID-** is used for structures that resemble the Egyptian pyramids. As we have already learned in previous chapters, the root **PAPILL-** is used for "nipples" or "nipple-like" structures.

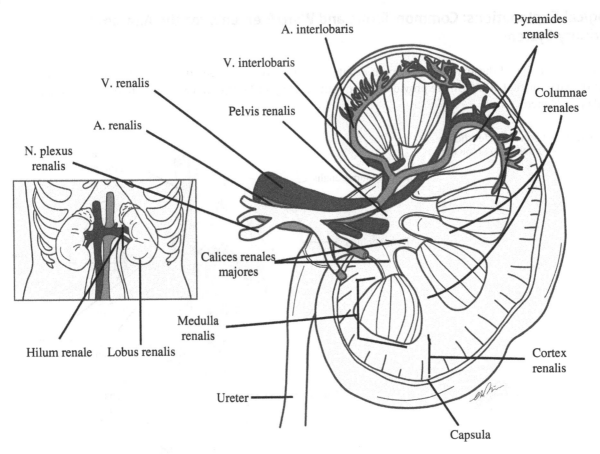

A. interlobaris
V. interlobaris
V. renalis
Pelvis renalis
A. renalis
N. plexus
renalis
Pyramides
renales
Columnae
renales
Calices renales
majores
Medulla
renalis
Hilum renale   Lobus renalis
Ureter
Cortex
renalis
Capsula

Fig. 14.2 Anatomical Latin terms for the kidney. *Source:* Drawing by Chloe Kim.

Renal calices (L. *calices renales*) and renal pelvis (L. *pelvis renalis*) – The renal papilla releases urine into a cup-like structure called the **calyx (L. *calyx, calicis*)**. The calices of the kidney empty into the renal pelvis. The roots used for the renal calices are **CALYC-** and **CALIC-**. Because the Greek word for *kalyx* refers to the cup-shaped part of the flower that holds the petals, these roots are also used for similar *kalyx*-shaped objects. Derived from the Greek word for "a basin," *pyelos*, the root used for the renal pelvis is **PYEL-**.

Ureter (L. *ureter, ureteris*) – The urine created in the kidneys contains waste products, excess fluids, and electrolytes that will be eliminated from the body with urination. The urine then moves from the kidneys to the urinary bladder via two urinary vessels called the ureters, whose root is **URETER-**. These musculo-membranous tubes are about 10–12 in. long. The urine travels down the ureters, assisted by peristaltic contractions. From the ureters, the urine enters the bladder via slit-like orifices called **ostia (L. *ostium, -i*)**, whose shape acts like a valve to prevent the backflow of urine into the ureters during bladder contraction.

Urinary bladder (L. *vesica urinaria*) – Urine is stored in the urinary bladder. The primary function of the urinary bladder is to store urine and expel it during urination. The roots used for the "urinary bladder" are **CYST-** and **VESIC-**. The anatomical Latin term for the "bladder" is **vesica**. The suffix **-CYST** is used for the 'urinary bladder' or a 'cyst', which is a closed sac or pouch that holds fluid or solid marterial. The urinary bladder is capable of distention due to its elasticity and the **rugae** (ridges, wrinkles) in its mucosal lining. The bladder has three openings: two for the ureters and one for the urethra. These three openings form a triangle, which is referred to as the **trigone (L. *trigonum, -i*)**. The trigone gets its name from the Greek word for "triangular," *trigonos* (three angles).

Urethra (L. *urethra, -ae*) – The urine stored in the bladder is emptied outside of the body via the urethra, whose root is **URETHR-**. The opening at the end of the urethra is the **meatus (L. *meatus, -us*)**, and the root for this opening of the urethra is **MEAT-**. In females, the urethra is rather straight and about 1 to 1 ½ inches long. Its meatus is located between the clitoris and the vagina's opening. The urethra in males is curved and about 8 inches long, and its meatus is located at the tip of the penis.

Nephron and filtration of the blood

Nephron – The modern understanding of the production of urine reveals it to be both mechanical and chemical processes that occur in a microscopic structure of the kidney called the nephron (Fig. 14.3). The nephron filters the blood, reabsorbs what is needed, then excretes the rest as urine. There are close to two million nephrons in the cortex of each kidney. The nephron is composed of the Bowman's capsule, the proximal convoluted tubule, the loop of Henle, and the distal convoluted tubule. The distal convoluted tubule excretes urine into the collecting duct, which descends and ultimately empties into the renal pelvis.

Filtration – Renal blood flow (RBF) and filtration occur as follows: the renal artery carries unfiltered blood into the kidney through the anatomical depression known as the **hilum (L. *hilum, -i*)**. The renal artery branches off into interlobular arteries. The interlobular arteries bring the unfiltered blood to the lobes of the kidney, where these arteries branch off into smaller and even smaller vessels, eventually becoming the afferent arteriole. The afferent arteriole enters Bowman's capsule, where it becomes the **glomerulus (L. *glomerulus, -i*)**. The glomerulus is a ball-like mass that filters the blood. The walls of the glomerulus allow smaller molecules, wastes, and fluids to pass into the proximal convoluted tubule. The filtered fluid moves from the proximal convoluted tubule through the loop of Henle and into the distal convoluted tubule. The larger molecules, particularly blood cells, and proteins, stay in the glomerulus and exit out via the efferent arteriole. The efferent arteriole becomes the renal vein, which ultimately carries the filtered blood out of the kidney. Prior to becoming the renal vein, this blood vessel moves along the tubules of the nephron, reabsorbing almost all of the water, along with minerals and nutrients the body needs. The remaining fluid and waste products in the proximal convoluted tubule form the urine that is excreted into the collecting duct.

Fig. 14.3 Nephron and blood vessels.
Source: OpenStax College, Anatomy & Physiology, Connexions Web, Jun 19, (2013)/Rice University/ CC by 4.0.

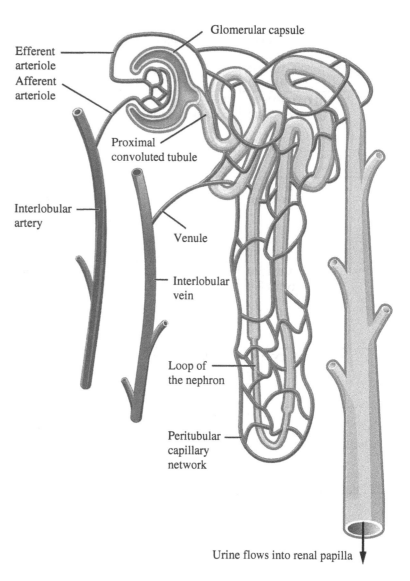

Glomerular capsule

Efferent arteriole

Afferent arteriole

Proximal convoluted tubule

Interlobular artery

Venule

Interlobular vein

Loop of the nephron

Peritubular capillary network

Urine flows into renal papilla

Greek or Latin word element	Current usage	Etymology	Examples
REN/O (rĕ-nō)	Kidney	L. *ren, renis*, m. kidney	**Ren**ogastric, ad**ren**al, supra**ren**al Loan word: **Ren** (rĕn) pl. **Renes** (rĕn′ēz″)
NEPHR/O (nef-rō)	Kidney	Gr. *nephros*, kidney	**Nephr**itis, **nephr**oabdominal, **nephr**oblastoma Loan word: **Nephros** (nĕf′rŏs)
HIL/O (hī-lō)	Hilum	L. *hilum, -i*, n. little thing, trifle	**Hil**itis, **hil**ar Loan word: **Hilum** (hī′lŭm) pl. **Hila** (hī′lă)
PYEL/O (pī-ĕ-lō)	Renal pelvis, basin	Gr. *pyelos*, basin	**Pyel**ocystitis, **pyel**ectasis, **pyel**ogram
CALYC/O (kăl-ĭ-kō) **CALIC/O** (kăl-ĭ-kō)	Renal calices, cup-like structure	L. *calyx, calicis*, m. calix fr. Gr. *kalyx, kalykos*, covering, shell; cup of flower	**Calyc**iform, **Calic**eal Loan word: **Calyx** (kā′lĭx) pl. **Calices** (kā′lĭ-sēz″)
GLOMERUL/O (glŏ-mer-yŭ-lō)	Glomerulus of the nephron, little ball	L. *glomerulus, -i*, m. little ball fr. L. *glomerare*, to form into a sphere	**Glomerul**opathy, **glomerul**itis, **glomerul**ar Loan word: **Glomerulus** (glŏ-mer′yŭ-lŭs) pl. **Glomeruli** (glŏ-mer′yŭ-lī″)
URETER/O (ū-rē-tĕr-ō)	Ureter	L. *ureter, ureteris*, m. ureter fr. Gr. *oureter*, ureter	**Ureter**olith, **ureter**ectasis, **ureter**algia Loan word: **Ureter** (ū-rēt′ĕr) pl. **Ureteres** (ū-rēt′ĕr-sēz″)
VESIC/O (vĕs-ĭ-kō)	Bladder, sac, vesicle	L. *vesica, -ae*, f. bladder, sac	Cervico**vesic**al, **vesic**oclysis, **vesic**ocele Loan word: **Vesica** (vĕ-sī′kă) pl. **Vesicae** (vĕ-sī′kē″)
CYST/O (sis-tō)	Bladder, sac, cyst	Gr. *kystis*, bladder	**Cyst**ocele, **cyst**ocentesis, **cyst**algia Loan word: **Cyst** (sist)
URETHR/O (ū-rē-thrō)	Urethra	L. *urethra, -ae*, f. urethra fr. Gr. *ourethra*, urethra	**Urethr**orrhaphy, **urethr**al, **urethr**ocystopexy Loan word: **Urethra** (ū-rē′thră) pl. **Urethrae** (ū-rē′thrē″)
MEAT/O (mē-ă-tō)	Opening, passageway	L. *meatus, -us*, m. a path or course	**Meat**ometer, **meat**itis, **meat**al Loan word: **Meatus** (mē-āt′ŭs) pl. **Meatus** (mē-āt′ŭs) / **Meatuses** (mē-āt′ŭs-es)

Review	Answers
The root for the opening of the urethra is _____. The anatomical Latin term is _____.	**MEAT-** **meatus**
The urinary vessel leading from the bladder is called the _____and its root is _____.	**urethra, URETHR-**
The urinary vessel leading from the kidney is called the _____, and its root is _____.	**ureter, URETER-**
The roots used for the "urinary bladder" are _____ and _____. The anatomical Latin term for the urinary bladder is _____.	**CYST-, VESIC-** **vesica**
The roots used for the "kidney" are _____ and _____. The anatomical Latin term for the "kidney" is _____. The Greek loan word for "kidney" is _____.	**NEPHR-, REN-** **ren** **nephros**
The root for the "renal pelvis" is _____.	**PYEL-**
The roots for the "cup-like" expansions connected to the renal pelvis are _____ and _____. The anatomical Latin term is _____, but the singular _____ is often used in medical English.	**CALYC-, CALIC-** **calix, calyx**
The "ball-like" cluster of capillaries formed inside Bowman's capsule is called the _____, and its root is _____.	**glomerulus, GLOMERUL-**

Lessons from History: Uroscopy and Urinalysis

Food for Thought as You Read:

What made uroscopy an attractive diagnostic technique to patients and physicians?
In what ways is modern urinalysis similarly attractive to patients and physicians?

Uroscopy is the visual inspection of urine for the purposes of diagnosis and prognosis. The practice of uroscopy is evident in the Hippocratic Corpus. For instance, in *Aphorism* IV.76, the presence of foreign material in the urine is a sign indicating which anatomical structure in the urinary system could be affected: "When small fleshy objects like hairs are discharged with thick urine, these substances come from the kidneys." In *Aphorism* IV.72, the color of the urine is indicative of a specific disease: "When the urine is transparent and white, it is bad; it appears principally in cases of phrenitis." The smell, type of material in the urine, its transparency, and color were factors taken into consideration by authors in the Hippocratic Corpus. Texts in the Hippocratic Corpus, such as *Aphorisms*, reveal that urine was just one of the many signs used by ancient Greek physicians to diagnose the presence of unobservable internal pathologies.

Thanks to Theophilus Protospatharius' (c. 7th century AD) *On Urine* (*De urinis*), uroscopy became a prominent practice in the diagnosis of specific diseases. The popularity of Theophilus' text is partly due to its systemization of previous material on urine, which made it a practical handbook for the practice of uroscopy. Theophilus' *On Urine* inspired other works on uroscopy that further developed the physiological concepts behind the appearance of urine, leading to a widened application of uroscopy as a primary tool for the diagnosis of non-urinary-related diseases. This fascination with uroscopy would continue for centuries, leading to it being considered a fundamental skill of a good physician and making it iconic for the practice of medicine in the artwork of the medieval and the Renaissance periods.

One of the developments of this fascination with uroscopy was the creation of the matula (L. *matula*, vessel, jar), which was a glass uroscopy flask (Fig. 14.4). Patients would urinate into the flask, and the physician would then make a diagnosis based on the appearance of the urine. Therefore, the transparency of the matula' glass was thought to be imperative since any deformation in the glass or issues with its hue could lead to a mistaken diagnosis. The matula itself became a part of the diagnostic process in which physicians would consider where in the matula the sediment or cloudiness of the urine appeared. The location in the matula was then equated to the area in the body being affected.

The Arabic treatise on urine, Kitab al-Baul, written by Isaac Israeli ben Solomon (c. 832–932), the Jewish philosopher and physician living in the Arabic world, contained a urine-hue classification chart for the purpose of diagnosis, which is an important precursor to the medieval development of the diagnostic tool called the urine wheel or uroscopy wheel (Fig. 14.5).

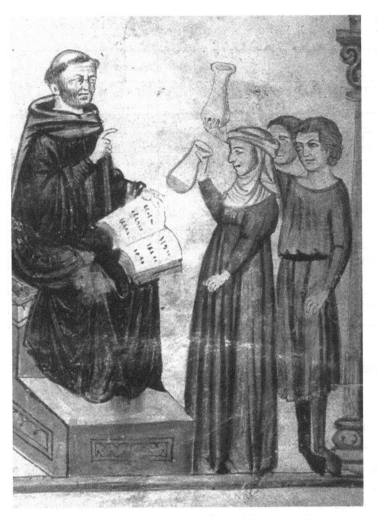

Fig. 14.4 Image of patients presenting their matulae full of urine to the physician Constantine the African. c. 14th century, Bodleian Library, MS. Rawl. C. 328, fol. 3r. *Source:* Unknown artist/Wikimedia Commons/ Public domain.

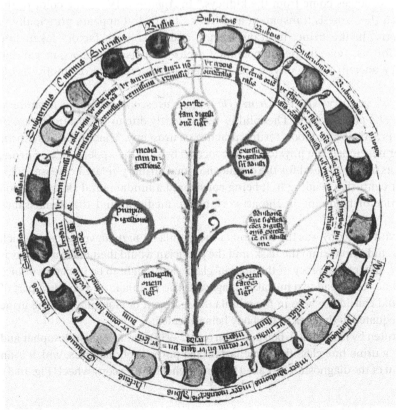

Fig. 14.5 Uroscopy wheel with twenty matulae containing urine of different colors. Image from Johannes de Kethem's *Fasciculus Medicinae*, 1491. *Source:* Johannes de Ketham/Wikimedia Commons/Public domain.

The uroscopy wheel was a diagram that typically had 20 colors of urine, often depicted in matulae. The colors of the urine were linked to particular pathologies. Gilles de Corbeil's *On Urine* (*De urinis*), a 13th-century medical poem on uroscopy, reveals that the colors of urine, such as green, white, livid, and wine-colored, on these wheels were used to speak to a patient's health. With respect to livid urine, he states the following: "If the urine is livid, the lividity is partial or total. If total, it means the mortification of a member or of its humors. Livid near the surface, it suggests various things: a mild form of hemitriteus fever; falling sickness; ascites; synochal fever; the rupture of a vein; catarrh, strangury; an ailment of the womb; a flux; a defect of the lungs; pain in the joints; consumptive phthisis; the extinction of natural heat. These are the causes of lividity – interpret them according to other symptoms." The belief that urine was a byproduct of the coction of blood and was connected therefore to the humors of the body was often the physiological justification used by physicians to explain the origins of the colors.

While the medieval pathological connections to the specific colors of urine are often quite erroneous, urine can indeed appear green, red, livid, brown, and black, and the color of urine can be indicative of specific pathologies and/or the health of the patient. Urochrome is the pigment that gives urine its color. The root **CHROM-** and **CHROMAT-** mean "color." The passing of colorless urine is termed **achromaturia** or **albinuria**, the root in the latter term meaning "white." When identifying colors of urine, the chemical substances that produce particular colors in urine will have the root for the color followed by the suffix **-IN**:

The brownish pigment in the urine with certain conditions is **urofuscin**.
A blue pigment present in the urine with certain conditions is **urocyanin**.
A black pigment present in the urine with certain conditions is **uromelanin**.
A strawy or pale-yellow pigment in the urine with certain conditions is **urolutein**.
A (fluorescent) bright yellow pigment in the urine with certain conditions is **uroflavin**.
A yellow pigment in the urine with certain conditions is **uroxanthin**.
A red pigment in the urine with certain conditions is **uroerythrin**.
A rose-colored pigment in the urine with certain conditions is **urorrhodin**.
A dark red (purple) pigment in the urine with certain conditions is **uroporphyrin**.
A grey pigment in the urine with certain conditions is **urophein** or **urophaein**.
A green pigment in the urine with certain conditions could be termed **urochlorin**.

While uroscopy is still used in modern medicine, it is a far less attractive approach to diagnosis in comparison to **urinalysis**, which is the primary way in which urine is used to diagnose disease and determine the health of a patient. Urinalysis is the chemical, physical, and microscopic examination of urine. Urinalysis commonly involves looking at the specific percentages of the contents of a urine sample that has been collected from a patient: the pH, specific gravity of urine, as well as the presence of glucose, albumin, protein, ketones, nitrites, bilirubin, urobilinogen, bacteria, blood, and blood cells. The suffix **-URIA** is used for pathological amounts of these constituents and qualities, for example:

The presence of protein, particularly albumin, in urine is termed **albuminuria**.
Excessive amount of glucose in the urine is termed **glucosuria** or **melituria**.
An excessive number of ketones in the urine is **ketonuria**.
Excessive concentration of calcium in the urine is **hypercalciuria**.
An increase in nitrogenous compounds in the urine is **azoturia**.
High levels of nitrites in the urine are **nitrituria**.
High pH (greater than 7) or basic urine is **alkalinuria**.
Low pH (lower than 7) or acidic urine is **aciduria**.
The high specific gravity of urine is **hypersthenuria**.
The low specific gravity of urine is **hyposthenuria**.

With ancient uroscopy and modern urinalysis, patients have willingly performed the uncomfortable act of urinating into a container and giving it to someone else based on their belief that this information will help their physician to diagnose their condition. In some respects, uroscopy and urinalysis are attractive because they allow the physician to "see" inside the patient's body.

Some Suggested Readings

Boxer, Carly B. "Uroscopy Diagrams, Judgment, and the Perception of Color in Late Medieval England." *Word & Image* 38, no. 4 (2022): 327–347.

Wallis, Faith. "Inventing Diagnosis: Theophilus' *De urinis* in the Classroom." *Dynamis* 20 (2000): 31–73.

Wallis, Faith. "Signs and Senses: Diagnosis and Prognosis in Early Medieval Pulse and Urine Texts." *Social History of Medicine* 13, no. 2 (2000): 265–278.

Etymological Explanations: Common Terms and Word Elements for Urine and Urination

Urine

Urine – Urine is liquid and dissolved solutes that the urinary system excretes. The word "urine" is ultimately derived from the Greek word for urine, *ouron*. The roots for urine are **UR-** and **URIN-**. **UR-** is a homomorph because it can also represent the Greek word for "a tail," *oura*, which is commonly used in biology. The average person excretes about 1.4l or 47.3 oz of urine a day. Urine is 95% water and 5% solid waste material. The bulk of the solid material is nitrogenous. The root used for nitrogen and nitrogenous waste in general is **AZOT-**, which comes from the Greek word for "lifeless."

Urea – The primary nitrogenous waste material in urine is called urea, and its root is **URE-**. Urea is formed in the liver from the deamination of amino acids.

Uric acid – Uric acid is the second highest percentage of nitrogenous waste products in urine; the root typically used for uric acid is **URIC-**. Uric acid is a crystalline substance formed from purine metabolism.

Creatine – Creatine is another nitrogenous waste product found in urine. The root for creatine is **CREATIN-**. Creatine is the waste product of muscle metabolism.

Urination and problems with urination

Urination – The passing of urine from the bladder is called urination. The suffixes **-URESIS** and **-URIA** are commonly used for urination (micturition).

Micturition – The other term used for urination is micturition. Derived from the Latin verb for urination, *micturire*, the roots for urination are also **MICT-** and **MICTUR-**.

Enuresis – Involuntary urination, which is termed **urinary incontinence** (L. *incontinentia*, inability to retain), is called **enuresis**. Urinary stress incontinence, which is also called **diurnal enuresis**, is the involuntary discharge of urine that often happens during physical activity and/or movement. **Nocturnal enuresis** is loosely termed "bedwetting." Nocturnal enuresis is the involuntary discharge of urine while sleeping by people past the age of bladder control.

Anuresis – The lack of ability to urinate is anuresis.

Diuresis – Increased excretion of urine by the kidneys is diuresis. Thus, a medication that causes urination is called a **diuretic**.

Polyuria – Frequent or excessive urination is termed polyuria.

Oliguria – Scanty amount of urine production is oliguria.

Hematuria – Blood in the urine is hematuria.

Pyuria – Pus in the urine is pyuria.

Nocturia – Excessive urination at night is nocturia.

Dysuria – Painful or difficult urination is dysuria.

Anuria – The absence of urine formation is anuria.

Ischuria – Derived from the root **ISCH-**, meaning "to hold back," ischuria (or uroschesis) is the suppression or retention of urine. This could be caused by stricture of the urinary tubules. A stricture/narrowing of the urethra is called urethrostenosis.

Uroplania – With respect to the flow of urine, **antegrade** is movement forward or with the flow, and **retrograde** is movement backward or against the flow. The root **PLAN-** and the suffix **-PLANIA** means "wandering." Hence, the presence or discharge of urine from parts other than the urinary tract is called uroplania. The term "planet" comes from this root. In ancient Greek astronomy, the visible planets were called *asteres planetai* "wandering stars" due to their irregular antegrade and retrograde movements in the heavens.

Greek or Latin word element	Current usage	Etymology	Examples
-URESIS (ū-rē-sĭs)	To urinate, involuntary urination	Gr. *ourein*, to urinate, to make water	En**uresis**, di**uresis**, kali**uresis** Loan word: **Uresis** (ū-rē′sĭs)
MICT/O (mĭk-tō) **MICTUR/O** (mĭk-tū-rō)	To urinate	L. *micturire* (*mictum*), to urinate	**Mict**ion, **mictur**ate Loan word: **Micturition** (mĭk-tū-rĭ′shŭn)
UR/O (ū-rō) **-URIA** (ū-rē-ă)	Urine	Gr. *ouron*, urine	Glucos**uria**, **ur**obilinemia, xanth**uria**
URIN/O (ū-rĭ-nō)	Urine	L. *urina*, *-ae*, f. urine	**Urin**ometer, **urin**ophil, **urin**ation Derivative: **Urine** (ūr′ĭn)
URE/O (ūr-ē-ō)	Urea (chief nitrogenous waste in urine)	Gr. *ouron*, urine	**Ure**ogenesis, **ure**otelic,
URIC/O (ū-rĭ-kō)	Uric acid (crystalline acid present in urine)	Gr. *ouron*, urine	**Uric**ocholia, **uric**opoiesis
PLAN/O (plă-nō) **PLANKT/O** (plangk-tō) **-PLANIA** (plă-nē-ă)	Wandering	Gr. *planos*, wandering; *planktos*, wandering	Uro**plania**, **plan**otopokinesia, meso**plankton**
GRAD/O (grăd-ō) **-GRADE** (grăd)	Step, walk, go	L. *gradi*, *gressum*, to step, walk, go	Retro**grade**, **grad**ient, **grad**uated
AZOT/O (ăz-ō-tō)	Nitrogenous waste; nitrogen	Gr. *azōtos*, lifeless	**Azot**uria, **azot**emia, **azot**obacter
KALI/O (kal-ē-ō) **KAL/O** (ka-lō)	Potassium	L. *kalium*, *-i*, n. potash	Hyper**kal**emia, **kali**openia, **kali**uresis
CALC/O (kal-kō)	Calcium, lime	L. *calx*, *calcis*, f. limestone, lime concretion	Hyper**calc**emia, **calc**itonin
NATRI/O (nă-trē-ō) **NATR/O** (nă-trō)	Sodium	L. *natrium*, *-i*, n. salt, fr. Gr. *nitron*, salt	Hyper**natr**emia, **natri**uresis
NITRIT/O (nī-trīt/ō)	Nitrite (a salt of nitrous acid)	Gr. *nitron*, salt	**Nitrit**uria, **nitrit**e
NITR/O (nī-trō)	Nitrogen, combination with nitrogen	Gr. *nitron*, salt	**Nitr**ification, **nitr**ocellulose

Greek or Latin word element	Current usage	Etymology	Examples
CREATIN/O (krĕ-ă-tin-ō)	Creatine	Creatine, a colorless crystalline substance in urine fr. Gr. *kreas*, *kreatos*, flesh, muscle	**Creatin**uria, **creatin**ase
ALBUMIN/O (al-bū-mĭ-nō)	Albumin, protein	L. *albumen*, *albuminis*, n. egg white	**Albumin**ocholia, **albumin**uria Loan word: **Albumin** (al-bū′mĭn) **Albumen** (al-bū′mĕn)
KET/O (kĕ-tō)	Ketone	Ketone *Ger. *Keton* fr. Ger. *Aceton*, fr. L. *acetum*, vinegar	**Keto**aciduria, **ket**ogenesis
GLUC/O (gloo-kō) **GLYC/O** (glī-kō)	Sugar, glucose	Gr. *glykys*, sweet; sugar, glucose	**Glyc**ogenic, **gluc**ogenesis, **glyc**osialia
MELIT/O (mel-ĭ-tō) **MELL/O** (mel-ō) **MEL/O** (mel-ō)	Honey, sugar, bees	Gr. *meli*, *melitos*, honey; sugar	**Melit**uria, **melitt**ology, **mell**iferous
ALKAL/O (al-kă-lō) **ALKALIN/O** (al-kă-lĭ-nō)	Basic, Alkali	L. *alkali* fr. Arabi *al-qali* burnt ashes, ashes of salt wort	**Alkalin**uria, **Alkal**emia Loan word: **Alkali** (al′kă-lī″)
ACID/O (as-ĭ-dō)	Acidic, acid	L. *acidus*, *-a*, *-um*, sour, sharp	**Acid**uria, keto**acid**osis, **acid**ophile Derivative: **Acid** (as′id)
STHEN/O (sthĕ-nō)	Strength, specific gravity	Gr. *sthenos*, strength	Mya**sthen**ia, hyper**sthen**uria, **asthen**opia
CHROM/O (krŏ-mō) **CHROMAT/O** (krŏ-măt-ō)	Color	Gr. *chroma*, *chromatos*, color	Uro**chrome**, **chromat**in, **chrom**osome
FLAV/O (flă-vō)	Yellow (bright yellow)	L. *flavus*, *-a*, *-um*, yellow	Uro**flavin**, **flav**escent, **flav**ism
XANTH/O (zan-thō)	Yellow	Gr. *xanthos*, yellow	Uro**xanth**in, **xanth**emia, **xanth**ene
LUTE/O (loo-tĕ-ō)	Yellow (pale or orangish)	L. *luteus*, *-a*, *-um*, yellow	Uro**lutein**, **lute**al Loan word: **Luteum** (lū′tĕ-ŭm)
ERYTHR/O (ĕ-rĭth-rō)	Red, redness (red blood cells)	Gr. *erythros*, red	Uro**erythr**in, **erythr**ocyte, **erythr**uria
RRHOD/O RHOD/O (rŏ-dō)	Rose color	Gr. *rhodon*, rose	Uro**rrhod**in, **rhod**opsin, **rhod**ogenesis
PORPHYR/O (por-fĭ-rō)	Purple, dark red	Gr. *porphyra*, purple	Uro**porphyr**in, **porphyr**ia
CYAN/O (sī-ă-nō)	Blue	Gr. *kyanos*, blue	Uro**cyan**in, **cyan**osis, **cyan**obacteria

Greek or Latin word element	Current usage	Etymology	Examples
CERUL/O (sĕ-roo-lŏ) **CAERUL/O** (sē-roo-lŏ)	sky-blue color; dark blue	L. *caerulus, -a, -um*, blue, sky-blue	**Cerul**oplasmin, **cerul**ean
FUSC/O (fŭs-kŏ)	Brown	L. *fuscare*, to darken, make dusky	Uro**fusc**in, **fusc**in
CHLOR/O (klŏ-rŏ)	Green, chlorine	Gr. *chloros*, green	**Chlor**osis, **chlor**ophyl
VIRID/O (vĭ-rĭ-dŏ)	Green	L. *viridis*, green	**Virid**escent, **virid**ity
MELAN/O (mĕl-ăn-ŏ)	Black	Gr. *melas, melanos*, black	Uro**melan**in, **melan**ocyte
PHAE/O (fē-ŏ) **PHE/O** (fē-ŏ)	Gray	Gr. *phaios*, gray	Uro**phe**in, uro**phae**in
ALBIN/O (al-bĭ-nŏ)	White	L. *albus, a, um*, white	**Albin**uria, **albin**ism

Review	Answers
The roots for urine are _____ and _____. The main nitrogenous waste product in urine is called urea, and its root is _____. Uric acid is another nitrogenous waste product; the root typically used for uric acid is _____. Creatine is another nitrogenous waste found in urine. The root for creatine is _____. The root used for nitrogen and nitrogenous waste in general is _____.	**UR-, URIN-** **URE-** **URIC-** **CREATIN-** **AZOT-**
The roots for urination are _____ and _____. The suffix _____ is commonly used for urination (micturition). Hence, involuntary urination (urinary incontinence) is termed _____, and the lack of ability to urinate is _____. Increased excretion of urine by the kidneys is _____. Consequently, a medication that increases urination is called a _____.	**MICTUR-,MICT-** **-URESIS** **enuresis** **anuresis** **diuresis** **diuretic**
The suffix _____ is used for pathological conditions/signs associated with urine and urination. Frequent or excessive urination is termed _____. A scanty amount of urine production is _____. Blood in the urine is _____. Pus in the urine is _____. The presence of protein, particularly albumin, in urine is termed _____. Excessive urination at night is _____. Painful or difficult urination is _____. Absence of urine formation is _____. Glucose in the urine is termed _____ or _____. Ketones in the urine are _____. Excessive concentration of calcium in the urine is _____. An increase in nitrogenous compounds in the urine is _____. High levels of nitrites in the urine are _____. High pH (greater than 7) or basic urine is _____. Low pH (lower than 7) or acidic urine is _____. High specific gravity of urine is _____.	**-URIA** **polyuria** **oliguria** **hematuria** **pyuria** **albuminuria** **nocturia** **dysuria** **anuria** **glusosuria,** **melituria** **ketonuria** **hypercalciuria** **azoturia** **nitrituria** **alkinuria** **aciduria** **hypersthenuria**
With respect to the flow of urine, _____ is movement forward or with the flow, and _____ is movement backward or against the flow.	**antegrade** **retrograde**

Review	Answers
The roots PLAN- and PLANKT- mean _____. Hence, the presence or discharge of urine from parts other than the urinary tract is called _____.	**wandering** **uroplania**
Urochrome is the pigment that gives urine its color. The root CHROM- and CHROMAT- mean _____. The passing of colorless urine is termed _____ or _____, the root in the latter term meaning "white."	**color** **achromaturia,** **albinuria**
The chemical substances that produce particular colors in urine will have the root for the color followed by the suffix -in. The brownish pigment in the urine with certain conditions is _____. A blue pigment present in the urine with certain conditions is _____. A black pigment present in the urine with certain conditions is _____. A strawy yellow pigment in the urine with certain conditions is _____. A (fluorescent) bright yellow pigment in the urine with certain conditions is _____. A yellow pigment in the urine with certain conditions is _____. A red pigment in the urine with certain conditions is _____. A rose-colored pigment in the urine with certain conditions is _____. A dark red (purple) pigment in the urine with certain conditions is _____. A grey pigment in the urine with certain conditions is _____. A green pigmen in the urine with certain conditions could be termed _____.	**urofuscin** **urocyanin** **uromelanin** **urolutein** **uroflavin** **uroxanthin** **uroerythrin** **urorrhodin** **uroporphyrin** **urophein** **(urophaein)** **urochlorin**

Lessons from History: Lithotomy and the Hippocratic Oath

Food for Thought as You Read:

What is the historical meaning of the Oath?
Does it speak to modern medical practices, such as the need for specialization?

I swear by Apollo the Physician and by Asclepius and by Health and Panacea and by all the gods as well as goddesses, making them judges [witnesses], to bring the following oath and written covenant to fulfillment, in accordance with my power and my judgment; to regard him who has taught me this *techne* as equal to my parents, and to share, in partnership, my livelihood with him and to give him a share when he is in need of necessities, and to judge the offspring [coming] from him equal to [my] male siblings, and to teach them this *techne*, should they desire to learn [it], without fee and written covenant, and to give a share both of rules and of lectures, and of all the rest of learning, to my sons and to the [sons]of him who has taught me and to the pupils who have both made a written contract and sworn by a medical convention but by no other.

And I will use regimens for the benefit of the ill in accordance with my ability and my judgment, but from [what is] to their harm or injustice I will keep [them]. And I will not give a drug that is deadly to anyone if asked [for it], nor will I suggest the way to such a counsel. And likewise, I will not give a woman a destructive pessary.

And in a pure and holy way, I will guard my life and my *techne*. **I will not cut, and certainly not those suffering from stone, but I will cede [this] to men [who are] practitioners of this activity.** Into as many houses as I may enter, I will go for the benefit of the ill, while being far from all voluntary and destructive injustice, especially from sexual acts both upon women's bodies and upon men's, both of the free and of the slaves. And about whatever I may see or hear in treatment, or even without treatment, in the life of human beings – things that should not ever be blurted out outside – I will remain silent, holding such things to be unutterable [sacred, not to be divulged].

If I render this oath fulfilled, and if I do not blur and confound it [making it to no effect] may it be [granted] to me to enjoy the benefits both of life and of *techne*, being held in good repute among all human beings for time eternal. If, however, I transgress and perjure myself, the opposite of these.

Translation by Heinrich von Staden in "'In a pure and holy way': Personal and
Professional Conduct in the Hippocratic Oath?" in Journal of the History of
Medicine and Allied Sciences, Volume 51, Issue 4, October 1996, pp. 406–408.

The statement in the Hippocratic Oath, "I will not cut, and certainly not those suffering from stone, but I will cede [this] to men [who are] practitioners of this activity," has been interpreted as Hippocrates' call for medical specialization, and therefore, the origins of **urology** in Hippocratic medicine. This interpretation of the Oath is rather problematic. There is insufficient evidence to prove that the Hippocratic Oath was written by Hippocrates, and therefore, it is probably best to refer to this original text simply as the Oath. Another problematic interpretation is that the Oath was written for all ancient Greek physicians for the practice of ethical medicine. The glaring problem with this interpretation is that no Hippocratic text or other ancient medical source ever mentions all Greek physicians having to swear the Oath. The earliest mention of the swearing of a "Hippocratic" Oath is in the *Life of Hippocrates*, which is an anonymous biography (c. 2nd–4th century AD) attributed to the physician Soranus. It is important to bear in mind that the "Life of Hippocrates" does not state that all physicians swore such an oath, rather it only states that Hippocrates made his disciples swear an oath, and it is quite clear from the famous physicians who were contemporaries of Hippocrates, that ancient Greek medicine did not begin with Hippocrates. Given no other source mentions such an Oath for over 600 years after the death of Hippocrates, and given Galen and many Greek physicians never mention swearing such an Oath to practice medicine, it's very unlikely that the Oath was written for all physicians.

If we divorce ourselves from the modern belief that the Oath was written for all physicians, and if we read the Oath strictly as a text from the 5th- and 4th-century BC, we begin to recognize a very different rhetorical situation for the swearing of the Oath. Based on the swearer of the oath pledging to treat the teacher as his father and his teacher's sons as his brothers, a historical reading of this text suggests that it is an oath made to a teacher of medicine by someone who is outside of the teacher's family guild. Such an interpretation of the rhetorical situation of the Oath is supported by the historical practice in ancient Greek culture of a father's trade being taught to his sons. Therefore, the Oath seems to represent an important transition in the teaching of medicine that involves opening up training to those outside the family medical guild.

The reference to "cutting for a stone" in the Oath is interpreted as the ancient practice of **lithotomy**, which was the cutting to remove a stone from the urinary tract. As to the concept of medical specialization, particularly the field of urology, being expressed by the phrase "ceding this to men who are practitioners of this activity," it is important to bear in mind that specialization was practically nonexistent in ancient Greek medicine of the 5th and 4th century BC. The ability to surgically treat specific conditions seems to be dependent on each physician's particular set of skills and what he had learned from his teacher(s). Because there were no medical universities or board certifications, an ancient Greek physician's reputation was based on his ability to cure and not harm a patient. Attempting something that was beyond one's skills or was quite dangerous to the patient would be a risk to one's reputation as an effective physician. Ancient medical descriptions of the lithotomies reveal that this surgery was perhaps one of the most dangerous of all surgeries undertaken by ancient Greek physicians. When describing the indications for a lithotomy in *On Medicine* (*De medicina* VII.26), Celsus (1st century AD) states the following:

> Now that mention has been made of the bladder and of stone, this seems the proper place to describe what treatment is to be adopted in cases of calculus, when it is impossible otherwise to afford relief; but it is most inadvisable to undertake it hastily, since it is very dangerous. This operation is not suitable for every season or at any age or for every lesion, but it must be used in the spring alone, in a boy who is not less than nine years of age and not more than fourteen, and if the disease is so bad that it cannot be relieved by medicaments, or endured by the patient without shortly bringing his life to a close.

The selection of such a young patient in this passage is interesting, given that kidney stones are more frequent in older patients than younger ones. The specificity of the young age and time of year to perform lithotomy suggests that these criteria are based on who could potentially survive such a dangerous surgery. In respect to the modern interpretation of the Oath speaking to all physicians, it is important to bear in mind that Celsus does not reference or pay attention to the Oath's injunction against lithotomy, which seems to speak to its limited influence on the ethics of ancient Greek medicine.

Like other Greek surgeries, lithotomies were performed without anesthesia. The patient lies on his back and two strong men then take hold of the patient's legs (Fig. 14.6). With his left hand, the surgeon inserts two fingers into the patient's rectum, and the surgeon's right hand rests on the hypogastrium. The physician then attempts to move the stone to the neck of the bladder manually. When the stone has been moved to the neck of the bladder, the surgeon is ready to perform the incision, which is described as follows: "When the stone has now got there, then the skin over the neck of the bladder next the anus should be incised by a semilunar cut, the horns of which point towards the hips; then a little lower down in that part of the incision which is concave, a second cut is to be made under the skin, at a right angle to the first, to open up the

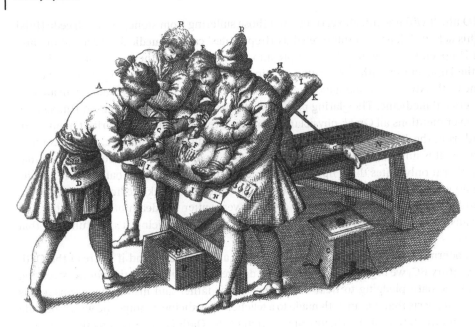

Fig. 14.6 Lithotomy scene from the early 18th century. The so-called term "lithotomy position" depicted here is used in gynecological, rectal, and urological procedures; the patient lies supine with his or her thighs abducted and flexed up toward the abdomen. Engraving from *Litotomia* by Tommaso Alghisi, 1707. *Source:* Litotomia; ovvero, del cavar la pietra / Wellcome Collection / Public domain.

neck of the bladder until the urinary passage is opened so that the wound is a little larger than the stone." The calculus was extracted from the opening by the fingers or by a hook. Despite how dangerous this surgery was, this ancient method of lithotomy, as described by Celsus, was performed for centuries by surgeons, which is why, to this day, the surgical removal of a stone by cutting is called lithotomy. Celsus does mention ancient Greek surgeons who were famous for their lithotomy techniques, but the same could be said about other surgical techniques. Thus, this was not a recognized specialization in the field of medicine, let alone the foundation of urology.

As to the rationale behind having an injunction against lithotomy in the Oath, it is important to consider the context in which this statement occurs. The other injunctions in the Oath that precede this statement are translated as, "And I will not give a drug that is deadly to anyone if asked [for it], nor will I suggest the way to such a counsel. And likewise, I will not give a woman a destructive pessary." The first sentence is commonly misunderstood as speaking to an injunction against euthanasia and the second against abortion. The interpretation that Hippocrates was speaking against "euthanasia" is problematic, considering that euthanasia was not commonly practiced by Greeks or Greek physicians of the Classical world. It would be better to take the statement at face value, namely, that a physician should not give a person information on how to make a poison. This interpretation is historically relevant given physicians were considered experts in *pharmaka*, and therefore, they were knowledgeable in regards to poisons and their antidotes. The fear of being poisoned by someone was a common sentiment expressed in Greek literature and law, particularly in respect to political figures, so it stands to reason that the author of The Oath is speaking of poisoning someone rather than assisting someone to end their life in as painless a manner as possible.

As to the interpretation of Hippocrates making an injunction against abortion, one should consider the use of the term destructive pessary (*phthorion*) in the Oath. A *phthorion* was a suppository/tampon that was impregnated with organic material that in fact could produce an abortion. Thus, the Oath is speaking strictly to just one of a number of ways in which an ancient physician could attempt to terminate a pregnancy. It is quite clear from the warnings about the use of a *phthorion* that it could harm the woman's vagina by causing inflammation. These warnings seem to reflect the caustic nature of the materia medica used. For example, rue, which is a common materia medica in a *phthorion*, can cause severe gastric pain, emesis, liver damage, and death if taken in large doses. In the Oath, the author links the injunction against poison to the injunction against using a *phthorion* with the Greek word ὁμοίως, which is translated "likewise." This seems to suggest that the author of the Oath sees the injunctions against poisons and the giving of a *phthorion* to a woman as speaking to a similar concept, namely, the avoidance of practices, particularly drugs, that are potentially deadly. Given how dangerous lithotomy was in ancient Greek medicine, and given how an ancient Greek physician's reputation was dependent on healing and not harming, much less killing, one's patient, the injunction against lithotomy seems to have served a similar purpose to the injunctions against poisons and the use of the *phthorion* in that the swearer of the Oath is to avoid practices that would bring disrepute to the family medical guild.

Some Suggested Readings

Orr, Robert D., et al. "Use of the Hippocratic Oath: A Review of Twentieth Century Practice and a Content Analysis of Oaths Administered in Medical Schools in the U.S. and Canada in 1993." *The Journal of Clinical Ethics* 8, no. 4 (1997): 377–388.

Rütten, Thomas. "*Receptions of the Hippocratic Oath in the Renaissance. The Prohibition of Abortion as a Case Study in Reception.*" *Journal of the History of Medicine and Allied Sciences* 51, no. 4 (1996): 456–483.

von Staden, Heinrich. "In a Pure and Holy Way: Personal and Professional Conduct in the Hippocratic Oath?" *Journal of the History of Medicine and Allied Sciences* 51, no. 4 (1996): 404–437.

Fig. 14.7 Kidney stones/renal calculi.
Source: Adapted from Blausen.com staff (2014). "Medical gallery of Blausen Medical 2014." WikiJournal of Medicine1 (2).

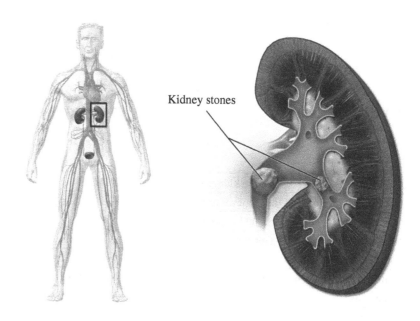

Kidney stones

Stones
Lithiasis – Derived from the Greek word for a stone, *lithos*, the formation of stones, particularly in the kidneys, is called lithiasis (Fig. 14.7). Hence, the presence or formation of stones in the kidneys is called nephrolithiasis, and the presence of stones in the ureters is termed **ureterolithiasis**. The Latin loan word for a stone is **calculus**, and its plural is **calculi**. The root **LITH-** for "stone" often appears as a suffix **-LITH**. Thus, a stone in the kidney is called a **nephrolith**; a stone located in the bladder would be a **cystolith**; and a stone in the ureter is a **ureterolith**.
Lithotomy – Although the surgical suffix **-TOMY** means "incision," due to its historical origins, the surgical procedure of cutting to remove a stone is called a lithotomy.
Lithotripsy – The surgical breaking of a stone, usually by sound waves, is called a lithotripsy. The loan word **tripsis** is used for "massaging, grinding, or crushing."
Lithoclasty – The surgical breaking of a stone with a forceps called a lithoclast is termed lithoclasty.
Litholapaxy – The breaking and immediate washing out of stone is a litholapaxy.
Catheter – A catheter is a flexible tubular device inserted into the body for removing or injecting fluids. Perhaps the most common type of catheter is a urinary catheter, which is typically introduced through the urethra into the bladder.

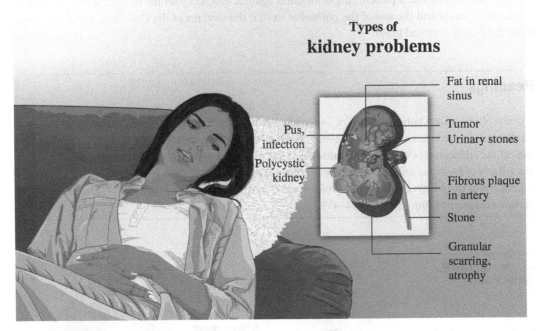

Fig. 14.8 Pathologies of the kidney. *Source:* Adapted from https://www.myupchar.com/en/last accessed on 19 January 2024.

Kidney pathologies

Nephroptosis – A prolapse of the kidney is termed nephroptosis.

Nephroma – A tumor of the kidney is termed a nephroma (Fig. 14.8).

Nephromegaly – An enlarged kidney is termed nephromegaly.

Nephropyosis – Nephropyosis is pus/purulence of the kidney (Fig. 14.8).

Polycystic kidney disease – PKD is an inherited kidney disease characterized by cystic degeneration of the kidney (Fig. 14.8).

Hydronephrosis – The distention of the renal pelvis and calyces due to obstructed outflow is called hydronephrosis.

Nephrosis – Nephrosis is a kidney disease that is characterized by the severe loss of protein leading to hypoproteinema and edema.

Nephrosclerosis – A disease causing the hardening of the kidney tissue, particularly renal tubules, is called nephrosclerosis.

Renal failure – The kidney's inability to properly filter and excrete nitrogenous wastes is called renal failure. The presence of nitrogenous waste in the blood is a sign of renal failure, and it is commonly called azotemia or uremia. Acute and chronic renal failures are commonly treated with **dialysis**, which involves the removal of waste and extra fluids by separating them from the blood via a semipermeable membrane. We have run into the suffix for "dissolution" or "breaking down," **-LYSIS**, in earlier chapters. That said, *dialysis* is an ancient Greek word that means "loosening one from another" or "separating."

Hypernatremia/Hyponatremia and Hyperkalemia/Hypokalemia – The concentration of sodium and potassium in the blood are signs of kidney dysfunction. Excessive sodium in the blood is termed **hypernatremia**, and a deficiency of sodium in the blood is **hyponatremia**. An excess of potassium in the blood is **hyperkalemia**; a deficiency in potassium in the blood is **hypokalemia**.

Inflammation

Nephritis – Inflammation of the kidney is called nephritis.

Glomerulitis – Inflammation of the glomeruli is called glomerulitis.

Pyelitis – Inflammation of the renal pelvis is called pyelitis.

Cystitis – Inflammation of the bladder is called cystitis.

Ureteritis – Inflammation of the ureters is called ureteritis.

Urethritis – Inflammation of the urethra is called urethritis.

Meatitis – Inflammation of the opening of the urethra is meatitis.

Hemorrhage

Cystorrhagia – A hemorrhage of the urinary bladder is called cystorrhagia.

Urethrorrhagia – A hemorrhage of the urethra is called urethrorrhagia.

Nephrorrhagia – Renal hemorrhage is called nephrorrhagia.

Greek or Latin word element	Current usage	Etymology	Examples
CALCUL/O (kăl-kū-lō)	Stone	L. *calculus, -i*, m. a little stone, pebble	**Calcul**ogenesis, **calcul**ous, **calcul**ation Loan word: **Calculus** (kal'kyŭ-lŭs) pl. **Calculi** (kal'kyŭ-lī")
LITH/O (lĭth-ō) **-LITH** (lĭth)	Stone, lithium	Gr. *lithos*, stone	**Lith**otripsy, **lith**emia, hystero**lith**
-TRIPSY (trip-sē)	To rub, crush	Gr. *tribein* (*trips-*), to rub, crush	Litho**tripsy**, neuro**tripsy**, omphalo**tripsy** Derivative: **Tripsis** (trip'sĭs)
-LAPAXY (lă-paks-ē)	Surgical evacuation (of a stone)	Gr. *lapaxis*, evacuation	Litho**lapaxy**
-CLASTY (klas-tē)	Surgical breaking (of a stone)	Gr. *klasis*, breaking	Litho**clasty**
CATHER/O (kath-ĕt-ĕr-ō)	Catheter	Gr. *catheter*, catheter * a surgical instrument for emptying the bladder, fr. Gr. *kathiemi*, send down	**Cather**ization Loan word: **Catheter** (kath'ĕt-ĕr)

Review	Answers
The formation of stones, particularly in the kidneys, is called _____. Hence, the presence or formation of stones in the ureters is termed _____. The loan word for a stone is _____, and its plural is _____. The root LITH- means _____. Hence, a stone in the kidney is called a _____; a stone located in the bladder would be a _____; and a stone in the ureter is a _____.	**lithiasis** **ureterolithiasis** **calculus, calculi** **stone** **nephrolith** **cystolith** **ureterolith**
The surgical procedure of cutting to remove a stone is called a _____. The surgical breaking of a stone, usually by sound waves, is called a _____. The surgical breaking of a stone with forceps called lithoclasts is termed _____. The breaking and immediate washing out of stone is a _____.	**lithotomy** **lithotripsy** **lithoclasty** **litholapaxy**
The flexible tubular device passed through an anatomical orifice into a body cavity, which is typically through the urethra to the bladder, is called a _____.	**catheter**
The presence of nitrogenous waste in the blood is called _____ or _____.	**azotemia, uremia**
Inflammation of the kidney is _____. Inflammation of the glomeruli is _____. Inflammation of the renal pelvis is _____. Inflammation of the bladder is _____. Inflammation of the urethra is _____. Inflammation of the opening of the urethra is _____. Inflammation of the ureters is _____.	**nephritis** **glomerulitis** **pyelitis** **cystitis** **urethritis** **meatitis** **ureteritis**

Review	Answers
A prolapse of the kidney is a _____.	**nephroptosis**
The distention of the renal pelvis and calyces due to obstructed outflow is called _____.	**hydronephrosis**
A disease causing the hardening of the kidney tissue is called _____.	**nephrosclerosis**
A hemorrhage of the urinary bladder is called a _____. A hemorrhage of the urethra is called a _____. Renal hemorrhage is a _____.	**cystorrhagia urethrorrhagia nephrorrhagia**
A stricture/narrowing of the urethra is called _____.	**urethrostenosis**
A medication that increases the secretion of urine is a _____.	**diuretic**
The concentration of sodium and potassium in the blood is a sign of kidney dysfunction. Excessive sodium in the blood is termed _____, and a deficiency of sodium in the blood is _____. A deficiency in potassium in the blood is _____; an excess of potassium in the blood is _____.	**hypernatremia, hyponatremia hypokalemia, hyperkalemia**
An enlarged kidney is called _____.	**Nephromegaly**
_____ is pus/purulence in the kidney.	**Nephropyosis**
Acute and chronic renal failure are commonly treated with _____, which involves the removal of waste and extra fluids by separating them from the blood via a semipermeable membrane.	**dialysis**

15

Male and Female Reproductive Systems

CHAPTER LEARNING OBJECTIVES
1) You will learn the word elements, loan words, and key terms associated with the male and female reproductive systems.
2) You will become familiar with the historical concepts associated with the male and female reproductive systems, as well as those associated with the formation of the fetus and childbirth.

Lessons from History: *Ancient Greek and Roman Conceptions of the Penis*

Food for Thought:

In what ways are ancient Greek and Roman conceptions of a normal penis different from our own? How are they similar?

To what extent did societal norms affect ancient Greek medicine's approach to the penis? Do societal norms have a similar effect on modern medicine's approach to the penis?

The term "penis" originally was a vulgar word rather than a technical term for the male sexual organ. Being derived from the verb *pendere*, "to hang," in classical Latin, *penis* originally meant "the tail" of an animal. In addition to *penis*, Romans had other words that they used as euphemisms and vulgar terms for the male sexual organ, such as *mentula* (little stalk) and *verenda (venerable things)*. The Latin medical term Celsus used in *De medicina* for the penis was *colis*, which is a Latin word meaning "the stalk of a plant." In the 17th century, "penis" started to be used as a technical term in human anatomy for the male sexual organ. The Greek word for the penis is *phallos*. The loan word **phallus** and its root **PHALL-** are commonly used for the "penis" in modern medical terminology. Although our technical terms for this organ are derived from Greek and Latin, ancient Greek and Roman sociocultural beliefs about the appearance, function, and symbolism of the penis are quite different from those of today.

Circumcision is the practice of removing the **preputium** or foreskin from the penis. Although it is natural for the penis to have a foreskin, a completely circumcised penis is the normal appearance of a penis in many countries, especially in America, where 80.5% of males from age 14 to 59 are circumcised. While circumcision may be considered normal in America, it is not, by any means, typical of all modern societies. Approximately 30% of males are estimated to be circumcised globally. Even among societies that have a long history of circumcision (e.g. subequatorial Africa, Egypt, and Arabia), the specific form and extent of circumcision has varied; for instance, some practice only partial removal of the foreskin. Religion and race offer two reasons why it is almost "uniformly practiced by Jews, Muslims, and the members of Coptic, Ethiopian, and Eritrean Orthodox Churches." However, contrary to popular belief, circumcision is not a tenet of Christianity. While Coptic, Ethiopian, and Eritrean Christians have a long history of practicing circumcision, early Christianity understood circumcision as a Jewish practice, and therefore, it was relevant only to Christians of Jewish decent. For the most part, the rise of Christianity led to circumcision falling into disregard, particularly among Europeans. In fact, the Catholic Church went so far as to condemn

Greek and Latin Roots of Medical and Scientific Terminologies, First Edition. Todd A. Curtis.
© 2025 John Wiley & Sons, Inc. Published 2025 by John Wiley & Sons, Inc.
Companion website: www.wiley.com/go/Curtis

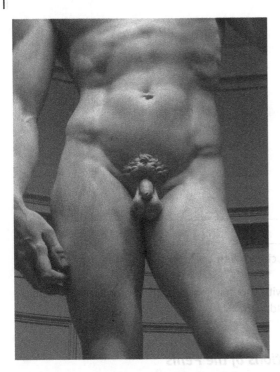

Fig. 15.1 Image of the uncircumcised penis in Michelangelo's sculpture of David. *Source:* Jörg Bittner Unna/Wikimedia Commons/CC BY 3.0.

circumcision as a moral sin at the Council of Basel–Florence in 1442. This foreignness of the circumcised penis can be observed in Michelangelo's statue *David* (1504), which is particularly interesting since it presents David, a Jewish man, as being uncircumcised (Fig. 15.1). The negative view of circumcision among Christians and non-Jewish Europeans continued well into the 19th century. However, by the late 19th century, circumcision became common among Christians and non-Christians in the English-speaking world. This change of attitude toward circumcision is partially due to the medical belief that circumcision is useful to prevent sexually transmitted diseases. The basis for this view was first articulated in 1855 by the English physician, Jonathan Hutchinson, who published a study that compared the presence of venereal diseases among gentile and Jewish populations in London. His study, which has largely been debunked, concluded that circumcision accounted for a lower incidence of sexually transmitted diseases in the Jewish population. That said, the argument for its health benefits continues. According to a study by the World Health Organization in 2007, "there is substantial evidence that male circumcision protects against several diseases, including urinary tract infections, syphilis, chancroid, and invasive penile cancer, as well as HIV." In addition to its health benefits, the belief that circumcision helped to prevent masturbation is said to be another reason for the rise in infant circumcision in the English-speaking world during the 19th century. Hutchinson again lent his medical voice to this use of circumcision when he published an article in 1893 entitled, *On Circumcision as a Preventive of Masturbation*. Thus, thanks to these beliefs, the medicalization of infant circumcision became prominent in English-speaking nations, thereby establishing what is considered to be a normal-looking penis in America today.

A circumcised penis was considered abnormal and somewhat barbaric by ancient Greeks and Romans. This is because, unlike in modern America, the practice of circumcision was largely understood as a marker of one's race and/or religion. Although a number of ancient groups of people other than Jews practiced circumcision (e.g. Samaritans, Egyptians, and Nabateans), circumcision was closely associated with the Jewish race and Judaism. Circumcision was a fundamental tenet of Judaism and Jewish culture. The practice of circumcision is based on the belief that God had Abraham, the patriarch of the Jewish nation, circumcise himself and all the males of his group prior to the promised birth of Isaac, his only son by Sarah. The act of circumcision was, therefore, considered part of Jewish custom because it was seen as a sign of God's covenant with Abraham, and by extension, the Jewish people. The stigmatization of the Jews for their practice of circumcision is evident in Greek and Roman literatures. For instance, in his *Satires* (XIV.96-106), Juvenal (c. 2nd century AD) criticized Romans who had adopted Judaism (i.e. proselytes). He sees the Jewish practice of circumcision as the final step of being proselytized by Jews. While there is much debate among scholars as to what Juvenal's actual opinions of the Jewish race were, it is quite clear that Juvenal deliberately used crude remarks regarding the religious beliefs of the proselytes, and therefore, he indirectly attacked the Jews, as he did many other groups of peoples in his satires about Roman life. Circumcision made Jews recognizable to their Greek and Roman rulers because hiding one's penis from the view of others was far less easy than it is today. In the Hellenistic world, as Jews exercised naked along with Greeks in the gymnasia and participated in the public baths of the Roman world, there were clearly opportunities for Jewish males to be recognized. Avoiding these cultural practices was not an option for a Jew who wanted to move in Greek and Roman societies. Consequently, some Jews tried to hide their circumcision, particularly during times of hostility and persecution. *I Maccabees* describes how Jews tried to hide their circumcision from their Hellenistic overlords by attempting to stretch the skin of their penis using a weight, and thereby, creating the appearance of a foreskin. The stigmatization Romans had toward Jews can also be seen Celsus' description (*De medicina* VII.25) of a cosmetic surgery that was used to reverse circumcision by creating a new foreskin for circumcised males and for those who were born without one. Celsus states that the purpose of such a surgery being performed on a boy or an adult male was "for the sake of what is fitting/proper (*causa decorum*)." Thus, whether it was natural, or on purpose, de-circumcision was for esthetic purposes, and undoubtedly, the sociocultural value of the appearance of an uncircumcised penis provided the impetus for an adult male to undergo such a painful surgery (Fig. 15.2).

Fig. 15.2 Depiction of one of the decircumcision surgeries that Celsus describes in *De medicina. Source:* Rubin, J. P. (1980)/with permission of Elsevier.

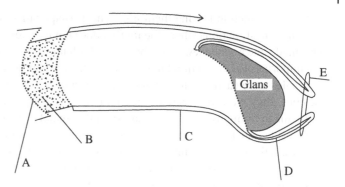

Achieving an erection is a sexual function of the penis. Much like today, this sexual function is closely tied to masculinity in the ancient world, and therefore, it has a greater meaning than its actual function. When describing the presence of Eunuchs among the Scythians, the author of the Hippocratic work *Airs, Waters, and Places*, relates how the Scythians' faulty understanding of anatomy and their practice of venesection led to them becoming **impotent**:

> Riding on horseback, swellings arise at their joints, because their legs are always hanging down from their horses; then they become lame, and develop lesions at their hips when the disease becomes serious. They cure themselves in the following way. At the beginning of the disease, they cut the vessel behind each ear. After the blood flows out, sleep comes over them from their weakness, and they go to bed. Later they wake up, some being cured and others not. Now, in my opinion, by this treatment their seed is destroyed; for by the side of the ear are vessels which, when someone cuts them, make the person cut sterile, and so I believe it is these vessels they are cutting. After this treatment, when the Scythians approach women and find themselves to be impotent, at first they take no notice and ignore it. But when on making two, three or even more attempts the same thing happens to them, thinking that they have wronged the divinity to which they attribute the cause, they put on women's clothing, admit that they have lost their manhood, and so play the woman and do the same work with women that they do.
>
> Translated by Paul Potter. *Loeb Classical Library* 147. Cambridge, MA: Harvard University Press, 2022, 132–133.

Rather than accepting a divine explanation for their impotence, the author of *Airs, Waters, and Places* attributes the cause to the Scythians cutting off the "seminal" vessels behind the ears. The erroneous notion that the seminal vessels lie behind a man's ear is also found in some other Hippocratic works and the writings of other ancient Greek physicians, particularly Diogenes of Apollonia (5th century BC). In Diogenes' reproductive system, there are two parallel vessels; each vessel serves one side of the body. Blood passes through these vessels into the spinal marrow, which finds its way to the spermatic vessels as semen. The Scythians' clumsy approach to venesection was understood as cutting off the blood supply necessary for the production of semen. Given that sexual desire and the ability to achieve an erection were commonly linked to the production of semen in ancient Greek medicine, the Scythians' malady is explained, albeit incorrectly, via nature and the customs of the people. With respect to the social value of achieving an erection, the author claims that the impotent Scythians no longer see themselves as men. Instead, they put on women's clothing and take on the role of women in the community. While it is unclear if the author has accurately portrayed the behavior of these Scythians, it does speak to the strong shame and stigmatization males feel about their masculinity based on a common sexual dysfunction. In these respects, modern and ancients have some similar, but regrettable, sociocultural beliefs.

It is important to bear in mind that the author of *Airs, Waters, and Places* also likens impotent Scythians to being Eunuchs. The term Eunuch comes from a Greek word meaning "bed-guard;" Eunuchs served as guards and attendants for women in royal and aristocratic courts, particularly those in the regions of the Levant and Mesopotamia, which is why in ancient Greek literature Eunuchs are associated with the foreign practices of the East. However, over time, Eunuchs became an important feature of Greek and Roman cultures. As Stevenson notes, based on Roman inheritance laws, there were four different types of Eunuchs in the Roman world: "*spadones, thlibiae, thladiae,* and *castrati* of whom all but the *castrati* could pass on an inheritance – the legal essence of Roman patriline." The latter three terms suggest the means by which their male genitalia was physically damaged: based on a reading of Soranus, *thlibiae* (pressed) seems to refer to those whose testicles did not descend after their birth (cryptorchidism); *thladiae* are those whose testicles were crushed leaving them impotent; and *castrati* are males whose testicles and/or penis were cutoff to make them a Eunuch. *Spadones* appear to be those who have a sexual dysfunction leaving them impotent. Perhaps our modern diagnoses of **hypospadias** and **epispadias**, which are congenital dysfunctions where the urethra does not exit out of the normal place on the penis, are dysfunctions that would have made one a *spadones*. Thus, there were both natural and man-made factors that led to one being considered a Eunuch. It is important to bear in mind that the term Eunuch applied to a wide variety of males, both heterosexual and homosexual, and males were castrated for religious reasons and for the slave trade. Although some Eunuchs held great power in their societies, they were considered a different class of people and somewhat despised. Thus, the author likening impotent Scythians to Eunuchs reveals to what extent the sexual function of one's penis determined his place in society.

On a side note to the discussion of Eunuchs, in the Roman world, the word *testis* was used both for the "testicle" and for "witness"; the latter meaning is where we get the word "testimony." Likewise, the statement of *testis unus, testis nullus* (one witness is no witness), which is a statement to the historical principle that a single piece of evidence in history cannot be trusted because it cannot be corroborated, also speaks to the nonanatomical meaning of the Latin word *testis*. There are numerous explanations for this odd pairing of meanings. Some have claimed that having one's testicles intact and functioning determined their ability to provide evidence in a Roman court. The rationale behind this interpretation is based on the mistaken belief that the testimony of Eunuchs was inadmissible in a Roman court. Some have argued that it speaks to the practice of swearing an oath that is evident in ancient Mediterranean literature, such as in the Bible. In some cases, the oath was taken by the oath-swearer placing his hand under the testicles of the one to whom he was swearing the oath. The word picture for this odd speech act seems to speak to the potential consequences of breaking one's oath. Perhaps the genitalia are symbolic of the progeny of the man, who will hold the swearer and his family accountable if the oath is broken. However, there is little to no evidence that this was a practice of oath-taking in the Roman world.

In modern culture, particularly in psychology and gender studies, almost any object that vaguely resembles a penis (e.g. a building, statue, or cigar) can be considered a phallic symbol. That said, one almost never sees a lifelike image of the penis in a public space in modern American culture. Perhaps, this is because a realistic image would be considered pornographic due to the strong sexual connotations of an image of a penis. Unlike in modern America, it was not uncommon for one to see a sculpture of a penis in a Greek public space. This is particularly true with respect to Greek sculptures of gods and men. Because Greek males exercised in the nude, it has been argued that these figures were understood in the context of the "athletic nude." A realistic image of a penis also commonly appeared on a type of statue called a "herm." A herm, which later became associated with the Greek god Hermes, was a rectangular pillar that had a sculpture of a bearded head placed at the top (Fig. 15.3). Often there was an erect penis carved somewhere on the front of herm; and in some cases, instead of a bearded head, a sculpture of a penis was featured on the top of the pillar. Herms were commonly found at crossroads, before temples, and in front of houses, where they served the purpose of boundary markers in the ancient Greek world. The herm warned people that they were about to cross into another area (e.g. moving from a public space to a sacred space). It has been hypothesized that the bearded head and the penis both symbolized power and virility, and therefore, they carried with them apotropaic qualities, which is the ability to avert evil.

In the ancient Greek world, an erect penis could also be considered a sexual symbol, albeit with a slightly different meaning than in the modern world. Satyrs are rustic lower deities associated with fertility and Dionysus, the god of wine. They were commonly depicted as bearded men with ears like a donkey, pug noses, long asinine tails, and large erect penises (Fig. 15.4). As followers of Dionysus, they are often portrayed in states of revelry and intoxication. The large erect penises on these creatures are symbolic of their lack of sexual continence, and coupled with their animalistic features, their hypersexuality is portrayed as being consistent with a bestial nature. Owing to the Satyrs' association with hypersexuality, ancient Greek medicine used the term **satyriasis** for an overactive sex drive in men. In ancient Greek medicine, the physiological cause for this excessive drive was thought to be the overproduction of semen. The term **satyriasis** is still used today for excessive sexual drive/activity among males. Thus, unlike the image of a penis being a sign of virility and power on a Herm, images of satyrs with large erect penises seem to connote sexual incontinence or hypersexual behavior of wild rather than civilized sexual behavior.

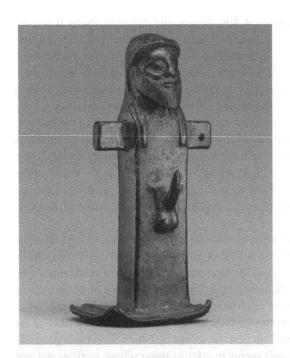

Fig. 15.3 Bronze statue of a Greek Herm (c. 490 BC). *Source:* The Metropolitan Museum of Art/Wikimedia Commons/CC0 1.0.

Today, the root **SATYR-** is used for "excessive sexual desire" and "satyr-like" characteristics. As to deities being associated with sex, medical terminology is full of such words. The name of the Greek goddess of eros, Aphrodite, supplies the root for "sex, sexual desire," **APHRODISI-**; a derivative from her Roman name, Venus, forms the root for "sex, sexual desire, and sexually transmitted diseases," **VENERE-**. The term syphilis and its corresponding root **SYPHIL-** is derived from the name of a character in the 16th-century poem, *Syphilis, sive Morbus Gallicus* (Syphilis or the French Disease) written by an Italian physician named Girolamo Fracastoro. In jest, the poem links the cause of this disease to a shepherd named Syphilus, who insulted the sun god of Haiti. In retaliation, the god sent a plague to Haiti and Syphilus was its first victim.

Priapus is another word used in modern medical terminology for "penis." In modern medicine, the condition of an abnormal, painful, and continued erection of the penis is termed a **priapism**. **Priapus** and its root **PRIAP-** are derived from the name of the Greek god of the gardens, Priapos (in Latin Priapus). Priapus is perhaps the most famous of the ithyphallic [Gr. *ithys*, straight + Gr. *phallos*, penis] deities found in ancient Greek myth and religion. Priapus was commonly depicted as looking like a rustic man with a very large erect penis. Rather than being entirely sexual, Priapus' penis symbolized the fertility and generative qualities of the garden. This can be observed in the well-known Pompeiian wall fresco, which depicts the god weighing his phallus against assumedly a bag of money that was derived from a fertile, and therefore, profitable garden (Fig. 15.5). As with many other mythological accounts of the parentage of lower deities, there are some variations as to the parents of Priapus. Depending on the ancient Greek accounts, he is said to be the child of Zeus and Aphrodite, Dionysus, and Aphrodite, or Dionysus and a nymph. In some later accounts, the origin of his enlarged penis is explained as a curse sent by Hera, the wife of Zeus in Greek myth. Supposedly, Hera cursed Priapus with enormous genitals out of spite for Aphrodite's promiscuity with Hera's husband. While in ancient Greek religious cults, Priapus was worshipped as a fertility deity, his erect penis also became the subject of sexual poetry collectively called *Carmina Priapia*. The poems that make up the *Carmina Priapia*, speak not only to Priapus' hypersexual escapades as a youth but also to his pitiful state as an old, impotent god. The impotence of Priapus suggests that the ancients understood impotence as a part of old age. However, unlike in modern American culture, which tends to fixate on the length of a man's penis as being a marker of his masculinity so much so that it borders on "brachyphallopobia," having an overly large penis could be viewed as both a curse and a sign of hypersexual behavior. This is also used as an explanation as to why Greek statues of gods and men, even mythological figures of masculine power, such as Herakles (Hercules), are not depicted with large penises. Humorously, it is the modern world's fixation on the length of a penis that has recognized and even measured this feature of Greek sculptures.

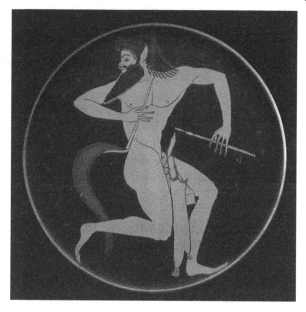

Fig. 15.4 Attic red-figure plate with an image of a Satyr with pipes and a pipe case hanging on his penis. 520–500 BC. *Source:* Bibi Saint-Pol/Wikimedia Commons/ Public domain.

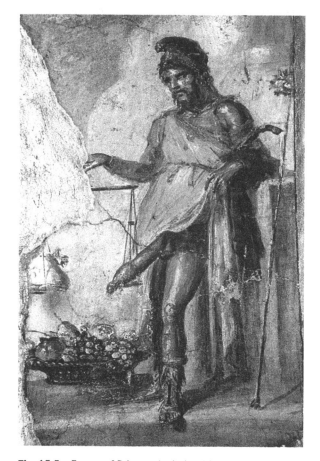

Fig. 15.5 Fresco of Priapus depicting him weighing his large penis against a bag of gold, assumedly for the sale of the fruit in the back of the image. c. 1st century BC. *Source:* Fer.filol/Wikimedia Commons/Public domain.

Some Suggested Readings

Hippocrates. *Ancient Medicine. Airs, Waters, Places. Epidemics 1 and 3. The Oath. Precepts. Nutriment.* Edited and translated by Paul Potter. Loeb Classical Library 147. Cambridge, MA: Harvard University Press, 2022.

Hankins, Catherine, *et al. Male circumcision: Global Trends and Determinants of Prevalence, Safety, and Acceptability.* Geneva: *World Health Organization,* 2007.

Hodges, Frederick. "The Ideal Prepuce in Ancient Greece and Rome." *Bulletin of the History of Medicine* 75 (2001): 375–405.

McNiven, Timothy J. "The Unheroic Penis: Otherness Exposed." *Source: Notes in the History of Art* 15, no. 1 (1995): 10–16.

Rubin, Jody P. "Celsus's Decircumcision Operation." *Urology* 16, no. 1 (1980):121–124.

Stevenson, Walter. "The Rise of Eunuchs in Greco-Roman Antiquity." *Journal of the History of Sexuality* 5, no. 4 (1995): 495–511.

Etymological Explanations: Common Terms and Word Elements for the Male Reproductive System

In the following discussion of the anatomical terms associated with the male reproductive system, the nominative and genitive singular form of the anatomical Latin term are provided in parenthesis. The Greek and Latin roots are formatted in all caps and emboldened.

Male external genitalia

Penis (L. *penis*, *-is*) – The male cylindrical organ of copulation and urination is the penis (Fig. 15.6). The roots for the "penis" are **PEN-**, **PHALL-**, and **PRIAP-**. The loan words for penis are **priapus** and **phallus**.

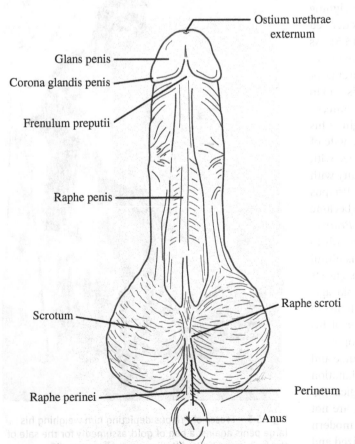

Ostium urethrae externum

Glans penis

Corona glandis penis

Frenulum preputii

Raphe penis

Scrotum

Raphe scroti

Raphe perinei

Perineum

Anus

Fig. 15.6 Anatomical Latin for the external male genitalia. *Source:* Drawing by Chloe Kim.

Glans penis (L. *glans penis*) – The bulbous end of the penis is termed the glans penis because it looks like an acorn. The root **GLAND-** is used for "gland" in modern medical terminology. The Latin *glans* (L. *glans, glandis*) was the Roman word for "acorn." This meaning corresponds to the Greek root commonly used for the glans penis in medicine, **BALAN-**. **BALAN-** is derived from the Greek word for an "acorn," *balanos*. Thus, depending on the context, **BALAN-** can mean "acorn" or "glans penis."

Foreskin (L. *preputium, -i*) – The foreskin that covers an uncircumcised penis is termed the **prepuce** or **preputium**. The root for "foreskin" is **PREPUTI-**.

Scrotum (L. *scrotum, -i*) – The last obvious external feature of the male genitalia is the sac-like structure called the scrotum. The scrotum is divided into two sacks, each containing a testicle and its epididymis. The roots used for the scrotum are **SCROT-** and **OSCHE-**. The Latin word scrotum meant "bag," and it began to be used for this anatomical part in the 15th century. Some have argued that scrotum was transposed from the Latin word for a "hide" or "skin," *scortum*. The root **OSCHE-** comes from the Greek word for the "scrotum," *oscheon*.

Perineum (L. *perineum, -i*) – The external region between the scrotum and the anus is termed the perineum. The root for perineum is **PERINE-**.

Internal male genitalia

Testicle (L. *testis, -is*) – As noted, the **testicles** lie inside the scrotum (Fig. 15.7). The testicles are two male reproductive glands that are responsible for the production of sperm and the male hormone testosterone. The anatomical Latin term for testicle is **testis**. The roots **TEST-** and **TESTICUL-** used for the "testicles" are clearly derived from the Latin word **testis**, which is also the loan word for testicle.

Derived from the Greek word for testicle (*orchis, orchidos*), the roots **ORCH-** and **ORCHID-** are also used today for "testicle." This root also refers to the plant called the orchid. The term orchid was first used in 1845 by John Lindley in the 3rd edition of his *School of Botany*. The plant is called an "orchid" not because of its beautiful flowers, but because of its tuberous roots that resemble testicles. The association of the word *orchis* for the flower extends back to the ancient world. In Ovid's *Metamorphoses*, Orchis was said to be the son of a nymph who was turned into an orchid after his death. Today the loan word **orchis** is also used for "the testicle."

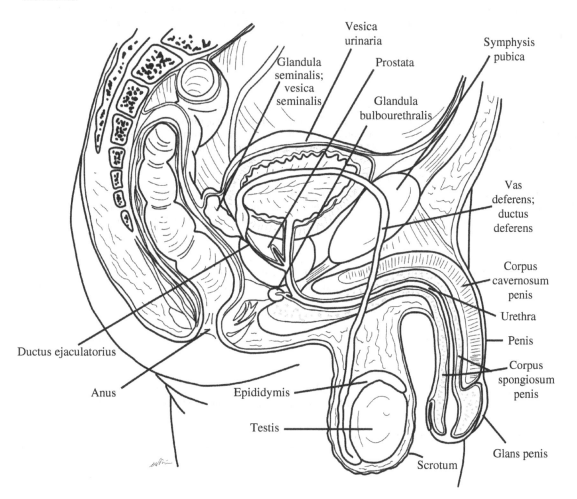

Fig. 15.7 Anatomical Latin for the internal male genitalia. *Source:* Drawing by Chloe Kim.

Internal male genitalia

Epididymis (L. *epididymis, epididymidis*) – The **epididymis** is the coiled spermatic vessel sitting on top and posterior to the testicle that serves the purpose of storing sperm before ejaculation. The compound root for this anatomical part is derived from the Greek word for a "twin," *didymos*. In ancient Greek astronomy, the constellation known today as Gemini was called the *Didymoi*, and this constellation was attached to the mythological twins, Castor and Pollux. Thus, **EPIDIDYM-** literally means "upon the twin." The twin that is being referred to is the testicle, and therefore, **DIDYM-** is sometimes used for "testicle." The suffix -**DIDYMUS**, as well as the suffix -**PAGUS** are used for conjoined twins. For example, a **gastrodidymus** refers to twins conjoined at the stomach/abdomen, and a **craniopagus** refers to twins conjoined at the cranium/head. **Didymus** is also used as a loan word today for "twin," particularly a conjoined twin.

Spermatic Cord (L. *funiculus spermaticus*) – The collection of vessels, nerves, muscles, and ducts that are connected to the testicles is termed the spermatic cord. The root **FUNICUL-**, which means "cord" or "small rope," is sometimes used for this structure. For example, **funiculitis** is an inflammation of the spermatic cord. The Cremaster muscle is associated with the spermatic cord and serves the purpose of raising the testicles. Cremaster is derived from a Greek word that means "the suspender."

Vas deferens (L. *vas deferens*; *ductus deferens*) – The vas deferens, which literally means "the carrying away vessel," is the spermatic vessel that carries the sperm away from the testicle. The vas deferens carries sperm cells to the other reproductive glands (seminal glands, prostate, and bulbourethral glands). The terms used for the surgical cutting of the vas deferens for the purpose of birth control are **vasectomy** and **gonangiectomy**. The reversal of this surgery is called a **vasovastostomy**.

Seminal gland (L. *glandula seminalis*) or seminal vesicle (L. *vesicula seminalis*) – A seminal gland is one of two sack-shaped glands that sit below the urinary bladder. The seminal glands produce a secretion that enhances the nourishing of the sperm and makes up 50–80% of the material in semen.

Prostate (L. *prostata, -ae*) – The prostate is a large trilobular gland that secretes an alkaline fluid into the semen. Derived from the Latin verb *prostare* ("to stand before"), the prostate derives its name from its location because it stands in front of the bladder. The root of the prostate is **PROSTAT-**. The prostate, seminal vesicles, and bulbourethral glands empty their contents into the seminal vessels that lead the semen out of the body via the urethra.

Bulbourethral gland (L. *glandula bulbourethralis*) or Cowper gland – The bulbourethral glands are two round glands that sit on each side of the prostate gland. These glands contribute a viscous fluid to semen that helps to lubricate the urethra. The root **BULB-** in this term indicates that they are "globe-shape" like a "plant bulb."

Sperm and semen

Sperm (L. *sperma, -ae*) – The terms that are used today for "semen" and "sperm" have an agrarian connotation to them in that they are derived from Greek and Latin words for "seed." Sperm is composed of the sex cells, also known as gametes, that are produced in the testicles. The roots for "sperm" are **SPERM-** and **SPERMAT-**. Depending on the context, these roots can also mean "seed," which is what the Greek word originally meant. A single sperm cell is called a **spermatozoon**; the root **ZO-** means "something living" and "animal." The plural of **spermatozoon** is **spermatozoa**.

Semen (L. *semen, seminis*) – The sperm and the rest of the fluid forming the ejaculate are termed **semen**. The associated root is **SEMIN-**. As in the case with sperm, depending on the context, **SEMIN-** can also mean "seed." Derived from the Greek word for "offspring" (*gone*), the root **GON-** can also mean "semen," as well as "genital" and "generation." **GON-** appears in the compound suffix -**GONY**, which is used for "generation" (e.g. agamogony, schizogony, cosmogony). **GON-** also forms the basis for the root **GONAD-**, which is used today for either the "testes" or the "ovaries." **Gonorrhea** is a sexually transmitted infection caused by the bacteria *Neisseria gonorrhoeae*. Its name is derived from the word elements **GON-** (semen, seed) and -**RRHEA** (discharge). Gonorrhea (**GONORRHE-**) was a term used in ancient medicine for a disease-causing uncontrolled, nonsexual discharge of semen. Although this is an actual pathology that some men experience, we do not call it gonorrhea. Instead of using the term gonorrhea, modern medicine uses **spermatorrhea** for "an abnormally frequent involuntary loss of semen without orgasm (Taber's)."

Sperm disorders

Azoospermia – Formed from the root for "dead" or "lack of living," **AZO-**, azoospermia is semen without living spermatozoa.

Oligospermia – Derived from the root for "few" or "scanty," **OLIG-**, oligospermia is a diminished number/count of spermatozoa in semen.

Aspermia – Aspermia is the inability to produce spermatozoa.

Prostate disorders

Hypertrophic or hyperplastic prostate – Formed from the root for "formation" **PLAST-** or the root for "nourishment/growth," **-TROPH**, benign hyperplastic or hypertrophic prostate (BPH) is a prostatic enlargement frequently occurring in older men that causes problems with urination (Fig. 15.8).

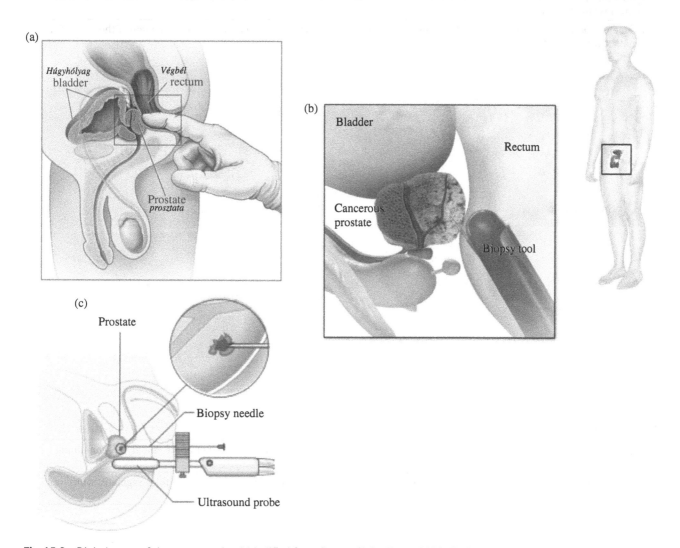

Fig. 15.8 Digital exam of the prostate gland. Modified from *Source:* Claire Tonry (2020)/Springer Nature/CC by 4.0.

Prostate cancer – Prostate cancer is a malignant tumor of the prostate gland, which is typically an **adenocarcinoma** (**ADEN-**, gland + **CARCIN-**, cancer + **-OMA**, tumor). Prostate cancer is often treated with **brachytherapy**. Brachytherapy is a form of radiation therapy in which the radiation is placed inside or close to the structure needing treatment. The Greek root **BRACHY-** means "short," and it commonly appears in numerous medical and scientific terms.

Prostatitis – Prostatitis is an inflammation of the prostate.

Scrotal and testicular pathologies

Seminoma – Derived from the root for "semen/seed" and the suffix for "tumor," a seminoma is a common type of testicular tumor that arises from male germ cells.

Cryptorchism – The condition in which there is an undescended testicle is called cryptorchism. The Greek root **CRYPT-** in this word means "hidden" or "covered."

Varicocele – Derived from the Latin root for "a swollen, twisted vein," **VARIC-**, a varicocele is an enlargement of the veins of the spermatic cord (Fig. 15.9).

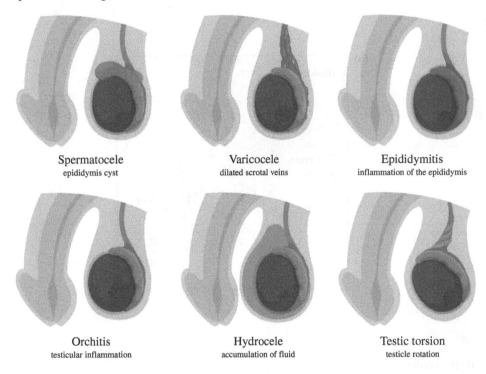

Spermatocele
epididymis cyst

Varicocele
dilated scrotal veins

Epididymitis
inflammation of the epididymis

Orchitis
testicular inflammation

Hydrocele
accumulation of fluid

Testic torsion
testicle rotation

Fig. 15.9   Image of various types of testicular pathologies.

Spermatocele – Derived from the root for "sperm/seed," **SPERMAT-**, a spermatocele is a tumor of the epididymis containing spermatozoa.

Hydrocele – Formed from the root for water, **HYDR-**, a hydrocele is an accumulation of fluid in the tunica vaginalis, which is a sheath-like structure of the testis.

Epididymitis – Epididymitis is an inflammation of the epididymis.

Orchitis – Orchitis is an inflammation of a testicle.

Scrotitis and oscheitis – Scrotitis and oscheitis refer to an inflammation of the scrotum.

Penis pathologies

Penischisis – Formed from the root for penis and the suffix for "split," **-SCHISIS**, penischisis is the term used for congenital defects in which the opening of the urethra occurs other than in its normal place (Fig. 15.10).

> **Hypospadias** means that it occurs on the undersurface of the penis.
> **Epispadias** means that it occurs on the top of the penis.
> **Paraspadias** means that it occurs on the side of the penis.

Ancient Greek physicians were familiar with this condition, and the origin of the term is from the Greek verb *spaein* which means "to tear, rend." Consequently, *spadon* was the Greek word for "a eunuch."

Fig. 15.10 Image of various types of hypospadias. *Source:* Adapted from Centers for Disease Control and Prevention.

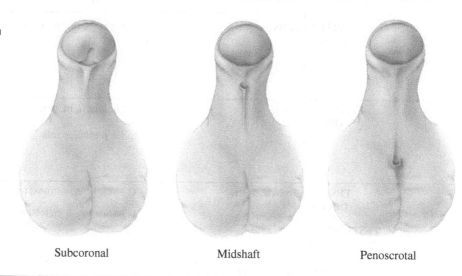

Subcoronal   Midshaft   Penoscrotal

Penis pathologies

Phimosis – Derived from a little used root for "muzzle," **PHIM**-, phimosis is a narrowing of the opening of the prepuce, which makes it difficult for the glans penis to move outside of the foreskin.

Phallitis, penitis, and priapitis – Derived from the roots for "penis," phallitis, penitis, and priapitis refer to an inflammation of the penis.

Balanitis – Formed from the root for "glans penis/acorn," balanitis is an inflammation of the glans penis.

Erectile dysfunction (ED) or impotence – Impotence is derived from the word elements *in*= not and *potis*= powerful, able. Impotence has been used for the condition in which a male cannot achieve an erection. Today, it is more commonly referred to as ED.

Phallocampsis – Formed from the suffix meaning "bent," **-CAMPSIS**, phallocampsis is a term for a pathologically bent penis during erection, which is usually associated with Peyronie disease (Fig. 15.11).

Fig. 15.11 Image of the Peyronie's disease.

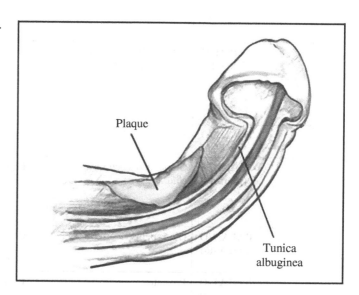

Plaque

Tunica albuginea

Greek or Latin word element	Current usage	Etymology	Examples
PEN/I (pē-nĭ)	Penis	L. *penis*, *-is*, m. tail, penis	**Pen**ial, **pen**ectomy, **pen**ischisis Loan word: **Penis** (pē'nĭs) pl. **Penes** (pē'nēz")
PHALL/O (făl-ō)	Penis	L. *phallus*, *-i*, m. penis fr. Gr. *phallos*, penis	**Phall**odynia, **phall**ocampsis, **phall**oncus, di**phall**ia, Loan word: **Phallus** (făl'ŭs) pl. **Phalli** (făl'ɪ")
TEST/O (tĕs-tō) **TESTICUL/O** (tĕs-tĭk-ū-lō)	Testicle, Testis	L. *testis*, *is*, m. witness, testicle L. *testiculus*, *-i*, m. testicle	**Test**algia, **testicul**ar, **test**imonial Loan word: **Testis** (tes'tĭs) pl. **Testes** (tes'tēz")
ORCH/O (or-kō) **ORCHID/O** (or-kĭ-dō)	Testicle; orchid (the flower)	Gr. *orchis*, *orchidos*, testicle	An**orch**ism, **orch**itis, crypt**orchid**ism, **orchid**ectomy
GONAD/O (gŏn-ă-dō)	Testicle or ovary	L. *gonas*, *gonadis*, f. gonad fr. Gr. *gone*, seed	**Gonad**opathy, hypo**gonad**ism, **gonad**arche, **gonad**al Derivative **Gonad** (gō'nad") pl. **Gonads** (gō'nadz")
DIDYM/O (did-ĭ-mō)	Testicle, twin, conjoined twin	L. *didymus*, *-i*, m. twin fr. Gr. *didymos*, twin	**Didym**algia, **didym**itis Loan word: **Didymus** (dĭd'ɪ-mŭs) pl. **Didymi** (dĭd'ɪ- mɪ")
EPIDIDYM/O (ep-ĭ-did-ĭ-mō)	Epididymis (Seminal organ resting on the posterior aspect of the testicle)	L. *epididymis*, *epididymidis*, n. epididymis fr. Gr. *didymos*, twin	**Epididym**ectomy, **epididym**al, **epididym**ography Loan word: **Epididymis** (ep"i-dĭd'ɪ-mĭs) pl. **Epididymides** (ep"i-dĭ-dim'ɪ-dēz")
SCROT/O (skrō-tō)	Scrotum (Pouch of skin containing the testicles)	L. *scrotum*, *-i*, n. bag	**Scrot**itis, **scrot**ectomy, **scrot**iform, perineo**scrot**al Loan word: **Scrotum** (skrō'tŭm) pl. **Scrota** (skrō't-ă)
OSCHE/O (ŏs-kē-ō)	Scrotum	Gr. *oscheon*, scrotum	Hemato**sche**ocele, **osche**itis, syn**osche**os
GLAND/O (glăn-dō)	Gland, *glans penis*, *glans clitoris*, acorn	L. *glans*, *glandis*, f. acorn	**Gland**iferous, **gland**ilemma Loan word: **Glans** (glanz) pl. **Glandes** (glan'dēz")
BALAN/O (bal-ă-nō)	Glans penis, acorn	Gr. *balanos*, acorn	**Balan**ocele, **balan**itis, **balan**opreputial, **balan**orrhagia
PROSTAT/O (pros-tă-tō)	Prostate	L. *prostata*, *-ae*, f. prostate *fr. prostare*, to stand before	**Prostat**itis, **prostat**ism, **prostat**ocystitis Derivative: **Prostate** (pros'tāt")

Greek or Latin word element	Current usage	Etymology	Examples
PREPUTI/O (prĕ-pū-tē-ō)	Foreskin	L. *preputium -i*, n. prepuce, foreskin	**Preputi**al, **preputi**otomy Loan word: **Preputium** (prĕ-pū′tē-ŭm) pl. **Preputia** (prĕ-pū′tē-ă)
PERINE/O (per-ĭ-nē-ō)	Perineum (area between the genitals and anus on males and females)	L. *perineum, -i*, n. perineum fr. Gr. *peraion*, perineum	**Perine**ocele, **perine**ometer, **perine**oplasty Loan word: **Perineum** (per″i-nē′ŭm) pl. **Perinea** (per″i-nē′ă)
VAS/O (vă-sō)	Vas deferens, any vessel (fluid carrying)	L. *vas, vasis*, n. vessel	**Vas**ectomy, **vasovas**ostomy, **vas**orrhaphy Loan word: **Vas** (vas) pl. **Vasa** (vā′să)
SEMIN/O (sĕm-ĭ-nō) **SEMEN/O** (sē-mĕ-nō)	Semen (male ejaculate), seed	L. *semen, seminis*, n. seed; semen	**Semin**iferous, **semin**oma, dis**semin**ate, **semen**arche Loan word: **Semen** (sē′mĕn) pl. **Semina** (sĕ′mĭ-nă)
SPERM/O (spĕr-mō) **SPERMAT/O** (spĕr-măt-ō)	Sperm (part of the male ejaculate), seed	L. *sperma, -ae*, f. sperm fr. Gr. *sperma, spermatos*, seed	Gymno**sperm**, **spermat**ocele, **sperm**acrasia, **sperm**arche Loan word: **Sperma** (spĕr′mă)
GON/O (gon-ō) **-GONY** (gŏn-ē)	Generation, genitals, semen	Gr. *gone*, seed, semen, generation	**Gon**ocyte, zoo**gony**, **gon**orrhea, **gon**angiectomy
GONORRHE/O (gon-ŏ-rē-ō)	Gonorrhea	Gr. *gonorrhea*, discharge of semen	**Gonorrhe**al Loan word: **Gonorrhea** (gon″ŏ-rē′ă)
ZO/O (zō-ō)	Something living; animal	Gr. *zoon*, a living being, animal	Spermato**zoo**n, a**zoo**spermia, **zoo**anthropy, proto**zoa**
PRIAP/O (prī-ă-pō)	Penis, erection	L. *priapus, -i*, m. penis fr. Gr. *Priapos*, the Greek god of gardens who is recognized by his large phallus	**Priap**ism, **priap**itis Loan word: **Priapus** (prī′ă-pŭs) pl. **Priapi** (prī′ă-pī″)
SATYR/O (săt-ĭ-rī-ō)	Satyr-like, sexual desire	Gr. *Satyros*, Satyr, anthropomorphic goat-tailed Greek mythical creature	**Satyr**iasis, **Satyr**idae, **satyr**ical
SYPHIL/O (sĭf-ĭl-ō)	Syphilis	L. *Syphilis*, title and character of a 16th-century poem, *Syphilis, sive Morbus Gallicus*	**Syphil**ophobia, **syphil**itic Loan word: **Syphilis** (sif′ĭ-lĭs)
APHRODISI/O (af-rŏ-dē-zē-ō)	Sex, sexual desire	Gr. *aphrodisiakos*, pert. to sexual love or desire, fr. *Aphrodite*, the Greek goddess of eros	**Aphrodisi**ac
VENERE/O (vĕ-nĕr-ē-ō)	Sex, sexual desire, sexually transmitted	L. *venereus, -a, um*, of Venus, the Roman goddess of eros	**Venere**al, anti**venere**al

Greek or Latin word element	Current usage	Etymology	Examples
CAMPT/O (kămp-tō) **CAMPYL/O** (kăm-pĭ-lō) **-CAMPSIA** (kamp-sē-ă) **-CAMPSIS** (kămp-sĭs)	Bent, crooked	Gr. *kamptos, kampylos*, bent	Phallo**campsis**, **campt**omelic, a**campsia**, **campyl**obacter
ITHY- (ĭth-ē)	Straight	Gr. *ithys*, straight	**Ithy**lordosis, **ithy**phallic, **ithy**kyphosis
BRACHY- (brăk-ē)	Short	Gr. *brachys*, short	**Brachy**cephalic, **brachy**therapy, **brachy**cardia

Review	Answers
The roots for the "testicles" are ___, ___, ___, ___, ___, and ___. The root ___ is also used for "twin." The root ___ can mean "testicle" or "ovary."	**TEST-, TESTICUL-, DIDYM-, ORCH-, ORCHID-, GONAD-**
The roots for the "penis" are ___, ___, and ___.	**PEN-, PHALL-, PRIAP-**
The roots for the "scrotum" are ___ and ___.	**SCROT-, OSCHE-**
The root for the "foreskin" is ___.	**PREPUTI-**
The root for the seminal gland that stands before the bladder is ___.	**PROSTAT-**
The bulbous end of the penis is called the ___ penis because it looks like an acorn. The roots for the glans penis are ___ and ___.	**glans GLAND-, BALAN-**
The ___ deferens is the vessel that carries the sperm away from the epididymis to the ejaculatory duct. The root for the vas deferens is ___.	**Vas VAS-**
The coiled spermatic vessel that rests upon each testicle is the epididymis. The root for this structure is ___.	**EPIDIDYM-**
The external region between the scrotum and the anus is termed the perineum. The root for perineum is ___.	**PERINE-**
The roots for "sperm" are ___ and ___. These roots can also mean ___. A single sperm cell is called a spermatozoon; the root ZO- means ___ and ___.	**SPERM-, SPERMAT- seed something living, animal**
Male reproductive ejaculate is collectively termed ___, and its associated root is ___. In addition to the male ejaculate, the root can also mean ___.	**semen, SEMIN- seed**
GON- can mean ___, ___, and ___.	**generation, genitals, semen**
Penischisis is a term used for congenital defects in which the opening of the urethra occurs other than in its normal place. ___ means that it occurs on the undersurface of the penis. ___ means that it occurs on the top of the penis. ___ means that it occurs on the side of the penis.	**hypospadias epispadias paraspadias**
The condition in which there is an undescended testicle is termed ___. The combining form CRYPT/O in this word means ___ or ___.	**cyptorchism hidden, covered**
An inflammation of the glans penis is termed ___. An inflammation of the prostate is termed ___. An inflammation of the scrotum is termed ___ or ___. An inflammation of the penis is termed ___, ___, or ___. Inflammation of the epididymis is termed ___.	**balanitis prostatitis scrotitis, oscheitis penitis, phallitis, priapitis epididymitis**

Review	Answers
A narrowing of the opening of the prepuce is termed _____.	**phimosis**
Impotence is derived from the word elements in= not and potis= powerful, able. Impotence has been used for the condition in which a male cannot achieve an erection. Today, it is more commonly known as _____.	**erectile dysfunction (ED)**
Named after a Greek fertility god, an abnormal, painful, and continued erection of the penis is called _____.	**priapism**
Named after a Greek mythological creature associated with the god Dionysus, _____ is the term used for "an excessive and often uncontrollable sexual drive among males."	**satyriasis**
An enlargement of the veins of the spermatic cord is called _____. A tumor of the epididymis containing spermatozoa is termed _____. An accumulation of fluid in the tunica vaginalis testis is termed _____.	**varicocele spermatocele hydrocele**
The terms used for the surgical cutting of the vas deferens as a means of birth control are _____ and _____. The reversal of this surgery is called a _____.	**vasectomy, gonangiectomy vasovasostomy**
A benign hypertrophic or hyperplastic prostate is a prostatic _____.	**enlargement/growth**
Phallocampsis is a term for a pathologically _____ penis during erection, which is usually associated with Peyronie disease.	**bent**
A _____ is a common type of testicular tumor.	**seminoma**
Semen without living spermatozoa is termed _____. A diminished number/count of spermatozoa in semen is termed _____. The inability to produce spermatozoa is termed _____.	**azoospermia oligospermia aspermia**

Lessons from History: *Society and Ancient Greek Medicine's Interpretation of the Female Genitalia*

Food for Thought:

How did sociocultural beliefs about gender affect ancient Greek interpretations of the female body, particularly their genitalia?

In what ways do society's views on gender and sex affect modern medicine's understanding of the female body?

The origin of gender being considered different than one's biological sex can be traced back to 1968, when Robert Stoller, a professor and psychiatrist, began to use the terms "sex" and "gender" as distinct categories in his study of people who felt "trapped in the wrong bodies." In this study, he used the term "sex" for biological traits and "gender" as a category by which he could judge the amount of femininity and masculinity a person exhibited. The distinction between gender and sex was picked up by the feminist movement, and by the 1990s, it became a cornerstone of gender studies and academic research into not only the perceived differences between males and females but also the spectrum of gender identities currently discussed in modern American culture. The distinction between gender and sex has provided a useful theoretical construct for examining both sociocultural and biological explanations for the perceived differences between males and females. Given medicine's perceived expertise in human anatomy and physiology, the physician's opinions on the differences and similarities between males and females are often perceived as scientific validation for the current construction of sex and gender. Unfortunately, history has shown that implanted cultural beliefs about the differences and similarities between males and females have had an effect on medical interpretations of human anatomy and physiology, and it stands to reason that this will continue to be the case. This bias is particularly true with respect to the long history of biological explanations for the female body in ancient Greek medicine. In the following discussion, we will consider some of the ways in which medical authors interpreted female external and internal genitalia through a sociocultural lens.

As Dean-Jones has pointed out in *Women's Bodies in Classical Greek Science*, sexual differentiation between males and females in ancient Greek medicine was far more dependent on external sexual characteristics than today. For the most part, female external genitalia were interpreted as being signs that a woman's body was qualitatively distinct from a man's body.

Although there was no consensus as to which qualities were inherently female and which were male, whatever quality was considered inherently female, the opposite quality was typically construed as being male (e.g. hot versus cold, wet versus dry). In general, women were considered to be moist, and this seems to be due to the phenomenon of menstruation. As Dean-Jones notes, the author of the Hippocratic text *Diseases of Women* attributes menstruation to the nature of a woman's flesh, which he describes as being loose and spongy, and thereby, it attracts blood from the stomach. Interestingly, this same author argues that one of the reasons for the production of menstrual blood is the fact that women do not do as much physical labor, and therefore, they do not use up all the nourishment in their bodies. Menstruation figures prominently in ancient Greek medical explanations about women's health, ability to conceive, and as physiological justification for the age of marriage. The woman's role in childbirth and the belief that the female body was qualitatively different than the male body resulted in a large collection of Hippocratic works being dedicated to this subject matter (*On Semen, On the Nature of the Child, On the Diseases of Women, On Sterile Women, On the Diseases of Young Women* or *Girls, On Superfetation*, and *On the Nature of the Woman*). Therefore, oddly enough, it could be argued that the "otherness" of the female body in ancient Greek medicine laid the foundation for the medical field of gynecology.

The belief in qualitative differences between males and females can be observed in Galen's highly influential explanation of male and female genitalia in his work *On the Use of the Parts*. In Galen's teleological approach to reproduction, he argues that Nature made women colder than men for the purpose of reproduction. In Galen's reasoning, this qualitative difference accounts for the different appearances between male and female external genitalia. Curiously, Galen argues that female reproductive parts are analogous to the male reproductive parts. In the following passage, he explains the female genitalia as being an inward projection constructed of the same parts as a male (II.297-298):

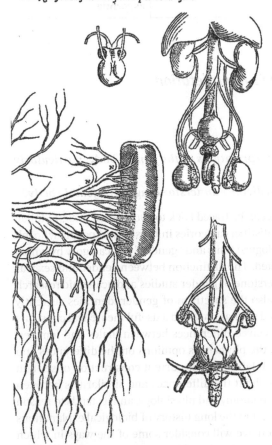

GENERATIONIS ORGA‑
NA, SVPERIVS VIRI, INFERIVS MVLIERIS.
Tertia figura semen deferentium vaforum implantationem refert.

Fig. 15.12 Male (above image) and female genitalia (below image) as depicted in Vesalius' *Tabulae anatomicae sex. Source:* Courtesy of the Wellcome Trust Collection/CC BY 4.0.

Then think first, please, of the man's [genitalia] turned in and extending inward between the rectum and the bladder. If this should happen, the scrotum would necessarily take the place of the uteri, with the testes being outside, next to it on either side, the penis of the male would become the neck of the cavity [the cervix] that had been formed, and the skin at the end of the penis, now called the prepuce, would become the female pudendum [vagina] itself.

Translation by Margaret May in *Galen On the Usefulness of the Parts*. Vol. 2. Ithaca, New York: Cornell University Press, 1968, 628–629.

Galen argues that the difference lies in the fact that Nature made men warmer, and therefore, this heat pushed out their reproductive parts, giving men visible external genitalia. The female genitalia remain on the inside of their bodies because of their cold nature. Galen claims the inward projection of the female genitalia is an intended imperfect that Nature has made so that reproduction can occur. In Galen's argument, cold is indicative of imperfection in that it means less activity and an inferior soul, particularly in the context of the Aristotelian theory of the relationship between heat and the soul. Thus, Galen's explanation for the different appearances of male and female genitalia serves to anatomically validate a common belief in his society that females were inherently inferior to males in respect to their vigor and intellectual abilities. Galen's understanding of the female genitalia had an effect on later anatomists. For instance, Vesalius *Tabulae anatomicae sex* (*Six Anatomical Tables*) contains an image of male and female genitalia that makes the female anatomical parts appear almost analogous to males. Knowing that the text and illustration were from the dissection table, and knowing that Vesalius dissected female bodies, it is quite conspicuous that Vesalius was influenced by Galen's isomorphic perspective of male and female genitalia (Fig. 15.12).

In modern medicine, breasts are considered a secondary sexual trait of females. In ancient Greek medicine, the presence of breasts was not only indicative of the sex of a person but they were also considered evidence of the nature of a female. In Hippocratic medicine, the breast's swollen appearance was considered to be a sign that females were inherently moister and softer than males, which in turn was used as a justification for why females were weaker than males and, therefore, not fit to participate in masculine activities such as athletics and battle. Interestingly, the breasts were central to Greek and Roman explanations for the Amazons in Greek mythology. According to the *Historical Library* (2.45-46) written by Diodorus of Sicily (1st century BC), the etymology of the Amazons' name (*a*- without + *mazos*, breast) reflects their practice of cauterizing the right breast of their female offspring so that it will not increase in size and create an annoyance when their bodies reach puberty. As for their male offspring, Diodorus claims that this mythological tribe of female warriors would maim the arms and legs of males so that they were useless in battle, and those who were not killed were assigned domestic work. It is generally believed that the term "Amazon" was formed from an unknown non-Indo-European word, and therefore, Diodorus' understanding of the origin of their name is a matter of speculation and folk etymology. The folk etymology that Diodorus provides for Amazons is also somewhat problematic considering all Greek artwork depicts Amazons having both of their breasts (Fig. 15.13). That said, Diodorus' false etymology seems to reflect the belief that breasts were a hindrance to the martial activities that Amazons engaged in. It is intriguing to consider, although not explicit in Diodorus' explanation, the ancient medical notion that cauterizing one's body could make it stronger. Following this line of reasoning, the Amazons' practice would have made them stronger, and therefore, more like men. It is also worthwhile mentioning that the Hippocratic author of *Airs, Waters, and Places* describes how a race of Scythians known as the Sauromatae, whose young women ride horses and fight in battle with their men, have no right breast because their mothers cauterized the breast of female girls. The rationale this medical author offers for this practice is that cauterization prevents the breast from growing, and therefore, all of the strength transfers to the right arm and shoulder of these girls so that they can hurl a javelin and shoot a bow.

The internal reproductive organs, particularly the uterus, were also interpreted by ancient Greek physicians through the lens of sociocultural beliefs about the characteristics and roles of females. As Dean-Jones points out, there are a variety of terms that Hippocratic authors used for the womb (*aggos*, "vessel"; *askos*, "wineskin bag") that seem to point to its "capacity to expand to contain a fetus during pregnancy." Likewise, the iconography for the uterus, as observed via the clay votives given to the god of medicine (Fig. 15.14), Asclepius, suggests that the uterus was likened to a bag. The wave-like features on these votives are interpreted as being rugae (wrinkles/folds) that symbolize the uterus' ability to expand during pregnancy. Thus, similar to the fundamental role of women in Greek and Roman societies, these votives seem to relay that the uterus' function was childbearing. The other common depiction of the uterus, particularly in Byzantine and medieval

Fig. 15.13 Image of 2nd century AD statue of a dying Amazon on horseback. As can be observed, both breasts are present. That said, it was typical to depict Amazons with at least one breast exposed. The exposed breast is a sign of masculinity since men are commonly depicted with their chests exposed. *Source:* Franz Robert Richard Brendámour / Wikimedia Commons / Public domain.

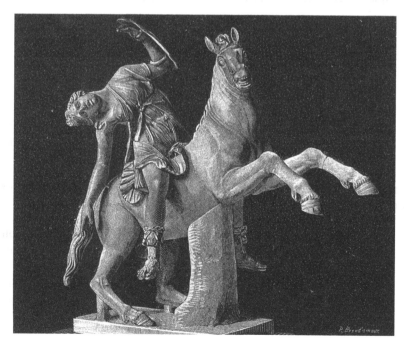

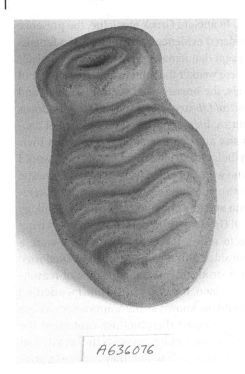

A636076

Fig. 15.14 Clay-backed uterus. Roman votive offering. *Source:* Clay-backed uterus/Wellcome Collection/Public domain.

illustrations of gynecology works, is that the uterus looks similar to a bag with two horns (Fig. 15.15). Dean-Jones suggests that the horned uterus can be traced back to the belief that the uterus contained two pockets, which was used to explain the phenomenon of twins. She points out how the Hippocratic author of *Superfetation*, which is a text that addresses the phenomenon of twins, describes these "pockets" as *kerata* (horns). Later authors, such as Galen and Herophilus, began to associate these horns with the uterine tubes, and they were thought to be orifices for female semen and menstrual fluid to enter the uterus.

One of the more famous misconceptions about the uterus in ancient Greek medicine is that it could move about within the female body. The belief in uterine movement came to be known as the "wandering womb," and it is evident in gynecological texts within the Hippocratic Corpus. It is important to bear in mind that Hippocratic authors never use the term "to wander" (*planein*) when describing the movement of the uterus. Instead, the uterus is often said "to turn," "rush," "moves swiftly," "touch," "leap upon," and "cling to." While it is tempting to attribute the origin of such wild speculations to men being ignorant about the female body due to their lack of experience, it is possible that Hippocratic authors derived this belief from observing anteverted, retroverted or prolapsed uteri, and therefore, they deduced that the uterus could move about in the body. That said, the cause of this movement is clearly based on preconceived ideas about the nature of females being inherently moist. In Hippocratic gynecological theory, the uterus was said to be naturally anchored, but when it became dry it was attracted to moisture, and therefore, it moved toward the moister organs and regions of the body. Interestingly, in Hippocratic medicine, there was a belief that inter-course was important to the health of females because this activity prevented the uterus from drying out and becoming displaced. Such a physiological explanation construed having sex as being therapeutic to females of childbearing age. Here again, it would appear that these authors' "biological" explanations for the physiology and pathophysiology of the uterus were influenced by the perception of childbearing being fundamental to the female identity.

Over time, the wandering womb took on different physiological and pathophysiological explanations. The 2nd-century-AD physician, Aretaeus of Cappadocia, describes the "wandering womb" in the following passage:

> In the middle of the flanks of women lies the womb, a female organ, closely resembling an animal; for it is moved of itself hither and thither in the flanks, also upwards in a direct line to below the cartilage of the thorax, and also obliquely to the right or to the left, either to the liver or the spleen, and it likewise is subject to prolapsus downwards, and in a word, it is altogether erratic. It delights also in fragrant smells, and advances towards them; and it has an aversion to fetid smells, and flees from them; and, on the whole, the womb is like an animal within an animal.
>
> Translation by Francis Adams in *The Extant Works of Aretaeus, the Cappadocian*. London: Printed for the Sydenham Society, 1856, 285.

Aretaeus' curious belief that the uterus was attracted to sweet-smelling things and fled from foul-smelling things appears to be linked to the practice of fumigation to entice or repulse the uterus, a practice that is evident in the following Hippocratic treatment in *Diseases of Women*:

> Another fumigation: it is necessary to dig a hole and roast grape stones in the amount of two Attic *choinikes*; let him throw some of this ash in the hole, continuously dropping sweet-smelling wine. Seating herself around <the hole> and taking her legs apart, let her be fumigated.
>
> Translation by Laurence Totelin, *Hippocratic Recipes. Oral and Written Transmission of Pharmacological Knowledge in Fifth- and Fourth-Century Greece*. Leiden: Brill, 2009, 253.

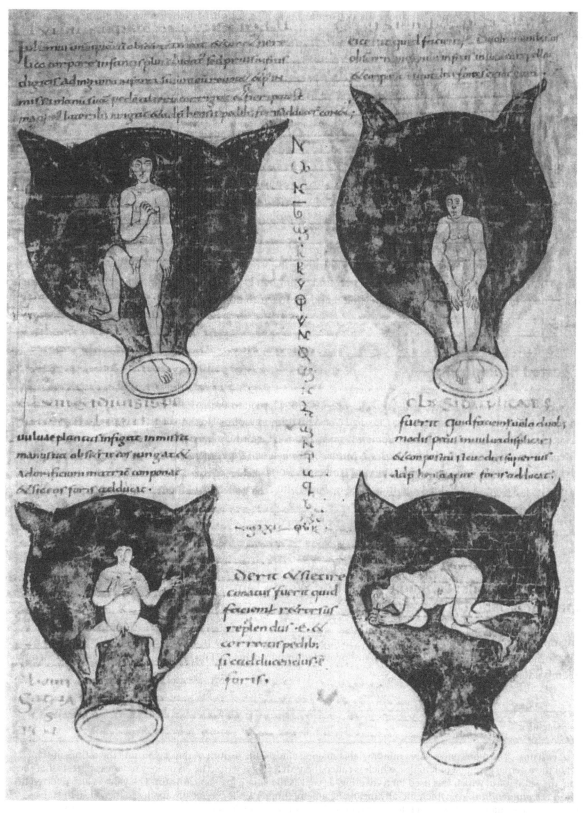

Fig. 15.15 Medieval illustrations (c. 900) of the fetuses in horned uteri. The illustrations appear to be for a Latin version of Soranus' *On Gynecology.* Brussels, Bibliothèque Royale, Codex 3714, fol. 28r. *Source:* Soranus of Ephesus/Wikimedia Commons/Public domain.

The medical practice of having women sit above heated material is also found in Babylonian medicine. Perhaps, the belief that the uterus responds to fragrant smells is a projection of the uterus sharing a similar behavior to humans, particularly females. That said, Hippocratic explanations for using fumigation treatments varied from mechanically filling a uterus full of air for the purpose of straightening it out to producing a drying effect for a uterus that had become overly moist. Aretaeus' description of the wandering womb is part of a larger discussion on the cause of the acute disease referred to as "hysterical suffocation." The Greek root in this term reveals that it was associated with the uterus (Gr. *hystera*, uterus), and therefore, in ancient Greek medicine, hysterical suffocation was a condition particular to women. According to Aretaeus, when the uterus moves upward and violently compresses "the intestines, the woman experiences a choking, after the form of epilepsy, but without convulsions. The liver, diaphragm, lungs, and heart are quickly squeezed within a narrow space; therefore, loss of breathing and speech seems to be present. And, moreover, the carotids are compressed from sympathy with the heart, and hence there is the heaviness of the head, loss of sensibility, and deep sleep." Although not all ancient Greek physicians thought the womb could move in such a way, the concept of the "wandering womb" was used as an explanatory model for centuries in medicine, and this concept is the origin of the term **hysteria**, which today is commonly associated with "widely fluctuating expression of emotions." While Aretaeus and other ancient Greek authors acknowledged that males could experience signs and symptoms similar to hysterical suffocation, hysteria has been historically an affliction associated with young women, which is evident in the writings of Sigmund Freud on hysteria. One explanation for this association may be that the experience of pregnancy and childbirth is linked to a litany of conditions that can affect both the mind and body of young women, such as perinatal and postpartum depression.

Some Suggested Readings

Dean-Jones, Lesley. *Women's Bodies in Classical Greek Science*. Oxford: Clarendon Press, 1994.

Demand, Nancy. *Birth, Death, and Motherhood in Classical Greece*. Baltimore: Johns Hopkins University Press, 1994.

Flemming, Rebecca. *Medicine and the Making of Roman Women*. Oxford: Oxford University Press, 2000.

Hippocrates. *Generation. Nature of the Child. Diseases 4. Nature of Women and Barrenness*. Edited and translated by Paul Potter. Loeb Classical Library 520. Cambridge: Harvard University Press, 2012.

Hippocrates. *Diseases of Women 1–2*. Edited and translated by Paul Potter. Loeb Classical Library 538. Cambridge: Harvard University Press, 2018.

King, Helen. *Hippocrates' Woman: Reading the Female Body in Ancient Greece*. London: Routledge, 1998.

Etymological Explanations: Common Terms and Word Elements for the Female Reproductive System

In the following discussion of the anatomical terms associated with the female reproductive system, the nominative and genitive singular forms of the anatomical Latin term are provided in parenthesis. The Greek and Latin roots are formatted in all caps and emboldened.

External female genitalia

Vulva (L. *vulva*, *vulvae*) – The mons pubis, labia minora, labia majora, clitoris, the ostium of the vagina, and the ostium of the urethra are part of the external genitalia of females, which is called the **vulva** (Fig. 15.16). The etymology of vulva suggests that the term comes from the Latin *volva*, which was used for a covering, as well as the womb in classical Latin. The vulva is also referred to as the **pudendum (L. *pundendum*, *-i*)**, which literally means "shameful thing." While it typically applies to the vulva, the term is also used for the external genitalia of males albeit less commonly. The roots used for "external female genitalia" are **VULV-**, **PUDEND-**, and **EPISI-**. The root **EPISI-** can also mean "the pubic region" in general. The root **EPISI-** comes from the Greek word for the "pubic region," *epision*.

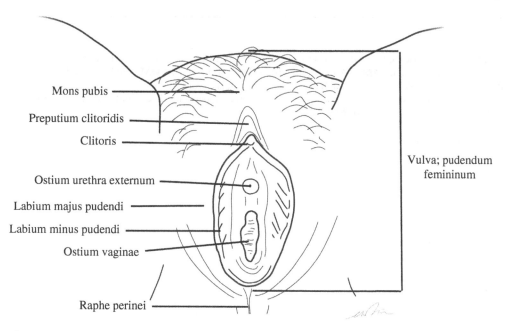

Mons pubis

Preputium clitoridis

Clitoris

Ostium urethra externum

Labium majus pudendi

Labium minus pudendi

Ostium vaginae

Raphe perinei

Vulva; pudendum femininum

Fig. 15.16 Latin terms for the female external genitalia. *Source:* Drawing by Chloe Kim.

Mons pubis (L. *mons pubis*) – The *mons pubis* is the fatty anatomical eminence above the genitalia of males and females. The nominative form of the genitive "pubis" is pubes and is used for the "pubic bone" in modern medical terminology. In classical Latin, *pubes* meant "the sign of puberty" which was attached to the growth of hair, particularly the hair associated with the male and female genitalia. Thus, the *mons pubis* means the "mound of puberty." This area is also called the *mons veneris* in medical terminology, which literally means the "mound of Venus." The Roman goddess, Venus, is commonly associated with sex. Thus, the *mons veneris* reflects the notion that puberty is an indication of the body's process of maturation for sex. The roots **PUB-** and **PUBI-** can refer to "puberty," "the pubic bone," and "the pubic region." **Puber** is the Latin loan word used today for "puberty," and **pubis** is the anatomical term for the pubic bone.

Labia majora and Labia minora (singular L. *labium majus/labium minus*) – The labia of the vulva are the folds of skin and adipose tissue on either side of the vaginal opening. The **labia majora** (greater lips) stand on the outside of the **labia minora** (lesser lips). Thus, the root for "lip," **LABI-**, is used for these folds of tissue on the sides of the vagina. The root **NYMPH-** is used for the labia minora. The root is derived from the Greek word for *nympha*, which was used for female deities commonly associated with waters in Greek myth. *Nympha* also could mean a "young marriageable female." **Nympha (L. *nympha, -ae*)** is used today as a loan word for one of the labia minora; **nymphae** is the plural form. In insect development, a nymph is an immature stage in which wings and genitalia have not fully developed. The term **nymphomania**, which is used in medicine as a colloquial term for excessive sexual desire in females, likely stems from Greek myth. In some Greek myths about nymphs, such as the rape of the young hero Hylas (depicted above in this Roman 4th-century-AD artwork), these Greek lower deities were associated with pursuing young males for the purpose of having a mate.

Clitoris (L. *clitoris, clitoridis*) – The female erectile organ is termed the **clitoris**. The roots derived from this word are **CLITOR-** and **CLITORID-**. The etymology of the clitoris is unclear. Perhaps the clitoris comes from the Greek verb *kleiein* "to sheathe" or "to shut" in reference to the clitoris being covered by the labia. The Greek *kleiein* is the source of a number of important word elements used in medicine and science. The root **CLEIST-** means "closed" or "shut." Thus, acleistocardia would be a pathological condition of the heart in which a normal closed off area is left patent. *Kleiein* is also linked to the surgical root **-CLEISIS**, which means "surgical occlusion or closing." Hence, a **colpocleisis** is a surgical occlusion/closure of the vagina.

Introitus (L. *introitus, -us*) – The entrance to the vagina is visible at the vulva. This entrance is referred to as the **ostium** (L. *ostium, -i*), which literally means "orifice," or the **introitus**, which literally means the "journey in."

Hymen (L. *hymen, hyminis*) – The mucous membrane that partially covers the entrance to the vagina is called the **hymen**; the root is **HYMEN-**. The hymen derives its name from the Greek god of weddings, Hymenaeus. Hymenaeus was often depicted as an intersexual deity, supposedly because he embodied the joining of males and females in ancient Greek marriages. The use of a hymen for the aforementioned membrane is problematic since it is linked to a mistaken belief that this membrane is an indicator of virginity. However, contrary to the folklore of ancient cultures, the presence or rupture of the hymen cannot be used to prove or disprove virginity or sexual intercourse. The hymen does not indicate a lack of sexual activity since pregnancies have been known to occur even when the hymen is intact, and conversely, the hymen can be broken without sexual intercourse. The hymen also speak to an ancient culture of inequality, where females alone were expected to remain virgins until marriage.

External female genitalia

Breast (L. *mamma*, -ae) – The breasts are considered a secondary female sex trait (Fig. 15.17). The anatomical Latin term for a breast is **mamma**. The roots used for "breast" are **MAMM-**, **MAST-**, and **MAZ-**. The Latin root **MAMM-** can be found in medical terms such as mammogram. It is also used in biological terms, such as mammal, which is a word that indicates these animals have breasts. The Greek roots **MAST-** and **MAZ-** are more commonly used for "breast," and are particularly evident in their appearance in the compound suffixes for breast pathologies, **-MASTIA** and **-MAZIA**.

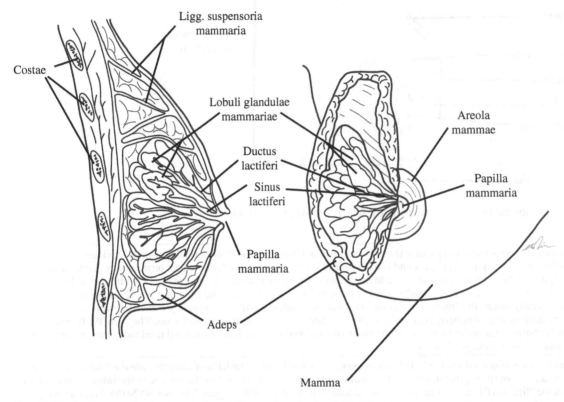

Costae

Ligg. suspensoria mammaria

Lobuli glandulae mammariae

Ductus lactiferi

Sinus lactiferi

Papilla mammaria

Adeps

Mamma

Areola mammae

Papilla mammaria

Fig. 15.17 Latin terms for the female breast. *Source:* Drawing by Chloe Kim.

Nipple (L. *papilla*, -ae) – The roots used for "a nipple" or a "nipple-like structure" are **THEL-**, **PAPILL-**, and **MAMMILL-**.

Internal female genitalia

Vagina (L. *vagina*, -ae) – Moving to the internal female genitalia (Fig. 15.18), the anatomical term **vagina** is used for the passageway from the vulva to the uterus. That said, the vagina comes from the Latin word for a scabbard/sheath. Thus, the root **VAGIN-** can refer to the female vagina or a sheath-like structure. The other root commonly used for the "vagina" is **COLP-** (or **KOLP-**). **COLP-** is derived from the Greek word for "a fold" or "a hollow," *kolpos*. It was not used specifically for the vagina in ancient Greek medicine. For example, Galen used *kolpos* for any sinus, and when he used it for the female genitalia, he felt the need to use the adjective for the female to specify which sinus he was speaking to.

Uterus (L. *uterus*, -i) – The **uterus** and its **adnexa** (i.e. ovaries and uterine tubes) play a central role in reproduction. The uterus is derived from a Latin word for the "womb," which etymologically is linked to words associated with "bags/sacs." The roots commonly used for the "uterus" are **UTER-**, **METR-**, and **HYSTER-**. The **neck of the uterus** (L. *cervix uteri*) is commonly referred to as the **cervix**. The vagina terminates into the cervix, which in turn leads into the **body of the uterus** (L. *corpus uteri*). The uterus is composed of multiple layers. The outer serous layer of the uterus is called the **perimetrium**. The muscular middle layer is called the **myometrium**. The mucous membrane that lines the inside of the uterus is termed the **endometrium**. This is also the location where the zygote must implant itself for a successful pregnancy. The root **METR-** appears to be derived ultimately from the Greek word for "a mother," *meter*, which is where the Latin word from mother (*mater*) is also derived. The root **HYSTER-** comes from the Greek word for "womb."

Adnexa (L. *adnexa*, -ae) – The **adnexa**, which is a term used for the accessory parts of an organ, is the uterine tubes and the ovaries.

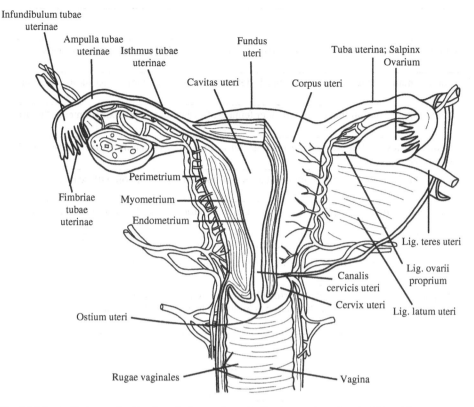

Infundibulum tubae uterinae

Ampulla tubae uterinae   Isthmus tubae uterinae

Fundus uteri

Cavitas uteri

Tuba uterina; Salpinx
Ovarium

Corpus uteri

Perimetrium

Myometrium

Endometrium

Fimbriae tubae uterinae

Lig. teres uteri

Lig. ovarii proprium

Canalis cervicis uteri

Cervix uteri

Lig. latum uteri

Ostium uteri

Rugae vaginales

Vagina

Fig. 15.18   Latin terms for the female internal genitalia. *Source:* Drawing by Chloe Kim.

Internal female genitalia

Uterine tube (L. *tuba uterina*) – The uterine tubes are two long cylindrical structures that extend from the lateral angle of the uterus and terminate at the ovary. Because these uterine tubes were "discovered" by the Italian anatomist Gabriel Fallopius (1523–1562), they are commonly referred to as the **Fallopian tubes**. Due to the uterine tube being quite long like the Eustachian tube, it is also called a **salpinx**. Thus, the root used for the "uterine tubes" is **SALPING-**, and its suffix is **-SALPINX**. Each uterine tube terminates at a fringe-like structure known as the **fimbria (L. *fimbria, -ae*)**. The term fimbria and its root **FIMBRI-** are used for any structure resembling a "fringe" or "border."

Ovary (L. *ovarium, -i*) – The roots for the ovaries, **OOPHOR-** and **OVARI-**, are derived from the Greek and Latin words for an "egg," which are *oon* and *ovum*, respectively. The notion that these structures were associated with the female gamete being linked to egg-like cells came with the invention of the microscope. In ancient Greek medicine, the term for a "testicle," *orchis*, was also used for the female ovary. The word **ovarium** is the anatomical Latin term for an "ovary." It is derived from the classical Latin word *ovarius* (egg holder/receptacle). An *ovarius* was a type of counting device that allowed the spectators at a chariot race to follow the progress of a chariot by looking at the number of eggs on the ovarius.

Ovum (L. *ovum, -i*) – The aforementioned roots for "egg" are used for the developmental stages of a female gamete. The Greek root **O-** for "egg" is used in the terms **oogonium** and **oocyte**. The oogonium is the primordial cell which becomes the oocyte. The **oocyte** is the stage of development before the ovum. The **ovum** is the mature sex cell, or gamete, that will join with the male gamete (i.e. the spermatozoon) to form a zygote. The Latin root **OV-** is used for the "ovum" and for "egg."

Gynecology and menstruation

Gynecology – Derived from the root for "female," **GYNEC-**, gynecology is the field of medicine dedicated to women's health, particularly reproduction and reproductive organs.

Menstruation – Menstruation is the cyclical discarding of the buildup of the endometrium, which is accompanied by a bloody vaginal discharge. Menstrual bleeding occurs around the period of a lunar month, every 21–35 days, and it typically lasts 2–7 days. The etymology of menstruation reveals that it is derived from the Latin word for "month," *mensis*. The root **MEN-** is used for "menstruation," and the loan word **menses** means "menstruation" in modern medical terminology.

Gynecology and menstruation

Amenorrhea – Formed from the root for menstruation, **MEN-** and the suffix for discharge, **-RRHEA**, amenorrhea is a lack of menstruation.

Polymenorrhea – Formed from the root for "many," **POLY-**, Polymenorrhea is defined as overly frequent menstruation (less than 21 days).

Menopause – Menopause is the cessation of menstruation that occurs in older females. In Classical Greek, *pauein* means "to bring to an end."

Menostasis – Formed from the Greek word for "a standing, stoppage, arresting," *stasis*, menostasis is a temporary suppression of menstruation, usually due to medication or loss of body fat.

Menostaxis – Derived from the Greek word for "a dripping," *staxis*, menostaxis is a prolonged menstruation with scanty bloody discharge.

Menoplania – Formed with the suffix for "wandering," **-PLANIA**, menoplania is menstruation through a place other than the normal outlet.

Menarche – Formed with the suffix meaning "beginning," **-ARCHE**, menarche is the beginning or first menstruation.

Menorrhagia – Formed with the suffix for "hemorrhage," **-RRHAGIA**, menorrhagia is an excessive menstrual bleeding or menstrual bleeding that lasts longer than 7 days.

Metrorrhagia – In contrast to menorrhagia, metrorrhagia is intermenstrual bleeding, which is associated with tumors and other pathological changes of the uterus rather than menstruation. This distinction is indicated by the use of the root for "uterus," **METR-**, in the term.

Inflammations

Vaginitis or Colpitis – Inflammation of the vagina is called vaginitis or colpitis.

Cervicitis – Inflammation of the neck of the uterus is called cervicitis.

Oophoritis – Inflammation of the ovary is called oophoritis.

Salpingitis – Inflammation of the uterine tubes (Fallopian tubes) is called salpingitis.

Mastitis – Inflammation of the breast is called mastitis.

Endometritis – Inflammation of the inner layer of the uterus is called endometritis.

Hernia, prolapse, and uterine displacement

Cystocele – Formed with the root for "bladder," **CYST-**, a bladder herniation into the vagina is called a cystocele.

Rectocele – A rectal herniation into the vagina is called a rectocele.

Enterocele – A hernia of the intestines into the vagina is called an enterocele.

Urethrocele – A hernia of the urethra into the vagina is called a urethrocele.

Hysteroptosis – A prolapse of the uterus is called hysteroptosis (Fig. 15.19).

Anteflexion – Formed from the root for "bend," **FLEX-**, the abnormal forward bending of the uterus in which the uterus is bent on itself is called anteflexion or an anteflexed uterus (Fig. 15.20).

Retroflexion – Formed from the root for "bend," **FLEX-**, the abnormal backward bending of the uterus in which the uterus is bent on itself is called retroflexion or a retroflexed uterus.

Anteversion – Formed with the roots for "turn," **VERS-** and **VERT-**, the abnormal turning forward of the whole uterus is called anteversion or an anteverted uterus.

Retroversion – Formed with the roots for "turn," **VERS-** and **VERT-**, the abnormal turning backward of the whole uterus is called retroversion or a retroverted uterus.

Fig. 15.19 Line drawing of a prolapsed uterus. *Source:* Adapted from original image found in Hewitt, G. *The Diagnosis, Pathology and Treatment of Diseases of Women Including the Diagnosis of Pregnancy,* (1868).

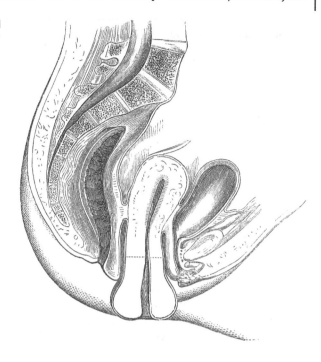

Fig. 15.20 Positions of the uterus.

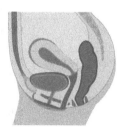
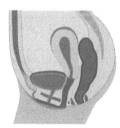
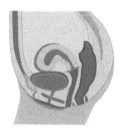
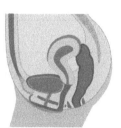

| Anteversion | Retroversion | Anteflexion | Retroflexion |

Fistula and endometriosis

Vesicovaginal fistula – Formed with the root for "bladder," **VESIC-**, a fistula that connects the bladder with the vagina is called a vesicovaginal fistula.

Rectovaginal fistula – Formed with the root for "rectum," **RECT-**, a fistula that connects the rectum with the vagina is called a rectovaginal fistula.

Endometriosis – Formed from the compound root for the endometrium, **ENDOMETRI-**, the proliferation of endometrial tissue outside the uterine cavity is called endometriosis.

Greek or Latin word element	Current usage	Etymology	Examples
GYN/O (jin-ō) or (gīn-ō)	Female, woman, pistil of a flower	Gr. *gyne, gynaikos,* woman	**Gynec**omastia, **gynec**ology, **gyn**oplasty, **gyn**ophobia
GYNEC/O (jin-ĕkō) or (gīn-ĕkō)			
THELY/O (thē-lĕ-ō)	Female	Gr. *thelys,* female	**Thely**genic, **thely**para

Greek or Latin word element	Current usage	Etymology	Examples
UTER/O (ūt-ĕ-rō)	Uterus	L. *uterus, -i,* m. womb; uterus	**Uter**ocervical, **uter**oabdominal, **uter**ocele Loan word: **Uterus** (ūt′ĕ-rŭs) pl. **Uteri** (ūt′ĕ-rī″)
HYSTER/O (his-tĕ-rō)	Uterus	Gr. *hystera,* womb	**Hyster**ectomy, **hyster**eurynter, **hyster**ic
METR/O (mē-trō)	Uterus	Gr. *metra,* womb	Endo**metrium**, myo**metrium**, peri**metrium**, **metr**itis
OVARI/O (ŏ-vă-rē-ō)	Ovary	L. *ovarium, -i,* n. egg holder; ovary	**Ovari**otomy, **ovari**algia, **ovari**an Loan word: **Ovarium** (ŏ-vă′rē-ŭm) pl. **Ovaria** (ŏ-vă′rē-ă)
OOPHOR/O (ŏ-ŏf-ŏ-rō)	Ovary	Gr. *oophoron,* egg carrier	**Oophor**ocystosis, **oophor**ectomy, **oophor**itis
OV/O (ŏ-vō)	Egg, Ovum	L. *ovum, -i,* n. egg; ovum	**Ov**iparous, **ov**ocyte, **ov**oflavin Loan word: **Ovum** (ŏ′vŭm) pl **Ova** (ŏ′vă)
O/O (ŏ-ō)	Egg, Ovum	Gr. *oon,* egg; ovum	**Oo**cyte, **oo**gonium, **oo**phagy
SALPING/O (săl-pĭng-gō) **-SALPINX** (sal-pingks)	Fallopian (Uterine) or Eustachian tube, a long tubular structure	L. *salpinx, salpingis,* f. uterine tube fr. Gr. *salpinx, salpingos,* long tubed trumpet	Meso**salpinx**, **salping**itis, **salping**emphraxis Loan word: **Salpinx** (sal′pingks) pl. **Salpinges** (sal-pin′jēz″)
FIMBRI/O (fim-brĕ-ō)	Fringe of the Fallopian tube, fringe, border	L. *fimbria, -ae,* f. fringe, border	**Fimbri**ated, **fimbri**ocele, **fimbri**ectomy Loan word: **Fimbria** (fim′brē-ă) pl. **Fimbriae** (fim′brē-ē″)
CERVIC/O (sĕr-vĭ-kō) **-CERVIX** (sĕr-viks)	Neck of the uterus, neck or neck-like structure	L. *cervix, cervicis,* f. neck	Utero**cervical**, **cervic**itis, endo**cervix** Loan word: **Cervix** (sĕr′viks) pl. **Cervices** (sĕr′vĭ-sēz″)
VAGIN/O (văj-ĭ-nō)	The female vagina, a sheath-like structure	L. *vagina, ae,* f. sheath, scabbard; the female vagina	**Vagin**ocele, **vagin**itis, extra**vagin**al Loan word: **Vagina** (vă-jī′nă) pl. **Vaginae** (vă-jī′nē″)
COLP/O (kol-pō)	The female vagina	Gr. *kolpos,* a hollow, fold, bay	**Colp**opexy, **colp**ocele, **colp**algia
VULV/O (vŭl-vō)	Vulva (external female genitalia), covering	L. *vulva, -ae,* f. a covering, shell, husk; external female genitalia	**Vulv**itis, **vulv**opathy, **vulv**ocrural Loan word: **Vulva** (vŭl′vă) pl. **Vulvae** (vŭl′vē″)

Greek or Latin word element	Current usage	Etymology	Examples
PUDEND/O (pūd-ĕn-dō)	External genitalia (esp. female), vulva	L. *pudendum, -i*, n. shameful thing; external genitalia	**Pundend**agra, **pudend**al Loan word: **Pudendum** (pū-dĕn'dŭm) pl. **Pudenda** (pū-dĕn'dă)
EPISI/O (i-piz-ē-ō)	Pubic region, vulva	Gr. *epision*, pubic region	**Episi**otomy, **episi**operineoplasty, **episi**ostenosis
PUBI/O (pū-bē-ō)	Pubic region, pubic bone	L. *puber, puberis*, m. signs of becoming an adult, puberty	**Pubi**otomy, **pub**algia, **pub**arche
PUB/O (pū-bō)		L. *pubis, -is*, f. pubic bone, pubic region	Loan word: **Puber** (pū'bĕr)
CLITOR/O (klit-ŏ-rō) **CLITORID/O** (kli-tō-rĭd-ō)	Clitoris (*female erectile organ)	L. *clitoris, clitoridis*, f. clitoris	**Clitor**itis, **clitorid**otomy, **clitor**ism Loan word: **Clitoris** (klĭt'ă-rĭs) pl. **Clitorides** (kli-tŏr'ĭd-ēz)
LABI/O (lă-bē-ō)	Labia of the vulva (i.e. Labia majora, Labia minora), lips	L. *labium,-i*, n. lip	**Labi**oplasty, **labi**oversion, **labi**al Loan word: **Labium** (lă'bē-ŭm) pl. **Labia** (lă'bē-ă)
NYMPH/O (nim-fō)	Labia minora; young female, developmental stage of insects	L. *nympha, -ae*, f. nymph; labium minus fr. Gr. *nymphe*, young bride, lower female deity	**Nymph**omania, **nymph**ectomy, **nymph**oncus Loan word: **Nympha** (nim'fă) Pl. **Nymphae** (nim'fē)
HYMEN/O (hī-mĕn-ō)	Membrane, the female hymen	L. *hymen, hyminis*, m. hymen fr. Gr. *hymen, hymenos* membrane, thin skin, Hymen the Greek god of marriages	**Hymen**otomy, **hymen**al, **hymen**itis Loan word: **Hymen** (hī'mĕn) pl. **Hymines** (hī'min-ēz)
MAMM/O (măm-ō)	Breast	L. *mamma, -ae*,f. breast	**Mamm**ography, **mamm**ogram, **mamm**al Loan word: **Mamma** (măm'ă) pl. **Mammae** (măm'ē'')
MAST/O (măst-ō)	Breast	Gr. *mastos*, breast	**Mast**ectomy, **mast**itis, **mast**ocarcinoma
MAZ/O (mā-zō)	Breast	Gr. *mazos*, breast	A**maz**ia, **maz**opexy, **maz**oplasia
MAMMILL/O (măm-mĭl-ō)	Nipple, nipple-like structure	L. *mamilla, -ae*, f. breast, nipple	**Mammill**itis, **mammill**ary, **mammill**ated Loan word: **Mammilla** (măm-mĭl'ă) pl. **Mammillae** (măm-mĭl'ē'')
PAPILL/O (păp-ĭl-ō)	Nipple, nipple-like structure	L. *papilla, -ae*, f. nipple	**Papill**oma, **papill**ary, **papill**itis Loan word: **Papilla** (pă-pil'ă) pl. **Papillae** (pă-pil'ē'')

Greek or Latin word element	Current usage	Etymology	Examples
THEL/O (thē-lō) **-THELE** (thē-lē)	Nipple, nipple-like structure	Gr. *thele*, nipple	**Thel**oncus, neuro**thele**, **thel**eplasty
MEN/O (mĕn-ō)	Menstruation	Gr. *men*, month L. *mensis, -is*, m. month; pl. menstruation	**Men**orrhagia, **men**ostasis, **men**ostaxis Loan word: **Menses** (mĕn′sēz)
MENSTRU/O (mĕn-stroo-ō)	Menstruation	L. *menstruare*, to discharge menses	Post**menstru**al, **menstru**ation
CLEIST/O (klīs-tō) **-CLEISIS** (klī-sĭs)	Closed *Suffix -surgical closure	Gr. *kleiein*, to close	A**cleist**ocardia, colpo**cleisis**, **cleist**ogamy

Review	Answers
The roots used for "menstruation" are _____ and _____. The loan word for menstruation is _____.	**MENSTRU-, MEN-** **menses**
The loan words used for "the external female genitalia" are _____ and _____. The roots used for "external female genitalia" are_____, _____, and _____.	**vulva, pudendum** **VULV-, PUDEND-, EPISI-**
The roots used for the "vagina" are _____ and _____.	**COLP- (KOLP-), VAGIN-**
The roots used for "nipple" are _____, _____, and _____.	**MAMMILL-, PAPILL-, THEL-**
The roots used for "ovary" are _____ and _____.	**OVARI-, OOPHOR-**
The roots used for "egg" are _____ and _____.	**OV-, O-**
The root used for the "uterine tubes" is _____, and its suffix is _____.	**SALPING-, -SALPINX**
The root used for "the fringe of the Fallopian tube" is _____.	**FIMBRI-**
The roots used for the "uterus" are _____, _____, and _____.	**UTER-, HYSTER-, METR-**
The root commonly used for the "neck of the uterus" is _____. The loan word for this part is _____.	**CERVIC-** **cervix**
The roots used for "female" are _____ and _____.	**GYNEC-, THELY-**
The roots used for "breast" are _____, _____, and _____.	**MAMM-, MAST-, MAZ-**
Named after the Greek god of marriage, the name of the membrane covering the entrance of the vagina is called the_____.	**hymen**
Named after lower female deities of the woods, the root for the labia minora is _____. The loan word for this anatomical structure is _____.	**NYMPH-** **nympha**
The root for "lip" and the folds of tissue on the sides of the vagina is _____. The loan word is _____.	**LABI-** **labium**
The roots for the "female erectile organ" are _____ and _____.	**CLITOR-, CLITORID-**
The root for the region just above the genitalia in which pubic hair grows is _____. The loan word for puberty is _____.	**PUBI-** **puber**
The root for the region between the vulva and the anus is _____. The loan word for this area is _____.	**PERINE-** **perineum**
The abnormal forward bending of the uterus in which the uterus is bent on itself is called _____. The abnormal backward bending of the uterus in which the uterus is bent on itself is called _____. The abnormal turning forward of the whole uterus is called _____. The abnormal turning backward of the whole uterus is called _____.	**anteflexion** **retroflexion** **anteversion** **retroversion**

Review	Answers
A prolapsed uterus is called a _____.	**hysteroptosis**
Inflammation of the vagina is called _____ or _____. Inflammation of the neck of the uterus is called _____. Inflammation of the ovary is called _____. Inflammation of the uterine tubes (Fallopian tubes) is called _____. Inflammation of the breast is called _____. Inflammation of the inner layer of the uterus is called _____.	**vaginitis, colpitis** **cervicitis** **oophoritis** **salpingitis** **mastitis** **endometritis**
_____ is the migration of endometrial tissue outside of the uterus.	**Endometriosis**
A bladder herniation into the vagina is a _____. A rectal herniation into the vagina is a _____. A hernia of intestines into the vagina is a _____. A hernia of the urethra into the vagina is a _____.	**cystocele** **rectocele** **enterocele** **urethrocele**
A vesicovaginal fistula is a fistula that connects the _____ with the _____. A rectovaginal fistula is a fistula that connects the _____ with the _____.	**bladder, vagina** **rectum, vagina**
Some aspects of menstruation are as follows: Lack of menstruation is termed _____. Cessation of menstruation that occurs in older females is called _____. A temporary suppression of menstruation, usually due to medication or loss of body fat, is called _____. A prolonged menstruation with scanty bloody discharge is called _____. Menstruation through an opening other than the normal outlet is called _____. The beginning or first menstruation is called _____. Overly frequent menstruation (less than 21 days) is called _____. Excessive menstrual bleeding or menstrual bleeding that lasts longer than seven days is called _____. Intermenstrual bleeding is called _____.	**amenorrhea** **menopause** **menostasis** **menostaxis** **menoplania** **menarche** **polymenorrhea** **menorrhagia** **metrorrhagia**
A surgical closure of the vagina is a _____.	**colpocleisis**

Lessons from History: *The Formation of the Fetus, Abortion, and Birth Defects in Ancient Greek Medicine and Society*

Food for Thought:

How would you characterize the interplay between Greek and Roman society and medicine with respect to the formation of the fetus and the value of infants with birth defects? What effect did this interplay have on medical ethics?

What is the interplay between modern society and medicine in respect to the formation of the fetus and the value of infants with birth defects? What effect does this interplay have on medical ethics?

The author of the Hippocratic text *On Seed* (*Peri gones*) claims that both men and women produce *gone* (semen) and that both of these ejaculates are necessary for reproduction in the uterus. Ancient Greek physicians often made use of a two-seed system to account for troubling questions of reproduction, such as: What accounts for a child having his mother's hands and his father's eyes? What determines the sex of a child during reproduction? Why does a particular illness of a parent show up in the child? The hereditary concept of pangenesis is employed by this author to explain some of these questions. Pangenesis is the theory of hereditary transmission in which all the parts of a person contribute to the formation of the child. Thus, the humors derived from all the parts of the parent make up the *gone*. In other words, the *gone* carries with it the fluids that formed the hands, feet, etc. of the parent. What determines which parent's part will manifest itself in the child has to do with the strength and volume of the parent's corresponding *gone*. If the hand part of the father's *gone* is stronger than the mother's hand part, then the child will have the father's hands, and vice versa. As to the sex of the child, this again has to do with the overall volume and/or strength of the *gone* of the parent. If the mother's *gone* is stronger, then the child will be female, and vice versa. In addition to the *gone*, concepts such as body heat, the shape of the womb, the impression of the soul, and other factors were used to explain the appearance and physiology of children in ancient Greek medicine and philosophy. The ancient Greek and Latin words used for male and female ejaculate (namely *gone*, *sperma*, and *semen*) are all terms used for plant seeds, which suggests that agrarian concepts shaped some of ancient Greek medicine's speculations about human conception and fetal development.

While there was no consensus among ancient Greek physicians as to the development of the prenatal human, there was a belief that human development occurred in different stages within the womb. In his work *On the Formation of the Fetus*, Galen used four different terms to denote specific stages in prenatal development. He used the term *gone*, for the first stage, which he linked to the first six days after intercourse. At this stage, the uterus is said to be retaining the male and female ejaculate, which is beginning to congeal. After these six days, he claims the amnion and chorion are formed, as well as the flesh. Galen calls this stage the *kuema*, which literally means "the thing conceived in the womb." The third stage of development he terms the *embryon*, which he links to the formation of the liver, heart, and brain. The last stage of development, when all the parts and limbs are differentiated, and there is movement in the limbs, he calls the *paidion* (little child thing). Galen's discussion of the formation of the liver, heart, and brain, which he links to the faculties of the soul, suggests that fetal development moves from the faculties of a plant to an animal and ultimately to a human being, albeit without a determinable gender.

It is important to bear in mind that Galen's discussion of the fetus was not directed toward improving the practice of obstetrics. Instead, the overarching purpose of Galen's detailed descriptions of these stages is to address a series of philosophical questions concerning the nature of semen and the soul's involvement in human development.

As is evident from this discussion, Greek medicine's understanding of the conception and development of the fetus is rather different from our own. Therefore, one should not expect their notions of abortion and contraception to be analogous to our own. In Soranus' *On Gynecology*, the following question is asked: "Whether one ought to make use of abortives and contraceptives and how?" He begins by saying that an *atokion* (contraceptive, literally "without labor") differs from a *phthorion* (abortive, literally "destructive thing") in that the *atokion* does not allow the seed to congeal and the *phthorion* destroys what has been conceived. He also discusses a third category, which he calls an *ekbolion* (expulsive, literally "what throws out"). Under the category of *atokion*, he lists a variety of medica materia (e.g. pine bark, alum, dried figs) that had the ability to prevent the seed from congealing. The rationale for this belief is that their styptic, clogging, and cooling effects caused the orifice of the uterus to shut before sex. He warns that this material can also destroy the seed in the uterus, and furthermore, can have deleterious effects on the woman's health. He notes that if the seed congeals in the uterus, then one must do everything opposite of what is advisable to retain the seed in the uterus. Thus, one should walk and leap about energetically, carry heavy things, take warm baths, use diuretic decoctions, receive vigorous massages, and sit in hot baths with various medica materia so as to separate the congealed seed from the uterus. This process appears to be what he means by *ekbolion*. In regard to a *phthorion*, he advised that the woman be bled off a large quantity of blood, shaken vigorously, and then given a suppository impregnated with medicament. He advises against using too strong of medication, as well as using a sharp instrument to separate the fetus from the womb because it may damage the uterus. That said, like other Greek physicians, he does not condone the use of an abortive. He notes that there was a disagreement among physicians of his time. One camp banishes the use of an abortive based on their interpretation of the Hippocratic Oath and based on medicine's task to guard and preserve life. The other camp only prescribes an abortive in the case of danger to the woman due to problems with parturition, such as a uterus that cannot accommodate a fetus. In some respects, Soranus' advice is in keeping with the laws of the ancient world, which typically did not allow a married woman to have an abortion, particularly without the consent of the husband. The reason for such prohibitions was that an abortion would deprive the father of a potential heir and the state of a potential citizen.

Greek and Latin terms for gross/large birth defects, such as *prodigium* (L. portent, ominous sign, unnatural thing) and *teras* (monster, sign, marvel) point to how birth defects were sometimes considered marvels, monstrosities, and signs of ill omens in the polytheistic Greco-Roman world. A variety of factors were used by ancient Greek physicians to explain birth defects: a misshapen womb, external trauma, disturbances of the pneuma during copulation, as well as problems with the *gone* itself. Such natural explanations for birth defects did not equate to better treatment of infants with birth defects. Although not universally condoned by all authors of antiquity, the practice of exposing children born with birth defects was considered a morally acceptable practice and was condoned by philosophers, physicians, and lawyers of antiquity. Soranus' *On Gynecology* has a discussion dedicated to deciding if a child is worth rearing: "How to recognize the newborn that is worth rearing?" He advised the midwife to examine and announce if the child was male or female. After doing this, the midwife should consider the following factors to advise the parents if the child is worth rearing: the health of the mother during pregnancy, the length of the pregnancy, if the child cries with vigor, if the child is perfect in all its parts and senses, and if the function of these parts is not sluggish. Anything contrary to these factors indicates the infant is not worth rearing. It is important to bear in mind that the father and mother will make the final decision as to whether or not the child lives or is abandoned, and the midwife and physician are only providing advice as to what constitutes a healthy infant. That said, Soranus does not exhibit any concern for the malformed infant's life.

Soranus' general prohibition or reluctance to perform an abortion coupled with his acceptance of the practice of infanticide is difficult for modern readers to understand because it does not conform to our ethical principles. It is possible that the practice of infanticide stems from the practical implications of living at a subsistence level in an agrarian society. Thus, raising a child who is unable to contribute to the production of crops equates to another burden on the limited supply of food that a family produces in a year. However, this argument does not fully account for why philosophers, such as Plato and Aristotle, saw no moral issue with infanticide and even advocated this practice to create and maintain an ideal state. The difference between modern and ancient notions of the value of a human being seems to explain ethical positions on infanticide and abortion. As Amundsen points out in his discussion of birth defects in antiquity, Greek and Roman evaluations of a human's worth were tied to what the individual could contribute to society. Thus, unlike today, human value is acquired rather than inherent. Following this line of thought, a birth defect revealed that an infant did not have the potential to fulfill its designated role in society, and therefore, it was of little or no value. With respect to abortion, there was no way to know if the fetus was malformed or "defective," and therefore, the child still had the potential to fulfill his or her role in society. Thus, aborting the fetus would potentially deprive the family of an heir and the state of a citizen. Amundsen argues that the origins of our current perspective on the inherent value of a human being can be traced back to the Judeo-Christian principle of the *imago Dei* (Image of God). The principle is that all humans are created in the image of God, and therefore, they should be understood as being valuable to God. To support this argument, Amundsen notes that the Roman prohibition against infanticide, which was established in 374 AD by Roman Emperor Valentinian, coincides with the Christianization of the Roman Empire. Amundsen points out that Christian philosophers such as Clement of Alexandria (2nd century AD) and Augustine of Hippo (354–430 AD) wrote against both abortion and infanticide based on the principle of the *imago Dei*. Augustine wrote specifically about birth defects in his *City of God* and *Enchiridion*, where he argues that everyone, including those society deems to be "defective" or "monstrosities," is created by God, and therefore, they are valuable to God. Augustine does not see these malformations as normal since he believes that birth defects will not be present in the spiritual bodies of believers in the afterlife. It should be noted that birth defects, particularly gross birth defects, were often stigmatized in the history of Christianity as signs of sin, demonic activity, and bad omens. This can be observed in the writings of the famous French surgeon, *Ambroise Paré* (c. 1510–1590), whose *On Monsters and Marvels* contains similar religious explanations for birth defects alongside the natural explanations found in Greek medicine (Fig. 15.21).

Fig. 15.21 Woodcut illustration (1628) of Ambroise Paré's discussion of conjoined twins, which is identified as a monstrosity. *Source:* Les œuvres d'Ambroise Paré Divisees en trente livres / Wellcome Collection / Public domain.

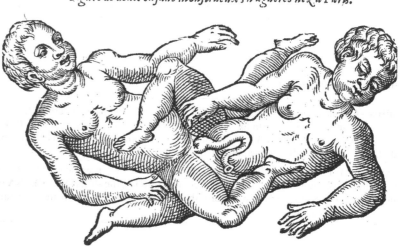

Figure de deux enfans monstrueux, n'agueres nez à Paris.

Some Suggested Readings

Amundsen, Darrel W. "*Medicine and the Birth of Defective Children.*" In *Medicine, Society, and Faith in the Ancient and Medieval Worlds*, 50–69. Baltimore: Johns Hopkins University Press, 1996.

Galen. "*On the Formation of the Fetus.*" In *Galen: Selected Works*, Translated by Peter N. Singer, 177–201. Oxford: Oxford University Press, 1997.

Flemming, Rebecca "*Galen's Generations of Seeds.*" In *Reproduction: Antiquity to the Present Day*, Edited by Nick Hopwood, Rebecca Flemming, and Lauren Kassell, 95–108. Cambridge: Cambridge University Press, 2018.

Pare, Ambroise. *Monsters and Marvels*. Translated by Janis Pallister. Chicago: University of Chicago Press, 1995.

Riddle, John R. *Contraception and Abortion from the Ancient World to the Renaissance*. Cambridge: Harvard University Press, 1992.

Soranus. *Soranus' Gynecology*. Translated by Owsei Temkin. Baltimore: Johns Hopkins University Press. 1956.

Etymological Explanations: Obstetrics

Practitioners and newborns

Obstetrics – Obstetrics is the field of medicine that is concerned with the management of pregnancy and childbirth. In Classical Latin, the term *obstetrix* was used specifically for "a midwife," w**ho** was a female practitioner associated with childbirth. The sex of the practitioner is evident by the suffix that is used to create this term; much like **-OR** is used for a male practitioner of something, the suffix **-TRIX** denotes a female practitioner (e.g. dominatrix, genetrix, etc.). The root **OBSTETR-** used today for obstetrics, ultimately comes from the Latin verb *obstare* (to stand before). The word element indicates the typical position that a Roman midwife took during childbirth (i.e. standing in front of the pregnant woman). Based on the information provided in Soranus' *On Gynecology*, it is understood that Roman women generally gave birth in a seated position and that they used chairs specifically designed for childbirth.

Pediatrics – The field of medicine that deals with the care of children and the treatment of their diseases is termed pediatrics. The root **PED-** in this term is derived from the Greek word for a "child," *pais, paidos*, and this root carries the meaning of "child" when used in modern medical and scientific terminology. The field of pediatrics is a modern development. That said, while there was not a pediatric specialization in ancient medicine, ancient Greek physicians often made a distinction between treatments for children and adults since they held that the nature of a child's body differed from an adult's body. The attention to these differences extends back to the content of works found in the Hippocratic Corpus, such as *On the Nature of the Child*.

Neonate – Technically, a **neonate** is an infant up to one month old. The root **NE-** means "new." Both **NAT-** and **NASC-** come from the Latin verb *nasci, natum,* which means "to give birth." Hence, a **neonatologist** is a physician who specializes in the treatment of the diseases of newborns.

Puerperium – Puerperium is defined as the first six weeks after childbirth. The term is derived from the Latin verb *puerperare*, which means "to give birth to a child, childbirth." The root **PUERPER-** is used for "childbirth" and "puerperium." Puerperium can be further broken down to the Latin root **PUER-**, which means "child" or "childlike."

Terms for sexual intercourse

Coitus – Coitus is a loan word that means "sexual intercourse." Being derived from *con*- together + *itus*, a going, the Latin word *coitus* was used as a euphemism for sexual intercourse. Consequently, the root **COIT-** is commonly used for "sexual intercourse" in modern medicine. The suffix **-ITUS**, denotes "a going," and it shows up in a collection of terms, for example: **introitus** (the entrance into the vagina) and **aditus** (an approach or entrance).

Pareunia – Pareunia is a medical term that is used for "sexual intercourse." The Greek word *pareunos,* which literally meant "lying alongside," was a euphemism for sexual intercourse. Today, the suffix **-PAREUNIA** commonly appears in medical terms for "sexual intercourse." For example, **dyspareunia** is the medical term used for "painful sexual intercourse," and **apareunia** is "an inability to have sexual intercourse".

Conception and human development

Gamete – The mature female sex cell, the **ovum**, and the mature male sex cell, the spermatozoon, are called gametes. The root **GAM-** is derived from the Greek word for "marriage," *gamos*. Today, the word elements **GAM-** and **-GAMY** are used for "sexual union, sexual reproduction, marriage." For example, **agamogenesis** is a term used for "asexual reproduction."

Zygote – The cell that is formed by the union of the male and female gametes is referred to as a zygote. The roots **ZYGOT-** and **ZYG-**, are commonly used for "zygote, joined." These roots ultimately come from Greek words associated with "a yoke." A yoke is a device, typically made of wood, that was used to join beasts of burden together. Thus, to be "yoked" means to be joined together.

Embryo – The embryo is the stage of human development from the fertilization of the ovum to the formation of the fetus (Fig. 15.22). This is the first eight weeks of the prenatal period. The root **EMBRY-** is used to refer to this stage of development. However, the Greek word *embryon* (*en*, inside + *bruein*, to swell) did not have the same meaning as today.

Fig. 15.22 Anatomical Latin for the fetus and the gravid mother. *Source:* Drawing by Chloe Kim.

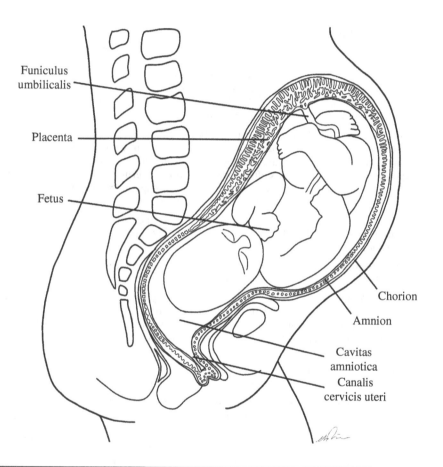

Funiculus umbilicalis

Placenta

Fetus

Chorion

Amnion

Cavitas amniotica

Canalis cervicis uteri

Fetus – A fetus is the stage of the prenatal human from the beginning of the 9th week to birth. The term fetus comes from the Latin word for "offspring." This usage of the "fetus" and its literal meaning in Latin reveals that this word was not delimited to a prenatal stage of human development. The root **FET-** is used today for the later stage of prenatal development in humans and animals.

Chorion – The chorion is the external membrane that surrounds the fetus. This loan word and its root **CHORI-** are derived from the ancient Greek word *chorion*. In ancient Greek, chorion could refer to the membrane that enclosed the fetus, as well as for structures that resemble a "membrane" or a "thin animal-hide." The root **CHORI-** is used today for similar structures, such as the choroid of the eye.

Amnion – The amnion is the inner membrane that surrounds the fetus. This loan word and its root **AMNI-** are derived from the ancient Greek word for "lamb skin." The 3rd-century-BC anatomist and physician, Herophilus, appears to be the first to use this term for the membrane of the fetus. Helen King, a modern medical historian, states that this term "recalls not only a word for soft lambskin, so indicating the protective function of the membrane, but also a Homeric term for a bowl used to collect the blood of an animal which has been sacrificed, reflecting the idea that a fetus is formed from the blood of its mother."

Conception and human development

Placenta – The placenta is a temporary, spongy structure in the uterus from which the fetus derives its oxygen and nourishment. The root for this structure is **PLACENT-**. The original meaning of the Latin word *placenta* was "a cake," which explains why the discoid shape and spongy nature of this structure in the womb led to the 16th-centuryItalian anatomist Realdo Colombo calling it the *placenta uterina* "uterine cake."

Umbilical cord – The umbilical cord is the attachment connecting the fetus to the placenta. The **umbilicus** is a term used for the "navel"/"bellybutton," which is the depressed point in the abdomen that marks the former attachment of the umbilical cord to the fetus. The Latin terms for a cord/rope *funis* and little rope/cord *funiculus* are used for the umbilical cord and other cord-like structures. Thus, the root **FUN-** in **funipuncture** refers to the umbilical cord, and likewise, the root **FUNIS-** in **funisitis** also refers to the umbilical cord.

Pregnancy and birth

Gravida – Derived from the Latin adjective for "heavy," *gravidus, -a, -um*, gravida is the medical term used for "pregnancy" or "a pregnant woman." The suffix **-GRAVIDA** often appears in obstetric terms, such as **primigravida** (first pregnancy), **secundigravida** (second pregnancy), and **multigravida** (multiple pregnancies), to denote the number of pregnancies a woman has had. The root **GRAVID-** also means "pregnancy." It shows up in terms such as **gravidity** (total number of pregnancies) and **gravidocardiac** (condition of the heart associated with pregnancy).

Para – Derived from the Latin verb "to give birth," *parere, partum*, **para** is an obstetric term used for "birth" or "a woman who has given birth." Taber's obstetric definition of para is "a woman who has produced a viable infant (weighing at least 500 g and more than 20 weeks' gestation) regardless of whether the infant is alive at birth. A multiple birth is considered to be a single parous experience." The suffix **-PARA** often appears in obstetric terms, such as **multipara** (multiple births), **primipara** (first birth), and nullipara (no births) to denote the number of birthing experiences that a woman has had. The roots **PAR-** and **PART-** carry the meaning of "to give birth or produce." Hence, an **oviparous** animal gives birth to eggs.

Abortus – Derived from the Latin word for "a miscarriage," abortus is an obstetric term used for "a fetus born before 20 weeks' gestation or weighing less than 500 g." The root **ABORT-** appears in terms such as **abortifacient** (something that makes/produces an abortion).

Parturition – Derived from the Latin word *parturio*, which meant "labor pains," parturition is the act of giving birth. The root **PARTUR-** is used in terms such as **parturient** to denote "labor" or "giving birth."

Cyesis – Coming from the Greek verb meaning "to be pregnant," *kyein*, cyesis is the obstetric term used for "pregnancy." Likewise, the suffix **-CYESIS** is commonly used in obstetrics to denote "pregnancy." For instance, an ectopic pregnancy is termed **eccyesis**, and a healthy implantation of the zygote on the endometrium is termed an **encyesis**. **Salpingocyesis** and **oocyesis** are two examples of ectopic pregnancies. A salpingocyesis is an ectopic pregnancy in which the zygote implants in the Fallopian tube. An oocyesis is an ectopic pregnancy in an ovary.

Tocus – **Tocus** is the Latinized Greek loan word used in obstetrics for "childbirth" or "parturition." Correspondingly, the root **TOC-** carries the meanings of "labor pains" and "childbirth," which is evident in medical words such as **tocography** and **oxytocin**.

Lochia – Coming from the Greek word for "childbirth," *lochia*, the obstetric term lochia is specifically used for the "puerperal discharge of blood, mucus, and tissue from the uterus." The root **LOCHI-** can be used for "childbirth" but most often it carries the aforementioned obstetric meaning of lochia.

Teras – Coming from the Greek word *teras*, which meant "marvel" or "monster," a **teras** is an obstetric term for "a severely deformed fetus." Derived from the Greek *teras*, the root **TERAT-** is used in medicine for "a severe birth defect" and "a monster." Hence, a **teratoma** is quite literally a "monster tumor," and a **teratogen** is something that "creates birth defects." There were Greek and Latin terms that seem to denote whether an infant had a minor or a major birth defect. The Latin term *prodigium* was used for major birth defects, and its original meaning reveals that it carried a similar connotation to the Greek word *teras*, in that it was used for an "unnatural wonder or something to be feared." Rather than preserving this negative denotation, its modern derivative "prodigy" is used today for "a person, particularly a youth, who has exceptional abilities." In ancient medicine, conjoined twins were considered *terata* and *prodigia*. In modern medicine, we use the suffixes **-PAGUS** and **-DIDYMUS**, which correspondingly mean "fixed" and "twin," to denote "conjoined twins." These suffixes are joined to an anatomical word element to indicate what part is shared by the conjoined twins (e.g. **craniodidymus**, **rachiopagus**). That said, the loan word **didymus** simply refers to "a twin."

Presentation – In obstetrics, the position of the fetus, particularly at childbirth, is referred to as the presentation of the fetus. Terms such as left sacrum, right mentum, and left occiput are used to indicate which part of the fetus is oriented toward the birthing canal. The term **breech presentation** is used for the fetal position in which the buttocks are coming first. The danger of this position and other non-cephalic presentations was not lost on ancient physicians.

Caesarian/Cesarian – Caesarian and Cesarian refer to the surgical procedure of cutting the abdomen to produce a nonvaginal delivery of the fetus, i.e. a cesarian section. The term "cesarian" is derived from the legend that such an operation was performed for the birth of Julius Caesar. Thus, the etymology of his cognomen, Caesar, is said to be from the Latin *caesus*, which is the perfect past participle of *caedere* "to cut" or "to kill" (see the appendix **–CIDE**). It is quite doubtful that Caesar was born this way since a mother would not have survived such a procedure in the ancient Roman world, and it is clear that Julius Caesar's mother, Aurelia, lived to see Caesar's adulthood. The inability to perform such surgery without killing the mother is perhaps the genesis for the Roman Law known as the *Lex Caesarea*, which mandated that a child be cut out of the mother's womb if she died during childbirth. Therefore, it has been speculated that Julius Caesar received his name because one of his ancestors was born via such an operation. Generally, some of the earliest accounts of successful cesarian sections are from the 15th century. That said, the first recorded successful cesarean section in which both mother and child survived may have occurred as early as 1337, in the court of John of Luxembourg, King of Bohemia.

Greek or Latin word element	Current usage	Etymology	Examples
OBSTETR/O (ŏb-ste-trō)	Branch of medicine associated with childbirth	L. *obstetrix, obstericis*, f. midwife	**Obstetr**ical, **obstetr**ics
PUERPER/O (pū-ĕr-pĕ-rō)	Childbirth, puerperium	L. *puerperare*, childbirth	**Puerper**ant, **puerper**al, **puerper**alism Loan word: **Puerperium** (pū″ĕr-pē′rē-ŭm)
PED/O (pĕd-ō)	Child	Gr. *pais, paidos*, child	**Ped**iatrics, **ped**iatrician, **ped**obaromacrometer
-CYESIS (sī-ē-sĭs)	To be pregnant	Gr. *kyein*, to swell, be pregnant	Oo**cyesis**, pseudo**cyesis** Loan word: **Cyesis** (sī-ē′sĭs)
-PAGUS (pă-gŭs)	Conjoined twins	Gr. *pagos*, something fixed or firmly set	Cranio**pagus**, pygo**pagus**, xipho**pagus**
-DIDYMUS (dĭd-ĭ-mŭs)	Conjoined twins, twin	Gr. *didymos*, double, twin	Cranio**didymus**, ischio**didymus** Loan word: **Didymus** (dĭd′ĭ-mŭs) pl. **Didymi** (dĭd′ĭ-mī″)
ZYG/O (zī-gō) **ZYGOT/O** (zī-gō-tō)	Zygote, yoke, joined	Gr. *zygon*, yoke, crossbar Gr. *zygotos*, yoked	**Zyg**odactyly, mono**zyg**otic, **zyg**oma Derivative: **Zygote** (zī′gōt″) pl. **zygotes** (zī′gōts″)
TERAT/O (tĕr-ă-tō)	Severely deformed fetus, monster	Gr. *teras, teratos*, a marvel, monster	**Terat**oma, **terat**ogenic, **terat**ism Loan word: **Teras** (tĕr′ăs) pl. **Terata** (tĕr′ă-tă)
FET/O (fĕt-ō)	Fetus (*unborn animal in the later stage of development)	L. *fetus, -us*, m. offspring	**Fet**oscopy, **fet**icide, **fet**al Loan word: **Fetus** (fĕt′ŭs) pl. **Fetus** (fĕt′ūs), **fetuses** (fĕt′ŭs-ez)

Greek or Latin word element	Current usage	Etymology	Examples
EMBRY/O (em-brē-ō)	Embryo (*unborn animal in the early stage of development)	Gr. *embryon*, young one, fetus	Dys**embry**oplasia, **embry**octony, **embry**ocardia Derivative: **Embryo** (em′brē-ō″) pl. **Embryos** (em′brē-ōz″)
AMNI/O (am-nē-ō)	Amnion (the innermost membrane enclosing the fetus)	L. *amnion*, *-i*, n. amnion fr. Gr. *amnion*, lamb skin	**Amni**otome, **amni**ocentesis, **amni**ogenesis Loan word: **Amnion** (am′nē-on″) pl. **Amnia** (am′nē-ă″)
CHORI/O (kō-rē-ō)	Chorion (the outermost membrane enclosing the fetus), tunic of eyeball	L. chorion, *-i*, n. chorion fr. Gr. *chorion*, animal hide	**Chori**ocele, **chori**oid, **chori**oadenoma Loan word: **Chorion** (kōr′ē-on″) pl. **Choria** (kōr′ē-ă″)
PLACENT/O (plas-ěn-tō)	Placenta	L. *placenta*, *-ae*, f. a cake, flat cake; placenta	**Placent**itis, **placent**ography Loan word: **Placenta** (plă-sent′ă) pl. **Placentae** (plă-sent′ē″)
GRAVID/O (grăv-ĭd-ō) -GRAVIDA (grav-ĭd-ă)	Pregnancy	L. *gravida*, *-ae*, f. a pregnant woman	**Gravid**ism, primi**gravida**, noni**gravida** Loan word: **Gravida** (grăv′ĭ-dă) pl. **Gravidae** (grăv′ĭ-dē″)
PAR/O (păr-ō) PART/O (păr-tō) -PARA (pă-ră)	Give birth, to bring forth	L. *parere*, *partum*, bring forth, bear	Bi**par**ous, ante**part**um, multi**para** Loan word: **Para** (păr′ă) pl. **Parae** (păr′ē″)
PARTUR- (păr-tū-rō)	Labor, to give birth	L. *parturire*, to have labor pains	**Partur**ient, **Partur**iphobia
ABORT/O (ă-bor-tō)	Miscarriage, abortion	L. *abortus*, *-us*, m. miscarriage	**Abort**ifacient, **abort**ion, **abort**ive Loan word: **Abortus** (ă-bor′tŭs)
TOC/O (tŏk-ō)	To be in labor, childbirth	Gr. *tokos*, labor, childbirth	Oxy**toc**in, dys**toc**ia, **toc**ography Loan word: **Tocus** (tō′kŭs)
NASC/O (năs-kō) NAT/O (nā-tō)	To be born	L. *nasci*, *natum*, to be born	**Nasc**ent, neo**nat**e, peri**nat**al

Greek or Latin word element	Current usage	Etymology	Examples
LOCHI/O (lō-kē-ō)	Childbirth, lochia (*vaginal discharge after childbirth)	Gr. *lochia*, childbirth	**Lochi**ometra, **lochi**al Loan word: **Lochia** (lō′kē-ă)
LACT/O (lak-tō)	Milk, lactose	L. *lac, lactis*, n. milk	**Lact**igerous, pro**lact**in, **lact**ose
UMBILIC/O (ŭm-bil-ĭ-kō)	Umbilical cord, navel	L. *umbilicus, -i*, m. the navel	**Umbilic**opubic, **umbilic**al Loan word: **Umbilicus** (ŭm-bĭ-lĭ′kŭs) pl. **Umbilici** (ŭm-bĭ-lĭ′sī″)
FUN/O (fū-nō) **FUNIS/O** (fū-nĭ-sō)	Umbilical cord, rope, rope-like	L. *funis, -is*, m. cord, rope	**Fun**ipuncture, **funis**itis

Review	Answers
The suffix meaning pregnancy is _____. An ectopic pregnancy in which a zygote implants in the Fallopian tube is a _____. An ectopic pregnancy in an ovary is called an_____.	**-CYESIS** **salpingocyesis** **oocyesis**
The suffixes used for conjoined twins are _____ and _____.	**-DIDYMUS, PAGUS**
The root NAT- in neonate means _____.	**born/birth**
Funisitis is an inflammation of the _____. The root UMBILIC- can be used for the "umbilical cord" and the _____.	**umbilical cord** **navel**
Based on its root LACT-, Prolactin is a hormone that prepares the breasts to produce _____.	**milk**
The vaginal discharge after the childbirth is called _____. The root of this word is _____.	**lochia** **LOCHI-**
The root for a "a severe birth defect" or "a monster" is _____. The loan word for this is _____.	**TERAT-** **teras**
Based on the root TOC-, tocography is the recording of _____. The loan word for labor/parturition/childbirth is _____.	**labor/parturition** **tocus**
The outer membrane surrounding the fetus is called the _____. The inner membrane surrounding the fetus is called the _____. The roots for these two parts are respectively _____ and _____.	**chorion** **amnion** **CHORI-, AMNI-**
The suffix _____ often appears in obstetric terms to denote the number of birthing experiences that a woman has had, for example: _____ (multiple births), _____ (first birth), and _____ (no births).	**-PARA, multipara, primipara, nullipara**
The suffix _____ often appears in obstetric terms, such as _____ (first pregnancy), _____ (second pregnancy), and _____ (multiple pregnancies), to denote the number of pregnancies a woman has had.	**-GRAVIDA, primigravida, secundigravida, multigravida**
_____ and _____ refer to the surgical procedure of cutting the abdomen to produce a nonvaginal delivery of the fetus, which is erroneously attributed to the way in which Julius Caesar was born.	**Caesarian, Cesarian**
The root PED- in pediatrician means _____.	**child**
The _____ is a temporary, spongy structure in the uterus from which the fetus derives its oxygen and nourishment.	**placenta**

Review	Answers
Two terms used for "sexual intercourse" in medical terminology are _____ and _____.	**coitus, pareunia**
The root PUERPER- means _____ and _____.	**childbirth, puerperium**
The branch of medicine that deals with childbirth is called _____. The corresponding root is _____.	**Obstetrics** **OBSTETR-**
The cell that is formed by the union of the male and female gametes is referred to as a _____. The roots _____ and _____, are commonly used for "zygote, joined."	**Zygote** **ZYGOT-, ZYG-**
The root PARTUR- means _____ or _____.	**labor, giving birth**
The word elements GAM- and -GAMY are used for _____, _____, and _____. Thus, mature male and female sex cells are called _____.	**sexual union, sexual reproduction, marriage gametes**
The _____ is the stage of human development from the fertilization of the ovum to the formation of the fetus.	**embryo**
The term _____ presentation is used for the fetal position in which the buttocks is coming first.	**breech**

Appendix A

Greek and Latin Word Elements

To be consistent with modern American pronunciations of medical terms, the phonetic spellings for the word elements are derived from those found in *Taber's Cyclopedic Medical Dictionary 24th Edition*. The phonetic spelling for a root beginning with a consonant cluster is based on this root being the first-word element in a compound term (see Chapter 2 for pronunciations).

Greek or Latin word element	Current usage	Etymology	Chapters
-A **(ă)**	State or condition of	Gr. *-a*, state or condition of	Chapter 2
A- **(a)** **AN-** **(an)**	Not, without	Gr. *a-*, *an-*, not, without	Chapter 2
AB- **(ab)**	Away, apart from	L. *ab-*, away, apart from	Chapter 2
ABDOMIN/O **(ab-dom-ĭ-nō)**	Abdomen	L. *abdomen, abdominis*, n. paunch, belly, abdomen	Chapters 3, 13
ABDUCT/O **(ab-dŭk-tō)**	To lead or convey away (midline)	L. *abductor, -oris*, m. abductor fr. L. *abductio*, a leading away	Chapter 7
ABORT/O **(ă-bor-tō)**	Miscarriage, abortion	L. *abortus, -us*, m. miscarriage	Chapter 15
-AC **(ak)**	Pertaining to	Gr. *-ac*, pertaining to	Chapter 2
ACANTH/O **(ă-kan-thō)**	Thorn, spine, spiny	Gr. *akantha*, thorn, spine	Chapter 8
-ACEOUS **(ă-shŭs)**	Made of, having the quality of, full of	L. *-aceus*, made of, having the quality of, full of	Chapter 2
ACID/O **(as-ĭ-dō)**	Acidic, acid	L. *acidus, -a, -um*, sour, sharp	Chapter 14
ACOUSMAT/O **(ă-kooz-măt-ō)**	Sound	Gr. *akousma, akousmatos*, a thing heard	Chapter 11
ACU/O **(ă-kū-ō)** **ACUT/O** **(ă-kū-tō)**	Needle, sharpness, pointed	L. *acus, -us*, f. needle, sharp L. *acutus, -a, -um*, sharp, pointed	Chapter 4

Greek and Latin Roots of Medical and Scientific Terminologies, First Edition. Todd A. Curtis.
© 2025 John Wiley & Sons, Inc. Published 2025 by John Wiley & Sons, Inc.
Companion website: www.wiley.com/go/Curtis

Greek or Latin word element	Current usage	Etymology	Chapters
ACUST/O (ă-koos-tō) **ACOUST/O** (ă-koos-tō) **-ACUSIS** (a-kū-sĭs) **-ACOUSIA** (ă-kū-sē-ă)	Listening, sense of hearing	Gr. *akouein*, to hear	Chapter 11
AD- (ăd) **AF-** (ăf) **-AD** (ăd)	Toward, to, near, -AD = indicates direction toward a part of the body	L. *ad-*, indicates direction toward a part of the body	Chapter 2
ADDUCT/O (ă-dŭk-tō)	To lead or convey toward (midline)	L. *adductor, -oris*, m. adductor fr. L. *adductio*, a leading toward	Chapter 7
ADEN/O (ad-ĕn-ō)	Gland	Gr. *aden, adenos*, gland	Chapters 3, 8, 12
ADIP/O (ad-ĭ-pō)	Fat	L. *adeps, adipis*, m. fat L. *adiposus, -a, -um*, fatty	Chapter 6
ADREN/O (ă-drē-nō)	Adrenal gland, suprarenal gland	L. *ad-* + L. *ren*, kidney = adren-, adrenal gland	Chapter 12
AER/O (ar-ō)	Air	Gr. *aer*, lower air, air	Chapters 5, 9
AETHER/O (ēth-ĕr-ō) **ETHER/O** (ēth-ĕr-ō)	Ether	Gr. *aither*, upper air, ether fr. *aithein*, to kindle, light, burn	Chapter 9
AGOG/O (ă-gŏg-ō) **-AGOGUE** (ă-gŏg)	Hormone that promotes something; leading forth	Gr. *agogos*, leading forth; promoting flow, expelling	Chapter 12
-AGRA (ag-ră)	Gout, attack (of severe pain)	Gr. *agra*, a taking, catching	Chapter 7
AKTIN/O (ak-ti-nō) **ACTIN/O** (ak-ti-nō)	Ray, ray-like, radiation, actinium	Gr. *aktinos*, ray	Chapter 5
-AL (ăl)	Pertaining to	L. *-alis*, pertaining to	Chapter 2
ALB/O (al-bō) **ALBIN/O** (al-bĭ-nō)	White	L. *albus, alba, album*, white Albino Portuguese fr. L. *albus*	Chapters 6, 14
ALBUMIN/O (al-bū-mĭ-nō)	Albumin, protein	L. *albumen, albuminis*, n. egg white; albumen protein	Chapters 13, 14

Greek or Latin word element	Current usage	Etymology	Chapters
ALG/O **(al-gō)** **-ALGIA** **(al-j(ē-)ă)** **-ALGESIA** **(al-jĕ′zē-ă)**	Pain; -ALGIA = Painful condition; -ALGESIA = Sense of pain	Gr. *algos*, pain	Chapter 4
ALIMENT/O **(al-ĭ-mĕnt-ō)**	Food	L. *alimentum*, *-i*, n. nourishment, food	Chapter 13
ALKAL/O **(al-kă-lō)** **ALKALIN/O** **(al-kă-lĭ-nō)**	Basic, Alkali	L. *alkali* fr. Arabi *al-qali* burnt ashes, ashes of salt wort	Chapter 14
ALL/O **(al-ō)**	Other, different, abnormal	Gr. *allos*, other (of a group), different, foreign	Chapters 5, 6
ALVEOL/O **(al-vē-ŏ-lō)** **ALVE/O** **(al-vē-ō)**	Alveolus, cavity, socket, sac	L. *alveolus*, *-i*, m. bucket, a little hollow	Chapter 9
AMBI- **(am-bi)**	Around, on both sides, both, twofold	L. *ambi-*, around, on both sides, both, twofold	Chapter 2
AMBLY/O **(am-blē-ō)**	Dull	Gr. *amblys*, blunt, dull	Chapter 11
AMNI/O **(am-nē-ō)**	Amnion (the innermost membrane enclosing the fetus)	L. *amnion*, *-i*, n. amnion fr. Gr. *amnion*, lamb skin	Chapter 15
AMPHI- **(am-fĭ)** **AMPHO-** **(am-fŏ)**	Around about, both, both sides, in two ways	Gr. *amphi-*, around about, both, both sides, in two ways	Chapter 2
AMYGDAL/O **(ă-mig-dă-lō)**	Amygdala (almond-shaped nuclei in the temporal lobe), almond, tonsil	L. *amygdala*, *-ae*, f. amygdala fr. Gr. *amygdale*, almond	Chapter 10
AMYL/O **(am-ĭ-lō)**	Starch	Gr. *amylon*, starch	Chapter 13
ANA- **(an-ă)** **ANO-** **(an-ō)**	Upward, back, against, again	Gr. *ana-*, upward, back, against, again	Chapter 2
ANCON/O **(ang-kō-nō)**	Elbow	Gr. *ankon*, elbow	Chapter 3
ANDR/O **(an-drō)**	Male, man, stamen of a flower	Gr. *aner*, *andros*, a man, male	Chapters 4, 12, 15
ANEM/O **(a-nĕ-mō)**	Wind	Gr. *anemos*, wind	Chapter 9
-ANEOUS **(ā-nē-ŭs)**	Made of, having the quality of, full of	L. *-aneus*, made of, having the quality of, full of	Chapter 2
ANEURYSM/O **(an-yŭ-rizm-ō)**	Abnormal widening of a vessel	Gr. *aneurysm*, dilation of a vessel	Chapter 8

Greek or Latin word element	Current usage	Etymology	Chapters
ANGI/O (an-jē-ō)	Vessel	Gr. *angeion*, vessel	Chapters 3, 8
ANGIN/O (an-jī-nō)	Angina pectoris, choking	L. *angina*, a choking, strangling	Chapter 8
ANIS/O (an-ĭ-sō)	Unequal	Gr. *anisos*, unequal	Chapter 8
ANKYL/O (ang-kĭ-lō)	Stiff, fused, crooked	Gr. *ankylos*, crooked, bent	Chapter 7
AN/O (ā-nō)	Anus	L. *anus*, -*i*, m. a ring, the anus	Chapter 13
-ANT (ănt)	Translated –ing added to the verb	L. -*ans*, translated –ing added to the verb	Chapter 2
ANTE- (ant-ē)	Before	L. *ante-*, before	Chapter 2
ANTEBRACHI/O (ant-ē-brăk-ē-ō)	Forearm	L. *antebrachium*, -*i*, n. forearm fr. Gr. *brachion*, arm	Chapter 3
ANTER/O (ant-ĕ-rō)	Front, anterior	L. *anterior*, -*ius*, more forward, anterior	Chapter 3
ANTHROP/O (an-thrŏ-pō)	Human	Gr. *anthropos*, a human being	Chapter 4
ANTI- (ant-i)	Against, opposed to	Gr. *anti-*, against, opposed to	Chapter 2
ANTR/O (an-trō)	Cave; cavity or sinus	L. *antrum*, -*i*, n. cave	Chapter 9
AORT/O (ā-or-tō)	Aorta	L. *aorta*, -*ae*, f. aorta fr. Gr. "what is lifts or hangs up"	Chapter 8
APHRODISI/O (af-rŏ-dē-zē-ō)	Sex, sexual desire	Gr. *aphrodisiakos*, pert. to sexual love or desire, fr. *Aphrodite*, the Greek goddess of eros	Chapter 15
APHTH/O (af-thō)	Ulcer of the mouth, thrush	Gr. *aphtha*, thrush, mouth ulcer	Chapter 13
APIC/O (ap-ĭ-kō)	Tip, summit, end	L. *apex*, *apicis*, m. tip, summit, end	Chapter 12
APO- (ap-ŏ)	Away/apart from, derived from	Gr. *apo-*, apart from, derived from	Chapter 2
APPEND/O (ap-ĕn-dō) APPENDIC/O (ă-pen-dĭ-kō)	Appendix (something hanging onto another part/body)	L. *appendix*, *appendicis*, f. hung to, appendage; appendix fr. L. *pendere*, *pensum*, to hang	Chapter 13
AQUE/O (ak-wē-ō) AQU/O (ak-wō)	Water, water-like	L. *aqua*, -*ae*, f. water	Chapter 11
-AR (ăr)	Pertaining to	L. -*aris*, pertaining to	Chapter 2
ARACHN/O (ă-rak-nō)	Arachnoid membrane, spider, spider-like	Gr. *arachne*, spider	Chapter 10
ARC/O (ar-kō)	Arch, a curved structure, a bow	L. *arcus*, -*us*, m. a bow, vault, arch	Chapter 8

Greek or Latin word element	Current usage	Etymology	Chapters
ARGENT/O (ar-jent-ō)	Silver	L. *argentum, -i,* n. silver	Chapter 5
ARTERI/O (ar-tēr-ē-ō)	Artery	L. *arteria, -ae,* f. artery fr. Gr. arteria, "air carrier," windpipe, artery	Chapters 3, 8
ARTERIOL/O (ar-tēr-ē-ō-lō)	Arteriole	L. *arteriola, -ae,* f. arteriole, little artery	Chapter 8
ARTHR/O (ar-thrō)	Joint	Gr. *arthron,* joint	Chapter 7
ARTICUL/O (ar-tik-yŭ-lō)	Joint, to join, to speak clearly	*L. articulatio, articulationis,* f. joint, knuckle fr. *articulare,* to segment, to speak distinctly	Chapter 7
-ARY (ā-rē)	Pertaining to, place of	L. *-arium,* pertaining to, place of	Chapter 2
ASC/O (as-kō)	Sac, saclike	Gr. *askos,* leather bag; bladder, sac	Chapter 13
-ASE (ās)	Enzyme	Suffix used for "enzyme"	Chapter 13
ASTHM/O (az-mō) **ASTHMAT/O** (az-mă-tō)	Asthma	Gr. *asthma, asthmatos,* panting, shortness of breath	Chapter 9
ASTRAGAL/O (ă-stra-gă-lō)	Talus bone	Gr. *astragalos,* talus, dice	Chapter 7
-ATE (āt)	To make, to cause, to act upon; having the form of, possessing	L. *-ate,* to make, to cause, to act upon; having the form of, possessing	Chapter 2
ATEL/O (at-ĕl-ō)	Incomplete, imperfect	Gr. *ateles,* without end, incomplete	Chapter 9
ATHER/O (ath-ĕ-rō)	Fatty plaque	Gr. *athere,* porridge, cereal, gruel	Chapter 8
ATM/O (at-mō)	Vapor, air, gas	Gr. *atmos,* steam, vapor	Chapter 9
ATRI/O (ā-trē-ō)	Atrium (a chamber of the heart), a central room	L. *atrium, -i,* n. a Roman foreroom; atrium (a chamber of the heart)	Chapter 8
AUDIT/O (od-ĭ-tō) **AUDI/O** (od-ē-ō)	Listening, sense of hearing	L. *audire, auditum,* to hear	Chapter 11
AUR/O (or-ō)	Ear	L. *auris, auris,* f. ear	Chapters 3, 11
AUR/O (or-ō)	Gold	L. *aurum, -i,* n. gold	Chapter 5
AURICUL/O (or-ik-yŭ-lō)	Auricle (visible external ear)	L. *auricula, -ae,* f. auricle, little ear	Chapter 11
AUSCULTAT/O (os-kŭl-tāt-ō)	To listen	L. *auscultare, auscultatum,* to listen to	Chapter 9
AUT/O (ot-ō)	Self, same	Gr. *autos,* self, by itself	Chapter 6

Greek or Latin word element	Current usage	Etymology	Chapters
AX/O (ak-sō)	Axon (long process of a neuron), axle, axis	Gr. *axon*, axle, axis	Chapter 10
AXILL/O (ak-sil-ō)	Armpit, axilla	L. *axilla, -ae*, f. armpit	Chapter 3
AZOT/O (ăz-ō-tō)	Nitrogenous waste; nitrogen	Gr. *azōtos*, lifeless	Chapter 14
BALAN/O (bal-ă-nō)	Glans penis, acorn	Gr. *balanos*, acorn	Chapter 15
BAR/O (bar-ō) **BARY/O** (bar-ĭ-ō)	Weight, pressure; Heavy, dull	Gr. *baros*, weight, pressure Gr. *barys*, heavy	Chapters 5, 11
BAS/O (bă-sō)	Base, foundation, step, a walking	L. *basis, -is*, f. fr. Gr. *basis*, foundation, base, step, a walking	Chapter 8
BATH/O (băth-ō) **BATHY/O** (băth-ē-ō)	Depth, deep	Gr. *bathys*, deep, inner; *bathos*, depth	Chapter 11
BI- (bī) **BIN-** (bī-n) before vowels	Twice, two, double, twofold	L. *bi-*, twice, two, double, twofold	Chapter 2
BIB/O (bī-bō)	To drink	L. *bibere*, to drink	Chapter 14
BIFID/O (bī-fĭd-ō)	Split in two	L. *bifĭdus, -a, -um*, split in two	Chapter 7
BIL/I (bil-ĭ)	Bile	L. *bilis, -is*, f. bile	Chapter 13
BIS- (bis)	Two times, two	L. *bis*, two times	Chapter 5
BLAST/O (blă-stō) **-BLAST** (blăst)	Embryonic cell, formative cell or layer, bud or shoot	Gr. *blastos*, a bud, shoot	Chapter 8
-BLE (bl)	Ability to	L. *-bilis*, ability to	Chapter 2
BLENN/O (blĕn-ō)	Mucus	Gr. *blennos*, mucus	Chapter 9
BLEPHAR/O (blĕf-ă-rō)	Eyelid	Gr. *blepharon*, eyelid	Chapter 11
BLEPS/O (blep-sō) **-BLEPSIA** (blep-sē-ă) **-BLEPSIS** (blep-sĭs)	Sense of sight	Gr. *blepsis*, sight	Chapter 11
BOL/O (bō-lō)	Mass of masticated food, lump, mass	Gr. *bolos*, rounded mass, lump, clod	Chapter 13

Greek or Latin word element	Current usage	Etymology	Chapters
BRACHI/O (brăk-ē-ō)	Upper arm, brachium, arm-like process	L. *brachium, -i,* n. upper arm fr. Gr. *brachion,* arm	Chapter 3
BRACHY- (brăk-ē)	Short	Gr. *brachys,* short	Chapter 15
BRADY- (brăd-ē)	Slow	Gr. *bradys,* slow	Chapters 8, 9
BROM/O (brŏ-mō)	Foul-smelling, bromine	Gr. *bromos,* foul-smelling	Chapter 5
BRONCH/O (brŏng-kō)	Bronchus	L. *bronchus, -i,* m. bronchus fr. Gr. *bronchos,* anatomical windpipe	Chapter 9
BRONCHIOL/O (brong-kē-ō-lō)	Bronchiole	L. *bronchiolus, -i,* m. bronchiole, small bronchus fr. Gr. *bronchos,* anatomical windpipe	Chapter 9
BUBON/O (boo-bŏn-ō)	Swollen lymph node(s)	Gr. *boubon,* a swollen gland	Chapter 8
BUCC/O (bŭk-ō)	Cheek	L. *bucca, -ae,* f. cheek	Chapters 3, 13
BULL/O (bŭl-ō)	Bulla, large blister	L. *bulla, -ae,* f. round swelling, amulet, water bubble	Chapter 6
BURS/O (bŭr-sō)	Bursa (anatomical), bag, pouch	*L. bursa, -ae,* f. a sack, purse; anatomical pad-like sac associated with joints	Chapter 7
CAL/O (kā-lō) **CALOR/O** (kă-lo-rō)	Heat, calorie	L. *calor, caloris,* m. heat; fr. *calere,* to heat	Chapters 4, 5
CALC/O (kal-kō)	Calcium, lime,	L. *calx, calcis,* f. limestone, lime concretion	Chapters 5, 14
CALC/O (kal-kō)	Heel	L. *calx, calcis,* f. the heel	Chapter 3
CALCANE/O (kal-kā-nē-ō)	Calcaneus bone	*L. calcaneus, -i,* m. heel, heel bone fr. L. *calx, calcis,* heel, *os calcis,* bone of the heel	Chapter 7
CALCUL/O (kăl-kū-lō)	Stone	L. *calculus, -i,* m. a little stone, pebble	Chapter 14
CALYC/O (kăl-ĭ-kō) **CALIC/O** (kăl-ĭ-kō)	Renal calices, cup-like structure	L. *calix, calicis,* m. calix fr. Gr. *kalyx, kalykos,* covering, shell; cup of flower	Chapter 14
CAMER/O (kăm-ĕr-ō)	Chamber, cavity	L. *camera, -ae,* f. camera, chamber fr. Gr. *kamara,* anything with an arched cover	Chapter 11
CAMPT/O (kămp-tō) **CAMPYL/O** (kăm-pĭ-lō) **-CAMPSIA** (kamp-sē-ă) **-CAMPSIS** (kămp-sĭs)	Bent, curved	Gr. *kamptos, kampylos,* bent	Chapters 7, 12

Greek or Latin word element	Current usage	Etymology	Chapters
CANCER/O (kan-ser-ō)	Cancer, crab	L. *cancer, cancri*, m. crab	Chapter 4
CANCR/O (kăng-krō)	Ulcer (rapidly spreading)	L. *cancrum, -i*, n. sore, lesion fr. L. *cancer, cancri*, m. crab, type of skin lesion	Chapter 6
CAPILLAR/O (kap-ĭ-ler-ō)	Capillary	L. *capillaris, -e*, hairlike; capillary fr. L. *capillus, -i*, m. a hair	Chapter 8
CAPIT/O (kap-ĭ-tō) **CIPIT/O** (sip-ĭ-tō) **-CIPUT** (sĭp-ŭt) **-CEPS** (seps)	Head, origin of a muscle	L. *caput, capitis*, n. head	Chapters 3, 7
CAPN/O (kap-nō)	Carbon dioxide, smoke	Gr. *kapnos*, smoke	Chapter 9
CAPSUL/O (kăp-sŭ-lŏ) **CAPS/O** (kă-'sŏ)	Capsule	L. *capsula, -ae*, f. little chest or box L. *capsa, -ae, f. box*	Chapter 7
CARB/O (kăr-bō) **CARBON/O** (kar-bŏ-nō)	Carbon dioxide, carbon	L. *carbo, carbonis*, m. charcoal	Chapters 5, 9
CARCIN/O (kar-sĭ-nō)	Cancer, crab	Gr. *karkinos*, crab, creeping ulcer; cancer	Chapter 4, 6
CARDI/O (kard-ē-ō)	Heart, the cardiac sphincter of the stomach	Gr. *kardia*, heart; the cardiac sphincter of the stomach	Chapters 8, 13
CARN/O (kar-nō)	Flesh	L. *caro, carnis*, f. flesh, fleshy pulp of fruit	Chapter 6
CAROTID/O (kă-rot-ĭd-ō)	Carotid	L. *carotis, carotidis*, f. carotid fr. Gr. *karodes*, causing stupor, soporific	Chapter 8
CARP/O (kăr-pō)	Wrist	L. *carpus, -i*, m. wrist	Chapters 3, 7
CARP/O (kăr-pō)	Fruit	Gr. *karpos*, fruit, seed	Chapter 13
CARTILAG/O (kăr-tĭ-lă-gō)	Cartilage	L. *cartilago, cartilaginis*, f. gristle, cartilage	Chapter 7
CATARACT/O (kăt-ă-răk-tō)	Cataract	L. *cataracta, -ae*, f. waterfall	Chapter 11
CATHART/O (kă-thart-ō)	Evacuation (of the bowels)	Gr. *katharis*, evacuation, purification	Chapter 13
CATHER/O (kath-ĕt-ĕr-ō)	Catheter	Gr. *catheter*, catheter; a surgical instrument for emptying the bladder fr. Gr. *kathiemi*, to send down	Chapter 14
CAUD/O (kowd-ō)	Tail, tail-like	L. *caudalis, -e*, pertaining to the tail, caudal L. *cauda, -ae*, f. tail	Chapter 3

Greek or Latin word element	Current usage	Etymology	Chapters
CAUS/O (kaw-sō) **CAUST/O** (kaw-stō) **CAUTER/O** (kaw-tĕr-ō)	To burn, burnt	Gr. *kausos*, burning heat; *kaustos*, burnt; *kauterion*, searing-iron	Chapter 13
CAV/O (kā-vō)	Hollow	L. *cavus, -a, -um*, hollow	Chapter 7
CAVIT/O (kăv-ĭ-tō)	Cavity	L. *cavitas, cavitatis*, f. cavity, hollow	Chapter 3
-CE (s)	State or condition of	L. *-ce*, state or condition of	Chapter 2
CEC/O (sē-kō)	Cecum (Caecum)	L. *caecum, -i*, n. cecum fr. Latin adjective for "blind"	Chapter 13
CEL/O (sē-lō) **KEL/O** (kē-lō) **-CELE** (sēl)	Hernia, protrusion	Gr. *kele*, tumor, hernia	Chapters 4, 13
CELL/O (se-lō) **CELLUL/O** (sĕl-ū-lō)	Cell	L. *cella, ae*, f. room, chamber L. *cellula, -ae*, f. little room, chamber	Chapter 4
CENT/O (sĕn-tō)	One hundred	L. *centum*, one hundred	Chapter 5
-CENTESIS (sen-tē-sĭs)	Surgical puncture for aspiration	Gr. *kenteein*, to goad, prick	Chapter 4
CEPHAL/O (sĕf-ă-lō)	Head	Gr. *kephale*, head	Chapters 3, 10
CER/O (sē-rō) **-CERE** (sēr)	Wax	L. *cera, -ae*, f. wax	Chapter 11
CEREBELL/O (sĕr-ĕ-bĕl-ō)	Cerebellum	L. *cerebellum, -i*, n. cerebellum, little brain	Chapter 10
CEREBR/O (sĕr-ĕ-brō)	Cerebrum (largest part of the brain), brain	L. *cerebrum, -i*, n. cerebrum, brain	Chapter 10
CERUL/O (sē-roo-lō) **CAERUL/O** (sē-roo-lō)	sky-blue color; dark blue	L. *caerulus, -a, -um*, blue, sky-blue	Chapter 14
CERUMIN/O (sĕ-roo-mĭ-nō)	Earwax	L. *cerumen, ceruminis*, n. earwax	Chapter 11
CERVIC/O (sĕr-vĭ-kō) **-CERVIX** (sĕr-viks)	Neck	L. *cervix, cervicis*, f. neck	Chapters 3, 7, 15

Greek or Latin word element	Current usage	Etymology	Chapters
CHALAS/O (kă-lā-sō) -CHALASIS (kă-lā-sĭs)	Relaxation (of sphincter), slack	Gr. *chalaein*, to slacken, relax	Chapters 11, 13
CHEIL/O (kī-lō) CHIL/O (kī-lō)	Lip	Gr. *cheilos*, lip	Chapter 13
CHEIR/O (kī-rō) CHIR/O (kī-rō)	Hand	Gr. *cheir, cheiros*, hand	Chapter 3
-CHEZIA (kē-zē-ă)	Defecation	Gr. *chezein*, to defecate	Chapter 13
CHILI/O (kil-i-ō) KIL/O (kil-ō)	One thousand	Gr. *chilioi*, one thousand	Chapter 5
CHIRURGIC/O (kī-rŭr-jĭ-kō)	Surgery	Gr. *chirurgia*, surgery	Chapter 4
CHLAMYD/O (klă-mid-ō)	Cape-like, Chlamydia	Gr. *chlamys, chlamydos*, a short mantle, cape	Chapter 15
CHLOR/O (klō-rō)	Green, chlorine	Gr. *chloros*, green	Chapters 5, 14
CHOL/E (kō-lē)	Bile	Gr. *chole*, bile, gall; bitter anger	Chapter 13
CHONDR/O (kŏn-drō)	Cartilage	Gr. *chondros*, granule	Chapter 7
CHORD/O (kor-dō)	Cord, tendon	Gr. *chorde*, cord, rope, musical string	Chapter 8
CHORE/O (kō-rē-ō)	Chorea (i.e. involuntary dancing/writhing movement), dance	Gr. *choreia*, dancing	Chapter 10
CHORI/O (kō-rē-ō)	Chorion (the outermost membrane enclosing the fetus)	L. *chorion, -i*, n. chorion fr. Gr. *chorion*, animal hide	Chapter 15
CHOROID/O (kō-roy-dō)	Choroid (*middle tunic of the eye)	L. *choroidea, -ae*, f. choroid fr. Gr. *chorion*, lambskin	Chapter 11
CHROMI/O (krō-mē-ō) CHROM/O (krō-mō) CHROMAT/O (krō-mă-tō)	Chromium; Color	Gr. *chroma, chromatos*, color	Chapters 5, 14
CHRON/O (kro-nō)	Time	Gr. *chronos*, time	Chapter 4
CHYL/O (kī-lō)	Chyle, fluid of the lymph system	Gr. *chylos*, humor	Chapter 13
CHYM/O (kī-mō)	Chyme (nearly liquid mass of digested foot)	Gr. *chymos*, humor	Chapter 13

Greek or Latin word element	Current usage	Etymology	Chapters
CIB/O (sī-bō)	Food, meal	L. *cibus*, *-i*, m. food	Chapter 13
CICATRIC/O (sĭk″ă-trĭ-kō)	Scar	L. *cicatrix*, *cicatricis*, f. scar	Chapter 6
CILI/O (sil-ē-ō)	Ciliary body, eyelash, hair-like process	L. *cilium*, *-i*, n. eyelash	Chapter 11
CINGUL/O (sing-gyŭ-lō)	Girdle	L. *cingulum*, *-i*, n. belt, girdle	Chapter 3
CIRCUM- (sĭr″kŭm)	Around	L. *circum-*, around	Chapter 2
CIRRH/O (sĭ-rō)	Cirrhosis, yellow	Gr. *kirrhos*, yellow; cirrhosis	Chapter 13
CIS- (sĭs)	On this side	L. *cis*, on this side	Chapter 5
CIS/O (sī-sō) **-CIDE** (sīd)	Kill, cut	L. *caedere*, *caesum*, to cut, kill	Chapters 4, 5
CLAST/O (klăs-tō) **-CLAST** (klăst) **-CLASIS** (klă-sĭs) **-CLASIA** (klă-zē-ă)	Broken, breaking; -CLAST = A breaker of things; -CLASIS and -CLASIA = A breaking of something	Gr. *klastos*, broken	Chapters 4, 14
-CLASTY (klas-tē)	A surgical breaking	Gr. *klastos*, broken	Chapters 4, 14
CLAUDIC/O (klod-ĭ-kō)	Limping	L. *claudicare*, to limp	Chapter 8
CLAVICUL/O (klă-vĭk′ū-lō) **CLAVIC/O** (klăv-ĭ-kō)	Clavicle, collar bone	L. *clavicula*, *-ae*, f. little key, collar bone	Chapter 7
-CLE (k-l)	Diminutive (little)	L. *-culus*, diminutive (little)	Chapter 2
CLEID/O (klī-dō)	Clavicle, collar bone	Gr. *kleis*, *kleidos*, key, collar bone	Chapter 7
CLEIST/O (klīs-tō) **-CLEISIS** (klī-sĭs)	Closed *Suffix = surgical closure	Gr. *kleiein*, to close	Chapter 15
CLITOR/O (klit-ŏ-rō) **CLITORID/O** (kli-tō-rĭd-ō)	Clitoris (female erectile organ)	L. *clitoris*, *clitoridis*, f. *clitoris*	Chapter 15
CLON/O (klō-nō)	Clonus (i.e. spasmadic alteration of muscle contractions)	Gr. *klonos*, a confused motion, turmoil	Chapter 10

Greek or Latin word element	Current usage	Etymology	Chapters
CLUN/O (klū-nō)	Buttocks, clunes	L. *clunes, -ium*, f. buttocks	Chapter 3
CLUS/O (kloo-sō) **CLAUD/O** (klod-ō)	Shut, closed off	L. *claudere, clausum*, to shut, close	Chapter 8
-CLYSIS (klī-sĭs)	Washing, lavage	Gr. *klysein*, to wash or rinse out	Chapter 13
CNEM/O (nē-mŏ)	Leg	Gr. *kneme*, leg, tibia	Chapter 7
COAGUL/O (kō-ag-yŭ-lō)	Thickening of liquid into a gel or solid	L. *coagulum, -i*, n. that which causes to curdle	Chapter 8
COARCT/O (kō-ărk-tō) **COARCTAT/O** (kō-ărk-tāt-ō)	To confine, stricture	L. *coarctare*, to confine, draw together	Chapter 8
COCCYG/O (kŏk-sĭ-gō) **COCCY/O** (kŏk-sē-ō)	Coccyx, tailbone	L. *coccyx, coccygis*, m. coccyx, cuckoo, tailbone fr. Gr. *kokkyx*, a cuckoo, particularly its beak, which is what the coccyx bone looks like	Chapter 7
COCHLE/O (kok-lē-ō)	Cochlea of the inner ear, spiral shell	L. *cochlea, -ae*, f. cochlea fr. Gr. *kochlias*, snail with a spiral shell	Chapter 11
COEL/O (sē-lō) **CEL/O** (sē-lō) **KOIL/O** (koy-lō) **CELI/O** (sē-lē-ō) **-COELE** (sēl) **-CELE** (sēl)	Cavity, hollow, abdomen	Gr. *koilia*, cavity, hollow, belly; abdomen	Chapters 3, 10, 13
COIT/O (kō-ĭt-ō)	Sexual intercourse	L. *coitus, -us*, m. sexual union fr. *con-* together, *itus*, a going	Chapter 15
COL/O (kŏ-lō) **COLON/O** (kō-lŏ-nō)	Colon	L. *colon, -i*, n. colon fr. Gr. *kolon*, colon	Chapter 13
COLL/O (kŏl-lō)	Neck, neck of a long bone	L. *collum, -i*, n. neck	Chapters 3, 7
COLP/O (kol-pō)	The female vagina	Gr. *kolpos*, a hollow, fold, bay	Chapter 15

Greek or Latin word element	Current usage	Etymology	Chapters
COMAT/O (kō-mă-tō) **-COMA** (kō-mă)	Coma (i.e. state of unconsciousness that cannot be aroused from)	Gr. *koma*, *kamatos*, deep sleep	Chapter 10
COMED/O (kŏm-ă-dō)	Pimple, blackhead, whitehead	L. *comedo*, *comedonis*, m. a glutton; comedone fr. L. *comedere*, to eat up	Chapter 6
CON- (kŏn) **COL-** (kŏl) before l **COM-** (kŏm) before b, m, p **CO-** (kŏ) before h **COR-** (kŏr) before r	With, together, complete	L. *con-*, with, together, complete	Chapter 2
CON/O (kō-nō)	Cone, pine cone	Gr. *konos*, pine cone, cone	Chapter 12
CONCH/O (kŏng-kō)	Auricle (visible external ear), shell, shell-like	L. *concha*, *-ae*, f. concha fr. Gr. *konche*, shell, cockle	Chapter 11
CONDYL/O (kon-dĭ-lō)	Rounded protuberance at the ends of bones, (condyle)	L. *condylus*, *-i*, m. condyle fr. Gr. *kondylos*, knuckle	Chapter 7
CONI/O (kō-nē-ō)	Dust	Gr. *konis*, *konios*, dust	Chapter 9
CONJUNCTIV/O (kŏn-jŭnk-tĭ-vō)	Conjunctiva	L. *conjunctiva*, *-ae*, f. conjunctiva	Chapter 11
CONTRA- (kon-tră)	Against, opposite	L. *contra-*, against, opposite	Chapter 2
COPR/O (kop-rō)	Feces	Gr. *kopros*, feces	Chapter 13
COR/O (kor-ō) **-CORIA** (kŏr-ē-ă)	Pupil of the eye	Gr. *kore*, maiden, doll	Chapter 11
CORD/O (kor-dō)	Heart	L. *cor*, *cordis*, n. heart	Chapters 3, 8
CORI/O (kō-rē-ō)	Skin, dermis	L. *corium*, *-i*, n. hide, skin	Chapter 6
CORN/O (kor-nō) **CORNE/O** (kor-nē-ō)	Horn, hard, horn-like, cornea	L. *cornea*, *-ae*, f. cornea fr. L. *cornu*, *cornus*, n. horn	Chapters 6, 11
CORON/O (kor-ō-nō)	On the coronal suture of the skull, crown, circular, coronary arteries	L. *corona*, *-ae*, f. a crown, garland, L. *corolla*, *-ae*, f. a crown	Chapters 3, 8

Greek or Latin word element	Current usage	Etymology	Chapters
CORPOR/O (kor-pǒ-rō)	Body	L. *corpus, corporis*, n. body	Chapters 3, 7
CORPUSCUL/O (kor-pǔs-kū-lō)	Corpuscle, small mass or body	L. *corpusculum, -i*, n. small body fr. L. *corpus, corporis*, n. body	Chapter 8
CORTIC/O (kor-tǐ-kō)	Cortex, outer layer of an organ or gland, bark	L. *cortex, corticis*, m. bark, outer layer	Chapters 10, 12
COSM/O (kŏz-mō) COSMET/O (kŏz-mě-tō)	Universe, world, beautification, cosmetic	Gr. *kosmos*, world, order, adornment Gr. *kosmetikos*, the art of dress and ornament	Chapter 6
COST/O (kŏs-tō)	Rib	L. *costa, -ae*, f. rib	Chapter 7
COX/O (kŏk-sō)	Hip	L. *coxa, -ae*, f. hip	Chapter 3
CRANI/O (krā-nē-ō)	Cranium (portion of the skull that encloses the brain)	L. *cranium, -i*, n. skull fr. Gr. *kranion*, skull	Chapters 3, 7, 10
CRAS/O (krā-sō) -CRASIA (krā-zē-ă)	Mixture, temperament	Gr. *krasis*, mixture, a mixing, temperament	Chapter 8
CRE/O (krē-ō) CREAT/O (krē-ăt-ō)	Flesh, muscle	Gr. *kreas, kreatos*, flesh, muscle	Chapter 6
CREATIN/O (krē-ă-tin-ō)	Creatine	Creatine, a colorless crystalline substance in urine, fr. Gr. *kreas, kreatos*, flesh, muscle	Chapter 14
CREPIT/O (krep-ǐ-tō)	Creak, crackle	L. *crepare, crepitatum*, rattle, creak, crackle	Chapter 7
CRESC/O (kres-ō)	Increasing, crescent	L. *crescere*, to grow, increase	Chapter 8
CRETIN/O (krět-ǐn-ō)	Cretinism	from French *crétin* (18th century)	Chapter 12
CRIN/O (krǐn-ō) -CRINE (krīn)	To secrete	Gr. *krinein*, to separate; to secrete	Chapter 12
CRIST/O (kris-tō)	Crest, ridge	L. *crista, -ae*, f. crest, ridge, comb of rooster	Chapter 7
CRIT/O (krit-ō) -CRIT (krǐt)	Separate, decide	Gr. *kritos*, fr. Gr. *krinein*, to separate, distinguish, judge	Chapter 8
CRUR/O (kroo-rō)	Leg, leg-like part	L. *crus, cruris*, n. leg	Chapter 3

Greek or Latin word element	Current usage	Etymology	Chapters
CRYPT/O (krĭp-tō) **KRYPT/O** (krĭp-tō)	Hidden, covered, krypton	Gr. *kryptos*, covered, hidden	Chapters 5, 6
CUBIT/O (kū-bĭ-tō)	Elbow	L. *cubitus, -i,* m. elbow fr. L. *cubitum, -i,* n. elbow	Chapter 3
CUPR/O (kū-prō)	Copper	L. *cuprum, -i,* n. copper	Chapter 5
CUSPID/O (kŭs-pĭ-dō)	Cuspid, point	L. *cuspis, cuspidis,* f. a point	Chapter 8
CUT/O (kū-tō) **CUTANE/O** (kū-tā-nē-ō)	Skin	L. *cutis, -is,* f. skin, hide	Chapter 6
CYAN/O (sī-ă-nō)	Blue	Gr. *kyanos,* blue	Chapter 14
CYCL/O (sī-klō)	Ciliary body of the eye, circle, wheel	Gr. *kyklos,* circle, wheel, ring	Chapter 11
-CYESIS (sī-ē-sĭs)	To be pregnant	Gr. *kyein,* to swell, be pregnant	Chapter 15
CYST/O (sĭs-tō)	Bladder, cyst, sac, cholecyst/o = gall bladder	Gr. *kystis,* bladder, cyst, sac	Chapters 3, 6, 13, 14
CYT/O (sī-tō) **-CYTE** (sīt)	Cell	Gr. *kytos,* a hollow receptacle, a vessel	Chapters 4, 8
DACRY/O (dak-rē-ŏ)	Tear	Gr. *dakryon,* tear	Chapter 11
DACTYL/O (dak-tĭ-lō) **-DACTYL** (dak-tĭl)	Finger or toe	Gr. *daktylos,* finger or toe	Chapters 3, 7
DE- (dē)	Down from, from, not	L. *de-,* down from, from, not	Chapter 2
DECIM/O (dĕs-ĭ-mō)	Tenth, ten	L. *decimus,* tenth	Chapter 5
DEC/A (dek-ă)	Ten	Gr. *deka,* ten	Chapter 5
DEM/O (de-mō)	People	Gr. *demos,* people of a country or land	Chapter 4
DEMI- (dĕm-ĭ-)	Half, part	L. *demi-,* half, part	Chapter 2
DENDR/O (dĕn-drō)	Tree, branched/treelike structure, dendrite (part of neuron)	Gr. *dendron,* tree	Chapter 10
DENT/O (dĕn-tō)	Tooth	L. *dens, dentis,* m. tooth	Chapter 13

Greek or Latin word element	Current usage	Etymology	Chapters
DEPRESS/O (dĕ-prĕs-ō)	To press down	*L. depressor, -oris*, m. depressor fr. *L. depressio*, f. a pressing down	Chapter 7
DERM/O (dĕr-mō) **DERMAT/O** (dĕr-mă-tō) **-DERM** (dĕrm)	Skin	*L. dermis, -is*, f. dermis fr. *Gr. derma, dermatos*, skin	Chapters 3, 6
-DESIS (dē-sĭs)	Surgical binding, fusion	*Gr. deein*, to bind	Chapter 4
DEUTER/O (doo-tĕr-ō)	Second, secondary (in vision, green blindness, i.e. secondary color)	*Gr. deuteros*, second	**Chapter 11**
DEXTR/O (deks-trō)	Right	*L. dexter, -tra, -trum*, right	**Chapter 3**
DI- (dī)	Twice, double, two	*Gr. di-*, twice, double two	**Chapter 2**
DIA- (dī-ă)	Through, across	*Gr. dia-*, through, across	**Chapter 2**
DIAPHRAGM/O (dī-ă-frăg-mō) **DIAPHRAGMAT/O** (dī-ă-frăg-ma-tō)	Diaphragm	*L. diaphragma, diaphragmatis*, n. diaphragm fr. *Gr. diaphragma*, partition, barrier	**Chapter 9**
DIASTOL/O (dī-as-tŏ-lō)	Expansion	*Gr. diastole*, expansion	**Chapter 8**
DICHO- (dī-kō)	In two, twofold	*Gr. dicho-*, in two, twofold	**Chapter 2**
DIDYM/O (did-ĭ-mō) **-DIDYMUS** (dĭd-ĭ-mŭs)	Conjoined twins, twin, testicle	*L. didymus, -i*, m. twin fr. *Gr. didymos*, double, twin	**Chapter 15**
DIET/O (dī-ĕ-tō)	Food	*Gr. diaita*, way of living/regimen; diet	**Chapter 4**
DIGIT/O (dij-ĭt-ō)	Finger, toe	*L. digitus, -i*, m. finger of toe	**Chapter 3**
DILAT/O (dī-lăt-ō)	To spread out, expand	*L. dilatator, -oris*, m. dilator fr. *L. dilatio*, f. a spreading out	**Chapter 8**
DIPHTHER/O (dif-thĕr-ē-ō)	Diphtheria	*Gr. diphthera*, leather, tanned skin	**Chapter 9**
DIPL/O (dĭp-lō)	Double	*Gr diploos*, twofold, double	**Chapter 11**
DIPS/O (dip-sō)	Thirst	*Gr. dipsa*, thirst	**Chapter 12**
DIS- (dĭs) **DIF-** (dĭf) before f	Apart from, separate	*L. dis-*, apart from, separate	**Chapter 2**

Greek or Latin word element	Current usage	Etymology	Chapters
DIST/O **(dĭs-tō)**	Farthest (from a given part of the center of the body)	L. *distalis, -e,* apart from, distal	**Chapter 3**
DIVERTICUL/O **(dī-vĕr-tik-yŭ-lō)**	Diverticulum (an outpouching of structure, particularly an intestine)	L. *diverticulum, -i,* n. turning out; a diverticulum	Chapter 13
DOCH/O **(dō-kō)**	Duct, receptacle choledoch/o = bile duct	Gr. *doche,* a receptacle	Chapter 13
DODEC/A **(dō-dek-ă)**	Twelve	Gr. *dodeka,* twelve	Chapter 5
DOLOR/O **(dō-lō-rō)**	Pain	L. *dolor, doloris,* m. pain	Chapter 4
DORS/O **(dor-sō)**	Back	L. *dorsum, -i,* n. back	Chapter 3
DU/O **(dū-ō)**	Two	L. *dou,* two	Chapter 5
DUC/O **(doo-kō)** **DUCT/O** **(dŭkt-ō)**	Duct, to draw, lead, or convey	L. *ductus, -us,* m. a duct fr. L. *ducere, ductus,* m. to lead, draw, convey L. *ducere, ductus,* to lead, draw or convey	Chapters 7, 13
DUODEN/O **(dū-ō-dē-nō)**	Duodenum (first part of the small intestine)	L. *duodenum, -i,* duodenum fr. Medieval Latin *duodenum digitorum* "space of twelve digits,"	Chapter 13
DUR/O **(dū-rō)**	Hard, dura mater membrane	L. *durus, -a, -um,* hard	Chapter 10
DY/O **(dī-ō)**	Two, a pair	Gr. *dyo,* two	Chapter 5
DYS- **(dis)**	Difficult, painful, faulty	Gr. *dys-,* difficult, faulty	Chapter 2
E- **(ē)** **EX-** **(eks)** **EF-** **(ef) before f**	Out of, off	L. *e-, ex-, ef-,* out of, off	Chapter 2
-EAL **(ē-ăl)**	Pertaining to	L. *-eal,* pertaining to	Chapter 2
EC- **(ek)** **EK-** **(ek)** **EX-** **(eks)**	Out of, outside	Gr. *-ek,* out of, outside	Chapter 2
ECCHYM/O **(ĕk-ĭ-mō)**	Broad bruising, ecchymosis	Gr. *ecchymosis,* bruise	Chapter 6
ECHIN/O **(ek-ĭ-nō)**	Spiny	Gr. *echinos,* sea urchin, hedgehog, spiny	Chapter 8

Greek or Latin word element	Current usage	Etymology	Chapters
-ECTASIS (ek-tă-sĭs) **-ECTASIA** (ek-tā-zhē-ă)	Dilation, expansion	Gr. *ektasis*, stretching out	Chapters 4, 8, 9
ECTO- (ĕk-tō)	On the outside	Gr. *ecto-*, on the outside	Chapter 2
EDEMAT/O (ĕ-dē-mă-tō) **-EDEMA** (ĕ-dē-mă)	Swelling	Gr. *oidema, oidematos*, swelling	Chapters 4, 8
ELECTR/O (ĕ-lek-trō)	Electricity	Gr. *elektron*, amber	Chapter 5
EMBOL/O (ĕm-bō-lō)	A moving clot in the blood (embolus), an interjection	L. *embolus, -i*, embolus Gr. *embolos*, that which is thrust into something, wedge, stopper	Chapter 8
EMBRY/O (em-brē-ō)	Embryo (*unborn animal in the early stage of development)	Gr. *embryon*, young one, fetus	Chapter 15
EMET/O (em-ĕ-tō) **-EMESIS** (ĕm-ĕ-sĭs)	Vomiting	Gr. *emetos*, vomit	Chapter 13
-EMIA (ē-mē-ă)	Condition of blood	Gr. *haima, haimatos*, blood	Chapter 8
EN- (en) **EM-** (em)	In, within	Gr. *en-*, in, within	Chapter 2
ENANTI/O (ĕn-ăn-tē-ō)	Opposite	Gr. *enanta*, opposite	Chapter 5
ENCEPHAL/O (ĕn-sef-ă-lō) **-ENCEPHALON** (en-sef-ă-lŏn)	Brain	L. *encephalon, -i*, n. encephalon, brain fr. Gr. *enkephalos*, brain	Chapters 3, 10
ENDO- (en-dō) **ENTO-** (ĕn-tō)	Within	Gr. *endo-*, within	Chapter 2
ENEM/O (en-ĕ-mō)	Enema	Gr. *enema, enematos*, a sending in	Chapter 13
ENNE/A (en-nē-ă)	Nine	Gr. *ennea*, nine	Chapter 5
-ENT (ĕnt)	Translated –ing added to the verb	L. *-ens*, translated –ing added to the verb	Chapter 2
ENTER/O (ent-ĕ-rō)	Intestine (usually the small intestine)	Gr. *enteron*, that within, intestine	Chapters 3, 13
-EOUS (ē-ŭs)	Made of, having the quality of, full of	L. *-eus*, made of, having the quality of, full of	Chapter 2

Greek or Latin word element	Current usage	Etymology	Chapters
EOS/O (ĕ-ōs-ō) **EO-** (ĕ-ō)	Dawn, early, morning red	Gr. *eos*, dawn	Chapter 8
EOSIN/O (ĕ-ō-sĭn-ō)	Red dyes used in histology (Eosine)	Gr. *eos*, dawn + chemical suffix -in	Chapter 8
EPI- (ep'ĭ-) **EPH-** (ĕf-)	Upon, on	Gr. *epi-*, upon, on	Chapter 2
EPIDIDYM/O (ep-ĭ-dĭd-ĭ-mō)	Epididymis (Seminal organ resting on the poster aspect of the testicle)	L. *epididymis, epididymidis,* n. epididymis fr. Gr. *didymos*, twin	Chapter 15
EPIGLOTT/O (ĕp-ĭ-glŏ-tō) **EPIGLOTTID/O** (ĕp-ĭ-glŏt-ĭd-ō)	Epiglottis	L. *epiglottis, epiglottidis,* f. epiglottis, valve covering the larynx fr. Gr. *epiglottis*	Chapter 9
EPISI/O (ĭ-pĭz-ē-ō)	Pubic region, vulva	Gr. *epision*, pubic region	Chapter 15
ERECT/O (ĕ-rek-tō) **ARRECT/O** (ă-rek-tō)	To lift up	L. *erector, -oris,* m. erector L. *erectio,* f. a raising	Chapter 7
ERG/O (ĕr-gō) **-ERGASIA** (ĕr-gā-sē-ă)	Work, function	Gr. *ergon*, work	Chapters 4, 5
EROT/O (ĕ-rōt-ō)	Sexual desire	Gr. *eros, erotos,* lust, love	Chapter 15
ERYTHEM/O (er-ĭ-thē-mō)	Erythema, a redness of skin	Gr. *erythema*, redness of skin	Chapter 6
ERYTHR/O (ĕ-rĭth-rō)	Red, redness (red blood cells)	Gr. *erythros*, red	Chapters 4, 6, 8, 14
-ESIS (ē-sĭs)	State or condition of	Gr. *-esis*, state or condition of	Chapter 2
ESO- (es-ŏ)	Inward, within	Gr. *eso-*, inward, within	Chapter 2
ESOPHAG/O (ĕ-sof-ă-gō)	Esophagus	L. *oesophagus, -i,* m. esophagus, fr. Gr. *oisaphgus*, esophagus, gullet	Chapter 13
ESTHESI/O (ĕs-thē-zē-ō) **ESTHET/O** (ĕs-thĕt-ō) **-ESTHESIA** (es-thē-zh-ē-ă)	Sensation, perception	Gr. *aisthesis*, feeling, sensation	Chapters 4, 10
ESTR/O (ĕs-trō)	Estrogen, estrus cycle (breeding period), sexual desire	Gr. *oistros*, gadfly; sexual desire, breeding period	Chapter 12

Greek or Latin word element	Current usage	Etymology	Chapters
ETHN/O (ĕth-nō)	Race, culture	Gr. *ethnos*, race, nation	Chapter 4
ETI/O (ĕt-ē-ō) **AETI/O** (ĕt-ē-ō)	Cause	Gr. *aitia*, cause	Chapter 4
EU- (ū)	Well, normal, good	Gr. *eu-*, well, normal, good	Chapter 2
EURY- (ū-rē)	Wide	Gr. *eurys*, wide	Chapter 8
EXANTHEM/O (eg-zan-thĕm-ō)	Rash	Gr. *exanthema*, eruption, pustule fr. Gr. *anthos*, flower fr. Gr. *anthein*, to blossom, erupt	Chapter 6
EXCRET- (ĕks-krē-tō)	Defecation	L. *excernere*, to separate	Chapter 13
EXO- (ek-sō)	Outside of, outward	Gr. *exo-*, outside of, outward	Chapter 2
EXTENS/O (ek-sten-sō)	To stretch out, straighten, extends	L. *extensor, -oris*, m. extensor fr. L. *extensio*, f. a stretching out, straighten	Chapter 7
EXTER/O (eks-tĕ-rō) **EXTERNAL/O** (ĕks-tĕr-nä-lō) **EXTREM/O** (ĕks-trĕm-ō)	Outside, outermost	L. *exter*, outward L. *externalis, -e* outside L. *extremus, -a, -um*, outermost	Chapter 3
EXTRA- (ĕks-trä) **EXTRO-** (eks-trō)	Outside, beyond	L. *extra-*, outside, beyond	Chapter 2
FAC/O (fak-ō) **FIC/O** (fik-ō) **FACT/O** (fak-tō) **FECT/O** (fek-tō)	To make, cause	L. *facere, factum*, to make, do	Chapter 4
FACI/O (fä-shē-ō)	Face, surface	L. *facies, -ei*, f. face, surface	Chapter 3
FASCI/O (fäsh-ē-ō)	Fascia, band	L. *fascia, -ae*, f. a broad band, bandage; a broad band of connective tissue enveloping muscle	Chapter 7
FASCICUL/O (fä-sik-yŭ-lō)	A small bundle of rod-like structures, fascicle	L. *fasciculus, -i*, m. small bundle of rods, fascicle	Chapters 7, 10
FEBR/O (fē-brō)	Fever	L. *febris, -is*, f. fever	Chapter 4

Greek or Latin word element	Current usage	Etymology	Chapters
FEC/O (fē-kō)	Feces	L. *faex, faecis*, f. dregs of wine; feces	Chapter 13
FEMIN/O (fem-ĭn-ō)	Female, feminine	L. *femina, -ae*, f. woman	Chapter 4
FEMOR/O (fem-ŏ-rō)	Femur bone, thigh	L. *femur, femoris*, n. thigh, bone of the thigh	Chapters 3, 7
FENESTR/O (fĕ-nes-trō)	Opening, window	L. *fenestra, -ae*, f. window	Chapter 11
FERR/O (fĕr-ō)	Iron	L. *ferrum, -i*, n. iron	Chapter 5
FET/O (fēt-ō)	Fetus (unborn animal in the later stage of development)	L. *fetus, -us*, m. offspring	Chapter 15
FIBR/O (fī-brō) **FIBRILL/O** (fī-bril-ō)	Fiber, fibril (muscle fiber), quivering of the heart	L. *fibra, -ae*, f. fiber, filament L. *fibrilla, -ae*, f. small fiber, fibril	Chapters 7, 8
FIBUL/O (fib-yŭ-lō)	Fibula bone	L. *fibula, -ae*, f. a brooch, pin, lateral bone of the lower leg	Chapter 7
FID/O (fī-dō) **FISS/O** (fī-sō)	Split, cleave	L. *findere, fissum*, to split, cleave	Chapter 10
FIMBRI/O (fim-brē-ō)	Fringe of the Fallopian tube, fringe, border	L. *fimbria, -ae*, f. fringe, border	Chapter 15
FISSUR/O (fi-shoor-ō)	Fissure, deep groove	L. *fissura, -ae*, f. cleft, fissure fr. L. *findere, fissum*, to split, cleave	Chapter 10
FISTUL/O (fish-chŭ-lō)	Fistula, tube, pipe-like	L. *fistula, fistulae*, f. pipe; a fistula (pipe-like ulcer)	Chapter 13
FLAT/O (flă-tō)	Gas in the GI, to blow	L. *flare, flatum*, to blow	Chapter 13
FLAV/O (flă-vō)	Yellow (bright yellow)	L. *flavus, flava, flavum*, yellow	Chapters 6, 14
FLEX/O (fleks-ō) **-FLEX** (fleks)	To bend, flex	L. *flexor, -oris*, m. flexor fr. L. *flexio*, f. a bending	Chapter 7
FOLLICUL/O (fŏ-lik-yŭ-lō)	Little bag, follicle	L. *folliculus, -i*, n. little bag fr. L. *follis*, bag, purse	Chapter 6
FORAMIN/O (fŏ-ram-ĭ-nō)	A hole or passageway in a bone (foramen)	L. *foramen, foraminis*, n. hole	Chapter 7
FOSS/O (fos-ō)	A shallow depression, something dug, ditch	L. *fossa, -ae*, f. a ditch	Chapter 7
FRANG/O (frăn-gō) **FRACT/O** (frak-tō)	Break, broken	L. *frangere, fractum*, to break	Chapter 7
FRONT/O (frŏn-tō)	Forehead, front	L. *frons, frontis*, f. forehead	Chapter 3

Greek or Latin word element	Current usage	Etymology	Chapters
FRUCT/O (frŭk-tō)	Fruit, fructose	L. *fructus, -us,* m. fruit	Chapter 13
FUNG/O (fŭng-gō)	Fungus	L. *fungus, -i,* m. mushroom, fungus	Chapter 6
FUNICUL/O (fū-nik-yŭ-lō) **FUN/O** (fū-nō) **FUNIS/O** (fū-nĭ-sō)	Funicle, rope-like	L. *funiculus, -i,* m. small rope, funiculus fr. L. *funis, -is,* m. rope, cord	Chapter 10
FURC/O (fŭr-kō) **FURCAT/O** (fŭr-kā-tō)	A forking, splitting	L. *furca, -ae,* f. a fork, prong	Chapter 8
FURUNCUL/O (fū-rŭng-kū-lō)	Furuncle, boil	L. *furunculus, -i,* m. boil, petty thief	Chapter 6
FUS/O (fū-sō)	A pouring, melting	L. *fundere, fusum,* to pour	Chapters 8, 9
FUSC/O (fŭs-kō)	Brown	L. *fuscare,* to darken, make dusky	Chapter 14
GALACT/O (gă-lăk-tō)	Milk, galactose, galaxy	Gr. *gala, galaktos,* milk; galactose, galaxy	Chapter 13
GAM/O (gam-ō) **-GAMY** (g-ă-mē)	Sexual union, union, marriage	Gr. *gamos,* marriage	Chapter 15
GANGLI/O (gang-glē-ō)	Ganglion (groups of nerve cells), cyst	L. *ganglion, -i,* n. ganglion fr. Gr. *ganglion,* tumor, cyst	Chapter 10
GASTR/O (gas-trō) **-GASTER** (găs-tĕr)	Stomach, belly	L. *gaster, gastris,* f. stomach fr. Gr. *gaster, gastros,* belly, stomach	Chapters 3, 13
GE/O (jē-ō)	Earth, land	Gr. *ge,* earth	Chapter 5
GEN/O (jē′nō) **-GEN** (jĕn)	To become, be produced	Gr. *–genes,* to be born, become; hormone that produces something fr. Gr. *gignomai,* to come into being	Chapters 4, 12
GEN/O (jē′nō)	Race, kind, hereditary, gene	Gr. *genos,* kind, race, descent; genea, stock, descent	Chapters 4, 12
GEN/O (jĕn-ō)	Knee	L. *genu, -us,* n. knee	Chapter 3
GENI/O (jē-nē-ō)	Chin	Gr. *geneion,* chin	Chapter 3
GER/O (jer-ō) **GERONT/O** (jer-ŏn-tō)	Elderly, old age	Gr. *geron, gerontos,* old person	Chapter 4

Greek or Latin word element	Current usage	Etymology	Chapters
GEST/O (jĕs-tō) GER/O (jĕr-ō) -GER (jĕr)	Hormone that helps with bearing; producing, carrying	L. *gerere*, *gestum*, to carry, produce, bear; progestin	Chapter 12
GEUS/O (gūs-ō) -GEUSIA (gū-zē-ă)	Tasting, sense of taste	Gr. *geusis*, taste	Chapter 11
GIGANT/O (jī-găn-tō)	Giant, large	Gr. *gigas*, *gigantos*, giant	Chapter 12
GINGIV/O (jĭn-jĭ-vō)	Gum	L. *gingiva*, *-ae*, f. the gum	Chapter 13
GLAND/O (glăn-dō) GLANDUL/O (glan-jŭ-lō)	Glandule, gland, *glans clitoris, glans penis*	L. *glandula*, *-ae*, f. little acorn; gland L. *glans*, *glandis*, f. acorn; gland	Chapters 3, 12, 15
GLAUC/O (glaw-kō)	Silver, gray, or bluish green	Gr. *glaukos*, gleaming, gray	Chapter 11
GLI/O (glī-ō)	Glia (supporting tissue of the nervous system), Glue	Gr. *glia*, glue	Chapter 10
GLOB/O (glō-bō) GLOBUL/O (glob-ū-lō)	Ball, sphere	L. *globulum*, *-i*, n. little ball fr. *globus*, ball or sphere	Chapter 8
GLOMERUL/O (glŏ-mer-yŭ-lō)	Glomerulus of the nephron, little ball	L. *glomerulus*, *-i*, m. little ball fr. L. *glomerare*, to form into a sphere	Chapter 14
GLOSS/O (glos-ō) GLOTT/O (glŏ-tō) -GLOT (glŏt)	Tongue, vocal cord	L. *glottis*, *-is*, f. glottis, vocal cord fr. Gr. *glossa; glotta*, tongue	Chapters 9, 13
GLUC/O (gloo-kō) GLYC/O (glī-kō)	Sugar, glucose	Gr. *glykys*, sweet; sugar, glucose	Chapters 12, 13, 14
GLUT/O (gloo-tō)	Buttock	Gr. *gloutos*, buttock	Chapter 3
GNATH/O (năth-ō)	Jaw	Gr. *gnathos*, jaw	Chapter 13

Greek or Latin word element	Current usage	Etymology	Chapters
GNOS/O (nō-sō) GNOST/O (gnos-tō) -GNOSIA (gnō-sē-ă) -GNOSIS (-gnō-sĭs) -GNOMY (gnō-mē)	Knowledge, knowing; -GNOMY = a means of knowing	Gr. *gnosis*, knowledge Gr. *gnomon*, judge, a means of knowing	Chapters 4, 10
GON/O (gon-ō) -GONY (gŏn-ē)	Generation, genitals, semen	Gr. *gone*, seed, semen, generation	Chapter 15
GONAD/O (gŏn-ă-dō)	Testicle or ovary	L. *gonas, gonadis,* f. gonad fr. Gr. *gone*, seed	Chapters 12, 15
GONI/O (gō-nē-ō) GON/O (go-nō) -GON (gon)	Angle	Gr. *gonia*, angle	Chapter 5
GONORRHE/O (gon-ŏ-rē-ō)	Gonorrhea	Gr. *gonorrhea*, discharge of semen	Chapter 15
GONY/O (gŏn-ĭ-ō) GONAT/O (gŏn-ăt-ō)	Knee	Gr. *gony, gonatos,* knee	Chapters 3, 7
GRAD/O (grăd-ō) -GRADE (grăd)	Step, walk, go	L. *gradi, gressum,* to step, walk, go	Chapter 14
-GRAFT (graft)	Tissue transplant	Gr. *graphis*, a stylus for writing, a needle for embroidering	Chapter 6
GRAMMAT/O (gra-mă-tō) GRAMM/O (gra-mō) -GRAM (gram)	Something written or drawn; A record or image of something	Gr. *gramma, grammatos,* something written or drawn	Chapter 4
GRANUL/O (gran-yŭ-lō)	Granule, small grain	L. *granulum, -i,* n. small grain, granule fr. L. *granum*, grain, seed	Chapter 8
GRAPH/O (gra-fō) -GRAPH (graf) -GRAPHY (gră-fē)	Writing; -GRAPH = A device for an image or written record, or the record itself; -GRAPHY = Process of recording, writing	Gr. *graphein*, to write, inscribe	Chapter 4

Greek or Latin word element	Current usage	Etymology	Chapters
GRAVID/O (grăv-ĭd-ō) -GRAVIDA (grav-ĭd-ă)	Pregnancy	L. *gravida, -ae*, f. pregnant woman	Chapter 15
GUST/O (gŭs-tō) GUSTAT/O (gŭs-tă-tō)	Tasting, sense of taste	L. *gustare, gustatum*, to taste	Chapter 11
GLUTIN/O (gloo-tĭn-ō)	Sticky, adhesive, gluten	L. *gluten, glutinis*, n. glue	Chapter 13
GYN/O (jin-ō) or (gīn-ō) GYNEC/O (jin-ĕkō) or (gīn-ĕkō)	Female, feminine, pistil of a flower (gynoecium)	Gr. *gyne, gynaikos*, woman	Chapters 4, 12, 15
GYR/O (jī-rō)	Gyrus (a convolution of the cerebrum), circle, ring	L. *gyrus, -i*, m. gyrus fr. Gr. *gyros*, circle, ring	Chapter 10
HALLIC/O (hal-ĭk-ō) HALLUC/O (hal-ŭk-ō)	Big toe	L. *hallux, hallucis* m. or *hallex, hallicis*, m. big toe	Chapter 3
HAL/O (hāl-ō) HALIT/O (hăl-ĭ-tō)	Breath, breathing	L. *halare, halitum*, to breathe	Chapters 9, 13
HALLUCIN/O (hă-loo-sĭ-nō)	A false sensory perception	L. *alucinari*, to wander in mind, to dream	Chapter 10
HAPT/O (hăp-tō)	Touching, sense of touch, to seize	Gr. *haptein*, to touch, to seize	Chapter 11
HEDON/O (hē-dō-nō)	Pleasure	Gr. *hedone*, pleasure	Chapter 10
HEDR/O (hē-drō)	Side	Gr. *hedra*, side	Chapter 5
HECAT/O (hĕk-ă-tō) HECT/O (hĕk-tō)	One hundred	Gr. *hekaton*, one hundred	Chapter 5
HELC/O (hĕl-kō)	Ulcer	Gr. *helkos*, skin lesion	Chapter 6
HELI/O (hē-lē-ō)	Sun, helium	Gr. *helios*, sun	Chapter 5
HEM/O (hē-mō) HEMAT/O (hēm-ă-tō) -EMIA (ēm-ē-ă) -HEMIA (hēm-ē-ă)	Blood; -EMIA = condition of blood	Gr. *haima, haimatos*, blood	Chapters 4, 8

Greek or Latin word element	Current usage	Etymology	Chapters
HEMI- (hĕm-ē)	Half, partly	Gr. *hemi-*, half, partly	Chapter 2
HEMORRHOID/O (hem-ŏ-royd-ō)	Hemorrhoid, pile	Gr. *haimorrhoïdes*, discharging blood	Chapter 13
HEN/O (hen-ō)	One	Gr. *hen*, one	Chapter 5
HENDEC/A (hen-dek-ă)	Eleven	Gr. *hendeka*, eleven	Chapter 5
HEPAT/O (hĕp-ă-tō) HEPAR/O (hep-ă-rō)	Liver; HEPATIC/O= pertaining to the liver; hepatic vessels	L. *hepar, hepatis*, n. liver fr. Gr. *hepar, hepatos*, liver	Chapters 3, 8, 13
HEPT/A (hĕp-tă)	Seven	Gr. *hepta*, seven	Chapter 5
HERNI/O (hĕr-nē-ō)	Hernia	L. *hernia*, rupture	Chapter 13
HERPET/O (hĕr-mĕt-ō)	Herpes, reptiles	Gr. *herpes, herpetos*, creeping thing (snake, lizards)	Chapter 6
HETER/O (hĕt-ĕr-ō)	Different, other	Gr. *heteros*, other (of two), different	Chapters 5, 6
HEX/A (heks-ă)	Six	Gr. *hex*, six	Chapter 5
HIAT/O (hī-āt-ō)	An opening, gap (hiatus of the diaphragm)	L. *hiatus, -us*, m. an opening or gap	Chapter 13
HIDR/O (hi-drō)	Sweat	Gr. *hidros*, sweat	Chapter 6
HIL/O (hī-lō)	Hilum	L. *hilum, -i*, n. little thing, trifle	Chapters 9, 14
HIPPOCAMP/O (hip-ŏ-kam-pō)	Hippocampus, seahorse	L. *hippocampus, -i*, m. hippocampus, seahorse fr. Gr. hippokampos, hippos "horse" + kampos "a sea monster"	Chapter 10
HIRSUT/O (hĭr-sŭ-tō)	Hairy	L. *hirsutus*, hairy, shaggy	Chapter 12
HISTI/O (hĭs-tē-ō) HIST/O (hĭs-tō)	Tissue	Gr. *histion*, web, sail	Chapter 6
HOD/O (hŏ-dō) OD/O (ŏd-ō) -ODE (ōd)	Road, path, traveling	Gr. *hodos*, road, path	Chapter 5
HOL/O (hŏl-ō)	Whole, entire	Gr. *holos*, whole, entire	Chapter 12
HOM/O (hŏ-mō) HOME/O (hŏ-mē-ō)	Same, like	Gr. *homos*, like, same Gr. *homoios*, like similar	Chapters 5, 6

Greek or Latin word element	Current usage	Etymology	Chapters
HOM/O (ho-mō) **HOMIN/O** (hŏm-ĭn-ō)	Human	L. *homo, hominis,* m. a human being	Chapter 4
HORMON/O (hor-mō-nō)	Hormone	Gr. *hormon, hormonos,* stimulating, arousing; hormone	Chapter 12
HUMER/O (hūmĕ-rō)	Humerus	L. *humerus, -i,* m. bone of the upper arm	Chapter 7
HYAL/O (hī-ă-lō)	Glass, glass-like (vitreous humor of the eye)	Gr. *hyalos,* glass	Chapter 11
HYDR/O (hī-drō)	Water, liquid, hydrogen	Gr. *hydros,* water	Chapter 5
HYDRARGYR/O (hī-dror-jĭ-rō)	Mercury	L. *hydrargyrum, -i,* n. mercury, liquid silver	Chapter 5
HYGIEN/O (hī-jĕn-ō) **HYGIEI/O** (hī-jē-ō)	Health	Gr. *hygieine,* healthful Gr. *hygieia,* health	Chapter 4
HYGR/O (hī-grō)	Moisture, wet, humidity	Gr. *hygros,* wet	Chapter 5
HYMEN/O (hī-mĕn-ō)	Membrane, the female hymen	L. *hymen, hyminis,* m. hymen fr. Gr. *hymen, hymenos* membrane, thin skin, Hymen the Greek god of marriages	Chapter 15
HYPER- (hī-pĕr)	Above, beyond, excessive	Gr. *hyper-,* above, beyond, excessive	Chapter 2
HYPN/O (hip-nō)	Sleep	Gr. *hypnos,* sleep	Chapter 10
HYPO- (hī-pō)	Under, below, deficient	Gr. *hypo-,* under, below, deficient	Chapter 2
HYPOPHYS/O (hī-pō-fĭz-ō)	Hypophysis, pituitary gland	Gr. *hypo + physis,* undergrowth; pituitary gland	Chapter 12
HYSTER/O (his-tĕ-rō)	Uterus	Gr. *hystera,* womb	Chapter 15
-IA (ē-ă)	State or condition of	Gr. *-ia,* state or condition of	Chapter 2
-IAC (ē-ăk)	One who is afflicted with (forms a noun or adjective) like, resembling, in the form of	Gr. *-iac,* one who is afflicted with, like, resembling, in the form of	Chapter 2
-IAN (ē-ăn)	Thing or person performing an action; practitioner of	L. *-ianus,* thing or person performing an action; practitioner of	Chapter 2
-IASIS (ĭ-ă-sĭs)	State or condition of	Gr. *-iasis,* state or condition of	Chapter 2
IATR/O (ĭ-a-trō) **-IATRY** (ĭ-ă-trē)	Medicine, physician; medical treatment	Gr. *iatros,* physician, healer; *iatreia,* medicine, healing	Chapter 4
-IC (ĭk)	Pertaining to	Gr. *-ic,* pertaining to	Chapter 2

Greek or Latin word element	Current usage	Etymology	Chapters
ICHTHY/O (ĭk-thē-ō)	Fish, fish-like (e.g. scaly)	Gr. *ichthys*, fish	Chapter 6
ICT/O (ik-tō) **-ICTAL** (ik-tăl)	Seizure, stroke (CVA), a blow/strike	L. *ictus*, *-us*, m. a strike, blow	Chapter 10
ICTER/O (ĭk-tĕr-ō)	Jaundice	Gr. *ikteros*, yellow; jaundice	Chapter 13
-ID (ĭd)	One who is afflicted with, like, resembling, in the form of	Gr. *-id*, one who is afflicted, like, resembling, in the form of	Chapter 2
-ID (ĭd)	In a state or condition of	L. *-idus*, in a state or condition of	Chapter 2
-IDA (ĭ-dă)	Zoologic "order" and "class"	Gr. *-ida*, zoologic "order" and "class"	Chapter 2
-IDAE (ĭ-dē)	Zoologic "family"	Gr. *-idae*, zoologic "family"	Chapter 2
-IDES (ĭ-dēz)	Zoologic "genus"	Gr. *-ides*, zoologic "genus"	Chapter 2
IDI/O (ĭd-ē-ō)	Individual, distinct	Gr. *idios*, private, personal, peculiar	Chapter 4
-IENT (ē-ĕnt)	Translated –ing added to the verb	L. *-iens*, translated –ing added to the verb	Chapter 2
-IL (ĭl)	Diminutive (little)	L. *-illus*, diminutive (little)	Chapter 2
-ILE (ĭl)	Pertaining to	L. *-ilis*, pertaining to	Chapter 2
ILE/O (il-ē-ō)	Ileum (third portion of the small intestine)	L. *ileum*, *-i*, n. ileum	Chapter 13
ILI/O (il-ē-ō)	Ilium (bone of the pelvis)	L. *ilium*, *-i*, n. groin, flank, upper bone of the pelvis	Chapter 7
-IN (ĭn) **-INE** (ēn) or (ĭn)	Substance, typically a chemical or hormone	Gr. *-in*, *-ine*, substance, typicaly a chemical or hormone	Chapters 2, 12
IMMUN/O (ĭm-ū-nō)	Free from, safe	L. *immunis*, exempt from duty, fees, taxation	Chapter 8
IN- (ĭn) **IM-** (ĭm) before b, m, p **IL-** (ĭl) before l **IR-** (ĭr) before r	Into, in, against, not	L. *in-*, into, in, against, not	Chapter 2
INCISUR/O (ĭn-sī-zhoor-ō)	Notch, indentation, incision	L. *incisura*, *-ae*, f. notch fr. L. *incidere*, *incisus*, to cut into	Chapter 7
INCUD/O (ing-kyŭ-dō)	Incus (one of the ossicles of the ear), anvil	L. *incus*, *incudis*, f. anvil	Chapter 11

Greek or Latin word element	Current usage	Etymology	Chapters
INFER/O (in-fĕr-ō)	Below, inferior	L. *inferior, -ius*, more below, inferior	Chapter 3
INFRA- (in-fră)	Below, lower	L. *infra-*, below, lower	Chapter 2
INGUIN/O (ing-gwĭ-nō)	Groin	L. *inguen, inguinis*, n. groin	Chapter 3
INTESTIN/O (in-tes-tĭn-ō)	Intestine	L. *intestinum, -i*, n. internal, intestine	Chapters 3, 13
INTRA- (ĭn-tră)	Within, during	L. *intra-*, within, during	Chapter 2
INTRO- (ĭn-trō)	Within, inward	L. *intro-*, within, inward	Chapter 2
INTUS- (ĭn-tŭs)	Within	L. *intus-*, within	Chapter 2
-ION (shŏn)	Action; condition resulting from an action	L. *-io*, action; condition resulting from an action	Chapter 2
IR/O (ī-rō) **IRID/O** (ir-ĭ-dō)	Iris of the eye, rainbow, rainbow-like	L. *iris, iridis*, f. iris fr. Gr. *iris, iridos*, rainbow	Chapter 11
IS/O (ī-sō)	Equal	Gr. *isos*, equal	Chapters 5, 6
ISCH/O (is-kō)	Hold back	Gr. *ischein*, to hold back	Chapter 8
ISCHI/O (is-kē-ō)	Hip, ischium bone	L. *ischium, -i*, n. lower, posterior bone of the pelvis fr. Gr. *ischion*, hip joint	Chapters 3, 7
-ISM (ĭzm)	State or condition of	Gr. *-ism*, state or condition of	Chapter 2
-IST (-ĭst)	Person interested in; a practitioner who specializes in	Gr. *-ist*, person interested in; a practitioner who specializes in	Chapter 2
-ITE (īt)	Belonging to, the nature of	Gr. *-ite*, belonging to, the nature of	Chapter 2
ITHY- (ĭth-ē)	Straight	Gr. *ithys*, straight	Chapter 15
-ITY (ĭ-tē)	State or condition of	L. *-itas*, state or condition of	Chapter 2
-IUM (ē-ŭm)	Tissue or part of the body	Gr. *-ium*, tissue or part of the body	Chapter 2
-IZE (īz)	To do; to become; to use; to engage in	Gr. *-ize*, to do; to become; to use; to engage in	Chapter 2
JEJUN/O (jĕ-joon-ō)	Jejunum (second portion of the small intestine)	L. *jejunum, -i*, n. jejunum fr. Latin adjective for "empty"	Chapter 13
JUG/O (jū-gō) **JUNCTUR/O** (jŭngk-too-rō)	Joint, a joining	L. *jungere (jugere), junctum*, to join L. *junctura, -ae*, f. a joining, joint	Chapters 7, 12
JUGUL/O (jŭg-yŭ-lō)	Jugular vein, throat	L. *jugulum, -i*, n. throat	Chapter 8

Greek or Latin word element	Current usage	Etymology	Chapters
JUXTA- (jŭks-tă)	Beside, near to	L. *juxta-*, beside, near to	Chapter 2
KAK/O (ka-kō) **CAC/O** (ka-kō)	Bad, faulty	Gr. *kakos*, bad	Chapter 4
KALI/O (kal-ē-ō) **KAL/O** (ka-lō)	Potassium	L. *kalium, -i*, n. potash	Chapters 5, 14
KARY/O (kar-ē-ō)	Center of cell (nucleus), nut, kernel	Gr. *karyon*, nut, kernel	Chapter 8
KATA- (kăt-ă) **CATA-** (kăt-ă) **CAT-** (kăt)	Down, downward, against, complete (intensive)	Gr. *kata-*, down, downward, against, complete (intensive)	Chapter 2
KERAT/O (kĕr-ăt-ō) **CERAT/O** (sĕr-ăt-ō)	Horn, hard, horn-like, keratin, cornea	Gr. *keras, keratos*, horn	Chapters 6, 11
KET/O (kē-tō)	Ketone	Ketone; Ger. *Keton*, fr. Ger. *Aceton*, fr. L. *acetum*, vinegar	Chapter 14
KIN/O (kĭ-nō) **CIN/O** (sĭ-nō) **KINESI/O** (kĭ-nē-sē-ō) **KINE/O** (kin-ĕ-ō) **KINESIS** (kĭ-nē-sĭs) **-CINESIS** (sĭ-nē-sĭs) **-KINESIA** (kĭ-nē-zhē-ă)	Movement, action	Gr. *kineein*, to move	Chapters 10, 12
KNEM/O (nē-mō) **CNEM/O** (nē-mō)	Lower leg	Gr. *kneme*, lower leg, shin	Chapter 3
KYPH/O (kĭ-fō)	Bent forward (convex posteriorly)	Gr. *kyphos*, bent forward	Chapter 7

Greek or Latin word element	Current usage	Etymology	Chapters
LABI/O (lă-bē-ō)	Lip, labia of the vulva (i.e. Labia majora, Labia minora)	L. *labium*, *-i*, n. lip	Chapters 13, 15
LABYRINTH/O (lab-ĭ-rin-thō)	Labyrinth of the ear, maze	L. *labyrinthus*, *-i*, m. labyrinth fr. Gr. *labyrinthos*, a maze	Chapter 11
LACRIM/O (lak-rĭ-mō)	Tear	L. *lacrima*, *-ae*, f. tear	Chapter 11
LACT/O (lak-tō)	Milk, lactose	L. *lac*, *lactis*, n. milk	Chapters 12, 13, 15
-LAGNIA (lăg-nē-ă)	Lust, sexual arousal	Gr. *lagneia*, lust	Chapter 10
LAL/O (lăl-ō) **-LALIA** (lă-lē-ă)	Speech	Gr. *lalein*, to talk, speak	Chapter 10
LAMIN/O (lă-mĭn-ō)	Plate (lamina)	L. *lamina*, *-ae*, f. plate	Chapter 7
LAPAR/O (lap-ă-rō)	Abdomen	Gr. *lapara*, loin, flank, abdomen	Chapters 3, 13
-LAPAXY (lă-paks-ē)	Surgical evacuation (of a stone)	Gr. *lapaxis*, evacuation	Chapter 14
LARYNG/O (lăr-ĭn-gō) **LARYNX** (lar-ingks)	Voice box, larynx	L. *larynx*, *laryngis*, m. larynx, organ of voices of the upper trachea fr. Gr. *larynx*	Chapter 9
LAT/O (lă-tō)	To bear, convey	L. *ferre*, *latum*, to bear, carry	Chapter 8
LATER/O (la-ĕ-rō)	Side	L. *lateralis*, *-e*, pertaining to the side, lateral fr. L. *latus*, *lateris*, side	Chapter 3
LAV/O (lă-vō) **LUT/O** (loo-tō) **LOT/O** (lō-tō)	Washing	L. *lavare*, *lotum*, to wash	Chapter 13
LAX/O (lăk-sō) **LAXAT/O** (lăk-să-tō)	Loosen, relax	L. *laxare*, to loosen	Chapter 13
LEI/O (lī-ō)	Smooth	Gr. *leios*, smooth	Chapter 7
LEMM/O (lĕm-ō) **-LEMMA** (lem-ă)	Membrane, husk, sheath-like structure	Gr. *lemma*, a peel, husk; a membrane	Chapter 7
-LENT (lĕnt)	Full of	L. *-lentus*, full of	Chapter 2

Greek or Latin word element	Current usage	Etymology	Chapters
LENT/O (lĕn-tō) **LENTICUL/O** (lĕn-tĭk-ū-lō)	Lens, lentil, lentil-shaped	L. *lens, lentis*, f. lentil; L. *lenticula, -ae*, f. lentil-shaped	Chapter 11
LEPID/O (lĕ-pĭd-ō)	Scaly	Gr. *lepis, lepidos*, scale, scaly	Chapter 6
LEPR/O (lĕp-rō)	Leprosy, scaly	Gr. *lepra*, scaly, scaly disease	Chapter 6
LEPS/O (lep-sō) **LEPT/O** (lĕp-tō) **-LEPSY** (lep-sē)	Seizure	Gr. *lepsis*, a taking, seizing	Chapter 10
LEPT/O (lĕp-tō)	Thin	Gr. *leptos*, thin, delicate	Chapter 10
LETH/O (lē-thō)	Forgetfulness	Gr. *lethe*, oblivion, forgetfulness	Chapter 10
LETHARG/O (lĕth-ăr-gō)	Mental sluggishness, drowsiness	Gr. *lethargos*, drowsiness	Chapter 10
LEUC/O (loo-kō) **LEUK/O** (loo-kō)	White	Gr. *leukos*, white	Chapters 6, 8
LEV/O (lē-vō)	Left	L. *laevus, -a, -um*, left	Chapters 3, 7
LEVAT/O (le-vă-tō)	To lift, raise	L. *levator, -oris*, m. levator L. *levatio*, f. a lifting up fr. *levare, levatum* to lift, raise	Chapter 7
LEX/O (lek-sō)	Word, speech, reading	Gr. *lexis*, speaking, diction	Chapter 10
LIBER/O (lĭ-buh-rō)	To free	L. *liberare*, to free	Chapter 12
LIEN/O (lĭ-ĕ-nō)	Spleen	L. *lien, lienis*, m. spleen	Chapter 8
LIGAT/O (lĭ-gă-tō) **LIGAMENT/O** (lig-ă-men-tō)	To bind, tie; ligament	L. *ligare, ligatum*, to bind, tie L. *ligamentum, -i*, n. ligament	Chapter 7
LIMB/O (lim-bō)	Limbic system, border	L. *limbus, -i*, m. border	Chapter 10
LINGU/O (lĭng-gwō)	Tongue	L. *lingua, -ae*, f. tongue	Chapter 13
LIP/O (lĭp-ō)	Fat	Gr. *lipos*, fat	Chapters 6,13
LITH/O (lĭth-ō) **-LITH** (lĭth)	Stone, lithium	Gr. *lithos*, stone	Chapters 5, 14

Greek or Latin word element	Current usage	Etymology	Chapters
LOB/O (lō-bō)	Lobe, pod	L. *lobus, -i,* m. lobe fr. Gr. *lobos,* a pod, lobe	Chapters 9, 10
LOCHI/O (lō-kē-ō)	Childbirth, lochia (vaginal discharge after child birth)	Gr. *lochia,* childbirth	Chapter 15
LOG/O (lŏg-ō) **-LOGY** (lŏ-jē)	Word, speech; -LOGY the study of	Gr. *logos,* word, speech, reason, thought of	Chapters 4, 10
-LOQUY (lō-kwē)	Voice, speach	L. *loqui,* to speak	Chapter 9
LORD/O (lor-dō)	Bent backward (convex anteriorly)	Gr. *lordos,* bent backward	Chapter 7
LUMB/O (lŭm-bō)	Loin, lumbar	L. *lumbus, -i,* loin, lumbar	Chapter 7
LUMIN/O (loo-mĭ-nō)	Light, lumen (the open space between walls of a vessel)	L. *lumen, luminis,* n. light	Chapters 8, 11
LUN/O (loo-nō)	Moon	L. *luna, -ae,* f. moon	Chapter 8
LUP/O (loo-pō)	Wolf, lupus	L. *lupus, -i,* m. wolf	Chapter 6
LUTE/O (loo-tē-ō)	Yellow (pale or orangish)	L. *luteus, -a, -um,* yellow	Chapter 14
LUX/O (lŭks-ō)	Dislocated	L. *luxare,* to dislocate	Chapter 7
LYMPH/O (lim-fō) **LYMPHAT/O** (lim-fa-tō)	Lymph, water	L. *lympha, -ae,* f. clear water; lymph	Chapter 8
LYS/O (lī-sō) **-LYSIS** (lī-sĭs)	Breakdown, dissolving	Gr. *lysis,* a loosening, setting free	Chapter 4
MACR/O (mak-rō)	Large, long	Gr. *makros,* long, large	Chapters 4, 8
MACUL/O (mak-yŭ-lō)	Spot, macule (macula lutea retina of the eye)	L. *macula, -ae,* f. spot, stain	Chapters 6, 11
MAL/O (măl-ō) **MALIGN/O** (mă-lig-nō)	Bad, faulty; MALIGN- = Cancerous, becoming worse	L. *malus, -a, -um,* bad L. *malignus, -a, -um,* ill-disposed, wicked	Chapter 4
MALAC/O (mal-ă-kō) **-MALACIA** (mă-lā-shē-ă)	Soft, abnormal softening	Gr. *malakos,* soft	Chapters 4, 7
MALLE/O (mal-ē-ō)	Malleus (one of the ossicles of the ear), hammer	L. *malleus, -i,* m. hammer	Chapter 11
MAMM/O (măm-ō)	Breast	L. *mamma, -ae,* f. breast	Chapter 15

Greek or Latin word element	Current usage	Etymology	Chapters
MAMMILL/O (măm-mĭl-ō)	Nipple, nipple-like structure	L. *mamilla, -ae*, f. breast, nipple	Chapter 15
MAN/O (mă-nō)	Hand	L. *manus, -us*, f. hand	Chapter 3
MANDIBUL/O (man-dib-yŭ-lō)	Mandible	L. *mandibula, -ae*, f. lower jaw	Chapters 7, 13
MANI/O (mă-nē-ō) -MANIA (mă-nē-ă)	Frenzy, madness, -MANIA = excessive fascination with something	Gr. *mania*, madness, frenzy	Chapter 10
MASCHAL/O (măs-kăl-ō)	Armpit	Gr. *maschale*, armpit	Chapter 3
MAST/O (măst-ō)	Breast	Gr. *mastos*, breast	Chapter 15
MASTOID/O (mas-toyd-ō)	Mastoid (process of the temporal bone)	Gr. *mastoeides*, like a breast	Chapter 11
MAXILL/O (mak-sil-ō)	Maxilla	L. *maxilla, -ae*, f. upper bone of jaw, maxilla	Chapters 7, 13
MAZ/O (mă-zō)	Breast	Gr. *mazos*, breast	Chapter 15
MEAT/O (mē-ă-tō)	Opening, passageway	L. *meatus, -us*, m. a path or course	Chapters 11, 14
MEDI/O (mĕd-ē-ō)	Middle	L. *medius, -a, -um*, middle	Chapter 3
MEDIASTIN/O (mē-dē-ăs-tī-nō) -MEDIASTINUM (mē-dē-ăs-tī-nŭm)	Mediastinum	L. *mediastinum, -i*, n. mediastinum fr. L. *mediastinus*, a middling, a lowly servant	Chapter 9
MEDIC/O (mĕd-ĭ-kō)	Medicine, medical treatment	L. *medicus, -i*, physician; medicine, healer	Chapter 4
MEDULL/O (mĕd-ū-lō)	Bone marrow, medulla oblongato, innermost part of an organ	L. *medulla, -ae*, f. marrow	Chapters 7, 10, 12
MEGA- (mĕg-ă) MEGAL/O (meg-ă-lō) -MEGALY (meg-ă-lē)	Enlargement, large	Gr. *megas, megalous*, large	Chapters 4, 8, 12
MEL/O (mĕl-ō)	Cheek, fruit	Gr. *melon*, cheek, fruit	Chapter 13
MEL/O (mĕl-ō)	Limb	Gr. *melos*, limb	Chapters 3, 12
MELAN/O (mĕl-ăn-ō)	Black	Gr. *melas, melanos*, black	Chapters 6, 14
MELIT/O (mel-ĭ-tō) MELL/O (mel-ō) MEL/O (mel-ō)	Honey, sugar, bees	Gr. *meli, melitos*, honey; sugar	Chapters 12, 13, 14

Greek or Latin word element	Current usage	Etymology	Chapters
MEMBR/O **(mem-brō)**	Limb	L. *membrum, -i,* n. limb	Chapter 3
MEN/O **(měn-ō)**	Menstruation	Gr. *men,* month L. *mensis, -is,* month; menstruation	Chapter 15
MENING/O **(měn-ĭn-gō)** **-MENINX** **(mē-ningks)**	Meninx (one of the three membranes enveloping the brain and spinal cord), membrane	L. *meninx, meningis,* f. meninx fr. Gr. *meninx, meningos,* membrane	Chapter 10
MENISC/O **(měn-ĭs-kō)**	Meniscus, crescent	L. *meniscus, -i,* m. meniscus fr. Gr. *meniskos,* crescent	Chapter 7
MENSTRU/O **(měn-stroo-ō)**	Menstruation	L. *menstruare,* to discharge menses	Chapter 15
-MENT **(měnt)**	Action; condition resulting from an action	L. *-mentum,* action; condition resulting from an action	Chapter 2
MENT/O **(men-tō)**	Chin	L. *mentum, -i,* n. chin	Chapter 3
MENT/O **(men-tō)**	Mind	L. *mens, mentis,* f. mind	Chapter 10
MER/O **(měr-ō)** **-MER** **(měr)** **-MERE** **(měr)**	Part, partial	Gr. *meros, mereos,* part	Chapters 3, 5, 12
MER/O **(měr-ō)**	Thigh	Gr. *meros,* thigh	Chapter 3
MESENTER/O **(měs-ěn-těr-ō)**	Mesentery	L. *mesenterium, -i,* n. the mesentery	Chapter 13
META- **(met-ă)** **MET-** **(met)**	After, beyond, change	Gr. *meta-,* after, beyond, change	Chapter 2
METACARP/O **(met-ă-kar-pō)**	Metacarpal bone(s)	L. *metacarpus, -i,* m. metacarpus, bone of the palm fr. Gr. *meta-,* beyond + *karpos,* wrist	Chapters 3, 7
METATARS/O **(met-ă-tar-sō)**	Metatarsus bone	L. *metatarsus, -i,* m. metatarsus fr. Gr. *meta-,* beyond + Gr. *tarsos,* flat of foot, ankle bones	Chapters 3, 7
METOP/O **(me-top-ō)**	Forehead	Gr. *metopon,* forehead	Chapter 3
METR/O **(mē-trō)**	Uterus	Gr. *metra,* womb	Chapter 15
METR/O **(mě-trō)** **-METER** **(mět-ěr)** **-METRY** **(mě-trē)**	Measure, measurement; -METER = measuring instrument; -METRY = the process of measuring something	Gr. *metron,* a measure	Chapters 4, 11

Greek or Latin word element	Current usage	Etymology	Chapters
MI/O (mī-ō)	Less, smaller	L. *meion*, less, smaller	Chapter 11
MEI/O (mī-ō)			
MICR/O (mī-krō)	Small	Gr. *mikros*, small	Chapters 4, 8
MICT/O (mĭk-tō)	To urinate	L. *micturire* (*mictum*), to urinate	Chapter 14
MICTUR/O (mĭk-tū-rō)			
MILL/I (mĭl-ĭ)	One thousand	L. *mille*, one thousand	Chapter 5
MITR/O (mī'trō)	Mitral valve	L. *mitralis, -e*, mitral fr. Gr. *mitre*, a two-pointed hat	Chapter 8
MITT/O (mĭt-tō)	To send, let go	L. *mittere*, *missum*, to send, let go	Chapter 11
MISS/O (mĭs-sō)			
MNEMON/O (nē-mŏn-ō)	Memory	Gr. *mneme*, memory	Chapter 10
-MNESIA (mnē-zhă)			
MOL/O (mŏl-ō)	Mass, mole; molecule	L. *moles, -is*, f. a mass L. *molecula, -ae*, f. little mass	Chapter 5
MOLECUL/O (mŏ-lek-yŭ-lō)			
MON/O (mŏn-ō)	One, alone	Gr. *monos*, alone, single	Chapter 5
MORB/O (mor-bō)	Disease	L. *morbus, -i*, m. disease	Chapter 4
MORPH/O (mŏr-fō)	Shape, form	Gr. *morphe*, shape, form, figure	Chapter 8
MORT/O (mor-tō)	Death	L. *mors, mortis*, f. death	Chapter 4
MOT/O (mōt-ō)	Movement	L. *movere*, *motum*, to move	Chapter 10
MUC/O (mū-kō)	Mucus	L. *mucus, -i*, m. mucus	Chapter 9
MULT/I (mŭl-tē)	Many	L. *multus, a, um*, many	Chapter 4
MUSCUL/O (mŭs-kyŭ-lō)	Muscle; mouse	L. *musculus, -i*, m. muscle, mouse	Chapters 3, 7
MY/O (mī-ō)	To close, shut	Gr. *myein*, to close, shut	Chapter 11
MY/O (mī-ō)	Muscle, mouse	Gr. *mys, myos*, muscle, mouse	Chapters 3, 7
MYOS/O (mī-ō-sō)			
MYS/O (mī-sō)			

Greek or Latin word element	Current usage	Etymology	Chapters
MYC/O (mĭ-kō) **MYCET/O** (mĭ-sĕ-tō)	Fungus, mold	Gr. *mykes, myketos,* mushroom	Chapter 6
MYDRIASIS (mĭ-drī-ă-sĭs)	Enlargement of the pupil	Gr. *mydriasis,* enlargement of the pupil	Chapter 11
MYEL/O (mĭ-ĕ-lō)	Spinal cord, marrow	Gr. *myelos,* marrow, bone marrow	Chapters 7, 10
MYRI/O (mĭr-ē-ō)	Ten thousand, innumerable	Gr. *myrioi,* ten thousand, innumerable	Chapter 5
MYRING/O (mĭ-ring-gō)	Eardrum, membrane	Gr. *myrinx, myringos,* a membrane	Chapter 11
MYX/O (mĭks-ō)	Mucus	Gr. *myxa,* slime; mucus	Chapter 12
NAN/O (nă-nō) **NANN/O** (nă-nō)	Dwarf, very small, one billionth	Gr. *nanos,* dwarf; one billionth	Chapter 12
NAR/I (nar-ē)	Nostril	L. *naris, -is,* f. nostril	Chapter 9
NARC/O (nar-kō)	Stupor, sleep	Gr. *narke,* numbness, deadness	Chapter 10
NARCISS/O (nar-sĭ-sō)	Self-love	Gr. *Narkissos,* a Greek mythological character who fell in love with his reflection	Chapter 10
NAS/O (nā-zō)	Nose	L. *nasus, -i,* m. nose	Chapters 3, 9
NASC/O (năs-kō) **NAT/O** (nā-tō)	To be born	L. *nasci, natum,* to be born	Chapter 15
NAT/O (nā-tō)	Buttocks, nates	L. *nates, -ium,* f. buttocks	Chapter 3
NATRI/O (nā-trē-ō) **NATR/O** (nā-trō)	Sodium	L. *natrium, -i,* n. salt fr. Gr. *nitron,* salt	Chapters 5, 14
NAUSE/O (naw-sē-ō) **NAUT/O** (naw-tō)	Nausea, NAUT/O = ship, sailor	Gr. *nausea,* sea sickness Gr. *nautes,* sea sailor	Chapter 13
NEBUL/O (neb-yŭ-lō)	Cloud, cloud-like, mist	L. *nebula, -ae,* f. cloud, mist	Chapter 9
NECR/O (nĕk-rō)	Dead body/tissue, dead	Gr. *nekros,* dead body; dead	Chapters 4, 6
NEON/O (nē-on-ō) **NE/O** (nē-ō)	Neon; NE/O = new, recent	Gr. *neos,* new, recent, young	Chapter 5

Greek or Latin word element	Current usage	Etymology	Chapters
NEPHR/O (nef-rŏ)	Kidney	Gr. *nephros*, kidney	Chapters 3, 14
NERV/O (něr-vŏ)	Nerve	L. *nervus, -i*, m. sinew; nerve	Chapters 3, 10
NEUR/O (nū-rŏ)	Nerve, sinew	Gr. *neuron*, nerve, sinew, tendon	Chapters 3, 10
NEUTR/O (nū-trŏ)	Neither, neutral	L. *neuter, neutra, neutrum*, neither	Chapters 5, 8
NEV/O (ně-vŏ)	Mole	L. *nevus, -i*, m. birthmark, mole	Chapter 6
NIGR/O (ni-grŏ)	Black, dark	L. *niger, nigra, nigrum*, black	Chapter 6
NITRIT/O (nĭ-trĭt/ŏ)	Nitrite (a salt of nitrous acid)	Gr. *nitron*, salt	Chapter 14
NITR/O (nĭ-trŏ)	Nitrogenous	Gr. *nitron*, salt	Chapter 5
NO/O (nŏ-ŏ)	Mind, thought	Gr. *noos*, mind; Gr. *noesis*, thought	Chapter 10
NOC/O (nŏ-kŏ) **NOXI/O** (nŏk-shŏ)	Pain	L. *nocere*, to harm, hurt L. *noxius, -a, -um*, hurtful	Chapter 4
NOCT/O (nok-tŏ)	Night	L. *nox, noctis*, f. night	Chapter 11
NOD/O (nŏ-dŏ) **NODUL/O** (nŏd-ū-lŏ)	Knot-like, node, nodule	L. *nodus, -i*, m. a knot L. *nodulus, -i*, m. a little knot	Chapters 6, 8
NOM- (nŏ-mŏ) **-NOMY** (nŏ-mē)	Law, custom; -NOMY = Knowledge of/laws of	Gr. *nomos*, law, custom	Chapter 4
NON- (non)	Not, without	L. *non-*, not, without	Chapter 2
NON/A (nŏn-ă)	Ninth, nine	L. *nonus*, ninth	Chapter 5
NOS/O (nŏ-sŏ) **-NOSIS** (nŏ-sĭs)	Disease	Gr. *nosos*, disease	Chapter 4
NOT/O (nŏt-ŏ)	The back, the spine	Gr. *noton*, the back, a ridge	Chapter 10
NOV/I (nŏ-vĭ)	Nine	L. *novem*, nine	Chapter 5
NUCLE/O (nū-klē-ŏ)	Core, little nut, or kernel nucleus of a cell, group of neuronal cell bodies	L. *nucleus, -i*, m. little nut, kernel, core; nucleus	Chapters 8, 10
NYCT/O (nik-tŏ)	Night	Gr. *nyx, nyktos*, night	Chapter 11

Greek or Latin word element	Current usage	Etymology	Chapters
NYMPH/O (nim-fŏ)	Labia minora; young female, developmental stage of insects	L. *nympha, -ae*, f. nymph; labia minora fr. Gr. *nymphe*, young bride, lower female deity	Chapter 15
NYSTAGM/O (nis-tag-mŏ)	Nystagmus (*disorder involving involuntary movement of the eye)	L. *nystagmus, -i*, m. nystagmus fr. Gr. *nystagmus*, nodding, drowsiness	Chapter 11
O/O (ŏ-ŏ)	Egg, ovum	Gr. *oon*, egg	Chapter 15
OB- (ŏb) OC- (ŏk) before c OP- (ŏp) before p	Against, in the way, facing	L. *ob-*, against, in the way, facing	Chapter 2
OBSTETR/O (ŏb-ste-trŏ)	Branch of medicine associated with childbirth	L. *obstetrix, obstericis*, f. midwife	Chapter 15
OCCIPIT/O (ŏk-sĭp-ĭ-tŏ)	Back of cranium, occiput	L. *occiput, occipitis*, n. back of head	Chapter 3
OCT/O (ŏk-tŏ)	Eight	L. *octo*, eight	Chapter 5
OCTAV/A (ŏk-tă-vă)	Eighth, eight	L. *octavus*, eighth	Chapter 5
OCUL/O (ŏk-ū-lŏ)	Eye	L. *oculus, -i*, m. eye	Chapters 3, 11
-ODE (ŏd)	One who is afflicted with, like, resembling, in the form of	Gr. *-ode*, one who is afflicted with, like, resembling, in the form of	Chapter 2
ODONT/O (ŏ-don-tŏ)	Tooth	Gr. *odous, ondontos*, tooth	Chapter 13
ODYN/O (ŏ-dĭn-ŏ) -ODYNIA (ŏ-dĭn-ē-ă)	Pain; -ODYNIA = Painful condition	Gr. *odyne*, pain	Chapter 4
-OID (oyd)	One who is afflicted with, like, resembling, in the form of	Gr. *-oid*, one who is afflicted with, like, resembling, in the form of	Chapter 2
OCT/A (ŏk-tă)	Eight	Gr. *okto*, eight	Chapter 5
-OLE (ōl)	Diminutive (little)	L. *-olus*, diminutive (little)	Chapter 2
OLECRAN/O (ŏ-lek-ră-nŏ)	Elbow	Gr. *olekranon*, elbow	Chapter 3
OLFACT/O (ol-fak-tŏ)	Smelling, sense of smell	L. *olfactare*, to smell	Chapter 11
-OLISTHESIS (ŏ-lis-thē-sĭs)	Slipping	Gr. *olisthesis*, a slipping	Chapter 7
OM/O (ŏ-mŏ)	Shoulder	Gr. *omos*, shoulder	Chapter 7
-OMA (ŏ-mă)	Tumor	Gr. *-oma*, tumor	Chapter 2

Greek or Latin word element	Current usage	Etymology	Chapters
OMENT/O (ō-měn'tō)	Omentum	L. *omentum, -i*, n. fat skin, caul; omentum	Chapter 13
OMPHAL/O (om-fă-lō)	Navel, umbilicus, center	Gr. *omphalos*, the navel, center	Chapter 13
ONC/O (ong-kō) -ONCUS (ong-kus)	Swelling, tumor, abnormal mass	Gr. *onkos*, mass, tumor	Chapters 4, 6
ONEIR/O (ō-nī-rō)	Dream	Gr. *oneiros*, dream	Chapter 10
ONYCH/O (ŏn-ĭ-kō)	Fingernail, toenail, claws, talon, hoof	Gr. *onyx, onychos*, fingernail, claw, hoof	Chapter 6
O/O (ō-ō)	Egg, ovum	Gr. *oon*, egg; ovum	Chapter 15
OOPHOR/O (ō-ŏf-ō-rō)	Ovary	Gr. *oophoron*, egg carrier; ovary	Chapter 15
OP/O (ŏp/ō) -OPIA (ō-pē-ă) OPS/O (ŏp-sō) -OPSIA (op-sē-ă) -OPSIS (op-sĭs)	Seeing, sense of sight	Gr. *ops, opos*, eye, face; Gr. *opsis*, a sight, vision	Chapter 11
OPHTHALM/O (of-thal-mō) -OPHTHALMUS (ŏf-thăl-mŭs)	Eye	Gr. *ophthalmos*, eye	Chapters 3, 11
OPISTHO- (ŏ-pis-thō)	Behind, backward	Gr. *opisthen*, behind, at the back, backward	Chapters 2, 10
OPPON/O (ŏ-pō-nō) OPPOS/O (ŏ-pō-sō)	To place opposite (oppose)	L. *opponens, -entis*, opponens fr. L. *opponere*, to place opposite, oppose	Chapter 7
OPT/O (ŏp-tō) OPTIC/O (ŏptĭ-kō)	Seeing, sense of sight	Gr. *optos*, seen, visible; Gr. *optikos*, pertaining to vision	Chapter 11
-OR (or)	Something (usually a muscle) that performs an action; quality of condition	L. *-or*, something (usually a muscle) that performs an action; quality of condition	Chapter 2
OR/O (ō-rō)	Mouth	L. *os, oris*, n. mouth	Chapters 3, 13
ORCH/O (or-kō) ORCHID/O (or-kĭ-dō)	Testicle; orchid (the flower)	Gr. *orchis, orchidos*, testicle	Chapters 12, 15

Greek or Latin word element	Current usage	Etymology	Chapters
OREX/O (ŏ-rek-tō) **-OREXIA** (ŏ-rek-sē-ă)	Appetite	Gr. *orexis*, desire for; appetite	Chapters 10, 12, 13
ORGAN/O (or-gă-nō)	Organ	L. *organum*, *-i*, n. organ fr. Gr. *organon*, tool, instrument	Chapter 3
ORTH/O (or-thō)	Upright, straight, correct, normal	Gr. *orthos*, straight	Chapters 7, 9
-ORY (ōr-ē)	Pertaining to; (also forms a noun) place of	L. *-ory*, pertaining to; (also forms a noun) place of	Chapter 2
-OSE (ōs)	Carbohydrate	Suffix used for "carbohydrate"	Chapter 13
-OSE (ōs)	Full of	L. *-osus*, full of	Chapter 2
-OSIS (ō-sĭs)	State or condition of	Gr. *-osis*, state or condition of	Chapter 2
OSM/O (oz-mō)	Impulse, push, osmosis	Gr. *osmos*, impulse, push	Chapter 5
OSM/O (oz-mō) **-OSMIA** (oz-mē-ă)	Smelling, sense of smell, osmium	Gr. *osme*, smell, sense of smell	Chapters 5, 11
OSPHRESI/O (ŏs-frē-zē-ō) **OSPHRESIS** (ŏs-frē-sĭs)	Smelling, sense of smell	Gr. *osphresis*, smell, sense of smell	Chapter 11
OSS/O (ŏs-ō) **OSSE/O** (ŏs-ē-ō)	Bone	L. *os*, *ossis*, n. bone L. *osseus*, *-a*, *-um*, bony	Chapters 3, 7
OSTE/O (os-tē-ō)	Bone	Gr. *osteon*, bone	Chapters 3, 7
OSTI/O (os-tē-ō)	Orifice, opening	L. *ostium*, *-i*, n. door, mouth	Chapter 8
OT/O (ō-tō) **-OTIA** (ō-shē-ă)	Ear	Gr. *ous*, *otos*, ear	Chapters 3, 11
OUL/O (oo-lō)	Gum	Gr. *oulon*, the gum	Chapter 13
OV/O (ō-vō)	Egg, ovum	L. *ovum*, *-i*, n. egg; ovum	Chapter 15
OVARI/O (ō-vă-rē-ō)	Ovary	L. *ovarium*, *-i*, n. egg holder; ovary	Chapters 12, 15
OX/O (oks-ō)	Oxygen	Gr. *oxys*, sharp, swift, sour, acid	Chapters 5, 8, 9
OXY/O (ŏk-sē-ō) **-OXIA** (ok-sē-ă)	Sharp, quick, acid, oxygen; -OXIA = oxygen condition	Gr. *oxys*, sharp, swift, sour, acid	Chapters 4, 5, 9

Greek or Latin word element	Current usage	Etymology	Chapters
PACHY- (pak-ē) PACH/O (pak-ō)	Thick	Gr. *pachys*, thick	Chapter 10
-PAGUS (pă-gŭs)	Conjoined twins	Gr. *pagos*, something fixed or firmly set	Chapter 15
PALAT/O (păl-ă-tŏ)	Palate	L. *palatum, -i*, n. palate, upper part of the mouth	Chapter 13
PALI- (păl-ĭ) PALIN- (păl-ĭn)	Again, once more, backward	Gr. *palin-*, again, once more, backward	Chapter 2
PALLID/O (păl-ĭ-dō)	Pale, globus pallidus	L. *pallidus, -a, -um*, pale	Chapter 6
PALM/O (pal-mō)	Palm of the hand	L. *palma, -ae*, f. palm	Chapter 3
PALPEBR/O (pal-pĕ-brō)	Eyelid	L. *palpebra, -ae*, f. eyelid	Chapter 11
PALPIT/O (păl-pĭ-tō)	Sensation of rapid beating of the heart	L. *palpitare*, to tremble, move quickly	Chapter 8
PALSY (pal-zē)	Paralysis	Gr. *paralysis*, loosening, disabling by the side	Chapter 10
PANCREAT/O (păn-krē-ă-tō)	Pancreas	L. *pancreas, pancreatis*, n. pancreas fr. Gr. *pankreas, pankreatos*, all flesh; pancreas	Chapters 12, 13
PANIC (pan-ik)	Panic	Gr. *panikos*, of or for Pan, the goat-legged Greek god of shepherds	Chapter 10
PAPILL/O (păp-ĭl-ō)	Nipple, nipple-like structure	L. *papilla, -ae*, f. nipple	Chapters 6, 15
PAPILLOMAT/O (păp-ĭ-lō-mă-tō)	Epithelial tumor, human papilloma virus (HPV)	fr. Gr./L. *papilloma*, epithelial tumor	Chapter 15
PAPUL/O (pap-yŭ-lō)	Papule	L. *papula, -ae*, f. pimple, pustule	Chapter 6
PAR/O (păr-ō) PART/O (păr-tō) -PARA (pă-ră)	Give birth, to bring forth	L. *parere, partum*, bring forth, bear	Chapter 15
PARA- (par-ă)	Alongside, beyond, opposite; abnormal	Gr. *para-*, alongside, beyond, opposite; abnormal	Chapter 2
PARATHYROID/O (par-ă-thī-royd-ō)	Parathyroid gland	Parathyroid gland	Chapter 12
-PARESIS (pă-rē-sĭs)	Partial paralysis	Gr. *paresis*, a letting go	Chapter 10
-PAREUNIA (păr-ĕ-ū-nē-ă)	Sexual intercourse	Gr. *pareunos*, lying alongside	Chapter 15
PARIET/O (pă-rī-ĕt-ō)	Wall	L. *paries, parietis*, m. wall	Chapter 8

Greek or Latin word element	Current usage	Etymology	Chapters
PART/O (par-tō)	Part	L. *pars, partis*, f. part	Chapter 3
PARTUR- (păr-tū-rō)	Labor, to give birth	L. *parturire*, to have labor pains	Chapter 15
PATELL/O (pă-tĕl-ō)	Patella bone, kneecap	L. *patella, -ae*, f. dish, platter, kneecap bone	Chapter 7
PATH/O (path-ō) **-PATHY** (pă-thē) **-PATH** (path)	Disease, feeling, suffering; -PATH = one affect by a disease, one who treats a disease	Gr. *pathos*, feeling, suffering, disease	Chapters 4, 10
PECTOR/O (pek-tŏ-rō)	Chest	L. *pectus, pectoris*, n. chest	Chapters 3, 9
PED/O (pē-dō) **-PEDIA** (pē-dē-ă)	Child -PEDIA = education in something	Gr. *pais, paidos*, child Gr. *paideia*, education	Chapters 4, 7, 15
PED/O (ped-ō)	Foot	L. *pes, pedis*, m. foot	Chapter 3
PEDICUL/O (pi-dik-yŭ-lō)	Louse, lice	L. *pediculus, -i*, m. a louse	Chapter 6
PELL/O (pĕ-lō)	Skin	L. *pellis, -is*, f. hide, skin	Chapter 6
PELV/O (pel-vō)	Pelvis	L. *pelvis, -is*, f. a basin, basin shaped cavity	Chapter 3
PEN/I (pē-nĭ)	Penis	L. *penis, -is*, m. tail, penis	Chapter 15
-PENIA (pē-nē-ă)	Decrease, deficiency	Gr. *penia*, poverty; deficiency	Chapters 4, 7, 8
PENT/A (pen-tă)	Five	Gr. *pente*, five	Chapter 5
PEPT/O (pĕp-tō) **PEPS/O** (pĕp-sō)	Digestion	Gr. *peptein*, to cook; digestion	Chapter 13
PER- (pĕr)	Through, throughout, (intensive)	L. *per-*, through, throughout, (intensive)	Chapter 2
PERI- (per-ĭ)	Around	Gr. *peri-*, around	Chapter 2
PERINE/O (per-ĭ-nē-ō)	Perineum (area between the genitals and anus on males and females)	L. *perineum, -i*, n. perineum fr. Gr. *perineon*	Chapter 15
PERITONE/O (per-it-ŏ-nē-ō) **PERITON/O** (per-it-ŏ-nō)	Peritoneum	L. *peritoneum, -i*, n. peritoneum fr. Gr. *peritonaion*, stretched around; peritoneum	Chapter 13
PERONE/O (pĕr-ō-nē-ō)	Fibula bone	Gr. *perone*, a pin or brooch	Chapter 7

Greek or Latin word element	Current usage	Etymology	Chapters
PETECHI/O (pē-tē′kē-ō)	Petechia, red spots	Ital. *petecchia*, skin spot	Chapter 6
PEX/O (pĕ-ksō) -**PEXIS** (pĕk-sĭs)	Fixation, binding	Gr. *pexis*, a fixing together of something	Chapter 4
-**PEXY** (pĕk-sē)	Surgical fixation	Gr. *pexis*, a fixing together of something	Chapter 4
PHAC/O (făk-ō) **PHAK/O** (făk-ō)	Lens, lentil	Gr. *phakos*, lentil	Chapter 11
PHAE/O (fē-ō) **PHE/O** (fē-ō)	Gray	Gr. *phaios*, gray	Chapter 14
PHAG/O (făg-ō)	Eat, swallow	Gr. *phagein*, to eat, swallow	Chapters 10, 12, 13
PHALANG/O (fal-ăn-gō)	Phalanx	*L. phalanx, phalangis*, f. phalanx, a finger or toe bone fr. Gr. *phalanx*, a finger and a finger-like battle formation	Chapter 7
PHALL/O (făl-ō)	Penis	*L. phallus, -i*, m. penis fr. Gr. *phallos*, penis	Chapter 15
PHANER/O (făn-ĕr-ō)	Evident, visible	Gr. *phaneros*, visible	Chapter 10
PHANT/O (fan-tō) **PHANTASM/O** (fan-taz-mō)	Illusion, hallucination	Gr. *phantasma*, image, vision	Chapter 10
PHARMAC/O (făr-mă-kō) **PHARMACEUTIC/O** (făr-mă-sū-tĭ-kō)	Drugs, medicine	Gr. *pharmakon*, a drug, poison Gr. *pharmakeutikos*, by means of a drug or poisons	Chapter 4
PHARYNG/O (fă-ring-gō) -**PHARYNX** (far-ingks)	Throat, pharynx	*L. pharynx, pharyngis*, f. throat fr. Gr. *pharynx*, throat	Chapter 9
PHAS/O (fā-zō) -**PHASIS** (f-ā-sĭs) -**PHASIA** (fā-z-ē-ă)	Speech	Gr. *phasis*, speech fr. Gr. *phanai*, to speak	Chapter 10

Greek or Latin word element	Current usage	Etymology	Chapters
PHIL/O (fĭ-lō) **-PHIL** (fĭl) **-PHILE** (fĭl) **-PHILIA** (fil-ē-ă)	Attraction, love, in psychology; -PHILIA = means sexual arousal	Gr. *philein*, to love, affinity for	Chapters 8, 10
PHLEB/O (flĕ-bō)	Vein	Gr. *phleps, phlebos*, vein	Chapters 3, 8
PHLEGMAT/O (fleg-ma-tō)	Phlegm	Gr. *phlegm*, a type of humor; fr. Gr. *phlegma*, flame, heat	Chapter 9
PHLEGMON/O (flĕg-mŏn-ō)	Inflammation	Gr. *phlegmasia; phlegmone*, inflammation	Chapter 9
PHLOG/O (flō-gō)	Inflammation	Gr. *phlogosis*, inflammation	Chapter 4
PHOB/O (fō-bō) **-PHOBIA** (fō-bē-ă)	Fear, avoidance	Gr. *phobos*, fear	Chapter 10
PHON/O (fō-nō)	Sound, voice	Gr. *phone*, sound, voice	Chapters 9, 11
PHOR/O (fŏ-rō) **-PHORESIS** (fŏ-rē-sĭs) **-PHORIA** (for-ē-ă)	To convey, bear, bearing (in psychology, a mental state in respect to emotional well-being); -PHORESIS = transmission	Gr. *phoros*, bearing, carrying, bringing	Chapters 8, 10
PHOSPH/O (fŏs-fō-rō)	Phosphorus	Gr. *phosophoros*, light bringer, morning star	Chapter 5
PHOT/O (fō-tō)	Light	Gr. *phos, photos*, light	Chapter 11
PHRAGM/O (frăg-maō) **PHRAGMAT/O** (frăg-ma-tō) **-EMPHRAXIS** (ĕm-frăks-ĭs)	Obstruction, wall	Gr. *phragma, phragmatos*, fence, partition; *emphrassein*, to block	Chapter 9
PHRAS/O (frā-zō) **-PHRASIA** (frā-zē-ă)	Speech, phrase	Gr. *phrasis*, speech, expression	Chapter 10
PHREN/O (frĕ-nō)	Mind, diaphragm, phrenic nerve	Gr. *phren*, midriff, mind, diaphragm, seat of thought/emotion	Chapters 9, 10

Greek or Latin word element	Current usage	Etymology	Chapters
PHTHISI/O (thĭ-sĭ-ō) **-PHTHISIS** (-f-thĭ-sĭs)	Wasting, tuberculosis	Gr. *phthisis*, a wasting	Chapter 9
-PHYMA (fī′mă)	A growth, tumor	Gr. *phyma*, tumor, growth	Chapter 7
PHYS/O (fĭ-sō)	Air, gas, air bubble	Gr. *physa*, bellows, wind, air bubble; related to *physema*, that which is produced by blowing	Chapter 9
PHYSI/O (fĭz-ē-ō) **PHYSIC/O** (fĭz-ĭ-kō-kō) **-PHYSIS** (fĭ-sĭs)	Nature, growth, function; PHYSIC/O = Physical, natural; -PHYSIS = growth plate of a bone	L. *physis*, *-is*, f. growth plate of a bone Gr. *physis*, nature, growth, function Gr. *physikos*, of nature	Chapters 4, 7
PHYT/O (fĭ-tō) **-PHYTE** (fĭt)	A growth, plant	Gr. *phyton*, growth, plant	Chapter 7
PIL/O (pĭ-lō)	Hair	L. *pilus*, *-i*, m. a hair	Chapter 6
PINE/O (pĭn-ē-ō) **PINEAL/O** (pĭn-ē-ăl-ō)	Pineal gland, pine cone	L. *pineus*; *pinealis*, of a pine cone; pineal gland	Chapter 12
PINN/O (pĭn-ō) **PENN/O** (pen-ō)	Auricle (visible external ear), feather, fin, wing	L. *pinna*, *-ae*, f. feather, fin, wing	Chapter 11
PITUI/O (pĭ-too-ō) **PITUITAR/O** (pĭ-tū-ĭt-ă-rō)	Pituitary gland, hypophysis	L. *pituita*, *pituitaries*, phlegm, mucus; pituitary gland	Chapter 12
PLACENT/O (plas-ĕn-tō)	Placenta	L. *placenta*, *-ae*, f. a cake, flat cake; placenta	Chapter 15
PLAN/O (plă-nō)	Flat	L. *planus*, *-a*, *-um*, flat	Chapter 7
PLAN/O (plă-nō) **PLANKT/O** (plangk-tō) **-PLANIA** (plă-nē-ă)	Wandering	Gr. *planos*, wandering; *planktos*, wandering	Chapter 14
PLANT/O (plan-tō)	Sole (of foot), sprout or cutting, plant	L. *planta*, *-ae*, f. sole (of foot) fr. L. *planta*, a sprout, seedling	Chapter 3
PLASM/O (plăz-mō) **-PLASM** (plă-zm)	Fluid portion of blood (plasma), something formed	Gr. *plasma*, anything formed or molded fr. *plassein*, to form, mold	Chapter 8

Greek or Latin word element	Current usage	Etymology	Chapters
PLAST/O (pla-stō) **-PLAST** (plast) **-PLASIA** (plă-zē-ă)	Formed, molded; -PLAST = Forming cell or organelle; -PLASIA = Condition of formation, growth	Gr. *plastos*, formed, molded	Chapters 4, 8
-PLASTY (plas-tē)	Surgical reconstruction	Gr. *plastos*, formed, molded	Chapters 4, 6
PLATY- (plă-tĭ) **PLAT/O** (plă-tō)	Flat, broad	Gr. *platys*, wide, broad	Chapter 9
PLE/O (plē-ō) **PLEI/O** (plī-ō) **PLI/O** (plī-ō)	More, increased	Gr. *pleion*, more, increase	Chapter 8
PLEG/O (plĕg-ō) **-PLEGIA** (plē-jē-ă) **PLECT/O** (plĕk-tō) **-PLEXY** (plĕks-ē)	Paralysis, stroke	Gr. *plessein*, to strike, hit, smite	Chapter 10
PLETH/O (plĕth-ō) **PLETHYSM/O** (pleth-iz-mō)	Excess, overfullness	Gr. *plethora*, overabundance of a humor Gr. *plethysmos*, an increase	Chapter 8
PLEUR/O (ploo-rō)	Pleura, rib, side	L. *pleura, -ae*, f. pleura fr. Gr. *pleuron*, rib, side	Chapter 9
PLEX/O (plek-sō)	Plexus (an interwoven network of vessels or nerves), to plait, interweave	L. *plexus, -us*, m. a braid, plexus fr. L. *plectere, plexum*, to plait, interweave	Chapters 8, 10
PLIC/O (plī-kō) **PLICAT/O** (plī-kā-tō)	To fold, a fold	L. *plicare*, to fold	Chapter 13
PNE/O (p-nē-ō) **-PNOEA** (p-nē-ă) **-PNEA** (p-nē-ă)	Breath, breathing	Gr. *pnoia, pnoe*, breath fr. Gr. *pneein*, to breath	Chapter 9

Greek or Latin word element	Current usage	Etymology	Chapters
PNEUM/O (nū-mō) **PNEUMAT/O** (nū-măt-ō)	Wind, gas, air	Gr. *pneuma, pneumatos,* a breeze, breath, spirit	Chapter 9
PNEUM/O (nū-mō) **PNEUMON/O** (noo-mŏ-nō)	Lung	Gr. *pneumon, pneumonos,* lung	Chapters 3, 9
POD/O (pŏ-dō) **-PUS** (pŭs) **-POD** (pod)	Foot, foot-like structure, stalk	Gr. *pous, podos,* foot	Chapter 3
POIET/O (poy-ē-tō) **-POIESIS** (poy-ē-sĭs)	To make, produce	Gr. *poieein,* to make, produce	Chapters 4, 8, 12
POIKIL/O (poy-kĭ-lō)	Irregular, varied, spotted, mottled	Gr. *poikilos,* spotted, changeful, various	Chapter 8
POLLIC/O (pŏl-ĭk-ō)	Thumb	L. *pollex, pollicis,* m. thumb	Chapter 3
POLI/O (pŏl-ē-ō)	Gray (gray matter of CNS)	Gr. *polios,* gray	Chapter 10
POLY- (pŏl-ĭ)	Many, much	Gr. *polys,* many, much	Chapters 4, 9
POLYP/O (pŏl-ĭ-pō)	Polyp	Gr. *polypous,* many footed, octopus	Chapter 13
PON/O (pō-nō) **POS/O** (pō-sō) **POSIT/O** (pŏ-zi-tō)	To place, put	L. *ponere, positum,* to place, put	Chapter 7
PONT/O (pŏn-tō)	Pons (of the brain), bridge-like structure	L. *pons, pontis,* m. pons, bridge	Chapter 10
POPLIT/O (pop-li-tō)	Hollow of the knee, poples	L. *poples, poplitis,* m. posterior thigh, hamstring	Chapter 3
POR/O (pō-rō)	Passage, pore	Gr. *poros,* passage	Chapter 7
PORPHYR/O (por-fĭ-rō)	Purple, dark red	Gr. *porphyra,* purple	Chapter 14
PORT/O (port-ō)	Gate, entrance (Port of entry of a vessel or nerve into an organ)	L. *porta, -ae,* f. gate, entrance	Chapter 8
POST- (pōst)	After, behind	L. *post-,* after, behind	Chapter 2
POSTER/O (pŏs-tĕr-ō)	Behind, posterior	L. *posterior, -ius,* more behind, posterior	Chapter 3

Greek or Latin word element	Current usage	Etymology	Chapters
PRAE- or PRE- (prĕ)	Before, in front of	L. *prae-*, before, in front of	Chapter 2
PRAX/O (prăk-sō) -**PRAXIA** (prak-sē-ă) -**PRAXIS** (prăk-sĭs)	Activity, doing, practice	Gr. *praxis*, a doing	Chapter 10
PREPUTI/O (prĕ-pū-tē-ō)	Foreskin	L. *preputium, -i*, n. prepuce, foreskin	Chapter 15
PRESBY/O (prez-bĭ-ō)	Elderly, old age	Gr. *presbys*, an old man, elder	Chapters 4, 11
PRESS/O (prĕs-ō)	To press	L. *premere, pressum*, to press	Chapter 7
PRIAP/O (prī-ă-pō)	Penis, erection	L. *priapus, -i*, m. penis fr. Gr. *Priapos*, the Greek god of gardens who is recognized by his large phallus	Chapter 15
PRIM/I (prī-mĭ)	First, one	L. *primus, -a, -um*. first	Chapter 5
PRIV/O (prĭv-ō) -**PRIVIA** (prĭv-ē-ă)	Deprived of; -PRIVIA = condition following the removal of an endocrine gland	L. *privare*, to stripe, deprive of	Chapter 12
PRO- (prō)	Before, in front of, forward	L. *pro-*, before, in front of, forward	Chapter 2
PROCT/O (prok-tol-ō)	Anus and rectum	Gr. *proktos*, anus; the rectum and anus	Chapter 13
PRON/O (prō-nō) -**PRONAT/O** (prō-nă-tō)	Face down, lying prone	L. *pronator, -oris*, m. pronator fr. L. *pronatio*, f. a facing down	Chapter 7
PROS- (pros)	Toward, in addition, near	Gr. *pros-*, toward, in addition, near	Chapter 2
PROSO- (pros-ŏ)	Forward, before	Gr. *proso-*, forward, before	Chapter 2
PROSOP/O (prŏ-sō-pō)	Face	Gr. *prosopon*, face	Chapter 3
PROSTAT/O (pros-tă-tō)	Prostate	L. *prostata, -ae*, f. *prostate*, fr. *prostare*, to stand before	Chapter 15
PROT/O (prŏ-tō)	First, primary (in vision, red blindness i.e. primary color)	Gr. *protos*, first	Chapters 5, 11
PROTE/O (prŏt-ē-ō)	Protein, first, primary	Gr. *proteios*, first; protein	Chapter 13
PROXIM/O (prok-sĭm-ō)	Nearest (to a given part or center of body)	L. *proximalis, -e*, proximal *proximus, -a, -um*, nearest, closest *Superlative from L. *propior*, nearer	Chapter 3

Greek or Latin word element	Current usage	Etymology	Chapters
PRURIT/O (proo-rĭ-tō)	Severe itch	L. *pruritus, -i,* m. itch	Chapter 6
PSOR/O (sŏ′rō) **PSORIAS/O** (sŏ-rī′ă-sō)	Itch, psoriasis	Gr. *psoros,* itch; Gr. *psoriasis,* itch, mange	Chapter 6
PSYCH/O (sī-kō)	Mind, soul	Gr. *psyche,* spirit, soul, breath of life	Chapter 10
PSYCHR/O (sī-krō)	Cold	Gr. *psychros,* cold	Chapter 5
PTERN/O (tĕr-nō)	Heel	Gr. *pterna,* heel	Chapters 3, 7
PTERYG/O (ter-ĭ-gō) **PTER/O** (ter′ō) **-PTERYX** (pter-iks)	Wing, wing-like	Gr. *pteryx, pterygos,* wing; Gr. *pteron,* wing	Chapter 11
-PTOSIS (ptō-sĭs)	Downward displacement, prolapse	Gr. *ptosis,* a dropping, falling	Chapters 4, 13
PTYAL/O (tī-ăl-ō) **-PTYSIS** (-ptĭ-sĭs)	Spit, spitting	Gr. *ptyein,* to spit	Chapter 9
PUB/O (pū-bō) **PUBI/O** (pū-bē-ō)	Pubic bone, pubic region, puberty	L. *pubis, -is,* f. pubic bone, anterior inferior bone of the pelvis fr. L. *puber, puberis* m. arrived at the age of puberty, adult,	Chapters 7, 15
PUDEND/O (pŭd-ĕn-dō)	External genitalia (esp. female), vulva	L. *pudendum, -i,* n. shameful thing; external genitalia	Chapter 15
PUERIL/O (pū-ĕ-rĭ-lō)	Child, child-like	L. *puerilis, -e* child-like fr. L. *puer, -i,* m. child	Chapter 4
PUERPER/O (pū-ĕr-pĕ-rō)	Childbirth	L. *puerperare,* childbirth	Chapter 15
PULM/O (pŭl-mō) **PULMON/O** (pul-mŏ-nō)	Lung	L. *pulmo, pulmonis,* m. lung	Chapters 3, 8, 9
PUPILL/O (pū-pĭl-ō)	Pupil of the eye	L. *pupilla, -ae,* f. pupil of the eye fr. L. *pupa, -ae,* f. doll, child	Chapter 11
PUP/O (pū-pō)	Pupa (developmental stage after a larva)	L. *pupa, -ae,* f. doll, child	Chapter 11
PUR/O (pū-rō) **PURUL/O** (pŭr-ū-lō)	Pus, consisting of pus	L. *pus, puris,* n. pus L. *purulentus,* full of pus	Chapters 4, 6
PURPUR/O (pŭr-pyŭ-rō)	Purple, purpura	L. *purpura, -ae,* f. purple	Chapter 6

Greek or Latin word element	Current usage	Etymology	Chapters
PUSTUL/O (pŭs-tū-lō)	Pustule	L. *pustula, -ae*, f. blister, pimple	Chapter 6
PY/O (pī-ō)	Pus	Gr. *pyon*, pus	Chapters 4, 6, 9
PYEL/O (pī-ĕ-lō)	Renal pelvis, basin	Gr. *pyelos*, basin	Chapter 14
PYG/O (pī-gō)	Buttocks	Gr. *pyge*, buttocks	Chapter 3
PYKN/O (pĭk-nō) **PYCN/O** (pĭk-nō)	Thick, dense, frequent	Gr. *pyknos*, thick, dense	Chapter 10
PYL/O (pī-lō)	Orifice, portal vein	Gr. *pyle*, gait; orifice esp. portal vein	Chapter 13
PYLOR/O (pī-lor-ō)	Pylorus	L. *pylorus, -i*, m. pylorus fr. Gr. *pyloros*, gatekeeper; the pylorus	Chapter 13
PYR/O (pī-rō)	Fire, fever	Gr. *pyr*, fever, fire, heat	Chapters 4, 5
PYRET/O (pī-rĕ-tō)	Fever	Gr. *pyretos*, fire, fever	Chapter 4
QUADR/I (kwŏd-rĭ)	Four	L. *quattuor*, four	Chapter 5
QUART/A (kwor-tă)	Forth, four	L. *quartus*, fourth	Chapter 5
QUATER- (kwŏ-tĕr)	Four times, four	L. *quater*, four times	Chapter 5
QUINQU/E (kwĭn-kwē)	Five	L. *quinque*, five	Chapter 5
QUINT/A (kwĭn-tă)	Fifth, five	L. *quintus*, fifth	Chapter 5
RACH/O (răk-ō) **RACHI/O** (ră-kē-ō)	Vertebral column, spine	Gr. *rachis*, backbone	Chapter 7
RADI/O (răd-ē-ō)	Radius, ray, radioactive	L. *radius, -i*, m. staff, rod, ray, outer bone of forearm	Chapter 7
RADICUL/O (ră-dĭk-ū-lō) **RADIC/O** (răd-ĭ-kō)	Nerve root, root	L. *radicula, radiculae*, f. little root fr. L. *radix, radicis*, f. root	Chapter 10
RAM/O (ră-mō)	Ramus (a branching of vessels), branch, branchlike	L. *ramus, -i*, m. branch	Chapters 8, 10
RE- (rē)	Again, back, (intensive)	L. *re-*, again, back, (intensive)	Chapter 2
RECT/O (rek-tō)	Straight, correct, the rectum	L. *rectum, -i*, n. rectum fr. L. *rectus, -a, -um*, straight	Chapters 7, 13
REN/O (rē-nō)	Kidney	L. *ren, renis*, m. kidney	Chapters 3, 14
RET/O (rē-tō)	Net, network	L. *rete, retis*, n. net	Chapter 8

Greek or Latin word element	Current usage	Etymology	Chapters
RETICUL/O (rĕ-tik-yŭ-lō)	Net, network	L. *reticulum, -i*, n. little net	Chapter 8
RETIN/O (rĕt-ĭ-nō)	Retina (innermost coat of the eye)	L. *retina, -ae*, f. retina fr. L. *rete, retis*, n. net, network	Chapter 11
RETRO- (rĕt-rō)	Backward, behind	L. *retro-*, backward, behind	Chapter 2
RHABD/O (răb-dō)	Striated, rod, rod-like	Gr. *rhabdos*, rod, wand	Chapter 7
RHAPH/O (rā-fō) **R(H)APHID/O** (rā-fĭ-dō)	Seam, suture; R(H)APHID/O = needle, needle-like	Gr. *raphe*, a suture, seam; Gr. *rhaphis, rhaphidos*, needle	Chapter 4
RHE/O (rē-ō) **-RRHEA** (rē-ă)	Flow; -RRHEA = a discharge (of a fluid)	Gr. *rheein*, to flow	Chapter 4
RHEUM/O (roo-mō) **RHEUMAT/O** (roo′mă-tō)	Flow, discharge, rheumatoid arthritis	Gr. *rheuma, rheumatos*, flow, current, stream	Chapter 7
-(R)RHEXIS (rek-sĭs)	A rupture	Gr. *rhexis*, burst, rupture	Chapters 4, 7, 8
RHIN/O (rī-nō)	Nose	Gr. *rhis, rhinos*, nose	Chapters 3, 9
RHIZ/O (rī-zŏt-ō)	Nerve root, root	Gr. *rhiza*, root	Chapter 10
RHOD/O (rō-dō)	Rose-colored, red, rhodium	Gr. *rhodon*, rose, rose-colored	Chapters 5, 14
RHONCH/O (rŏng-kō) **RHONC/O** (rŏng-kō)	Wheezing, snoring, or squeaking sound heard during auscultation	L. *rhonchus, -i*, m. a snore fr. Gr. *rhonchos*, a snore	Chapter 9
RHYTHM/O (rith-mō)	Rhythm	Gr. *rhythmos*, regular, measure, rhythm	Chapter 8
RHYTID/O (rit-ĭ-dō)	Wrinkle	Gr. *rhytis, rhytidos*, wrinkle	Chapter 6
ROSTR/O (rŏs-trō)	Snout, beak	L. *rostralis, -e*, pertaining to the snout or beak, rostral fr. L. *rostrum, -i*, n. snout, beak	Chapter 3
ROT/O (rōt-ō) **ROTAT/O** (rō-tā-tō)	To turn around	L. *rotare, rotatum*, to cause to go around L. *rotator, -oris*, m. rotator fr. L. *rotatio*, f. a turning	Chapter 7
-RRHAGIA (rā-jē-ă) **-RRHAGE** (răj) **-RRHAGY** (rā-jē)	Rupture with profuse discharge of a fluid (typically blood)	Gr. *rhegnynai*, to break, burst forth	Chapters 4, 8

Greek or Latin word element	Current usage	Etymology	Chapters
RHAGAD/O (răg-ă-dō)	Tear, fissure, cleft	Gr. *rhagas, rhagados*, cleft, fissure	Chapter 4
-RRHAPHY (ră-fē)	Surgical suturing	Gr. *rhaptein*, to sew, stitch	Chapter 4
RUBR/O (roo-brō)	Red, redness	L. *ruber, rubra, rubrum*, red	Chapters 4, 6
RUG/O (roo-gō)	A crease, fold	L. *ruga, -ae*, f. crease, wrinkle	Chapter 6
SACCHAR/O (sak-ă-rō)	Sugar	Gr. *sakchar*, sugar	Chapter 13
SACCUL/O (sak-yŭ-lō)	Saccule of the inner ear, bag, sack	L. *sacculus, -i*, m. saccule fr. L. *saccus, -i*, m. sack, bag	Chapter 11
SACR/O (să-krō)	Sacrum bone, sacred	L. *sacrum, -i*, n. posterior triangular bone of the pelvis fr. L. *os sacrum*, holy bone	Chapter 7
SAGITT/O (să-jĭ-tō)	On or parallel to the sagittal suture of the skull, arrow	L. *sagittalis, -e*, pert. to an arrow; the sagittal suture fr. L. *sagitta, -ae*, f. arrow	Chapter 3
SALIV/O (să-lī-vō)	Saliva	L. *saliva, -ae*, f. saliva	Chapter 13
SALPING/O (săl-pĭng-gō) **-SALPINX** (sal-pingks)	Eustachian tube, or Fallopian tube (uterine tube), a long tubular structure	L. *salpinx, salpingis*, f. Eustachian tube, Fallopian tube fr. Gr. *salpinx, salpingos*, long tubed trumpet	Chapters 11, 15
SAN/O (să-nō) **SANIT/O** (san-ĭ-tō)	Health	L. *sanus, -a, -um*, healthy L. *sanitas, sanitatis*, f. health	Chapter 4
SANGUIN/O (sang-gwi-nō)	Blood	L. *sanguis, sanguinis*, m. blood	Chapter 8
SAPHEN/O (săf-ĕ-nō)	Saphenous vein	L. *saphena, -ae*, f. saphenous vein fr. Gr. *saphenes*, clear, manifest	Chapter 8
SARC/O (săr-kō)	Flesh, muscle	Gr. *sarx, sarkos*, flesh, fleshy pulp of fruit	Chapters 6, 7
SATYR/O (săt-ĭ-rī-ō)	Satyr-like, sexual desire	Gr. *Satyros*, Satyr, anthropomorphic goat-tailed Greek mythical creature	Chapter 15
SCABI/O (skā-bē-ō)	Scabies	L. *scabies, -ei*, f. scabies/itch	Chapter 6
SCAPH/O (skaf-ō)	Scaphoid, shaped like the hull of a boat	Gr. *skaphe*, boat	Chapter 7
SCAPUL/O (skăp-ū-lō)	Scapula, shoulder blade	L. *scapula, -ae*, f. scapula, shoulder blade	Chapter 7
SCAT/O (skă-tō)	Feces	Gr *skor, skatos*, feces	Chapter 13
SCHIST/O (skĭs-tō) **SCHIZ/O** (skĭz-ō) **-SCHISIS** (skĭ-sĭs)	Split, cleft	Gr. *schizein*, to split, cleave; Gr. *schistos*, cleft	Chapters 4, 7, 11

Greek or Latin word element	Current usage	Etymology	Chapters
SCLER/O (sklĕ-rō)	Hard, sclera of the eye	L. *sclera, -ae,* f. sclera fr. Gr. *skleros,* hard	Chapters 8, 11
SCOLI/O (skō-lē-ō)	Bent sideways, crooked	Gr. *skolios,* twisted, curved	Chapter 7
SCOP/O (skō-pō)	To view	Gr. *skopeein,* to look at, view	Chapter 4
-SCOPY (skŏ-pē) **-SCOPE** (skōp)	Examination, esp. with a device; -SCOPE = a device for looking into a body part	Gr. *skopeein,* to look at, view	Chapter 4
SCOT/O (skō-tō)	Darkness	Gr. *skotos,* darkness	Chapter 11
SCROT/O (skrŏ-tō)	Scrotum (pouch of skin containing the testicles)	L. *scrotum, -i,* n. bag	Chapter 15
SE- (sĕ)	Aside, apart from	L. *se-,* aside, apart from	Chapter 2
SEB/O (se-bō, or sē-bō)	Sebum	L. *sebum, -i,* n. tallow, fat; sebum	Chapter 6
SECT/O (sĕk-tō) **SEC/O** (sē-kō)	Cut, a section	L. *secare, sectum,* to cut	Chapter 4
-SECTION (sek-shŏn)	A cutting	L. *secare, sectum,* to cut	Chapter 4
SECUND/I (sē-kŭn-dĭ)	Second, two	L. *secundus,* second	Chapter 5
SELENI/O (sĕ-lĕ-nē-ō) **SELEN/O** (sĕ-lĕ-nō)	Selenium, SELEN/O = moon, crescent-shaped	Gr. *selene,* moon	Chapter 5
SEMI- (sem-ē)	Half	L. *semi-,* half	Chapter 2
SEMIN/O (sĕm-ĭ-nō) **SEMEN/O** (sē-mĕ-nō)	Semen (male ejaculate), seed	L. *semen, seminis,* n. seed	Chapter 15
SEN/O (sĕ-nō) **SENIL/O** (sē-nĭ-lō)	Elderly, old age	L. *senex, senis,* n. old, old person L. *senilis, -e,* old	Chapter 4
SEPT/I (sĕp-tĭ)	Seven	L. *septem,* seven	Chapter 5
SEPT/O (sĕp-tō)	A wall dividing two cavities	L. *septum, -i,* n. a wall, barrier, an enclosure fr. L. *saepire,* to hedge, separate	Chapter 8
SEPTIC/O (sĕp-tĭ-kō)	Sepsis	Gr. *septikos,* putrid fr. *sepsis,* rotting, putrefaction	Chapter 8
SEPTIM/A (sĕp-tĭ-mă)	Seventh, seven	L. *septimus,* seventh	Chapter 5

Greek or Latin word element	Current usage	Etymology	Chapters
SEQUESTR/O (sĕ-kwes-trŏ)	Fragment of bone/tissue	L. *sequestrum, i,* n. a deposit	Chapter 7
SER/O (sĕr-ŏ)	Fluid left over after blood clotting (blood serum), a watery fluid	L. *serum, -i,* n. watery part of curdled milk (whey)	Chapter 8
SESQUI- (sĕs-kwĭ)	One and a half	L. *sesqui,* one and a half	Chapter 5
SEX/A (sĕks-ă)	Six	L. *sex,* six	Chapter 5
SEXT/I (sĕks-tĭ)	Sixth, six	L. *sextus,* sixth	Chapter 5
-SIA (shă, sē-ă)	State or condition of	Gr. *-sia,* state or condition of	Chapter 2
SIAL/O (sĭ-al-ŏ)	Saliva	Gr. *sialon,* saliva	Chapters 12, 13
SICC/O (sĭk-ŏ)	Dry	L. *siccus, sicca, siccum,* dry	Chapter 6
SIGMOID/O (sĭg-moyd-ŏ)	Sigmoid colon	Gr. *sigmoeides,* shaped like the capital sigma Σ; sigmoid colon	Chapter 13
SILIC/O (sĭl-ĭ-kŏ)	Silica, silicon	L. *silex, silicis,* m. flint; silica	Chapter 5
SIN/O (sĭn-ŏ)	Curve; cavity, socket, or sinus	L. *sinus, sinus,* m. bending, curve, fold	Chapter 9
SINCIPIT/O (sĭn-sĭp-ĭ-tŏ)	Front of cranium, sinciput	L. *sinciput, sincipitis,* n. forehead	Chapter 3
SINISTR/O (sĭn-ĭs-trŏ)	Left	L. *sinister, -tra, -trum,* left	Chapter 3
SIT/O (sĭ-tŏ)	Food, grain	Gr. *sitos,* grain; food	Chapter 13
SKELET/O (skĕl-ĕ-tŏ)	Skeleton	L. *skeleton, -i,* skeleton fr. Gr. *skeletos,* dried-up	Chapter 7
SOMAT/O (sŏ-măt-ŏ) **SOM/O** (sŏ-mŏ) **-SOME** (sŏm)	Body, body of neuron	Gr. *soma, somatos,* body	Chapters 3, 10
SOMN/O (som-nŏ)	Sleep	L. *somnus, -i,* m. sleep	Chapter 10
SON/O (sŏ-nŏ)	Sound	L. *sonus, -i,* m. sound	Chapter 11
SOPOR/O (sŏ-pŏ-rŏ)	Sleep	L. *sopor, soporis,* m. sleep	Chapter 10
SPASM/O (spaz-mŏ) **SPAST/O** (spas-tŏ) **SPASMOD/O** (spaz-mŏ-dŏ)	Convulsion, spasm	L. *spasmus, -i,* m. spasm fr. Gr. *spasmos,* a wrenching	Chapters 7, 8, 10

Greek or Latin word element	Current usage	Etymology	Chapters
SPERM/O (spĕr-mō) SPERMAT/O (spĕr-măt-ō)	Sperm (part of the male ejaculate), seed	L. *sperma, -ae*, f. sperm fr. Gr. *sperma, spermatos*, seed	Chapter 15
SPHINCTER/O (sfĭngk-tĕr-ō)	Shincter (ringlike muscle of an orifice)	L. *sphincter, -eris*, m. sphincter fr. Gr. *sphinkter*, anything that binds tight, constricts	Chapters 7, 13
SPHYGM/O (sfĭg-mō) -SPHYGMIA (sfĭg-mē-ă)	Pulse	Gr. *sphygmos*, pulse	Chapter 8
SPIN/O (spī-nō)	Spine, thorn, vertebral column	L. *spina, -ae*, f. thorn	Chapters 7, 10
SPIR/O (spī-rō) SPIRAT/O (s-pĭ-răt-ō)	Breath, breathing	L. *spirare, spiratum*, to breathe, blow	Chapter 9
SPLANCHN/O (splangk-nō)	Viscera (internal organs enclosed in a cavity, particularly the abdominal cavity)	Gr. *splanchna*, innards, viscera	Chapter 13
SPLEN/O (splē-nō)	Spleen	Gr. *splen*, spleen	Chapter 8
SPONDYL/O (spŏn-dĭ-lō)	Vertebra	Gr. *spondylos*, vertebra	Chapters 7, 10
SPUT/O (spū-tō)	Sputum, spit	L. *sputum, -i*, n. spit	Chapter 9
SQUAM/O (skwă-mō) SQUAMAT/O (skwă-mă-tō)	Scale, scaly	L. *squama, -ae*, f. a scale (i.e. of a fish/reptile)	Chapter 6
STANN/O (stan-ō)	Tin	L. *stannum, -i*, n. tin	Chapter 5
STAPED/O (stă-pĕd-ō)	Stapes (one of the ossicles of the ear), stirrup	L. *stapes, stapedis*, m. stirrup	Chapter 11
STAPHYL/O (staf-ĭ-lō)	Uvula, staphlycoccus bacteria, grape-like	Gr. *staphyle*, bunch of grapes, uvula	Chapter 13
STAS/O (stă-sō) STAT/O (stă-tō) -STASIS (stă-sĭs) -STAT (stăt)	A standing, stoppage, cause to stand; -STAT = a device for stopping, ceasing something	Gr. *stasis*, standing, stoppage	Chapters 4, 8, 12
-STAXIS (stăk-sĭs)	Dripping, oozing	Gr. *staxis*, a dripping, oozing	Chapters 8, 9

Greek or Latin word element	Current usage	Etymology	Chapters
STEAR/O (stē-ă-rō) **STEAT/O** (stē-ă-tō)	Sebum, fat	Gr. *stear, steatos*, tallow, fat	Chapters 6, 13
STERC/O (stĕr-kō) **STERCOR/O** (stĕr-kō-rō)	Feces	L. *stercus, stercoris*, n. feces	Chapter 13
STERE/O (ster-ē-ō)	Solid, three-dimensional	Gr. *stereos*, solid	Chapters 5, 10
STERN/O (stĕr-nō)	Sternum, breastbone	L. *sternum, -i*, n. sternum, breast bone fr. Gr. *sternon*, chest	Chapter 7
STERTOR/O (stĕr-tor-ō)	Snoring or snorting sound with laborious breathing heard during auscultation	L. *stertor, -oris*, m. a snore	Chapter 9
STETH/O (steth-ō)	Chest	Gr. *stethos*, chest, breast	Chapters 8, 9
STHEN/O (sthĕ-nō)	Strength, specific gravity	Gr. *sthenos*, strength	Chapters 10, 14
STIGMAT/O (stĭg-măt-ō)	Spot, point, shame/disgrace	Gr. *stigma, stigmatos*, a mark of a pointed instrument, brand, tattoo-mark	Chapter 11
STOICHI/O (stoy-kē-ō)	Element	Gr. *stoicheion*, element	Chapter 5
STOMAT/O (stō-măt-ō) **STOM/O** (stō-mō)	Mouth, outlet, opening	Gr. *stoma, stomatos*, mouth	Chapters 3, 4, 13
-STOMY (stō-mē)	Surgical creation of an opening (stoma)	Gr. *stoma, stomatos*, mouth, opening	Chapter 4
STRABISM/O (stră-biz-mō)	Strabismus (disorder of the eye in respect to the optic axis)	L. *strabismus, -i*, m. strabismus fr. Gr. *strabismos*, a squinting	Chapter 11
STRAT/O (stră-tō)	layer	L. *stratum, -i*, n. covering fr. L. *sternere*, to spread out	Chapter 6
STRICT/O (strĭk-tō) **STRING/O** (strĭn-gō)	Narrowing	L. *stringere, strictum*, to draw tight, press together	Chapter 8
STRID/O (strĭ-dō) **STRIDUL/O** (strĭd-ū-lō)	A high-pitched, harsh sound occurring during inspiration heard during auscultation	L. *stridor, -oris*, m. a creaking, grating	Chapter 9
STYL/O (stĭ-lō) **-STYLE** (stĭl)	Column-shaped bone, pillar	Gr. *stylos*, pillar, column, peg	Chapter 7

Greek or Latin word element	Current usage	Etymology	Chapters
SUB- (sŭb) **SUC-** (sŭk) before c **SUF-** (sŭf) before f **SUG-** (sŭg) before g **SUP-** (sŭp) before p **SUR-** (sŭr) before r	Under, below, less than normal	L. *sub-*, under, below, less than normal	Chapter 2
SUD/O (sood-ō) **SUDOR/O** (sood-ŏ-rō)	Sweat	L. *sudor, sudoris*, m. sweat	Chapter 6
SULC/O (sŭl-kō)	Sulcus (groove of brain), furrow, groove	L. *sulcus, -i*, m. furrow, groove	Chapters 7, 10
SUPER- (soo-pĕr)	Over, above, excessive	L. *super-*, over, above, excessive	Chapter 2
SUPER/O (soo-pĕr-ō)	Above, superior	L. *superior, -ius*, more above, superior	Chapter 3
SUPIN/O (soo-pĭn-ō) **SUPINAT/O** (soo-pĭ-nāt-ō)	Face up, lying supine	L. *supinator, -oris*, m. supinator fr. L. *supernatio*, f. a facing up	Chapter 7
SUPRA- (soo-pră)	Above, upon	L. *supra-*, above, upon	Chapter 2
SUPRAREN/O (soo-pră-rē-nō)	Suprarenal gland, adrenal gland	L. *supra* + L. *ren*, kidney = supraren-, adrenal gland	Chapter 12
SUR/O (sū'rō)	Calf	L. *sura, surae*, f. calf	Chapter 3
SYN- (sin) **SYM-** (sim) before b or p	Together, with	Gr. *syn-*, together, with	Chapter 2
SYNOVI/O (sĭ-nō-vē-ŏ) **SYNOV/O** (sĭn-ō-vŏ)	Synovial fluid	L. *synovia, -ae*, f. synovial fluid (new L. *synovia*, albuminous joint fluid)	Chapter 7
SYPHIL/O (sĭf-ĭl-ō)	Syphilis	L. *Syphilis*, title and character of a 16th century poem, *Syphilis, sive Morbus Gallicus*	Chapter 15
SYRING/O (sĭr-ĭng-ō) **-SYRINX** (sir-inks)	Fistula, short tube, pipe-like	Gr. *syrinx, syringos*, pipe, fistula	Chapter 13

Greek or Latin word element	Current usage	Etymology	Chapters
SYSTOL/O (sis-tŏ-lō)	Contraction	Gr. *systole*, contraction	Chapter 8
TABET/O (tă-be-tō)	Wasting	L. *tabes*, *-is*, f. wasting away, decay	Chapter 4
TACHY- (tak-i) TACH/O (tak-ō)	Rapid, quick, speed	Gr. *tachys*, fast; *tachos*, speed	Chapters 8, 9
TACT/O (tak-tō) TAG/O (tag-gō) TANG/O (tang-gō)	Touching, sense of touch	L. *tangere*, *tactum*, to touch	Chapter 11
TAL/O (tā-lō)	Talus bone, ankle	L. *talus*, *-i*, m. talus, the ankle bone	Chapter 7
TALIP/O (tal-ĭ-pō)	Deformity of foot and ankle	L. *talus*, ankle + *pes*, foot	Chapter 7
TARS/O (tar-sō)	Ankle, flat of the foot, edge of the eyelid	L. *tarsus*, *-i*, m. ankle fr. Gr. *tarsos*, flat of foot	Chapter 3
TAX/O (tak-sō)	Coordination, order	Gr. *taxis*, order, arrangement	Chapter 10
TECHN/O (tek-nō)	Art, skill	Gr. *techne*, art, skill, craft	Chapter 4
TEL/O (tĕl-ō)	End, complete, purpose	Gr. *telos*, end, fulfillment, purpose	Chapter 6
TELE- (tel-ĕ)	Distant	Gr. *tele*, distant, far off	Chapter 6
TEN/O (ten-ō) TENONT/O (tĕn-ŏn-tō)	Tendon	Gr. *tenon*, *tenontos*, tendon, sinew	Chapter 7
TENDIN/O (ten-dĭ-nō)	Tendon	L. *tendo*, *tendinis*, m. tendon fr. L. *tenere* to stretch	Chapter 7
TENS/O (tĕn-sō)	Stretch	L. *tendere*, *tensum*, to stretch	Chapter 8
TERAT/O (tĕr-ă-tō)	Severely deformed fetus, monster	Gr. *teras*, *teratos*, a marvel, monster	Chapter 15
TERTI/A (tĕr-shē-a)	Third, three	L. *tertius*, third	Chapter 5
TEST/O (tĕs-tō) TESTICUL/O (tĕs-tĭk-ū-lō)	Testicle, testis	L. *testis*, *is*, m. witness, testicle L. *testiculus*, *-i*, m. testicle	Chapters 12, 15
TETART/O (te-tar-tō)	Fourth, one-fourth	Gr. *tetartos*, fourth	Chapter 5
TETR/A (tĕt-ră)	Four	Gr. *tetra*, four	Chapter 5
TETRAKIS- (tĕ-tră-kis)	Four times, four	Gr. *tetatrakis*, four times	Chapter 5

Greek or Latin word element	Current usage	Etymology	Chapters
THALAM/O (thăl-ăm-ō)	Thalamus (mass of gray matter located in the diencephalon), chamber, inner room	L. *thalamus, -i*, m. thalamus fr. Gr. *thalamos*, inner room, chamber	Chapter 10
THALL/O (thăl-lō)	Young branch, shoot, simple plants (i.e fungi, lichens, algae) thallium	Gr. *thallos*, young shoot or branch	Chapter 5
THANAT/O (thă-nă-tō) -THANASIA (thă-nā-zē-ă)	Death	Gr. *thanatos*, death	Chapter 4
THEL/O (thē-lō) -THELE (thē-lē)	Nipple, nipple-like structure	Gr. *thele*, nipple	Chapters 6, 15
THELY/O (thē-lē-ō)	Female	Gr. *thelys*, female	Chapter 15
THERAP/O (thĕr-ă-pō) THERAPEUT/O (thĕr-ă-pū-tō) -THERAPY (ther-ă-pē)	Treatment	Gr. *therapeuein*, to take care of, to heal, to treat Gr. *therapeutike*, treatment, therapy, treatment	Chapter 4
THERM/O (thĕr-mō) -THERM (thĕrm)	Heat, temperature	Gr. *thermos*, heat	Chapter 5
THORAC/O (thō-ră-kō) -THORAX (thōr-aks)	Thorax	L. *thorax, thoracis*, m. thorax fr. Gr. *thorax*, breastplate	Chapters 3, 7, 9
THROMB/O (thrŏm-bō)	A clot	L. *thrombus, -i*, m. a clot fr. Gr. *thrombos*, clot	Chapter 8
THYM/O (thī-mō)	Emotion, state of mind	Gr. *thymos*, spirit, soul, mind, anger, strong feeling	Chapter 10
THYM/O (thī-mō)	Thymus gland	L. *thymus, -i*, m. thymus fr. Gr. *thymos*, warty excrescence; thymus gland	Chapters 8, 12
THYR/O (thī-rō) THYROID/O (thī-royd-ō)	Thyroid gland	Gr. *thyreos*, shield in the shape of door; thyroid gland	Chapter 12
-TIA (shē-ă)	State or condition of	L. *-tia*, state or condition of	Chapter 2
TIBI/O (tib-ē-ō)	Tibia bone	L. *tibia, -ae*, f. pipe, flute, medial bone of the lower leg	Chapter 7
-TIC (t-ik)	Pertaining to	Gr. *-tic*, pertaining to	Chapter 2
TOC/O (tŏk-ō)	To be in labor, childbirth	Gr. *tokos*, labor, childbirth	Chapters 12, 15

Greek or Latin word element	Current usage	Etymology	Chapters
TOM/O (tŏ-mō)	Cut, a section	Gr. *tomos*, cutting	Chapter 4
-TOMY (tŏ-mē) **-ECTOMY** (ek-tŏ-mē) **-TOME** (tōm)	-TOMY = Incision; -ECTOMY = Excision; -TOME =Device for making an incision	Gr. *tome*, a cutting Gr. *ek*, out + *tome*, a cutting	Chapter 4
TON/O (ton-ō)	Tension, stretching, tone (esp. in muscles)	Gr. *tonos*, that which is stretched, cord, rope	Chapters 7, 10, 12
TONSILL/O (tŏn-sĭl-ō)	Tonsil	L. *tonsilla, -ae*, f. tonsil, almond	Chapters 8, 13
TOP/O (tŏ-pō) **-TOPE** (tōp)	Place	Gr. *topos*, place	Chapters 5, 10
TORS/O (tor-sō) **TORT/O** (tort-ō)	Twist, turn	L. *torquere, tortum, torsum*, to twist, turn	Chapter 7
TOX/O (tok-sō)	Poison, bow and arrow	Gr. *toxon*, a bow and arrows	Chapter 8
TRACH/O (tră-kō) **TRACHY-** (tră-kĭ)	Rough	Gr. *trachys*, rough	Chapter 9
TRACHE/O (tră-kē-ō)	Trachea	L. *trachea, -ae*, f. trachea, windpipe, fr. Gr. *traxeia arteria*	Chapter 9
TRACHEL/O (trak-ĕ-lō)	Neck, cervix	Gr. *trachelos*, neck, throat	Chapters 3, 9
TRACT/O (trak-tō)	To draw, pull	L. *trahere, tractum*, to draw, drag	Chapter 7
TRANS- (trăns)	Across, through	L. *trans-*, across, through	Chapters 2, 5
TREM/O (tre-mō) **TREMUL/O** (trĕm-ū-lō)	Shaking, trembling	L. *tremor, -oris*, m. a shaking	Chapter 10
TREPAN/O (trĕ-păn-ō) **TREPHIN/O** (trĕ-fī-nō) **TRYPAN/O** (trĭ-pă-nō)	Borer, drilling; TRYPAN- = borer; a genus of parasitic protozoa called Trypanosomes	L. *trepanum, -i*, fr. Gr. *trypanon*, a borer	Chapter 4
TRET/O (trē-tō) **-TRESIA** (trē-zē-ă)	Perforated, bored	Gr. *tresis*, perforation; Gr. *tretos*, bored, perforated	Chapter 11

Greek or Latin word element	Current usage	Etymology	Chapters
TRI- (trĭ)	Three	L. *tres*, *tria*, three Gr. *treis*, three	Chapter 5
TRICH/O (trĭk-ō) **-THRIX** (thrĭks)	Hair	Gr. *thrix*, *trichos*, hair	Chapter 6
TRICHOMON/O (trĭk-ō-mōn-ō)	Trichomonas (particularly *trichomonas vaginalis*)	Gr. *trichomonas*, family flagellate parasites	Chapter 15
TRIPS/O (trip-sō) **TRIPT/O** (trip-tō)	Crushing, grinding	Gr. *tripsis*, a rubbing, friction, massage	Chapters 4, 14
-TRIPSY (trip-sē)	Surgical crushing	Gr. *tripsis*, a rubbing, friction, massage	Chapters 4, 14
TRIS- (tris) **TER-** (tĕr)	Three times, three	Gr. *tris*, three times L. *ter*, three times	Chapter 5
TRIT/O (trĭt-ō)	Third	Gr. *tritos*, third	Chapter 5
TROP/O (trŏ-pō) **-TROPIA** (trŏ-pē-ă) **-TROPION** (trŏ-pē-ŏn)	Turning, change, stimulating; -TROPIA = deviation of eyes from the visual axis; -TROPION = turning the edge or margin, particular of the eyelid)	Gr. *trope*, turning, change	Chapters 5, 11, 12
TROPH/O (trŏ-fō) **-TROPHY** (trŏ-fē)	Nourishment, growth	Gr. *trophe*, nourishment	Chapters 4, 12
TRUNC/O (trŭn-kō)	Trunk, cut off	L. *truncus*, *-i*, m. trunk of a tree, lopped off part fr. L. *truncare*, to cut off	Chapter 3
-TRYPESIS (trĭ-pē-sis)	A surgical boring	Gr. *trype*, a piercing, a hole	Chapter 4
TUBER/O (tū-bĕ-rō)	An elevated process of bone (tuberosity), tubercle, nodule, swelling	L. *tuber*, *tuberis*, n. a swelling, hump	Chapter 9
TUBERCUL/O (tū-bĕr-kū-lō)	Tubercle, tuberculosis	L. *tuberculus*, *-i*, m. a little swelling, tubercle	Chapter 9
-TUDE (tood)	State or condition of	L. *-tudo*, state or condition of	Chapter 2
TUM/O (tū-mō)	Swelling, tumor, abnormal mass	L. *tumor*, *tumoris*, m. tumor, swelling	Chapters 4, 6
TUSS/O (tŭs-sō) **-TUSSIS** (tŭs-ĭs)	A cough, coughing	L. *tussis*, *-is*, f. a cough	Chapter 9

Greek or Latin word element	Current usage	Etymology	Chapters
TYMPAN/O (tĭm-pă-nō)	Eardrum, drum	L. *tympanum, -i*, n. tympanum fr. Gr. *tympanon*, a drum	Chapter 11
TYPHL/O (tĭf-lō)	Cecum (Caecum), blindness	Gr. *typhlos*, blind; the cecum	Chapter 13
ULCER/O (ŭl-sĕ-rō)	Ulcer	L. *ulcus, ulceris*, n. open sore; ulcer	Chapters 6, 13
-ULE (ūl)	Diminutive (little)	L. *-ulus*, diminutive (little)	Chapter 2
ULN/O (ŭl-nō)	Ulna	L. *ulna, -ae*, f. elbow, inner bone of the forearm	Chapter 7
ULTRA- (ŭl-tră)	Beyond, excessive	L. *ultra-*, beyond, excessive	Chapter 2
UMBILIC/O (ŭm-bil-ĭ-kō)	Navel, umbilical cord	L. *umbilicus, -i*, m. the navel	Chapters 13, 15
UN/I (ū-ni)	One	L. *unus*, one	Chapter 5
-UNCLE (ŭng-kĕl)	Diminutive (little)	L. *-unculus*, diminutive (little)	Chapter 2
UNGU/O (ŭng-gwō, or ŭng-gyō)	Fingernail, toenail, claws, talon, hoof	L. *unguis, -is*, m. fingernail, talon, hoof	Chapter 6
UR/O (ū-rō) **-URIA** (ū-rē-ă)	Urine	Gr. *ouron*, urine	Chapters 12, 14
-URE (ŭr)	Action; condition resulting from an action	L. *-ura*, action; condition resulting from an action	Chapter 2
URE/O (ŭr-ē-ō)	Urea	Gr. *ouron*, urine	Chapter 14
-URESIS (ū-rē-sĭs)	To urinate, involuntary urination	Gr. *ourein*, to urinate, to make water	Chapter 14
URETER/O (ū-rē-tĕr-ō)	Ureter	L. *ureter, ureteris*, m. ureter fr. Gr. *oureter*, ureter	Chapter 14
URETHR/O (ū-rē-thrō)	Urethra	L. *urethra, -ae*, f. urethra fr. Gr. *ourethra*, urethra	Chapter 14
-URGY (ŭr-jē)	Work	Gr. *ergon*, work	Chapters 4, 5
URIC/O (ū-rĭ-kō)	Uric acid	Gr. *ouron*, urine	Chapter 14
URIN/O (ū-rĭ-nō)	Urine	L. *urina, -ae*, f. urine	Chapter 14
URTIC/O (ŭrt-i-kō)	Wheal, hive	L. *urtica, -ae*, f. stinging nettle	Chapter 6
UTER/O (ūt-ĕ-rō)	Uterus	L. *uterus, -i*, m. womb	Chapter 15
UTRICUL/O (ū-trik-yŭ-lō)	Utricle of the inner ear, bag, sack	L. *utriculus, -i*, m. utricle fr. L. *uter, utris*, m. a bag or bottle	Chapter 11
UVUL/O (ū-vyŭ-lō)	Uvula	L. *uvula, -ae*, f. small grape, uvula, fr. L. *uva*, grape	Chapter 13

Greek or Latin word element	Current usage	Etymology	Chapters
VAGIN/O (văj-ĭ-nō)	The female vagina, a sheath-like structure	L. *vagina, -ae*, f. sheath, scabbard; the female vagina	Chapter 15
VAL/O (va-lō) or (vā-lō)	Strength	L. *valere*, to be strong	Chapter 5
VALG/O (val-gō)	Bent outward	L. *valgus, -a, um*, bent outward	Chapter 7
VALV/O (val-vot-ō)	Valve	L. *valva, -ae*, f. a Roman folding door; valve	Chapter 8
VALVUL/O (val-vyŭ-lō)	Valvule	L. *valvula, -ae*, f. a small valve, valvule	Chapter 8
VAR/O (vă-rō)	Bent inward	L. *varus, -a, um*, bent	Chapter 7
VARIC/O (var-ĭ-kō)	A swollen, tortuous vein	L. *varix, varicis*, f. enlarged vein	Chapter 8
VAS/O (vă-zō) **VASCUL/O** (vas-kyŭ-ō)	Vessel (carrying fluids)	L. *vas, vasis*, n. vessel L. *vasculum, -i*, n. a small vessel	Chapters 3, 8, 15
VEN/O (vē-nō)	Vein	L. *vena, -ae*, f. vein	Chapters 3, 8
VENERE/O (vē-nĕr-ē-ō)	Sex, sexual desire	L. *venereus, -a, um*, of Venus, the Roman goddess of eros	Chapter 15
VENTR/O (ven-trō)	Belly, abdomen, cavity	L. *venter, ventris*, m. belly, cavity	Chapters 3, 7, 9
VENTRICUL/O (ven-trik-yŭ-lō)	Ventricle, cavity	L. *ventriculus, -i*, m. ventricle, little belly fr. L. *venter, ventris*, m. belly, cavity	Chapters 8, 10
VENUL/O (ven-yŭ-lō)	Venule	L. *venula, -ae*, f. venule, little vein	Chapter 8
VERRUC/O (vĕr-roo-kō)	Wart	L. *verruca, -ae*, f. wart	Chapter 6
VERT/O (vĕr-tō) **VERS/O** (vĕr-sō)	Turning	L. *vertere, versum*, to turn	Chapter 10
VERTEBR/O (vĕr-tĕ-brō)	Vertebra, back bone	L. *vertebra, -ae*, f. a joint, vertebra	Chapters 7, 10
VERTIC/O (vĕr-tĭ-kō)	Crown of the cranium, summit	L. *vertex, verticis*, m. summit	Chapter 3
VESIC/O (vĕ-sĭ-kō) **VESICUL/O** (vĕ-sĭk-ū-lō)	Bladder, blister, VESICUL- = small blister/ vesicle	L. *vesica, -ae*, f. bladder, sack L. *vesicula, -ae*, f. little bladder, sack	Chapters 3, 6, 13, 14
VESTIBUL/O (vĕs-tĭb-ū-lō)	Vestibule of the inner ear, an entrance	L. *vestibulum, -i*, n. an entrance-court, entrance to a place	Chapter 11
VIRID/O (vĭ-rĭ-dō)	Green	L. *viridis*, green	Chapter 14
VIRIL/O (vĭr-ĭl-ō)	Male, masculine	L. *virilis, -e*, male fr. L. *vir, viri*, m. man, male	Chapter 4

Greek or Latin word element	Current usage	Etymology	Chapters
VIS/O (vĭ-zō)	Seeing, sense of sight	L. *videre*, *visum*, to see	Chapter 11
VISCER/O (vis-ĕ-rō)	Organ	L. *viscus*, *visceris*, n. organ	Chapter 8
VITRE/O (vi-trē-ō)	Glass, glass-like (vitreous humor of the eye)	L. *vitrum*, *-i*, n. glass	Chapter 11
VOL/O (vŏ-lō)	Palm of the hand	L. *vola*, *-ae*, f. palm	Chapter 3
VOLV/O (vŏl-vō)	To roll	L. *volvere*, to roll	Chapter 13
VOR/O (vŏ-rō)	To devour, eat	L. *vorare*, to devour	Chapter 13
VULV/O (vŭl-vō)	Vulva (external female genitalia), covering	L. *vulva*, *-ae*, f. a covering, shell, husk	Chapter 15
XANTH/O (zan-thō)	Yellow	Gr. *xanthos*, yellow	Chapters 6, 14
XEN/O (zen-ō)	Foreign, strange, xenon	Gr. *xenon*, foreign, strange	Chapters 5, 6
XER/O (zer-ō)	Dry	Gr. *xeros*, dry	Chapters 5, 6
XIPH/O (zif-ō)	Xiphoid process, sword-like	Gr. *xiphos*, sword	Chapter 7
-Y (ē)	State or condition of, the act of	Gr. *-y*, state or condition of, the act of	Chapter 2
ZO/O (zō-ō)	Something living; animal	Gr. *zoon*, a living being, animal	Chapter 15
ZYG/O (zī-gō) **ZYGOT/O** (zī-gō-tō)	Zygote, yoke, joined	Gr. *zygon*, yoke, crossbar fr. Gr. *zygotos*, yoked	Chapter 15
ZYM/O (zī-mō) **-ZYME** (zīm)	Enzyme, fermentation	Gr. *zyme*, ferment; enzyme	Chapter 13

Appendix B

Latin Grammar for Anatomical Latin

Abbreviated Paradigms for Nouns Used in Anatomical Latin

Declension	Nom. Sing.	Gen. Sing.	Nom. Pl.	Gen. Pl.
First Declension	-a	-ae	-ae	-arum
Second Declension	-us	-i	-i	-orum
Second Declension Neuter	-um	-i	-a	-orum
Third Declension Consonant Stem	Various	-is	-es	-um
Third Declension Consonant Stem Neuter	Various	-is	-a	-um
Third Declension I-stem	Various	-is	-es	-ium
Third Declension I-stem Neuter	Various	-is	- ia	-ium
Fourth Declension	-us	-us	-us	-uum
Fourth Declension Neuter	-u	-us	-ua	-uum
Fifth Declension	-es	-ei	-es	-erum

Abbreviated Paradigms for Adjectives Commonly Used in Anatomical Latin

First and Second Declension Adjectives

	Singular			Plural		
	Masc.	Fem.	Neut.	Masc.	Fem.	Neut.
Nom.	-us (-er)	-a	-um	-i	-ae	-a
Gen.	-i	-ae	-i	-orum	-arum	-orum

Third Declension Adjectives of Two Termination

	Singular		Plural	
	Masc. and Fem.	Neut.	Masc. and Fem.	Neut.
Nom.	-is	-e	-es	-ia
Gen.	-is	-is	-ium	-ium

Comparative Adjectives

	Singular		Plural	
	Masc. and Fem.	Neut.	Masc. and Fem.	Neut.
Nom.	-ior (-or)	-ius (-us)	-es	-a
Gen.	-is	-is	-um	-um

Greek and Latin Roots of Medical and Scientific Terminologies, First Edition. Todd A. Curtis.
© 2025 John Wiley & Sons, Inc. Published 2025 by John Wiley & Sons, Inc.
Companion website: www.wiley.com/go/Curtis